# Textbook of Ventilation, Fluids, Electrolytes and Blood Gases

# Textbook of Ventilation, Fluids, Electrolytes and Blood Gases

*Editor*

**Mohan Gurjar** MD PDCC FICCM
Additional Professor
Department of Critical Care Medicine
Sanjay Gandhi Postgraduate Institute of Medical Sciences (SGPGIMS)
Lucknow, Uttar Pradesh, India

*Forewords*

**Arvind Kumar Baronia**
**Jean-Louis Vincent**

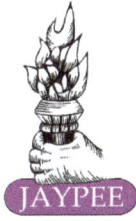

## JAYPEE BROTHERS MEDICAL PUBLISHERS
*The Health Sciences Publisher*
New Delhi | London | Panama

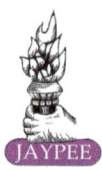
### Jaypee Brothers Medical Publishers (P) Ltd

### Headquarters
Jaypee Brothers Medical Publishers (P) Ltd
4838/24, Ansari Road, Daryaganj
New Delhi 110 002, India
Phone: +91-11-43574357
Fax: +91-11-43574314
Email: jaypee@jaypeebrothers.com

### Overseas Offices
J.P. Medical Ltd
83 Victoria Street, London
SW1H 0HW (UK)
Phone: +44 20 3170 8910
Fax: +44 (0)20 3008 6180
Email: info@jpmedpub.com

Jaypee-Highlights Medical Publishers Inc
City of Knowledge, Bld. 235, 2nd Floor
Clayton, Panama City, Panama
Phone: +1 507-301-0496
Fax: +1 507-301-0499
Email: cservice@jphmedical.com

Jaypee Brothers Medical Publishers (P) Ltd
Bhotahity, Kathmandu, Nepal
Phone: +977-9741283608
Email: kathmandu@jaypeebrothers.com

Website: www.jaypeebrothers.com
Website: www.jaypeedigital.com

© 2020, Jaypee Brothers Medical Publishers

The views and opinions expressed in this book are solely those of the original contributor(s)/author(s) and do not necessarily represent those of editor(s) of the book.

All rights reserved. No part of this publication may be reproduced, stored or transmitted in any form or by any means, electronic, mechanical, photocopying, recording or otherwise, without the prior permission in writing of the publishers.

All brand names and product names used in this book are trade names, service marks, trademarks or registered trademarks of their respective owners. The publisher is not associated with any product or vendor mentioned in this book.

Medical knowledge and practice change constantly. This book is designed to provide accurate, authoritative information about the subject matter in question. However, readers are advised to check the most current information available on procedures included and check information from the manufacturer of each product to be administered, to verify the recommended dose, formula, method and duration of administration, adverse effects and contraindications. It is the responsibility of the practitioner to take all appropriate safety precautions. Neither the publisher nor the author(s)/editor(s) assume any liability for any injury and/or damage to persons or property arising from or related to use of material in this book.

This book is sold on the understanding that the publisher is not engaged in providing professional medical services. If such advice or services are required, the services of a competent medical professional should be sought.

Every effort has been made where necessary to contact holders of copyright to obtain permission to reproduce copyright material. If any have been inadvertently overlooked, the publisher will be pleased to make the necessary arrangements at the first opportunity. The **CD/DVD-ROM** (if any) provided in the sealed envelope with this book is complimentary and free of cost. **Not meant for sale.**

**Inquiries for bulk sales may be solicited at:** jaypee@jaypeebrothers.com

*Textbook of Ventilation, Fluids, Electrolytes and Blood Gases*

*First Edition:* 2020

ISBN 978-93-89188-05-9

*Printed at*

**Dedicated to**
*Teachers who carry lamp of knowledge and
spread it through their fellows to serve humanity*

# Contributors

**A Sachdeva** MBBS
Director, Interventional Pulmonology
Division of Pulmonary, Critical Care and Sleep Medicine
University of Maryland School of Medicine
Baltimore, MD, USA

**Aaron Lim** MD
Assistant Professor
Department of Anesthesiology
Virginia Commonwealth University Health System
Richmond, Virginia, USA

**Abdul Wahab** MD
Resident Physician/Research Collaborator
Department of Internal Medicine
Unity Hospital
Rochester, NY, USA
METRIC Research Group
Department of Pulmonary and Critical Care Medicine
Mayo Clinic, Rochester, MN, USA

**Abhay Vakil** MD
Assistant Professor
Department of Pulmonary Critical Care Medicine
Corpus Christi Medical Center
Corpus Christi, TX, USA

**Addy Yh Tan** MBBS (S'pore) MMed Anesthesiology (S'pore) EDIC
Senior Consultant and Assistant Professor
Department of Anesthesia
National University Health System
Singapore

**Afzal Azim** MD PDCC FICCM
Professor
Department of Critical Care Medicine
Sanjay Gandhi Postgraduate Institute of Medical Sciences (SGPGIMS)
Lucknow, Uttar Pradesh, India

**Alan D Kaye** MD PhD
Professor, Program Director, and Chairman
Department of Anesthesiology
The Louisiana State University Health Sciences Center
New Orleans, LA, USA
Professor, Department of Pharmacology
The Louisiana State University Health Sciences Center
New Orleans, Louisiana, LA, USA

**Albert Phan Nguyen** MD
Assistant Professor
Department of Anesthesiology
University of California San Diego
San Diego, California, USA

**Alex Yartsev** MBBS BApp Sci (MRS) FCICM
Staff Specialist (Intensive Care Medicine)
Department of Intensive Care
Westmead Hospital
Sydney, New South Wales, Australia

**András Lovas** MD PhD EDIC EDAIC
Consultant
Department of Anesthesiology and Intensive Therapy
Faculty of Medicine
University of Szeged
Szeged, Hungary

**Andrew Davenport** MD FRCP
Consultant Nephrologist and Professor of Dialysis and ICU Nephrology
UCL Centre for Nephrology
The Royal Free London NHS Foundation Trust
London, NW3 2QG, UK

**Anjali Agarwal** MBBS
Research Trainee
Department of Critical Care Medicine
Mayo Clinic
Florida, USA

**Antonio M Esquinas** MD PhD FCCP
International Fellow
American Association for Respiratory Care
Intensive Care Unit
Hospital General Universitario Morales Meseguer
Murcia, Spain

**Anumeha Bhagat** MD DNB FAIMER Fellow
Associate Professor and MEU Faculty
Department of Physiology
Government Medical College and Hospital
Chandigarh, India

**Armin Ahmed** MD PDCC
Assistant Professor
Department of Critical Care Medicine
King George Medical University
Lucknow, Uttar Pradesh, India

**Audrey De Jong** MD PhD
Associate Professor
Department of Anesthesiology and Intensive Care
Saint Eloi Teaching Hospital
Centre Hospitalier Universitaire Montpellier
Montpellier, France

**Banwari Agarwal** MBBS MD FRCA FRCP EDIC FFICM
Consultant (Critical Care Medicine) and Associate Professor
Department of Intensive Care Unit
The Royal Free London NHS Foundation Trust
London, NW3 2QG, UK

**Bethany Menard** MD
Assistant Professor
Department of Anesthesiology
The Louisiana State University Health Sciences Center
New Orleans, Louisiana, LA, USA

**Bhuvana Krishna** MD IDCCM IFCCM
Professor and Head
Department of Critical Care Medicine
St John's Medical College and Hospital
Bengaluru, Karnataka, India

**Bogdan Tiru** MD
Assistant Professor of Medicine
Tufts University School of Medicine
Co-Director Medical ICU
Division of Pulmonary and Critical Care Medicine
Baystate Medical Center
Springfield, MA, USA

**Bryan Anderson** DO
Clinical Fellow
Department of Pulmonary Critical Care Medicine
Corpus Christi Medical Center
Corpus Christi, TX, USA

**Char Ogborn** PhD
Research Project Coordinator
Department of Pediatrics
McLane Children's Hospital
Baylor Scott and White
Texas A & M University
Temple, Texas, USA

**Cody M Koress** MD
Research Associate and Senior Medical Student
Department of Anesthesiology
The Louisiana State University Health Sciences Center
New Orleans, Louisiana, LA, USA

**Daniel Arellano Sepúlveda** MSc
Adjunct Professor
Critical Care Unit
Hospital Clínico Universidad de Chile
Santiago of Chile
Department of Physical Therapy
Faculty of Medicine
University of Chile
Santiago, Chile

**Devang Sanghavi** MBBS MD
Senior Associate Consultant
Department of Critical Care Medicine
Mayo Clinic
Florida, USA

**Dharmendra Bhadauria** MD DM
Additional Professor
Department of Nephrology and Renal Transplant
Sanjay Gandhi Postgraduate Institute of Medical Sciences
Lucknow, Uttar Pradesh, India

**Dharshan Rangaswamy** MD DM
Associate Professor
Department of Nephrology
Kasturba Hospital and Medical College
Manipal Academy of Higher Education
Manipal, Karnataka, India

**Diego Luis Carrillo-Pérez** MD
Clinical Assistant Professor
Department of Internal Medicine
Instituto Nacional de Ciencias Médicas y Nutrición
Salvador Zubirán
Mexico City, Mexico

**Elena Spinelli** MD
Staff Physician
Maggiore Policlinico Hospital
Milan, Italy
Department of Anesthesia, Critical Care and Emergency
Fondazione IRCCS Ca'Granda Ospedale Maggiore Policlinico
Milan, Italy

Contributors

**Ewan C Goligher** MD PhD
Assistant Professor of Medicine
Interdepartmental Division of Critical Care Medicine
University of Toronto
Scientist, Toronto General Hospital Research Institute
Critical Care Medicine
University Health Network
Toronto General Hospital
Toronto, Canada

**Fabrice Galia** PhD
Engineer
Department of Anesthesiology and Intensive Care
Saint Eloi Teaching Hospital
Centre Hospitalier Universitaire Montpellier
Montpellier, France

**Gerardo Gamba** MD PhD
Professor and Director of Research
Instituto Nacional de Ciencias Médicas y Nutrición
Salvador Zubirán
Head, Molecular Physiology Unit
Instituto de Investigaciones Biomédicas
Universidad Nacional Autónoma de México
Mexico City, Mexico

**Harsh Vardhan** MD DM
Associate Professor
Department of Nephrology and Renal Transplant
Indira Gandhi Institute of Medical Sciences
Patna, Bihar, India

**Ivan Ramírez Venegas** RT
Kinesiólogo (Physical Therapist)
Division of Critical Care Medicine
Hospital Clinico Universidad de Chile, Santiago
Faculty of Health Sciences
Universidad de Los Andes
Santiago, Chile

**Jacob George Pulinilkunnathil** MD IDCCM EDIC FCCP
Senior Resident
Department of Anesthesia, Critical Care and Pain
Tata Memorial Hospital
Mumbai, Maharashtra, India

**Jan Van der Mullen** MD
Registrar Emergency Medicine
Department of Emergency Medicine
University Hospitals of Leuven
Leuven, Belgium

**Jeroen Tahon** MD
Resident Internal Medicine
Department of Intensive Care Medicine
Ziekenhuis Netwerk Antwerpen Campus Stuivenberg
Antwerp, Belgium

**John Botha**
MBChB MMed FCP (SA) FRACP FCICM Dip Neph (London) PG Dip Echo
Director
Department of Intensive Care Medicine
Frankston Hospital
Frankston, Victoria, Australia

**JV Divatia** MD FICCM FCCM
Professor and Head
Department of Anesthesia, Critical Care and Pain
Tata Memorial Hospital
Mumbai, Maharashtra, India
Past-President
Indian Society of Critical Care Medicine

**Kapil Dev Soni** MD
Associate Professor
Critical and Intensive Care
JPN Apex Trauma Centre
All India Institute of Medical Sciences
New Delhi, India

**Kirtivardhan Vashistha** MBBS
Research Scholar
Department of Infectious Disease
Mayo Clinic, Rochester
METRIC Research Team
Mayo Clinic
Rochester, MN, USA

**Louis Anzalone** MD
Resident Physician
Department of Anesthesiology
University of Pennsylvania
Philadelphia, PA, USA

**Malvika Sagar** MD FAAP
Assistant Professor
Department of Pediatrics
McLane Children's Hospital
Baylor Scott and White
Texas A & M University
Temple, Texas, USA

**Manu Malbrain** MD PhD
Head
Department of Critical Care Medicine
University Hospital Brussels (UZB)
Brussels, Belgium

**Marco Albanese** MD
Resident
Department of Anesthesia, Critical Care and Emergency
Fondazione IRCCS Ca'Granda Ospedale Maggiore Policlinico
Milan, Italy

**Mark R Jones** MD
Senior Resident
Department of Anesthesia, Critical Care and Pain Medicine
Beth Israel Deaconess Medical Center
Harvard Medical School
Boston, MA, USA

**Mark W Motejunas** MD
Resident Physician
Department of Anesthesiology
The Louisiana State University Health Sciences Center
New Orleans, Louisiana, LA, USA

**MG Allison** MD
Assistant Director, ICU
Critical Care Medicine
Saint Agnes Hospital Center
Baltimore, MD, USA

**Nadia Corcione** MD
Staff Physician
Pulmonary Medicine
Maggiore Policlinico Hospital
Milan, Italy
Department of Anesthesia, Critical Care and Emergency
Fondazione IRCCS Ca' Granda Ospedale Maggiore Policlinico
Milan, Italy

**Nasirul J Ekbal** PhD MRCP FFICM
Consultant in Intensive Care and Renal Medicine
Department of Intensive Care Medicine and Nephrology
The Royal Free London NHS Foundation Trust
London, NW3 2QG, UK

**Niels Van Regenmortel** MD
ICU Director
Department of Intensive Care Medicine
Ziekenhuis Netwerk Antwerpen Campus Stuivenberg
Antwerp, Belgium

**Nilanchal Chakraborty** MD PDCC EDIC
Clinical Fellow
Department of Critical Care Medicine
Sunnybrook Health Sciences Centre
University of Toronto
Toronto, Ontario, Canada

**Nirvik Pal** MBBS MD
Assistant Professor
Division of Cardiothoracic Anesthesiology
Department of Anesthesiology
Virginia Commonwealth University
Richmond, VA, USA

**O Kalchiem-Dekel** MD
Fellow, Pulmonary Diseases and Critical Care Medicine
Division of Pulmonary, Critical Care, and Sleep Medicine
University of Maryland School of Medicine
Baltimore, MD, USA

**Paolo Pelosi** MD FERS
Full Professor
Anesthesiology and Intensive Care Medicine
Department of Surgical Sciences and Integrated Diagnostics (DISC)
San Martino Policlinico Hospital, IRCCS for Oncology and Neurosciences
University of Genoa
Genoa, Italy

**Patricia A Nicolato** DO
Assistant Professor
Director of ECMO Program
Division of Cardiothoracic Surgery
Department of Surgery
Virginia Commonwealth University
Richmond, VA, USA

**Patricia RM Rocco** MD PhD
Full Professor
Head, Laboratory of Pulmonary Investigation
Carlos Chagas Filho Institute of Biophysics
Federal University of Rio de Janeiro
Rio de Janeiro, Brazil

**Pedro Leme Silva** PhD
Associate Professor of Physiology
Laboratory of Pulmonary Investigation
Carlos Chagas Filho Institute of Biophysics
Federal University of Rio de Janeiro
Rio de Janeiro, Brazil

**Pramod K Guru** MBBS MD FASN
Assistant Professor of Medicine
Director, Adult ECMO Practice and Medical ICU
Department of Critical Care Medicine
Mayo Clinic
Florida, USA

**Pranav Jetley** MD DESA
Clinical Fellow (Anesthesiology)
West Middlesex University Hospital
Chelsea and Westminster Hospital NHS Trust
London, UK

**Rahul Kashyap** MBBS MBA
Assistant Professor
Department of Anesthesiology and Perioperative Medicine
Mayo Clinic, Rochester
METRIC Research Team
Mayo Clinic
Rochester, MN, USA

**Rahul Nanchal** MD MS
Professor of Medicine
Director, Medical Intensive Care Unit
Director, Critical Care Fellowship Program
Medical College of Wisconsin
Milwaukee, WI, USA

**Ram Baalachandran** MD
Fellow Physician
Division of Pulmonary and Critical Care
University of Maryland
Baltimore, Maryland, USA

**Ravindranath Tiruvoipati** MBBS MS FRCSEd MCh MSc FCICM EDIC
Director of Intensive Care Research
Department of Intensive Care Medicine
Frankston Hospital
Frankston, Victoria, Australia

**Renata de Souza Mendes** MD PhD
Nephrologist
Federal University of Rio de Janeiro
Post-doc Laboratory of Pulmonary Investigation
Carlos Chagas Filho Institute of Biophysics
Federal University of Rio de Janeiro
Rio de Janeiro, Brazil

**Robert Wise** MBChB MMed FCA Cert Crit Care
Clinical Fellow
Discipline of Anesthesia and Critical Care
Nelson Mandela School of Medicine
University of KwaZulu-Natal
Durban, South Africa

**Roop Kishen** MBBS DA MD FRCA
Consultant in Intensive Care Medicine and Anesthesia (Retd)
Hope Hospital, Salford Royal NHS Foundation Trust
Manchester, UK
Honorary Lecture (Retd)
Anesthesia, Translational Medicine and Clinical Neurosciences
Victoria University of Manchester
Manchester, UK

**Sai Saran PV** MD DM IDCCM EDIC
Assistant Professor
Department of Critical Care Medicine
Cancer Superspeciality Institute and Hospital
Lucknow, Uttar Pradesh, India

**Salim Surani** MD
Adjunct Clinical Professor of Medicine
Division of Pulmonary, Critical Care and Sleep Medicine
Texas A&M University, Health Science Center
Program Director, Pulmonary and Critical Care Fellowship Program
Bay Area Medical Center
Corpus Christi, TX, USA

**Samir Jaber** MD PhD
University Professor and Head
Department of Anesthesiology and Intensive Care
Saint Eloi Teaching Hospital
Centre Hospitalier Universitaire Montpellier
Montpellier, France

**Samir Samal** MD IDCC
Assistant Professor
Department of Critical Care Medicine
Institute of Medical Sciences and SUM Hospital
Bhubaneswar, Odisha, India

**Sarah L Wachter** MD
Clinical Instructor in Anesthesiology
R Adams Cowley Shock Trauma Center
University of Maryland
Baltimore, MD, USA

**Saurabh Saigal** MD PDCC EDIC
Associate Professor
Critical Care Medicine
All India Institute of Medical Sciences
Bhopal, Madhya Pradesh, India

**Saurabh Vig** MD DM
Assistant Professor
Department of Anesthesia
Super Specialty Cancer Institute and Hospital
Lucknow, Uttar Pradesh, India

**Shakti Bedanta Mishra** MD DM
Associate Professor
Department of Critical Care Medicine
Institute of Medical Sciences and SUM Hospital
Bhubaneswar, Odisha, India

**Shalini Donthi** MD
Research Trainee
METRIC Research Group
Department of Pulmonary and Critical Care Medicine
Mayo Clinic
Rochester, MN, USA

**Shekhar Ghamande** MD FCCP FAASM
Clinical Associate Professor
Department of Internal Medicine
Division of Pulmonary and Critical Care
Baylor Scott and White
Texas A & M University
Temple, Texas, USA

**Snigdha Ipsita** MD
Senior Resident
Department of Critical Care Medicine
Institute of Medical Sciences and SUM Hospital
Bhubaneswar, Odisha, India

**Sriram Sampath** MD
Professor
Department of Critical Care Medicine
St John's Medical College and Hospital
Bengaluru, Karnataka, India

**Tom Carmeliet** MD
Cardiology Resident
Department of Intensive Care (Cardiology)
University Hospital Brussels (UZB)
Brussels, Belgium

**Tom Schepens** MD PhD
PICU Staff Physician
Department of Critical Care Medicine
Antwerp University Hospital
Antwerp, Belgium

**Tommaso Mauri** MD
Assistant Professor
Department of Anesthesia, Critical Care and Emergency
Fondazione IRCCS Ca' Granda Ospedale Maggiore Policlinico
Milan, Italy
Department of Pathophysiology and Transplantation
University of Milan
Milan, Italy

**Ulrich H Schmidt** MD PhD MBA
Clinical Professor of Anesthesiology
Vice Chair Critical Care Medicine
Department of Anesthesiology
University of California San Diego
San Diego, California, USA

**Yugan Mudaliar**
MBChB FCP (SA) FANZCA FRACP FCICM ACPSEM AIP (Aus) IOP (UK)
Clinical Associate Professor
Senior Staff Specialist
Department of Intensive Care
Westmead Hospital
Sydney, New South Wales, Australia

**Zbigniew Szkulmowski** MD
Specialist in Anesthesiology and Intensive Care
Clinical Unit of Anesthesiology and Intensive Care
University Hospital No. 1 in Bydgoszcz
Collegium Medicum in Bydgoszcz
Nicolaus Copernicus University in Toruń
Bydgoszcz, Poland

**Zsolt Molnár** MD PhD EDAIC
Head
Department of Anesthesiology and Intensive Therapy
Faculty of Medicine
University of Szeged
Szeged, Hungary

# Foreword

Foundation of the globally expanding specialty of Critical Care Medicine is constructed by the basic elements like ventilation, fluids, electrolytes, and blood gas. The *Textbook of Ventilation, Fluids, Electrolytes and Blood Gases* deals with these fundamental subjects in a very creative and enthusiastic manner. The intricately linked information flows seamlessly from one chapter to the other. The composition of the first edition of the book shall take its place as one of the most comprehensive textbooks on the basic clinical management practices of intensive care units (ICUs) and reminds me that in the era of digital information, the printed textbooks are still extremely valuable to the students and practitioners in the field of medicine.

Dr Mohan Gurjar has done a commendable job by maintaining the uniformity in the content and style of all the chapters. The book lays more emphasis on information than on existing guidelines. Keeping in the mind that the chapters of this book are written by outstanding specialist practitioners and researchers who are also internationally acclaimed authors from around the world including UK, European Union, Australia, and North America, this book comprehensively addresses pertinent clinical challenges in each chapter and provides a balanced view where differences do exist.

The book has an international standard character and, therefore, it is expected to serve immensely to the students, residents, fellows, and attending physicians who cover the ICUs or emergency medicine wards across the world. Having said that, I believe the book is getting introduced at a very crucial time in the developing countries like India, where the younger generation of intensivists includes an ever-increasing number of doctors who had only recently started enjoying fully structured training program with clinical rotations, courses, and well-designed exit examinations conducted under the watchful eyes of the medical regulatory boards and councils.

**Arvind Kumar Baronia** MD
Professor and Head
Department of Critical Care Medicine
Sanjay Gandhi Postgraduate Institute of Medical Sciences
Lucknow, Uttar Pradesh, India

# Foreword

I am delighted to have been asked to write the foreword for *Textbook of Ventilation, Fluids, Electrolytes and Blood Gases*, edited by Dr Mohan Gurjar. The topics covered in this comprehensive book are important not only in critical care medicine, but also for all specialists taking care of acutely ill patients. The book is divided into three key sections—"Ventilation", "Fluids and Electrolytes", and "Blood Gases". Each section starts with chapters covering the essential physiology and pathophysiology of the field and then includes chapters on relevant practical considerations and subjects. Each chapter is clearly laid out, easy to read and understand, and supported by adequate and appropriate illustrations. A list of "salient points" at the end of each chapter provides a useful summary of the key points of each chapter. In a small fourth section "Miscellaneous", chapters are included on other important associated issues, notably nutrition, transfusion, and organ donation. The textbook chapters are written by an international group of authors providing a wealth of experience and knowledge from around the world.

Textbooks provide an abundance of information in one easy-to-reference volume. As medicine advances, so new, up-to-date books such as this are needed to provide the very latest evidence and guidance. I am sure that this book will be of value both to medical students and to practicing clinicians, and congratulate Dr Mohan Gurjar on his excellent effort.

**Jean-Louis Vincent** MD PhD
Professor
Department of Intensive Care Medicine
Université Libre de Bruxelles
Bruxelles, Belgium
Consultant, Department of Intensive Care
Erasme University Hospital
Bruxelles, Belgium

# Preface

In managing critically ill patients, the understanding of pathophysiological abnormalities, monitoring of clinical variables, and timely intervention makes an impact on patient outcome. The *Textbook of Ventilation, Fluids, Electrolytes and Blood Gases* encompasses essential topics for which thorough education and training is a must for any clinician who manages these patients. This concept makes it a unique book, in a sense that readers will not need to go through various books or sources, despite easily available information on individual topic in current era.

This book has four sections, each for ventilation, fluids and electrolytes, blood gases, and miscellaneous. Each section starts with applied physiology and then covers routine as well as advance topics related to ventilation, fluids, and electrolytes in critically ill adult patients. Miscellaneous section covers enteral and parenteral nutrition, immunonutrition, blood product transfusion, and care of potential organ donor in the intensive care unit (ICU). Also, there are chapters based on common problems like approach to the patient having hypoxemia, hypercapnia, hypovolemia, electrolyte abnormalities, and acid–base disturbances. These chapters start with a case scenario, then structured description of the problem, and in the last again discussion about the index case, which makes better understanding of commonly encountered problems in critically ill patients.

The splendid chapters are written by experts from across the world, with their vast experience and knowledge. In the background of rapid changes in evidences in medicine and the advancement of technology, all authors tried their best to keep the content of the chapter up-to-date and as practical as possible. For better clarity on given topics, appropriate Figures, Tables, and Flowcharts have been used throughout the chapters. At the end of each chapter, there are a few salient points to emphasis on the important area of that particular topic.

I hope that the book will be useful for trainees as well as consultants of various clinical specialties who manage critically ill adult patients, including critical care medicine, emergency medicine, pulmonary medicine, and anesthesiology.

**Mohan Gurjar**

# Acknowledgments

The concept of having *Textbook of Ventilation, Fluids, Electrolytes and Blood Gases* is the result of feedback from trainees in critical care medicine about the need of such a book, which covers ventilation, fluids, electrolytes, and blood gases; as these topics are backbone in managing any critically ill patient.

I am very much thankful for supports from Professor Arvind Kumar Baronia (India), Dr Chithambaram Veerappan (United Kingdom), Dr Nirvik Pal (USA), Dr Vishal Kant Tiwari (USA), and Dr Tommaso Mauri (Italy) on various aspects during this project.

I am indebted to all contributors from various institutes across the world, without their contribution, the book was not possible. They kept patience with me while making changes in the chapter for improvement.

I would like to sincerely thank to Shri Jitendar P Vij (Group Chairman), Mr Ankit Vij (Managing Director) of M/s Jaypee Brothers Medical Publishers (P) Ltd, New Delhi, India and the production team members, especially Ms Chetna Malhotra Vohra (Associate Director—Content Strategy) and Dr Savleen Kaur (Development Editor), for their efforts to make the book in present form.

Throughout this project, I received much needed moral support from my colleagues, friends, staffs and students of my department, and Sanjay Gandhi Postgraduate Institute of Medical Sciences (SGPGIMS), Lucknow, Uttar Pradesh, India.

I owe for blessings from my parents, Dr Ganga Bishan Gurjar and Dr Gulab Gurjar, and also best wishes from my sister Divya Kasana.

Finally, I acknowledge the tolerance and support of my wife, Dr Sheetal Gurjar and daughters Ishani and Bhavya during this endeavor, without whom the book could never have been completed.

# Contents

## SECTION 1: VENTILATION

### 1. RESPIRATION: APPLIED ANATOMY AND PATHOPHYSIOLOGICAL CONSIDERATIONS — 3
*Alex Yartsev, Yugan Mudaliar*

Macroscopic and Microscopic Structural Elements of the Respiratory Tract  3
Oral Cavity and the Pharynx  3
Applied Anatomy and Pathophysiology of the Pulmonary Circulation  9
Lung Volume and Capacities  11
Applied Anatomy and Pathophysiology of Respiratory Mechanics  12

### 2. OXYGEN DELIVERY DEVICES — 17
*Bogdan Tiru*

History of Oxygen Therapy  17
Oxygen as a Drug  17
Goals of Oxygen Therapy  17
Indications for Oxygen Use  17
Oxygen Delivery  18
Oxygen Delivery Devices  18

### 3. APPROACH TO THE PATIENT WITH HYPOXEMIA — 27
*Aaron Lim*

Case  27
Hypoxia and Hypoxemia  27
Oxygenation: Normal Physiology  27
Mechanism of Hypoxemia  29
Management  31

### 4. APPROACH TO THE PATIENT WITH HYPERCAPNIA — 35
*Malvika Sagar, Char Ogborn, Shekhar Ghamande*

Case  35
Definition  35
Pathophysiology  36
Causes  37
Clinical Features  37
Advantages and Disadvantages of Hypercapnia  38
Evaluation of Hypercapnia  39
Management  41
Impact of Hypercapnia on Outcome  43
Future Implications  44

### 5. NONINVASIVE VENTILATION — 47
*Zbigniew Szkulmowski, Antonio M Esquinas*

Basic Principle for Noninvasive Ventilation Use  47
Noninvasive Ventilation Use in Clinical Conditions  48

Equipment Used in Noninvasive Ventilation  51
Ventilation Modes Used in Noninvasive Ventilation  53
Implementation Technique  53
Monitoring  54
Causes of Noninvasive Ventilation Failure  54
Humidification of Inspiratory Air  58
Rebreathing during Noninvasive Ventilation  58
Oxygen Therapy during Noninvasive Ventilation  60
Contraindications for Noninvasive Ventilation  60

### 6. MECHANICAL VENTILATORS 65
*Fabrice Galia, Samir Jaber, Audrey De Jong*
Brief Historical Recall of Ventilation  65
Basic Principle of Mechanical Ventilation  65
Gas Supply  66
Turbine or Wall Gas  66
Triggering  67
Cycling  68
Circuit  68
Ventilation in ICU  68
Ventilation Apart ICU  71
Evolution of Mechanical Ventilation  73
NAVA® and PAV+®  73
Intellivent-ASV® and SmartCare®  74
Usability  74

### 7. MECHANICAL VENTILATION IN SPECIFIC CLINICAL SCENARIOS 77
*Afzal Azim*
Obstructive Airway Diseases  77
Bronchial Asthma  77
Chronic Obstructive Pulmonary Disease  82
Bronchopleural Fistula  83
Severe Metabolic Acidosis  84
Acute Respiratory Distress Syndrome  85

### 8. GRAPHIC ANALYSIS OF MECHANICAL VENTILATION 90
*Daniel Arellano Sepúlveda*
Basic Concepts  90
Curves  90
Loops  91
Nomenclature  91
Curves Interpretation  93
Loops Analysis  100

### 9. PATIENT-VENTILATOR ASYNCHRONY 107
*Daniel Arellano Sepúlveda, Ivan Ramírez Venegas*
Asynchrony Index  107
Impact of Asynchrony on Patient Outcome  107
Types of Asynchrony  108

## 10. MONITORING $O_2$ AND $CO_2$ DURING MECHANICAL VENTILATION   114
*András Lovas, Zsolt Molnár*

Oxygen Measurement   *114*
Carbion Dioxide Measurement   *117*

## 11. LUNG RECRUITMENT MANEUVERS   121
*Abdul Wahab, Shalini Donthi, Salim Surani, Rahul Kashyap*

Definition of Recruitment Maneuvers   *121*
Methods of Recruitment Maneuvers   *121*
Advantages and Disadvantages of Recruitment Maneuvers   *123*
Recruitment Maneuvers and Peep Titration   *123*
Derecruitment   *124*
Recruitment Maneuvers and Ventilator-induced Lung Injury   *124*
Future Trials and Future Directions   *124*

## 12. HEART LUNG INTERACTIONS DURING MECHANICAL VENTILATION   128
*JV Divatia, Jacob George Pulinilkunnathil*

Case   *128*
Determinants of Heart-lung Interaction   *128*
Hemodynamic Effects due to Changes in Intrathoracic Pressure   *129*
Hemodynamic Effects due to Changes in Lung Volume   *130*
Hemodynamic Effects due to Ventricular Interdependence   *131*
Clinical Applications of Heart-lung Interaction   *131*

## 13. MONITORING PRESSURES DURING MECHANICAL VENTILATION   137
*Nadia Corcione, Marco Albanese, Elena Spinelli, Tommaso Mauri*

Airway Pressure   *137*
Peak and Plateau Pressure   *137*
Mean Airway Pressure   *138*
Positive End-expiratory Pressure   *138*
Driving Pressure   *141*
Esophageal and Transpulmonary Pressure   *141*
Lung Stress and Strain   *141*
Inspiratory Pressure during Spontaneous Breathing   *142*

## 14. INSPIRATORY EFFORT ASSESSMENT IN VENTILATED PATIENT   144
*Sai Saran PV*

Assessment of Inspiratory Efforts in Ventilated Patients   *144*

## 15. VENTILATOR-INDUCED LUNG INJURY   151
*Renata de Souza Mendes, Pedro Leme Silva, Paolo Pelosi, Patricia RM Rocco*

Spontaneous Breathing: How does it Work?   *151*
Pathophysiology of Vili: Stress, Strain, and Stress Raisers   *152*
Principles of Mechanical Ventilation and Potential Mechanisms of Injury   *153*

## 16. VENTILATOR-INDUCED DIAPHRAGM DYSFUNCTION   161
*Tom Schepens, Ewan C Goligher*

Diaphragm Anatomy and Function   *161*
Diaphragm Dysfunction in the ICU   *162*
Pathophysiology of Ventilator-induced Diaphragm Dysfunction   *163*

Clinical Presentation and Diagnosis of Ventilator-induced Diaphragm Dysfunction  165
Prevention of Ventilator-induced Diaphragm Dysfunction  166
Recovery From Ventilator-induced Diaphragm Dysfunction  167

### 17. WEANING FROM MECHANICAL VENTILATION  172
*Abhay Vakil, Bryan Anderson, Kirtivardhan Vashistha, Rahul Kashyap*

Definitions  172
General Approach  172
Weaning after Prolong Mechanical Ventilation  178

### 18. AEROSOL DRUG DELIVERY IN VENTILATED PATIENT  181
*O Kalchiem-Dekel, MG Allison, A Sachdeva*

Factors Affecting Adequate Aerosol Delivery in Mechanical Ventilated Patients  181
Aerosol Delivery Devices and their Integration into the Ventilator Circuit  184
Aerosolized Drugs and their Use in Ventilator-supported Patients  188
Aerosolized Therapy in Patients Receiving Noninvasive Ventilation  191
Aerosolized Therapy in Patients Receiving High-flow Nasal Cannula  192

### 19. EXTRACORPOREAL MEMBRANE OXYGENATION  196
*Nirvik Pal, Patricia A Nicolato, Sarah L Wachter*

History  196
Indications  196
Pathophysiology of Gas Exchange  197
Types and Basic Principles of Extracorporeal Membrane Oxygenation  200
Management of Extracorporeal Membrane Oxygenation  202
Troubleshooting during Conduct of Extracorporeal Membrane Oxygenation  206
Weaning  207
Complications  207
How I do it—By Dr P Nicolato  207

### 20. EXTRACORPOREAL MEMBRANE CARBON DIOXIDE REMOVAL  213
*Pramod K Guru, Anjali Agarwal, Devang Sanghavi*

Extracorporeal Principles and Types  213
Unmet Needs: Problems in Relation to the Current Standard of Care  216
Clinical Application of Extracorporeal $CO_2$ Removal  217
Challenges of the Current Devices and Methods  218

### 21. HIGH FREQUENCY OSCILLATORY VENTILATION  220
*Albert Phan Nguyen, Ulrich H Schmidt*

Principles and Clinical Applications  220
Advantages and Disadvantages of HFOV  222
HFOV in Adult and Pediatric Population  222

### 22. DOMICILIARY AND PALLIATIVE VENTILATION  224
*Saurabh Vig*

Patient Selection for Domiciliary Ventilation  224
Setting Up the Hardware—Ventilator Selection  225
Preparation for Discharge at Home  227
Follow-up and Evaluation  230

## SECTION 2: FLUIDS AND ELECTROLYTES

**23. BODY FLUID HOMEOSTASIS** — 235
*Anumeha Bhagat*
- Daily Water Flux in the Body  235
- Body Fluid Compartments  235
- Measurement of Body Fluid Spaces  237
- Regulation of Extracellular Fluid Composition and Volume  238

**24. INTRAVENOUS FLUIDS** — 243
*Nilanchal Chakraborty, Addy Yh Tan*
- Classification of Fluids  243
- Crystalloids  243
- Colloids  247

**25. APPROACH TO THE PATIENT WITH HYPOVOLEMIA** — 251
*Tom Carmeliet, Robert Wise, Jan Van der Mullen, Manu Malbrain*
- Case  251
- Definitions  252
- Etiology of Hypovolemia  253
- Consequences of Hypovolemia  253
- Approach to Hypovolemic Patient  253

**26. FLUID THERAPY FOR SPECIFIC CLINICAL CONDITIONS** — 266
*Ram Baalachandran, Rahul Nanchal*
- Pathophysiology  266
- Adverse Effects of Fluids  268
- Choices of Intravenous Fluids  269
- Infusion Strategies—Bolus versus Maintenance  269
- Fluid Therapy in Specific Circumstances  270

**27. APPROACH TO THE PATIENT WITH HYPONATREMIA AND HYPERNATREMIA** — 275
*Dharmendra Bhadauria, Harsh Vardhan*
- Sodium Homeostasis  275
- Water Balance  276
- Hyponatremia  276
- Hypernatremia  283

**28. APPROACH TO THE PATIENT WITH HYPOKALEMIA AND HYPERKALEMIA** — 288
*Diego Luis Carrillo-Pérez, Gerardo Gamba*
- Potassium Homeostasis  288
- Hypokalemia  288
- Hyperkalemia  291

**29. APPROACH TO THE PATIENT WITH HYPOCALCEMIA AND HYPERCALCEMIA** — 296
*Bhuvana Krishna, Sriram Sampath*
- Calcium Homeostasis  296
- Hypocalcemia  297
- Hypercalcemia  302

## 30. APPROACH TO THE PATIENT WITH HYPOPHOSPHATEMIA AND HYPERPHOSPHATEMIA  307
*Nasirul J Ekbal, Andrew Davenport, Banwari Agarwal*
- Phosphate Homeostasis  307
- Hypophosphatemia  307
- Hyperphosphatemia  310

## 31. APPROACH TO THE PATIENT WITH HYPOMAGNESEMIA AND HYPERMAGNESEMIA  314
*Dharshan Rangaswamy*
- Magnesium Homeostasis  314
- Hypomagnesemia  315
- Hypermagnesemia  318

# SECTION 3: BLOOD GASES

## 32. ACID-BASE HOMEOSTASIS  325
*Saurabh Saigal*
- Acid-base Homeostasis  325
- Normal Physiological Response for Respiratory Disorders  326
- Normal Physiological Response for Metabolic Disorders  328

## 33. APPROACH TO THE PATIENT WITH METABOLIC ACIDOSIS AND ALKALOSIS  329
*Jeroen Tahon, Niels Van Regenmortel*
- Approach to the Patient with Metabolic Acid-base Disorders  329
- Metabolic Acidosis  333
- Metabolic Alkalosis  337

## 34. APPROACH TO THE PATIENT WITH RESPIRATORY ACIDOSIS AND ALKALOSIS  342
*John Botha, Ravindranath Tiruvoipati*
- Respiratory Acidosis  342
- Respiratory Alkalosis  345

## 35. BASICS OF ARTERIAL BLOOD GAS INTERPRETATION  348
*Roop Kishen*
- Why Measure ABG?  348
- General Principles and Technical Aspects  348
- Interpreting ABG (With Emphasis on Interpreting Acid-base Disturbances)  349
- Corrections and Concordance: Do we Really Need them?  353

## 36. ARTERIAL BLOOD GAS INTERPRETATION IN CLINICAL PRACTICE  355
*Roop Kishen*
- Arterial Blood Gas Interpretation in Clinical Practice  355
- Steps in Interpreting Arterial Blood Gas Results  355
- Do we Need Different Approaches for Arterial Blood Gas Interpretation?  360

# SECTION 4: MISCELLANEOUS

## 37. ENTERAL AND PARENTERAL NUTRITION IN THE ICU  365
*Mark W Motejunas, Bethany Menard, Louis Anzalone, Cody M Koress, Mark R Jones, Alan D Kaye*
- Indications for Therapy  365
- Enteral Nutrition  366

Parenteral Nutrition  *368*
Adjunctive Therapies  *368*
Drug Interactions  *369*
Side Effects and Complications  *370*

### 38. IMMUNONUTRITION, VITAMINS, AND TRACE ELEMENTS IN THE ICU  373
*Samir Samal, Shakti Bedanta Mishra, Snigdha Ipsita*

Immunonutrition  *373*
Macronutrients  *374*
Micronutrients: Vitamins  *377*
Trace Elements  *381*

### 39. TRANSFUSION OF BLOOD PRODUCTS IN CRITICALLY ILL ADULT PATIENTS  387
*Armin Ahmed*

Packed Red Blood Cells  *387*
Fresh Frozen Plasma  *389*
Cryoprecipitate  *391*
Prothrombin Complex Concentrate  *391*
Platelet Transfusion  *392*
Massive Transfusion  *393*
Blood Transfusion Reaction  *393*

### 40. CARE FOR THE POTENTIAL ORGAN DONOR IN THE ICU  396
*Pranav Jetley, Kapil Dev Soni*

Donation after Neurological (Brain) Death  *396*
Donation after Cardiac Death  *398*
Effects of Brain Death  *399*
Management of Potential Organ Donor after Brain Death  *400*

### INDEX  405

# SECTION 1

# Ventilation

1. Respiration: Applied Anatomy and Pathophysiological Considerations
2. Oxygen Delivery Devices
3. Approach to the Patient with Hypoxemia
4. Approach to the Patient with Hypercapnia
5. Noninvasive Ventilation
6. Mechanical Ventilators
7. Mechanical Ventilation in Specific Clinical Scenarios
8. Graphic Analysis of Mechanical Ventilation
9. Patient-Ventilator Asynchrony
10. Monitoring $O_2$ and $CO_2$ during Mechanical Ventilation
11. Lung Recruitment Maneuvers
12. Heart Lung Interactions during Mechanical Ventilation
13. Monitoring Pressures during Mechanical Ventilation
14. Inspiratory Effort Assessment in Ventilated Patient
15. Ventilator-induced Lung Injury
16. Ventilator-induced Diaphragm Dysfunction
17. Weaning from Mechanical Ventilation
18. Aerosol Drug Delivery in Ventilated Patient
19. Extracorporeal Membrane Oxygenation
20. Extracorporeal Membrane Carbon Dioxide Removal
21. High Frequency Oscillatory Ventilation
22. Domiciliary and Palliative Ventilation

# CHAPTER 1

# Respiration: Applied Anatomy and Pathophysiological Considerations

*Alex Yartsev, Yugan Mudaliar*

## INTRODUCTION

The macroscopic and microscopic anatomy of the respiratory tract is inseparable from its physiological function, and has significant relevance to the study of human respiratory pathophysiology. Applied respiratory anatomy and physiology is of fundamental importance to critical care, given the prevalence of respiratory conditions and complications among critically ill patients, and the frequency of the need for interventions directed at the respiratory system. This chapter focuses on those aspects of respiratory tract anatomy and physiology which are most relevant to the routine practice of critical care medicine, and which have the greatest impact on the management of a patient with severe respiratory pathology.

## MACROSCOPIC AND MICROSCOPIC STRUCTURAL ELEMENTS OF THE RESPIRATORY TRACT

The respiratory tract consists of mouth, nose, pharynx, larynx, trachea, bronchi, alveoli, and pulmonary vessels. Of these structural components, many have important roles which are not directly involved in respiration and gas exchange. For instance, the mouth and tongue have important roles in speech and swallowing, the nose in humidification, the trachea in the cough reflex, and the alveoli in the synthesis of angiotensin-converting enzyme (ACE).

The upper airway trachea and bronchi form the "conductive portion" of the respiratory system, so named because the function of these structures is not directly related to gas exchange. The macroscopic and microscopic structure of these components bears a direct relationship to their role as rigid conduits for gas, and the defenders of the delicate lower structures from thermal and physical insult. The "respiratory portion" of the respiratory tract consists of respiratory bronchioles and alveoli. These structures serve to maintain a low resistance to airflow as well as participating directly in gas exchange.

The histological structure of the respiratory tract is no less relevant to function and also calls for a detailed discussion. The mucosa of the upper respiratory tract is well-supplied with capillary blood flow and is an important route of drug delivery. Moreover, its epithelial layer harbors immunoglobulin molecules (predominantly IgA), numerous quiescent lymphocytes, and dendritic antigen-presenting cells (APCs), playing an important role in specific cellular and humoral immunity. Mucous glands and Bowman's glands in the epithelium produce secretions which moisturize the cellular layer and contribute to the humidification of the inspired gas. Lower airways are well-supplied with ciliated columnar epithelium to promote the outward movement of mucus, assisting in the clearance of small particles (Figs. 1A to C).

The respiratory portion of the respiratory tract consists of microscopic respiratory bronchioles and alveoli, the histology of which bears a direct relationship to the function of gas exchange. Respiratory bronchioles contain the smooth muscle, which acts as an important target for bronchodilators. Understanding the cellular structure of alveoli is of paramount importance to the understanding of gas exchange. The physical properties of alveoli and the actions of alveolar surfactant (secreted by Type 2 alveolar cells) are vital to the understanding of clinical approaches to the mechanical ventilation for acute respiratory distress syndrome (ARDS), as well as complications of mechanical ventilation such as barotrauma and biotrauma.

## ORAL CAVITY AND THE PHARYNX

The evolution of the human airway from precursor structures in earlier animals and fish has led to a single cavity that serves the purposes of speech, air intake, and swallowing.[1]

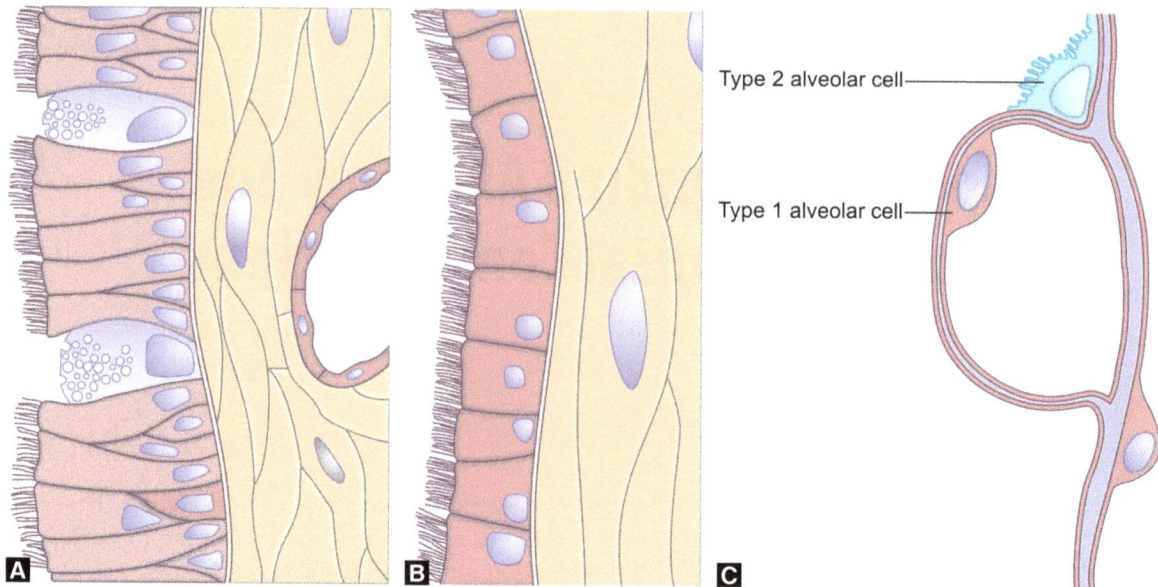

**Figs. 1A to C:** Microscopic structure of the respiratory epithelia. (A) The upper respiratory tract is lined with pseudostratified columnar epithelium; (B) The bronchioles are lined with ciliated cuboid epithelium; (C) The alveolar epithelial lining consists of Type 1 and Type 2 alveolar cells.

As such this cavity is a complex organ complete with multiple motor and sensory systems, which permit the isolation of these functions, with the resulting inability of human beings to speak, swallow, and breathe at the same time. The motor innervation of the oral cavity and pharynx enjoys a significant amount of central control. From the point of view of the critical care physician, the most important pathophysiological implications of this control is the loss of protective airway reflexes and pharyngeal muscle tone which is associated with a decreased level of consciousness.

### The Effect of Depressed Consciousness on Oropharyngeal Patency

The fact that a depressed level of consciousness can give rise to asphyxia due to airway obstruction is a well-recognized feature of advanced life support training. The pathophysiological mechanism underlying such airway obstruction is complex. Though relaxation of the tongue plays a role in obstruction at the level of the pharynx, closure of the laryngeal entrance by the epiglottis is the main cause of airway closure associated with unconsciousness. Cadaveric studies where the tongue was removed had demonstrated that an airtight seal could be achieved by the closure of the epiglottis alone.[2] The most important implication of this finding in critical care is the observation that elevation of the mandible-hyoid apparatus by jaw thrust relieves both causes of obstruction.

### Nasopharynx

The nasal cavity turbinates serve to increase the turbulence of air flow, thereby increasing the contact of inspired air with the nasal mucosa. The effect of this is to increase the temperature and humidity of inspired air, protecting the mucosa of lower passages from dehydration.

The anterior nares feature coarse hairs, called vibrissae (though the term usually applies to mammalian sensory hairs from which human nasal hair differs in both structure and function). These hairs arise from follicles which are similar to hair follicles elsewhere on the skin, and are neither richly innervated nor mapped onto the somatosensory cortex, in contrast to the mystacial vibrissae of mammals. These hairs are thought to serve the purpose of increasing the turbulence of nasal airflow as well as trapping inhaled macroscopic particles. The importance of these hairs in the critical care environment is seen in the context of airway burns; singed vibrissae are a signal that inhaled gas or smoke was sufficiently hot to be associated with a high risk of airway burns.[3]

### The Role of the Upper Airway in Humidification

The upper airway is able to warm and humidify inspired air over an enviable range of temperatures and ambient humidity levels. By the time it reaches the carina, inspired gas may be heated by 20–30°C during its passage through the upper airways, and inspired air as cold as –100°C achieves *core body temperature* and 100% humidity by the time it reaches the alveoli.[4] This exchange of heat and moisture occurs in both directions: On expiration, heat and moisture are reclaimed by the mucosa, and expired air has its temperature reduced from 37°C at the alveoli to 32°C at the nares. The expired air remains 100% saturated with water vapor, but as its temperature decreases, so does its absolute water content.[5]

The efficiency of heat and moisture exchange in the nasopharynx is increased by means of turbulent convection. Turbulence increases the contact between inspired air and nasopharyngeal mucosa, promoting increased heat exchange. At the same time, increased contact with inspired air promotes the evaporation of water from the mucosa. As heat is exchanged and inspired air increases in temperature, its capacity to "hold" water vapor also increases, until an equilibrium is reached where the inspired air is isothermic with the mucosa, and 100% saturated. This occurs at the "isothermic saturation boundary", at a level just below the carina during normal quiet breathing. At this level, the absolute humidity is 47 g/m$^3$.

The importance of maintaining humidification of the respiratory gases is twofold. It maintains the health and barrier integrity of the respiratory mucosa, and allows effective gas exchange. This has implications for the critical care environment, where mechanical ventilation often requires the use of piped gas supplies. The administration of dry cold gas (for instance, oxygen directly from the compressed gas storage system) leads to the inspissation of secretions, dehydration of the nasal mucosa, failure of the mucosal barrier function, an increased risk of epistaxis, as well as the thickening of the lower respiratory tract mucus layer, and the impairment of mucosal ciliary motility.[6]

For these reasons, in mechanically ventilated patients, humidification of inspired gas mixtures needs to be maintained, particularly if the upper airways have been bypassed by endotracheal intubation or tracheostomy. This can be accomplished by means of passive heat and moisture exchange filters which replicate the functions of the upper airway mucosa, or by active humidifiers which pass the inspired gas mixture across a heated water bath. In order to maintain mucosal integrity and enhance secretion clearance, a humidity output of 30 g/m$^3$ is recommended for long-term intensive care unit (ICU) use and 20 g/m$^3$ for short-term perioperative ventilation.[7]

## Larynx

The larynx is a cartilaginous tubular structure which acts as the entrance to the trachea and functions to occlude the airway. In evolutionary terms, it had developed from the airways of the lungfish, and had served to protect the air-filled cavities of the respiratory system during feeding and perfusion of the gills with water.[8] Similarly, the human larynx has multiple functions all of which in some way involve occluding or obstructing the flow of air in and out of the trachea. These functions include phonation (the laryngeal component of speech), effort closure (for forceful expulsion of lung air, as in coughing), and swallowing (where the larynx is elevated and epiglottis closes the laryngeal inlet, directing the food bolus backward into the esophagus).

The anatomy of the larynx as relevant to the practice of gaining airway access has paramount importance to the critical care physician. Figure 2 demonstrates the anatomical features of the adult larynx from the point of view of direct laryngoscopy. Anatomically, the larynx extends from the tip of the epiglottis to the inferior border of the cricoid cartilage. It is suspended from the hyoid bone, and is found at the level of the C3–C6 cervical vertebrae. Its rigid structural components consist of three single cartilages (thyroid, epiglottic, and cricoid) and three paired cartilages (arytenoid, cuneiform, and corniculate). In terms of importance to airway access, the most important cartilaginous structure is the epiglottic cartilage, a long teardrop-shaped cartilage which is attached anteriorly to the hyoid bone by the hyoepiglottic ligament.[9] Pressure in the vallecula during direct laryngoscopy elevates the epiglottis and affords a direct view of the vocal cords. Position of the epiglottis during laryngoscopy describes the difficulty of intubation by the Cormack–Lehane descriptive system,[10] ranging from Grade 4 (where not even the epiglottis is visible) to Grade 1 (where the epiglottis is completely elevated and most of the glottis can be visualized).

The larynx moves under the influence of intrinsic muscles that control the vocal cords and the extrinsic muscles which change the position of the larynx in relation to the hyoid and sternum to assist in swallowing.[9] Of the intrinsic muscles, all receive motor innervation from the recurrent laryngeal nerve except for the cricothyroid muscle (which increases tension on the vocal cords, and for which is motor innervation is supplied by the external branch of the superior laryngeal nerve). Damage to the recurrent laryngeal nerve produces paralysis of the ipsilateral intrinsic muscles, sparing the cricothyroid muscle. The resulting unopposed tension on the vocal cords can give rise to hoarseness or stridor with unilateral lesions and airway obstruction with bilateral recurrent laryngeal nerve injuries. Outside of surgical scenarios such

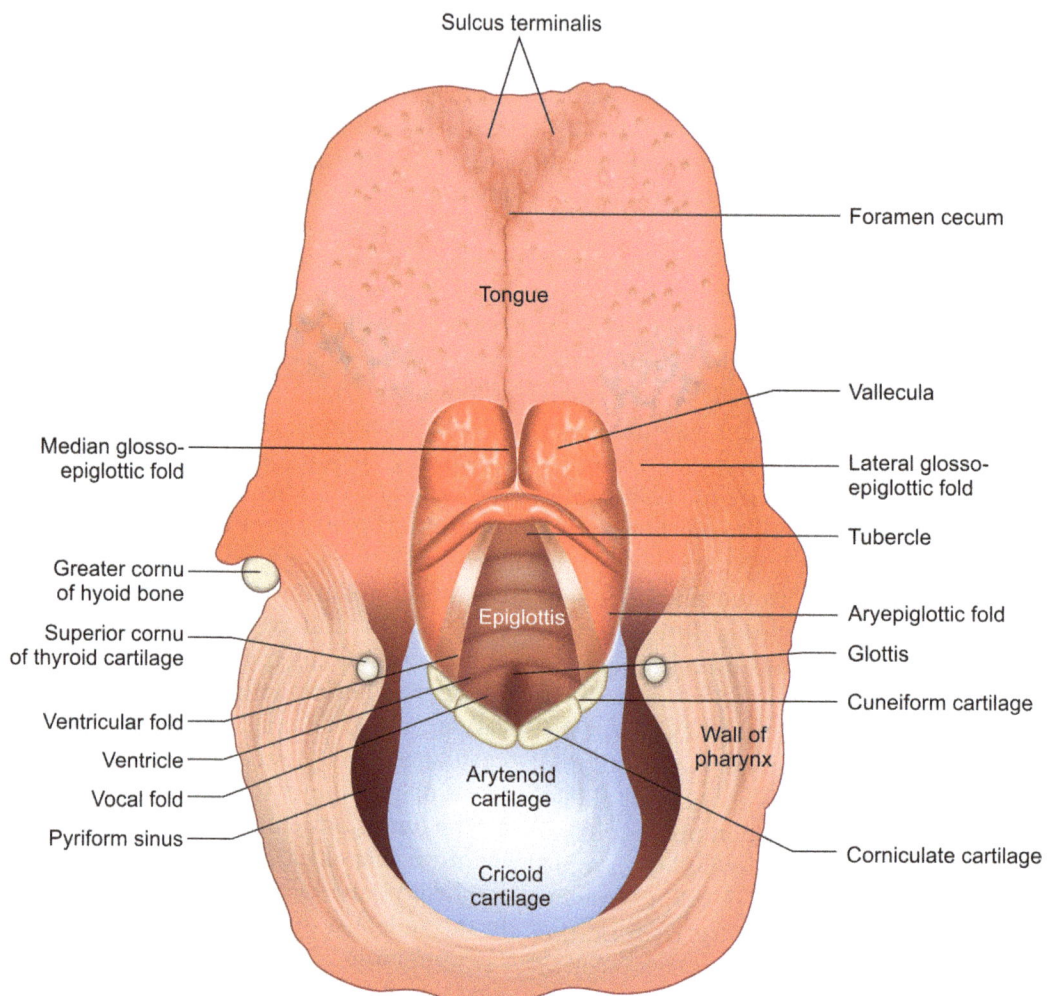

**Fig. 2:** Anatomy of the larynx as viewed for laryngoscopy.

as thyroid surgery, a likely cause of recurrent laryngeal nerve injury in the ICU is an endotracheal tube cuff which has been inflated in the subglottic larynx. The recurrent laryngeal nerve enters this area between the cricoid and the thyroid cartilage, and is susceptible to injury where an inflated cuff can compress it against the overlying thyroid cartilage.[11]

### Laryngospasm and Protection from Aspiration

The larynx is richly innervated by the superior laryngeal nerve and the recurrent laryngeal nerve, both are the branches of the vagus nerve.[12] Sensory innervation to the glottis and the glottic vestibule is supplied by the internal branch of the superior laryngeal nerve. The lower glottis sensory and motor innervation comes from the recurrent laryngeal nerve. The density of laryngeal sensory chemoreceptors and mechanoreceptors is greatest at the laryngeal opening, which allows rapid protective responses.

The stimulation of these receptors leads to the reflexive closure of the glottis by adduction of the vocal cords, which functions to protect the lower airways from foreign material. When this adduction response is long-lived, it may render ventilation impossible. Such a sustained closure of the true vocal cords (or both true and false cords) is described as "laryngospasm".[13] Failure of the afferent or efferent components of the laryngeal closure reflex (e.g. following stroke) may give rise to aspiration of upper airway secretions and subsequent pneumonitis.

### The Effect of Endotracheal Intubation on Cough

A normal cough sequence consists of deep inspiration, glottic closure, increase in transpulmonary pressure by forceful contraction of respiratory muscles, and ultimately glottis opening with an abrupt increase in airway gas flow. The tracheal lumen collapses and in the narrowed trachea the high peak air flow results in the expulsion of tracheal secretions. In the intubated state, glottis closure is not available, and normal cough efficiency is altered by the disruption of normal flow and pressure timing. The intubated patient is still able to transport secretions to the trachea, but failure of the trachea to collapse prevents the necessary high flows from being generated, with the resulting accumulation of secretions near the distal end of the endotracheal tube.[14] This has significant implications for secretion control and management of pulmonary infection in intubated patients.

### The Effect of Tracheostomy on Swallowing Function

A key function of the laryngeal apparatus is to permit airway closure during swallowing by the elevation of the larynx. The laryngeal inlet is both closed and physically removed from the path of the food bolus by action of a number of muscles, which are grouped under the term "laryngeal strap muscles" and which contribute to the suspension of the larynx.[15] This movement is permitted by the natural elasticity and mobility of the trachea. The presence of a tracheostomy tethers the larynx by immobilizing the trachea against the skin and strap muscles of the neck, inhibiting the normal upward excursion of the larynx.[16]

### Trachea and Bronchi—The Conductive Airways

The tracheobronchial tree is a series of tubular respiratory passages consisting of complete and incomplete cartilaginous rings as well as smooth muscle and the striated *trachealis* muscle. The tree branches into 23 "generations" of successively narrower airways with a progressive increase in the total cross-sectional area, from the 1.8 cm diameter of the trachea (generation 0) to the respiratory bronchioles (generations 17–19), which are approximately 0.4 mm in diameter (Fig. 3). As the total cross-sectional area of the lower airways may be up to 100 times that of the upper airways, the resistance to air flow in these regions is usually minimal.

Among the functions and structural properties of the tracheobronchial tree, of greatest pathophysiological importance to the critical care physician is the immune function of the mucociliary escalator and the role of bronchial smooth muscle tone in generating resistance to air flow.

### Mucociliary Escalator

The "mucociliary escalator" consists of a ciliated epithelial layer, which extends from the larynx to the terminal bronchioles (the 16th division of the tracheobronchial tree). This ciliated layer is the primary defense mechanism of the lower respiratory tract against inhaled particulate matter. The cells of this layer consist of ciliated columnar epithelial cells (each featuring approximately 200 cilia) and mucus-secreting goblet cells (Fig. 4). The secretions of the cells (4% mucus and 96% water by weight) form a layer over the ciliated epithelium. Rather than a continuous mucus layer that covers the epithelium like a blanket, discrete

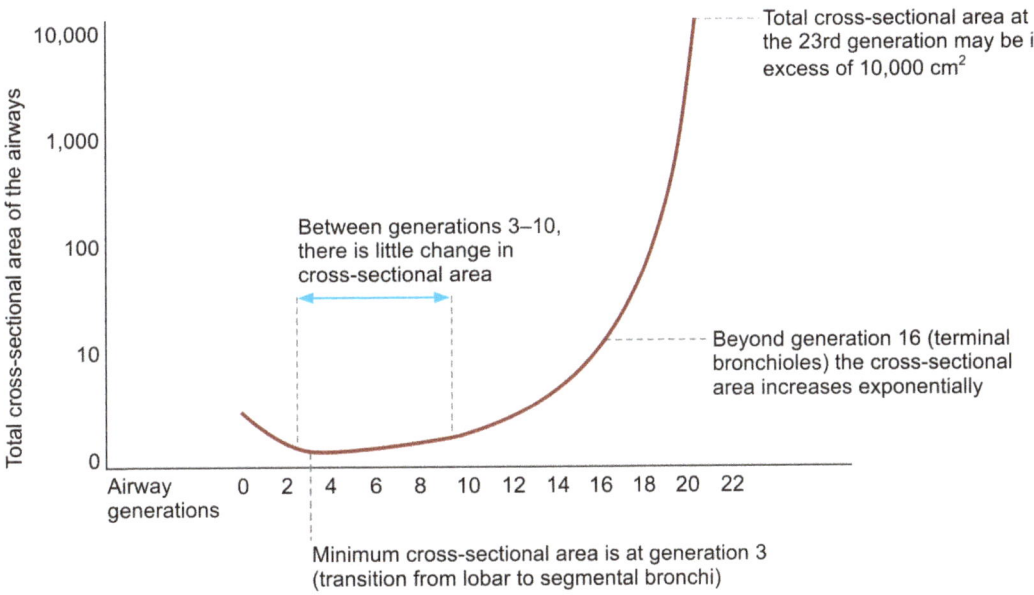

**Fig. 3:** The cross-sectional area of the airways is narrowest at the junction between the lobar and segmental bronchi, and increases exponentially in the lower airways.

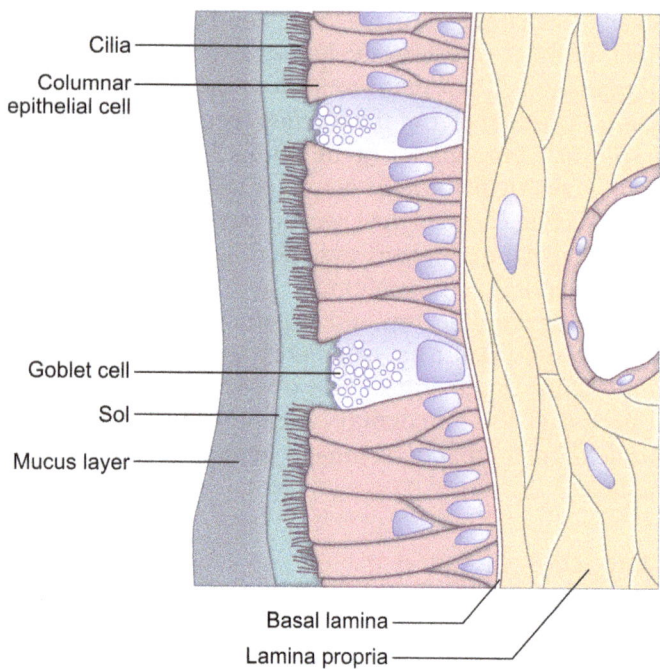

**Fig. 4:** Respiratory pseudostratified columnar epithelium of the trachea. The mucus layer sits atop an aqueous sol, in which the mobile cilia are situated.

islands of respiratory mucus float on a layer of periciliary sol like lilies on water; the sol forms a thinner fluid that allows the cilia to beat and thus propel the mucus islands up the airway.[17] The coordinated movement of the cilia is a surprisingly powerful force and can carry masses up to 10 g cm$^{-2}$ against gravity,[18] at velocities of approximately 5–20 mm per minute.

Increased susceptibility to pneumonia among ventilated patients has been attributed an impairment of the mucociliary escalator action. Intubated patients have slowed mucociliary clearance (down to 1 mm/min), and mucous flow may even be reversed in the semirecumbent position, which may contribute to the pathogenesis of atelectasis and ventilator-associated pneumonia.[19,20] High oxygen concentrations, poor humidification, systemic inflammatory response, colonization by bacteria, suction catheter damage to the mucosa, and bacterial colonization have all been implicated as possible causes of this mucociliary clearance impairment.

### The Role of Bronchial Smooth Muscle in Bronchospasm

Bronchi and bronchioles (generations 4–14) feature crisscrossing helical bands of muscle, the thickness of which is proportionally greatest at the level of the bronchioles.[21] These bands of muscle can alter the diameter of the small airways in response to local cellular factors, mechanical and chemical stimuli, and neural control or humoral circulating factors. The cross-sectional area of the distal bronchi may decrease by 50–80% at maximal bronchoconstriction; the degree of bronchoconstriction increases with increasing bronchial generations,[22] which has implications for drug delivery. Inhaled bronchodilator particle size needs to be sufficiently small in order to penetrate to these deeper structures.

### Alveolar Ducts and Alveoli

The terminal bronchioles are the last generation of conductive airways. Beyond these, the airway branches into respiratory bronchioles, alveolar ducts, and alveolar sacs. Like the terminal bronchioles, the respiratory bronchioles have a well-defined smooth muscle layer; however, with increasing generations respiratory bronchiole walls gradually increase in the number of mural alveoli. The alveolar ducts differ from respiratory bronchioles by having no walls (i.e. their walls consist only of the openings of mural alveoli). Alveolar sacs are the terminal branches of the respiratory tract. Approximately half of all alveoli take their origin from alveolar sacs, the other half originating from alveolar ducts. The total number of the alveoli is on average approximately 480 million, and each is approximately 0.2 mm in diameter at functional residual capacity (FRC). Each alveolus is usually polyhedral rather than spherical; the septa between alveoli are stretched tight by the tension of the elastic fibers they contain as well as by the surface tension created by the air–fluid interface. These septa contain pores of Kohn, microscopic fenestrations which permit the movement of gas between alveoli (Fig. 5). The alveolar septa also contain the pulmonary capillaries, which bulge into the airspace. The thickness of the active membrane here is 0.2–0.3 µm, and there is virtually no interstitial space.

Alveolar epithelial cells (Type I cells) have a flat sheet-like structure, mostly devoid of organelles and of approximately 0.1 µm in thickness. They are joined together by tight junctions, which prevent the escape of large proteins into the alveolar space. These cells do not have the capacity to undergo mitosis. Type II cells are the stem cells from which Type I cells arise; these serve to replenish the alveolar epithelium as well as being sources of alveolar surfactant.

### Alveolar Surfactant

Alveolar surfactant is a surface-active material, which is responsible for maintaining the low surface tension of alveolar fluid. Surfactant consists of one main active ingredient

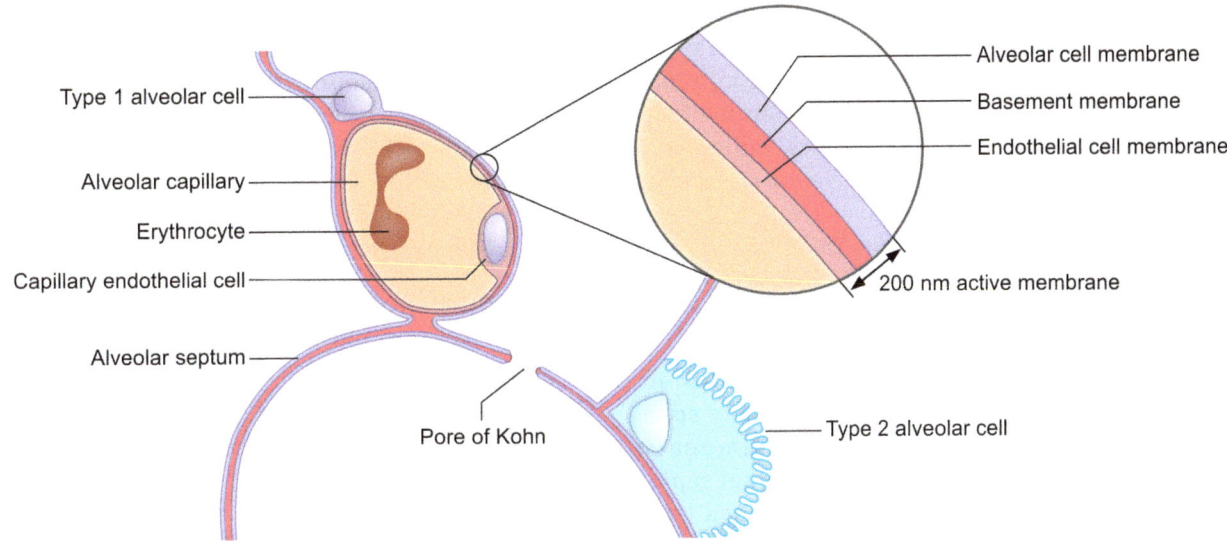

**Fig. 5:** Functional cellular anatomy of the alveoli.

(dipalmitoylphosphatidylcholine, a phospholipid) as well as carbohydrates and a small amount of surfactant proteins (2% by weight). Surfactant is released by Type II cells, has a half-life of 15–30 hours, and is degraded by reuptake into Type II cells. The clinical relevance of surfactant is apparent in surfactant-deficient pathological states, of which the prototypic model is a preterm neonatal lung. Severe respiratory failure with atelectasis tends to develop in premature infants who are yet to secrete enough surfactant[23] and those suffering from hereditary disorders of surfactant protein synthesis.[24] The presence of surfactant in bronchoalveolar lavage fluid can be confirmed by the presence of foam in the retrieved fluid, and indicates a deep lavage. However, the excessive washout of surfactant can give rise to postlavage hypoxia and atelectasis. Lastly, pulmonary surfactant interacts destructively with lipopeptide antibiotics such as daptomycin, resulting in their deactivation.[25]

### Ventilator-associated Lung Injury at the Alveolar Level

The alveolar septa derive their durability from a basement membrane layer (the lamina densa) composed of Type IV collagen fibers. This layer is approximately 50 nm thick and is adherent to the epithelial (respiratory) and endothelial (vascular) cells on either side by a network of attachment proteins called laminins. These proteins interact with the cytoskeleton of endothelial and epithelial cells, regulating the permeability of the membrane.

Mechanical ventilation with high pressures can damage the alveolar septa. Microscopically, there is damage to both alveolar epithelium and pulmonary capillary endothelium. At ventilation with pressures greater than 30 cm $H_2O$, there is flattening of alveolar capillaries, and visible disruption of the epithelial and endothelial layers. The basement membrane usually remains intact (and may be the sole remaining barrier between gas and blood). However, the diffusion of gases is still impaired because the membrane is usually thickened (up to 1 µm) due to cellular damage and resulting interstitial edema. At higher pressures (up to 50 cm $H_2O$) the basement membrane can also be damaged, and microscopy of alveoli ventilated at such pressures reveals a full-thickness of red blood cells in the alveolar spaces.[26] It would appear that the elastic collagen-rich basement membrane has a greater tolerance for mechanical stress, but the damage to endothelial and epithelial cells manifests at lower pressures. This cellular damage then gives rise not only to a degraded gas diffusion due to increasing membrane thickness, but also to a release of proinflammatory mediators into the systemic circulation. The systemic effects of such cytokine release are seen in mechanically ventilated patients with ARDS; the phenomenon has been called "biotrauma" and can lead to multi-organ dysfunction.[27]

## APPLIED ANATOMY AND PATHOPHYSIOLOGY OF THE PULMONARY CIRCULATION

The anatomical distinction between the pulmonary and systemic circulation lies in the different pressures between these two systems. The blood pressure within the pulmonary circulation is approximately 15–20% of the systemic arterial blood pressure. Consequently, pulmonary vessels have significantly less smooth muscle; in fact, the larger vessels are composed mainly of elastic connective tissue. Muscular layers become dominant in pulmonary arteries below 1mm diameter. In contrast to systemic arterioles, pulmonary arterioles have minimal smooth muscle tissue in their walls, and are structurally indistinguishable from pulmonary venules. Pulmonary arterioles and venules frequently have small (25-50 µm) anastomoses which remain closed under normal conditions and only open into shunts under conditions of increased cardiac output or with the use of inotrope agents.[28] Shunt, pulmonary hypertension, and their management are discussed in greater detail elsewhere.

Pulmonary capillaries form a dense network in the alveolar septa, and a capillary network may span several alveoli before emptying into a pulmonary venule. Pulmonary venules run along segmental septa. Pulmonary vessels and bronchi are surrounded by a network of pulmonary lymphatics, which occupy potential spaces between these structures and the rest of the lung parenchyma. During episodes of pulmonary edema, these potential spaces become distended with fluid, giving rise to the characteristic peribronchial cuffing seen on chest radiographs. Lymphatic drainage occurs in the direction of the hilum, also giving rise to the perihilar hazing and "bat-wing" appearance of acute pulmonary edema. Tracheobronchial lymph nodes accept drainage from pulmonary lymphatics, and these groups of nodes (particularly the subcarinal nodes) become attractive targets for bronchoscopic biopsy sampling.

## Ventilation and Perfusion Relationship

In ideal circumstances, alveolar ventilation (V) and alveolar capillary perfusion (Q) would be perfectly matched; i.e. the ideal alveolus is ventilated with the perfect amount of air in order to completely saturate all hemoglobin molecules passing through its capillaries. In reality, there is a regional variation of blood flow and ventilation which varies with posture, disease states, drug effects, and mechanical ventilation.

Perfusion is maximal in dependent regions of lung, which in the upright position are the lung bases. According to this "gravitational model", in upright man the perfusion of the lung apices can be attributed to the difference in hydrostatic pressure between the apices and the bases, which may be 30-40 cm $H_2O$.[29]

Ventilation is also maximal in the bases of the lungs, where the rib cage expands to the greatest extent in inspiration, and where diaphragmatic excursion contributes to the change in volume. Furthermore, lung tissue has a significant mass and therefore the weight of the tissue above compresses the tissue below; the dependent lung is therefore more compressed, has higher compliance and therefore better ventilation. In the upright position, the measured ratio of apical to basal ventilation is approximately 1:1.5 by volume at resting ventilation, and 1:3 at inspiration to full vital capacity.

## Zones of the Lung, Dead Space and Shunt

Regional differences in ventilation and perfusion give rise to three distinct patterns, which are known as Wests' Zones. Because the pulmonary circulation is a low pressure system, in the apices the pulmonary capillary pressure may be lower than alveolar pressure; this results in areas of lung which are ventilated but not perfused, referred to as *alveolar dead space*. This region is referred to as Wests Zone 1; the pattern of V/Q mismatch described by this zone does not occur in normal physiological states, but may be seen in critically ill patients suffering from extreme hypovolemia or hemorrhagic shock.[30] It can also be seen in circumstances where alveolar pressure is artificially increased, for instance in the context of mechanical ventilation with high pressures.

Wests Zone 2 describes a region which has pulsatile blood flow which is generated by the fact that pulmonary venous pressure is lower than pulmonary arterial pressure. In this region, flow occurs intermittently, when arterial pressure cyclically increases to a point where it overcomes the obstruction to venous flow. After the pressure is relieved, the system returns to a low pressure state and flow ceases again.

Wests Zone 3 describes an area of the lung where the capillaries enjoy constant blood flow because both arterial and venous pressure is higher than the alveolar pressure. This relationship describes blood flow in the dependent basal regions of the lung. Because there is an uninterrupted column of blood between the pulmonary arteries and the pulmonary veins in this region, Zone 3 makes an ideal position for measuring pulmonary capillary wedge pressures using a pulmonary artery catheter.

In disease states such as atelectasis or pneumonia, regions of lung will have minimal ventilation due to physical compression, bronchial obstruction, or copious secretions. In this case, the affected regions of lung will have perfusion, but no ventilation. Pulmonary veins returning from such regions will carry hypoxic blood back into the systemic circulation, and the addition of this hypoxic blood will reduce the oxygen saturation of arterial blood in the systemic circulation. This phenomenon is referred to as *intrapulmonary shunting,* and the resulting incompletely oxygenated percentage of cardiac output is described as the *shunt fraction*.

## LUNG VOLUME AND CAPACITIES

Static lung volumes and capacities have standard definitions (Fig. 6), where a "capacity" refers to a measurement consisting of more than one "volume".

The total lung capacity (TLS) is the volume of gas in the lungs at the end of a maximal inspiration. The residual volume (RV) is the volume which remains after a maximal expiration. The functional residual capacity (FRC) is the volume of gas which remains in the lungs after an expiration during normal breathing. Lung volumes are affected by age, gender, ethnicity, posture, obesity, and pregnancy; they change in linear proportion with the height of a patient. During mechanical ventilation, tidal volume is usually calculated with reference to the ideal body weight, which is indexed to height.

### Volume-Related Airway Collapse and Closing Capacity

Lung volumes influence the diameter of smaller airways, particularly those beyond generation 11 (as these have minimal cartilage and rely instead on the traction from lung tissue for their patency). As lung volume decreases in expiration, the volume of all air-filled cavities and passages decreases proportionally, which includes the smaller airways. As lung volume decreased toward RV, some of these smaller airways begin to close, which results in an increase in their resistance to airflow.[32] At some critical volume, these small airways collapse completely; the volume at which this occurs is referred to as *closing capacity*, and the effect of lung volume on increasing airway resistance is referred to as *volume-related airway collapse*. Closing capacity increases with age; it is well below the FRC in young patients, but becomes equal to FRC in patients over 70, even in the upright posture.[33] With the closing capacity exceeding FRC, during a period of expiration some of the alveoli will be perfused with pulmonary blood but not ventilated because of airway closure, which represents a shunt by definition. This is most marked in dependent regions of lung and in situations where the FRC is decreased (e.g. in obese patients, in pregnancy or when the patient is in a supine position). One of the effects of positive end-expiratory pressure (PEEP) is to increase the FRC above closing capacity, thereby decreasing shunt and improving oxygenation.

### Flow-Related Airway Collapse and Closing Capacity

Gas flow influences the diameter of smaller airways; even the trachea changes diameter with high expiratory gas flow velocity.[34] During forceful expiration, the normally negative intrathoracic pressure becomes positive with the effort of expiratory muscles, resulting in a high velocity gas flow out of the lung. Along the path of gas flow out of the lung, there is a pressure drop (as the resistance to airflow decreases with decreasing generations of airways). Therefore, at a point in the airway, the airway pressure will be equal to the intrathoracic pressure (this point is referred to as *the equal pressure point*). Beyond that point, intrathoracic pressure may be greater than the airway pressure, which (unless

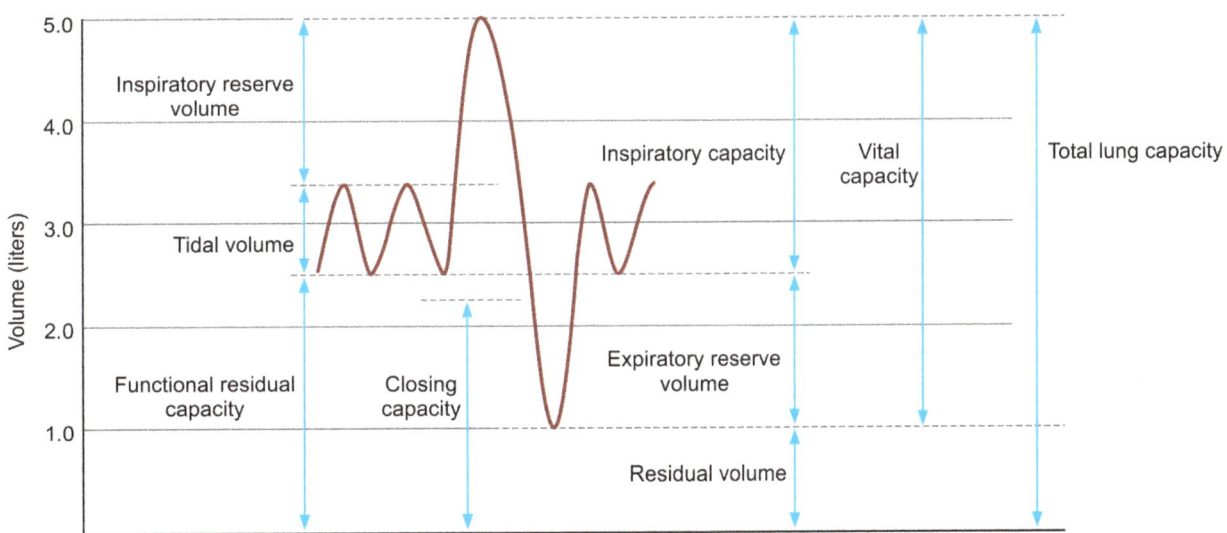

**Fig. 6:** Static lung volumes.[31]

the airway is endowed with rigidity by structural cartilage) will result in airway collapse. This effect is most prominent in airways already narrowed by disease (e.g. asthma), in dependent regions of lung, and at small lung volumes near closing capacity, where airway diameter is already decreased. One of the effects of PEEP is to oppose positive intrathoracic pressure (e.g. due to "intrinsic PEEP" in asthma), thereby allowing airways to remain open.

## APPLIED ANATOMY AND PATHOPHYSIOLOGY OF RESPIRATORY MECHANICS

"Respiratory mechanics" is a term conventionally applied to the interaction of pressure and flow in determining respiratory function. Pressure and flow are determinants from which a variety of indices may be derived, such as volume, compliance, resistance, and work of breathing. These parameters are of substantial importance in the critical care setting, where they are amenable to manipulation by means of mechanical ventilation.[35]

The respiratory system is composed of several interacting anatomical components, which can be functionally divided into airways, lungs, chest wall, and abdomen. Gas flow through the respiratory system is determined by pressure gradients, which are generated by the interaction of these anatomical elements. In order for gas flow to occur there needs to be a pressure gradient between the atmosphere and the alveoli. This pressure gradient across the lung ($P_L$) represents the difference between pressure at the airway ($P_{ao}$) and pressure in the pleural space ($P_{pl}$). As there is no convenient method to monitor pleural pressure directly, esophageal balloon manometry may be used as an acceptable surrogate.[36] For the intents and purposes of bedside physiology, $P_{pl} = P_{es}$. Thus,

$$P_L = P_{ao} - P_{es}$$

Thus, a negative pleural pressure must be generated by the respiratory muscles in order to produce a flow of atmospheric gas into the system. In the mechanically ventilated patient, positive pressure applied at the airway opening produces a positive pressure gradient which drives the flow of gas. Outward flow during expiration occurs passively, and is the consequence of elastic structures recoiling into their resting state (these structures include the lung parenchyma, chest wall, and the abdomen). The amount of pressure which needs to be generated by the patient (or applied by the ventilator) in order to produce gas flow is determined by pulmonary compliance and respiratory system resistance.

## Compliance

Respiratory system compliance is determined by the equation,

$$C = \frac{\Delta V}{P_{plat}}$$

where $\Delta V$ is the change in volume, $P_{plat}$ is the plateau airway pressure, and C is compliance expressed in terms of volume per unit pressure (classically as mL/cm $H_2O$). Normal static compliance in a mechanically ventilated patient is generally held to be 50–100 mL/cm $H_2O$.

Response of the respiratory system to distending pressure is nonlinear, and can be represented by a sigmoid curve. Ventilation typically occurs in the range of tidal volumes where compliance of the respiratory system is high (the "steep" portion of the pressure–volume curve); ventilation with higher volumes or higher pressures may lead to overdistension and a loss of lung compliance is seen, i.e. higher pressures produce a smaller increase in volume (Fig. 7).

Compliance may be further divided into static and dynamic compliance. Conventionally, discussions of compliance address static compliance alone, in the context of a respiratory system inflated with a static volume of gas. However, the process of mechanical ventilation is a dynamic process where inward and outward flow is constantly alternating. The compliance of this system is described by the term "dynamic compliance", which is described by the equation,

$$C_{dyn} = \frac{\Delta V}{P_{peak}}$$

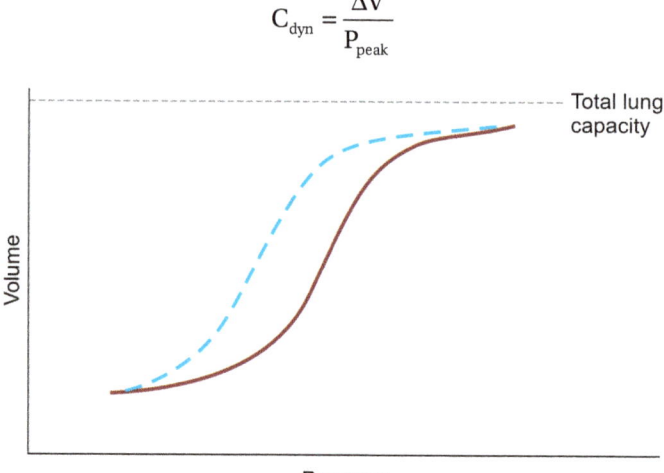

**Fig. 7:** Pressure and volume relationships in the respiratory system. The dashed line represents expiratory pressure and volume relationships. Note that as the tidal volume approaches total lung capacity, incremental increases in pressure produce ever-diminishing increases in volume.

where $P_{peak}$ represents the peak inspiratory pressure. Peak inspiratory pressure is the sum of pressure generated in overcoming lung compliance and pressure generated in overcoming respiratory resistance.

The anatomical and physiological determinants of static compliance are the elasticity of lung tissue and alveolar surface tension. These may be altered in disease states. For instance, decreased respiratory compliance is seen in states of surfactant deficiency (for instance, in premature neonates, or in patients recovering from bronchoscopic lavage). Pulmonary disease which decreases compliance may do so in a diffuse manner (e.g. the effects of ARDS) or by decreasing the total lung capacity by obliterating aeration of whole regions of lung (e.g. the effects of lung consolidation). Destructive pulmonary parenchymal disease may also have the effect of increasing lung compliance, as in the case of emphysema. Unique approaches to the management of mechanical ventilation in states of extremely poor lung compliance (such as ARDS) are discussed in later chapters.

## Resistance

Resistance, broadly speaking, is a resistance to motion. The respiratory system is resistant to the flow of gas. The determinants of this resistance and their proportional contributions are friction against airway surfaces (80%), tissue resistance (19%), and forces of inertia (1%). The resistance to airflow is, therefore, determined largely by the resistance of airways.

The relationship of airway diameter to airway resistance and the pressure generated thereby is described by Poiseuille's Law:

$$\Delta P = \frac{8L\eta Q}{\pi r^4}$$

where $\Delta P$ is the change in pressure generated by the resistance, Q is the flow rate of the gas, $\eta$ is the viscosity of the gas, L is the length of the airway, and *r* is the radius of the airway (which is assumed to be cylindrical in cross-section). By this relationship, the greatest airway resistance is to be expected at the transition point between lobar and segmental bronchi (generations 3, 4, and 5) where the total cross-section of the airways is the smallest (Fig. 3). Measurement and imaging of airways[37] has confirmed that 80% of total airway resistance is generated at this level.

Physiological changes in the respiratory system can influence airway resistance. For instance, airway resistance is inversely proportional to lung volume. Beyond the conducting airways, airflow resistance becomes dependent on lung volume. In inspiration, the expanding lung also puts distending pressure on the smallest airways by traction, therefore increasing their diameter and decreasing their resistance. Conversely, forced expiration increases airflow resistance by increasing pressure on these small airways, forming flow-limiting segments.

Pathological states can also influence airway resistance. Notably, asthma and anaphylaxis can give rise to marked reversible increases in airway resistance. Irreversible or incompletely reversible increases in airway resistance are associated with disease states such as chronic obstructive pulmonary disease (COPD). Unique approaches to the management of bronchospasm and mechanical ventilation in states of extremely high airway resistance are discussed in later chapters.

## Time Constant

Idealised models of lung function behold the lung as a perfectly elastic solid, which instantly expands by a volume ($\Delta V$) in response to the distending pressure ($\Delta P$). The properties of lung *in vivo* are not ideal, and lung tissue takes some time to distend to $\Delta V$. The time required to distend the lung up to 63% of the maximal inflation or deflation is referred to as the *time constant* ($\tau$), and is described mathematically as:

$$\tau = C \times R$$

where C represents compliance and R represents resistance. The value of this constant varies across lung units, and between inspiration and expiration. Lung units with a high compliance and high resistance (e.g. emphysema and COPD) fill slowly, empty even more slowly, and this is represented by a longer time constant ($\tau$) value. Conversely, lung units with poor compliance and low resistance (e.g. pulmonary fibrosis, ARDS) have a quick $\tau$ value, filling and emptying rapidly.

The concept of time constant has relevance with relation to positive pressure ventilation. As the lung is distended during a mechanical breath, the greatest part of the tidal volume will be distributed into lung units with the lowest (quickest) $\tau$ value. Even if the ventilator has cycled to inspiratory pause or expiration, gas may continue to redistribute from these "quick" lung units into "slow" lung units, a process referred to as *pendelluft*. This has the effect of reducing dynamic lung compliance and worsening oxygenation. As lung units with poor compliance and low airflow resistance fill the fastest, they will contribute to a rapid rise in pressure with the initiation of the mechanical breath. Gas, which subsequently redistributes from these units, has already participated in gas exchange and therefore will have a higher $PCO_2$ and a lower $PO_2$, diluting fresh gas and thereby impairing effective gas exchange.[38] Though likely to have minimal adverse influence on gas exchange physiology in the healthy subject, time constant may play a significant role in the physiology of the critically ill patient, particularly hypoxemic patients with severe COPD. This has implications for the approach to ventilation in such patients; classically a prolonged expiratory phase is programmed into the ventilator in order to allow for the lung units with low time constant to empty.

## Work of Breathing

The definition of work is the product of force and distance, or in the case of the respiratory system the product of pressure and volume. The commonly used term "work of breathing" is something of a misnomer as it is usually used to describe the *power* of breathing, which is defined as work per unit time, and where the respiratory rate is also incorporated. Work of breathing can be expressed in joules per liter, which is energy required during one breath cycle divided by the tidal volume in liters. Alternatively, power of breathing can be expressed in joules per minute, which is the energy in joules per breath cycle multiplied by the minute respiratory rate. The work and power of breathing of a normal healthy patient is approximately 0.35 J/L, or 2.4 J/min.[39] The main determinants of the work of breathing are elastic recoil of the respiratory system and the resistance to airflow.[40]

Work against the elastic recoil of the respiratory system is used to expand the chest and distend the lung parenchyma. During normal quiet breathing, approximately half of the energy is spent on this (and is stored as potential energy, to be used during the passive expiratory phase) and the other half is dissipated as heat in the process of overcoming frictional forces.

Work against airway resistance is spent to overcome the frictional resistance to airflow. Additional negative intrathoracic pressure needs to be generated in order to create a sufficient pressure gradient and overcome resistance to inspiratory flow.

Under normal conditions, only the inspiratory muscles perform any work (by storing the work against elastic recoil in elastic tissues, the work of expiration is completely transferred to expiratory muscles). Work against elastic recoil increases with slow and deep breathing, whereas work against airway resistance increases with rapid shallow breathing (i.e. where flow rates are increased). Patients with normal lung physiology who are at rest will trend toward a respiratory rate which is a compromise between these two competing sources of impedance, and which minimizes the work of breathing.

With normal quiet breathing the total oxygen consumption of the respiratory muscles is approximately 1 mL per liter of minute volume or 2% of the total body oxygen consumption.[31] When the minute volume increases to 10 L/min in the absence of lung pathology, the oxygen cost of work of breathing accounts for 5% of total body oxygen consumption. In disease states which affect pulmonary compliance or airway resistance the oxygen cost of breathing can increase markedly. In COPD patients with poor lung function, the oxygen cost of the work of breathing at rest has been found to be in excess of 16 mL/L, or up to 50% of the total body oxygen consumption.[41] Mechanical ventilation can significantly decrease the demands on a failing heart by assuming some or all of the respiratory workload.

The work of breathing can be measured by integrating the area under the pressure/volume diagram of a breath, where the measured pressure is the pleural pressure or next most convenient surrogate, e.g. esophageal pressure as measured by esophageal manometry.[42] Measurement of pleural pressure and esophageal manometry are not often available at the bedside, but the pressure and volume graphics of a mechanical ventilator are effective surrogate measures for ventilated patients on volume control mode of ventilation with a constant inspiratory gas flow.[43] During a mechanical breath a patient may perform part of the work of breathing, with the remainder being performed by the ventilator device. It is possible to calculate the level of ventilator dependence by comparing the work of breathing required for unsupported breaths and assisted breaths.

## SALIENT POINTS

- The respiratory tract consists of conductive (upper airway trachea and bronchi) and respiratory portions (respiratory bronchioles and alveoli), of which only the latter participate in gas exchange.
- The roles of the upper airway include humidification and heating of inspired gas, protection of the lower airway from foreign material, phonation, swallowing, immune defence, and the maintenance of low resistance to air flow.
- The gas exchange surface of the lower respiratory tract is made up of alveolar epithelial cells (Type I cells) and Type II cells which differentiate into Type I cells and secrete alveolar surfactant.

- Alveolar surfactant is a surface-active material, which is responsible for maintaining the low surface tension of alveolar fluid and thereby preventing alveolar atelectasis.
- The pulmonary circulation is a low-resistance system, where the pressure is 15–20% of the systemic pressure and the vessels have significantly less smooth muscle.
- The relationships of pressure volume and flow describe the mechanical properties of the respiratory system, such that compliance is the change in volume per unit pressure and resistance is the change in pressure per unit flow.
- The relationship of compliance and resistance describe the time constant ($\tau$), defined as the time required to distend the lung up to 63% of the maximal inflation.
- The work of breathing is the energy required to generate a tidal volume, and can expressed in joules per liter of breath volume, or as power of breathing in Joules per minute.

## REFERENCES

1. Massey BT. (2006). Physiology of oral cavity, pharynx and upper esophageal sphincter. GI Motility. [online] Available from: http://www.nature.com/gimo/contents/pt1/full/gimo2.html. [Accessed Jan. 2019].
2. Boidin MP. Airway patency in the unconscious patient. Br J Anaesth. 1985;57(3):306-10.
3. Achauer BM, Allyn PA, Furnas DW, et al. Pulmonary complications of burns: The major threat to the burn patient. Ann Surg. 1973;177(3):311-9.
4. Moritz AR, Weisiger JR. Effects of cold air on the air passages and lungs. An experimental investigation. Arch Intern Med. 1945;75:233-40.
5. Walker JE, Wells RE Jr, Merrill EW. Heat and water exchange in the respiratory tract. Am J Med. 1961;30:259-67.
6. Williams R, Rankin N, Smith T, et al. Relationship between the humidity and temperature of inspired gas and the function of the airway mucosa. Crit Care Med. 1996;24(11):1920-9.
7. Wilkes AR. Heat and moisture exchangers and breathing system filters: Their use in anesthesia and intensive care. Part 2–practical use, including problems, and their use with pediatric patients. Anaesthesia. 2011;66(1):40-51.
8. Kirchner JA. Functional evolution of the human larynx: variations among the vertebrates. In: Fujimura O (Ed). Vocal physiology: voice production mechanism, and functions. New York, NY: Raven Press; 1988. pp. 129-34.
9. Roberts JT. Functional anatomy of the larynx. Int Anesthesiol Clin. 1990;28(2):101-5.
10. Cormack RS, Lehane J. Difficult tracheal intubation in obstetrics. Anaesthesia. 1984;39(11):1105-11.
11. Lobo EP, Pellegrini F, Pusceddu E. Anesthesia Complications in Head and Neck Surgery. In: Eisele DW, Smith RV (Eds). Complications in Head and Neck Surgery, 2nd edition. Philadelphia, PA: Mosby Elsevier; 2009. pp. 3-27.
12. Ludlow CL. Laryngeal reflexes: Physiology, technique and clinical use. J Clin Neurophysiol. 2015;32(4):284-93.
13. Landsman IS. Mechanisms and treatment of laryngospasm. Int Anesthesiol Clin. 1997;35(3):67-73.
14. Gal TJ. Effects of endotracheal intubation on normal cough performance. Anesthesiology. 1980;52(4):324-9.
15. Kahrilas PJ. Pharyngeal structure and function. Dysphagia. 1993;8(4):303-7.
16. Bonanno PC. Swallowing dysfunction after tracheostomy. Ann Surg. 1971;174(1):29-33.
17. Clarke SW, Pavia D. Lung mucus production and mucociliary clearance: Methods of assessment. In: Methods in Clinical Pharmacology—Respiratory System. UK: Macmillan Education; 1981. pp. 85-94.
18. Maxwell SS. The effect of salt-solutions on ciliary activity. Am J Physiol. 1905;13(2):154-70.
19. Li Bassi G, Zanella A, Cressoni M, et al. Following tracheal intubation, mucus flow is reversed in the semirecumbent position: Possible role in the pathogenesis of ventilator-associated pneumonia. Crit Care Med. 2008;36(2):518-25.
20. Konrad F, Schreiber T, Brecht-Kraus D, et al. Mucociliary transport in ICU patients. Chest. 1994;105(1):237-41.
21. James A, Carroll N. Airway smooth muscle in health and disease; methods of measurement and relation to function. Eur Respir J. 2000;15(4):782-9.
22. Noble PB, McLaughlin RA, West AR, et al. Distribution of airway narrowing responses across generations and at branching points, assessed in vitro by anatomical optical coherence tomography. Respir Res. 2010;11:9.
23. Enhorning G, Shennan A, Possmayer F, et al. Prevention of neonatal respiratory distress syndrome by tracheal instillation of surfactant: a randomized clinical trial. Pediatrics. 1985;76(2):145-53.
24. Whitsett JA, Wert SE, Weaver TE. Alveolar surfactant homeostasis and the pathogenesis of pulmonary disease. Annu Rev Med. 2010;61:105-19.
25. Silverman JA, Mortin LI, VanPraagh AD, et al. Inhibition of daptomycin by pulmonary surfactant: In vitro modeling and clinical impact. J Infect Dis. 2005;191(12):2149-52.
26. Tsukimoto K, Mathieu-Costello O, Prediletto R, et al. Ultrastructural appearances of pulmonary capillaries at high transmural pressures. J Appl Physiol (1985). 1991;71(2):573-82.
27. Santos CC, Zhang H, Liu M, et al. Bench-to-bedside review: Biotrauma and modulation of the innate immune response. Crit Care. 2005;9(3):280-6.
28. Bryan TL, Van Diepen S, Bhutani M, et al. The effects of dobutamine and dopamine on intrapulmonary shunt and gas exchange in healthy humans. J Appl Physiol (1985). 2012;113(4):541-8.

29. Anthonisen NR, Milic-Emili J. Distribution of pulmonary perfusion in erect man. J Appl Physiol. 1966;21(3):760-6.
30. Naimark A, Dugard A, Rangno RE. Regional pulmonary blood flow and gas exchange in hemorrhagic shock. J Appl Physiol. 1968;25(3):301-9.
31. Lumb AB. Nunn's Applied Respiratory Physiology, 8th edition. Elsevier Health Sciences; 2016. pp. 1-560.
32. Webster IW. Airway collapse related to the subdivisions of lung volume. Respiration. 1970;27(4):384-95.
33. Leblanc P, Ruff F, Milic-Emili J. Effects of age and body position on "airway closure" in man. J Appl Physiol. 1970;28(4):448-51.
34. Aljuri N, Venegas JG, Freitag L. Viscoelasticity of the trachea and its effects on flow limitation. J Appl Physiol (1985). 2006;100(2):384-9.
35. Hess DR. Respiratory mechanics in mechanically ventilated patients. Respir Care. 2014;59(11):1773-94.
36. Mauri T, Yoshida T, Bellani G, et al. PLeUral pressure working Group (PLUG—Acute Respiratory Failure section of the European Society of Intensive Care Medicine). Esophageal and transpulmonary pressure in the clinical setting: Meaning, usefulness and perspectives. Intensive Care Med. 2016;42(9):1360-73.
37. Thien F. Measuring and imaging small airways dysfunction in asthma. Asia Pac Allergy. 2013;3(4):224-30.
38. Bates JH, Irvin CG. Time dependence of recruitment and derecruitment in the lung: a theoretical model. J Appl Physiol (1985). 2002;93(2):705-13.
39. Mancebo J, Isabey D, Lorino H, et al. Comparative effects of pressure support ventilation and intermittent positive pressure breathing (IPPB) in nonintubated healthy subjects. Eur Respir J. 1995;8(11):1901-9.
40. Milic-Emili J, Rocca E, D'Angelo E. Work of breathing. In: Basics of Respiratory Mechanics and Artificial Ventilation. Milan: Springer; 1999. pp. 165-75.
41. Mannix ET, Manfredi F, Farber MO. Elevated $O_2$ cost of ventilation contributes to tissue wasting in COPD. Chest. 1999;115(3):708-13.
42. Belen C, Mancebo J. Work of breathing. In: Applied Physiology in Intensive Care Medicine 1. Berlin, Heidelberg: Springer; 2012. pp. 11-4.
43. Grinnan DC, Truwit JD. Clinical review: respiratory mechanics in spontaneous and assisted ventilation. Crit Care. 2005;9(5):472-84.

# CHAPTER 2

# Oxygen Delivery Devices

*Bogdan Tiru*

## HISTORY OF OXYGEN THERAPY

The discovery of oxygen goes back to 1772 when the Swedish pharmacist Karl Scheele obtained a gas that caused candles to burn more brightly.[1] Working independently in 1774, Joseph Priestley, an English theologian-chemist, described the "dephlogisticated air"—an experiment which he reported in 1775.[2] The gas discovered by Scheele and Priestley was oxygen, but it is Antoine Lavoisier, who named the gas *oxygène,* meaning acid former, in 1778.

The first therapeutic use of oxygen in 1783 is credited to the French physician Caillens who treated a young woman with phthisis (tuberculosis) who "very much benefited" from daily inhalations of oxygen.

In the 1800s, oxygen administered in short spells was widely touted as a panacea. *The Lancet* and the *British Medical Journal* published many papers in the mid-1800s by Dr S B Birch, commending the role of oxygen.

The first continuous oxygen use was described by Albert Blodgett in 1890 in a case of pneumonia.[3] John Scott Haldane is considered the "Father of Oxygen Therapy"[4] due to his systematic approach and discoveries in understanding of the physiology of respiration made in the early 1900s.[5] The publication by Haldane of his book "Respiration"[6] in 1922 brought further understanding of oxygen therapy. While Haldane was one of the first to advocate for the use of continuous oxygen therapy, the understanding of the detrimental effects of intermittent use came only in 1962, when Massaro and Katz[7] demonstrated worsening hypoxemia with intermittent treatment. The first long-term oxygen therapy investigation, given for up to 41 months for chronic bronchitis patients living in Denver, Colorado, was published in 1968.[8]

## OXYGEN AS A DRUG

Currently, supplemental oxygen is routinely used in outpatient, prehospital and hospital care in the management of respiratory distress and the treatment of many acute and chronic medical conditions. Its use in the hospital setting is so frequent that it is often taken for granted; yet we must not forget that above atmospheric concentrations, oxygen should be considered a drug and prescribed accordingly.

Oxygen prescription should have written in: the indication, the dose, the rate, the target oxygen saturation, and the method of delivery. Monitoring via pulse oximetry should be available in all clinical situations in which oxygen is used.

## GOALS OF OXYGEN THERAPY

The goals of oxygen therapy are:
- Correction of hypoxemia by increasing alveolar and blood level of oxygen
- To relieve symptoms of hypoxemia such as dyspnea or shortness of breath
- To minimize the cardiopulmonary workload through increase in oxygen availability and decrease in ventilatory demand and the work of breathing in patients with hypoxemia.

## INDICATIONS FOR OXYGEN USE

The indication for oxygen therapy should always be hypoxemia and not breathlessness. The use of supplemental oxygen in patients with breathlessness without hypoxemia is not currently supported by evidence. In the absence of hypoxemia, oxygen therapy is not indicated in the treatment of acute coronary syndrome or stroke, conditions associated with reversible ischemia. In stroke, routine administration of continuous or nocturnal oxygen therapy does not improve outcomes.[9,10] However there is increasing evidence of harm in myocardial infarction, where high concentration oxygen therapy is associated with greater infarct size, when compared with room air or titrated oxygen therapy if required to avoid hypoxemia.[11,12]

Other side effects described with use of oxygen—nasal dryness and bleeding, headaches, pulmonary oxygen toxicity,[13] retinopathy, and increased risk of death[14] (in premature infants and neonates), and seizures[15] (with hyperbaric oxygen therapy). The mechanism proposed for these side effects is due to increase in oxidative stress by an increase in oxygen free radicals.

In 2018 clinical practice guidelines for oxygen therapy in acute medical patients[16] have been published with the following recommendations:

- Maintaining an oxygen saturation of no more than 96% in acutely ill medical patients (upper limit). Strong Recommendation. This recommendation does not apply to patients with carbon monoxide poisoning, cluster headaches, and sickle cell crisis or pneumothorax.
- No recommendations were made on when to start (the lower limit) for all medical patients because there was not enough evidence.
- Patients with acute stroke or myocardial infarction and a $SpO_2$ (oxygen saturation) more than or equal to 90% should not receive supplemental oxygen (a weak recommendation if $SpO_2$ is 90–92% and a strong recommendation if 93–100%).

The guidelines note that while it is reasonable to extend these recommendations to pre-hospital care the evidence available to extend it to other patient groups—surgical or obstetric patients is lacking. In addition, the panel did not review the evidence on postoperative healing and infections and therefore decided not to comment on these patients. Similarly, the panel did not review the evidence on oxygen therapy in neonates and infants.

## OXYGEN DELIVERY

To further understand the rationale for oxygen administration it is important to discuss about the oxygen delivery to the tissues. The amount of oxygen delivered to tissues ($DO_2$) depends on the amount of oxygen in the blood—$CaO_2$ (oxygen content in arterial blood) and the cardiac output (CO) and is easily understood through the following equations:

$CaO_2 = Hb \times 1.39 \times SaO_2 + PaO_2 \times 0.0003$

Hb—hemoglobin concentration; $SaO_2$—arterial saturation of oxygen; $PaO_2$—partial pressure of dissolved oxygen in blood

$DO_2 = CO \times CaO_2$ where $CO = SV \times HR$

SV—stroke volume; HR—heart rate

$DO_2 = SV \times HR \times (Hb \times 1.39 \times SaO_2 + PaO_2 \times 0.0003)$

The oxygen delivery to the tissues is mostly influenced by the cardiac output, hemoglobin level, and oxygen saturation. When hemoglobin level is very low or when the oxygen carrying capacity is affected (methemoglobinemia, carbon monoxide poisoning), increasing the amount of dissolved oxygen may provide an increased percentage of delivered oxygen to the tissues.

We refer therefore to hypoxemia (low concentration of oxygen in blood) and hypoxia (low delivery of oxygen to tissues). Tables 1 and 2 further define and describe these concepts.

## OXYGEN DELIVERY DEVICES

The use of oxygen needs to be individualized based on patient demand and the delivery of oxygen depends on availability of oxygen delivery devices, flow and monitoring capabilities. Healthcare providers need to understand the underlying pathophysiology when selecting the best available device (Table 3) for delivering treatment interventions.

### Low-flow Devices

#### Nasal Prongs/Cannula

Nasal cannula (Fig. 1) is probably the most widely used oxygen therapy device in the outpatient and hospital setting. It is usually used in non-acute situations where the degree of hypoxemia is mild-moderate. It delivers a constant flow of oxygen to the nasopharynx and oropharynx, acting as a small reservoir of approximately 50 cc (cubic centimeter) (or one-third of the anatomical dead space) of 100% fraction of inspired oxygen ($FiO_2$). Its main advantages are—ease of use, low cost, and good

**Table 1:** Classification of hypoxemia.

| Classification | $PaO_2$—Partial pressure of dissolved oxygen in blood (room air at sea level) |
|---|---|
| Normal | 80–100 mm Hg |
| Mild hypoxemia | 60–80 mm Hg |
| Moderate hypoxemia | 40–60 mm Hg |
| Severe hypoxemia | <40 mm Hg |

**Table 2:** Types of hypoxia and common causes.

| Types of hypoxia | Definition | Typical cases |
|---|---|---|
| Hypoxic | Inadequate oxygen at the tissue cells caused by low arterial oxygen tension ($PaO_2$) | Low $PaO_2$ caused by<br>• Hypoventilation (increased $CO_2$ in alveolus displaces oxygen)<br>• High altitude (low barometric pressure<br>• Decreases partial pressure of oxygen in the alveolus)<br>Diffusion defects<br>Ventilation–perfusion mismatch (most common cause)<br>Pulmonary shunting (right to left shunts) |
| Hypoxemic/ anemic | Decreased $O_2$ content ($CaO_2$) | Decreased hemoglobin<br>• Anemia<br>• Hemorrhage<br>Abnormal hemoglobin<br>Carboxyhemoglobinemia<br>Methemoglobinemia |
| Circulatory | Hypoperfusion or inadequate blood flow to the tissue cells<br>– systemic = shock<br>– ischemia = local lack of perfusion | Slow or stagnant (pooling) peripheral blood flow<br>Arterial-venous shunts<br>Decreased cardiac output |
| Histotoxic | Impaired ability of the tissue cells to metabolize oxygen | Cyanide poisoning<br>Shifting hemoglobin dissociation curve<br>Dysoxia—sepsis alters tissues ability to utilize oxygen |

**Table 3:** Types and characteristics of oxygen delivery devices.

| Types of oxygen delivery devices | | Device characteristics | | |
|---|---|---|---|---|
| | | Flow (LPM) | Patient Effort | Delivered Oxygen ($FiO_2$) |
| Low flow | Nasal cannula | 1–6 | Low–moderate | 22–40%<br>Variable |
| | Nasal catheter | 1–5 | Low–moderate | 22–45%<br>Variable |
| | Transtracheal catheter | 1–4 | Low–moderate | 22–35%<br>Variable |
| Low-flow reservoir devices | Reservoir cannula | 1–4 | Low–moderate | 22–35%<br>Variable |
| | Simple mask | 5–10 | Low–moderate<br>Mouth breathing | 22–50%<br>Variable |
| | Partial rebreathing mask | >10 | Low–high | 40–70%<br>Variable |
| | Non-rebreathing mask | >10 | Low–high | 60–90%<br>Variable |
| High Flow | Air entrainment mask (Venturi) | Variable based on $FiO_2$ | Low–high | 24–60%<br>Stable |
| | High flow nasal cannula | 30–60 | Low–high | 21–100%<br>Stable |
| | Bag mask ventilation | Variable | None–high | Near 100%<br>Stable |
| | Noninvasive ventilation | Up to 120 | Low–high | 21–100%<br>Stable |
| | Mechanical ventilation | Up to 150 | None–high | 21–100%<br>Stable |
| Enclosure | Oxyhood (infants) | >7 | Low–moderate | Fixed<br>stable |
| | Tent (toddlers – small kids) | 12–15 | Low–moderate | 40–50%<br>Variable |
| | Hyperbaric oxygen therapy | Variable | None–high | 100% |

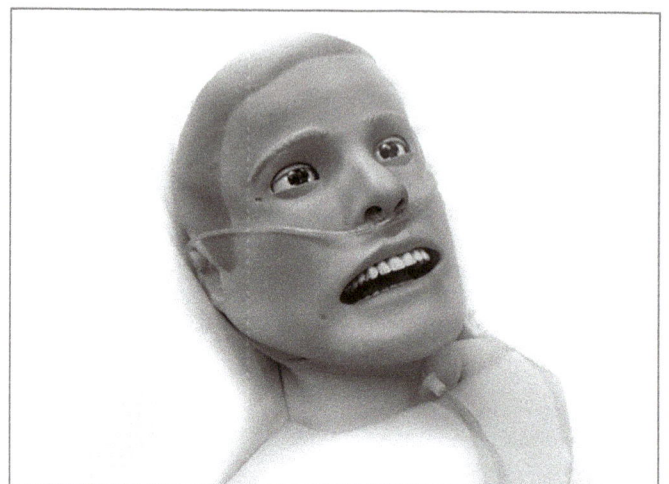

**Fig. 1:** Nasal cannula.

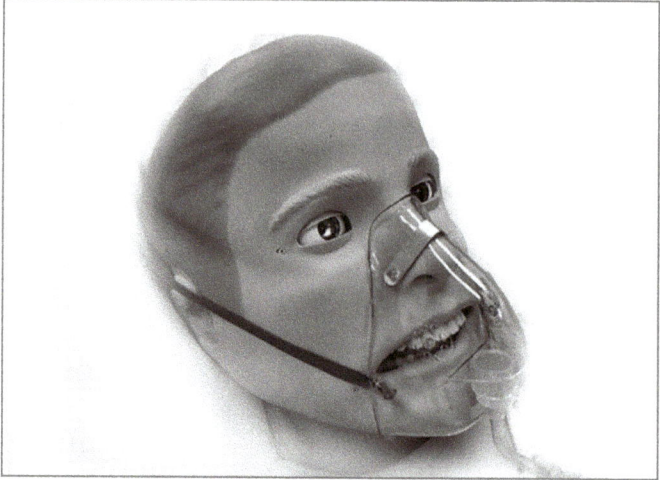

**Fig. 2:** Simple face mask.

tolerability. Some of the disadvantages are—can become dislodged, can cause dryness and bleeding especially at flows over 4 liters per minute (LPM) for which a humidifier should be used.

The nasal cannula is best used in patients who are not very sick and need low $FiO_2$. For patients with a normal rate and depth of breathing each 1 LPM of nasal oxygen increases $FiO_2$ by approximately 4%. So a 3 LPM flow will approximately deliver 33% $FiO_2$ (21 + 12). The actual $FiO_2$ delivered will vary greatly based on patient's minute ventilation, inspiration: expiration (I:E) ratio, rate of breathing, depth of breathing and anatomic reservoir.[17]

### Nasal Catheter and Transtracheal Catheter

The nasal catheter and transtracheal catheters are rarely utilized in adults due to being more invasive, with lower tolerability and higher risks (infection, bleeding) associated with placement. Being low-flow devices they share the same disadvantages of variability in delivered $FiO_2$.

### Low-flow Reservoir Devices

Reservoir systems incorporate a mechanism for storing oxygen between patient breaths. Whenever inspiratory flow exceeds the available oxygen flow the device reservoir allows the stored oxygen to be used, thus these devices generally provide higher $FiO_2$ than low-flow systems. This allows a decrease in oxygen use by providing the same $FiO_2$ at a lower flow. Reservoir systems currently in use include the reservoir cannulas, masks, and non-rebreathing circuits.

Reservoir cannulas are designed to conserve oxygen and are alternative to the pulse dose or on demand flow oxygen systems. A nasal reservoir cannula operates by storing approximately 20 cc of oxygen in a small membrane reservoir during exhalation. The patient draws on this stored oxygen during early inspiration. The amount of oxygen available increases with each breath and decreases the flow needed for given $FiO_2$. At low flow, reservoir cannulas can reduce oxygen use by 50-75%.[18] Although the device is comfortable to wear, many patients object to its appearance and may not be always compliant with the prescribed therapy. The performance of these devices is dependent on nasal anatomy, breathing pattern, and excess moisture. They are used predominantly in the outpatient setting.

Masks are the most commonly used reservoir systems. There are three types of reservoir masks: (1) simple mask, (2) partial rebreathing mask, and (3) non-rebreathing mask.

### Simple Mask

The simple mask (Fig. 2) is a disposable plastic unit designed to cover both the mouth and the nose which stores oxygen between patient breaths. The patient exhales directly through the open holes on ports in the mask. If oxygen input is insufficient the patient can draw an air through these holes and around the edge. These masks have an input flow between 5 LPM and 10 LPM. When greater than 10 LPM flow is needed to achieve satisfactory oxygenation, the prescriber should consider using a device capable of a higher $FiO_2$. At the flow less than 5 LPM the mask volume acts as dead space and can cause carbon dioxide rebreathing. These masks provide a variable $FiO_2$, which depends on the oxygen flow, the mask volume, the extent of air leakage, and the patient breathing pattern/minute ventilation.

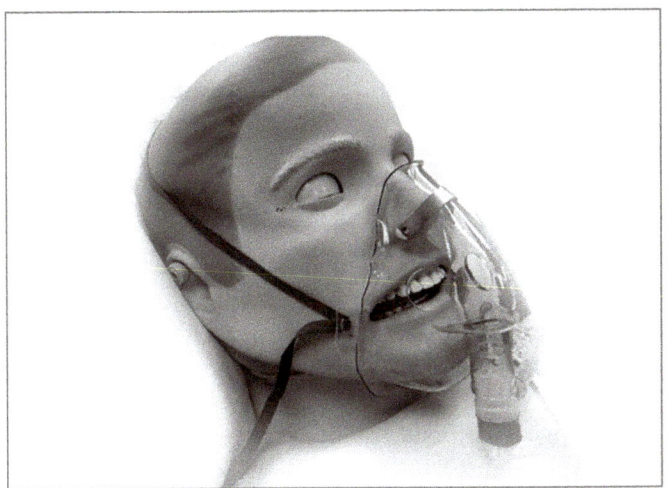

**Fig. 3:** Partial rebreathing mask.

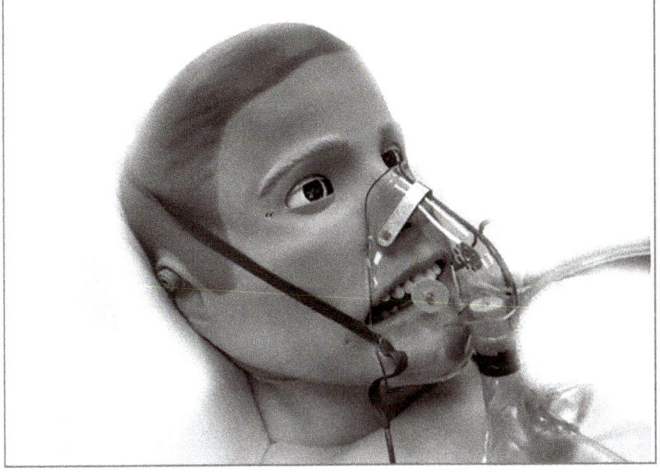

**Fig. 4:** Non-rebreather mask.

### *Partial Rebreathing Mask and a Non-rebreathing Mask*

Partial rebreathing mask (Fig. 3) and a non-rebreathing mask (Fig. 4) have a similar design, with a 1-liter flexible reservoir bag. The difference between the two consists on the presence of one way valves in the non-rebreathing masks, providing them with the ability to increase the amount of oxygen delivered. Both types of masks need higher flows of oxygen of over 10 liters to assure the adequate washout of carbon dioxide ($CO_2$). There masks have a significant variability in the $FiO_2$ delivered, based on patient characteristics (tidal volume, respiratory rate, pattern of breathing, etc.), as well as mask fit. Their main advantages are relatively straight forward use and ubiquitous presence in both pre-hospital and hospital settings. For these reasons they are widely used in emergencies or short-term situations where higher $FiO_2$ is needed.

The non-rebreathing circuit allows for a step-up in delivery of oxygen therapy and is capable of more precise titration and can deliver a full range of $FiO_2$ (21–100%).[19] It does require a flow of at least three times the patient's minute ventilation. With the higher flows humidification is necessary for better tolerability. Common problems with all masks systems are related to the removal of masks by patients either due to claustrophobia or inadequate ventilatory support.

## High-flow Devices

High-flow devices are devices capable of delivering at least 60 LPM total flow. They achieve these flows by mixing air and oxygen through a blender system or by air-entrainment. The following equation:

$$V_F C_F = V_1 C_1 + V_2 C_2$$

$V_F$ = Volume of gas mixture, $C_F$ = concentration of gas mixture,
$V_1$ = volume of gas 1, $C_1$ = concentration of gas 1,
$V_2$ = volume of gas 2, $C_2$ = concentration of gas 2

Can be used to determine
1. The delivered $FiO_2$
   $\%O_2 = [(Airflow \times 21) + (O_2\ Flow \times 100)]/Total\ flow$
2. The ratio of air to oxygen required to achieve a desired $FiO_2$
   Liters Air/Liters $O_2 = (100 - \%O_2)/(\%O_2 - 21)$, where $\%O_2$ is the desired oxygen $FiO_2$
3. The total output flow from an air entrainment device
   Total flow = $O_2$ flow $\times\ 79/(\%O_2 - 21)$,
4. The amount of air required to achieve a desired $FiO_2$
   Airflow = Liters $O_2 * (100 - \%O_2)/(\%O_2 - 21)$, where $\%O_2$ is the desired $FiO_2$.

### *Air Entrainment Devices*

Air entrainment devices (Fig. 5) are simple devices that use pressurized oxygen pushed through a restricted orifice (jet nozzle). Lateral shear forces cause air entrainment through ports located near the jet site.[20] The amount of air entrained at these ports is directly proportional to the velocity of oxygen at the jet. The smaller the jet the greater the velocity of oxygen and more air is entrained (Fig. 6).

Using the Formula 2 and 3, one can determine the necessary mixing ratios for a desired $FiO_2$ and approximating on patient's effort, the respiratory rate (RR), tidal volume ($V_T$), and minute ventilation (MV = RR $\times\ V_T$) (Table 4).

It can be easily observed that for a patient with minute ventilation of 20 liters, the maximum FiO$_2$ that can be achieved using 15 LPM oxygen is 40%. Lower FiO$_2$ needs can be achieved with lower oxygen flows. In theory at lower FiO$_2$ needs, these air entrainment devices assure relative constant and fairly reliable oxygen delivery with lower needed oxygen flows. However in clinical practice, different masks designs, especially regarding to reservoir volume, as well as positioning of the mask can have significant variation of delivered FiO$_2$.[21] Real life use of these systems can assure accurate delivery of FiO$_2$ less than 35%.[22]

### Air Entrainment Nebulizers

Air entrainment nebulizers (or jet nebulizers or large volume nebulizers) have additional benefits and capabilities like humidification and temperature control (though a separate/optional heating element). By delivering particulate water to the airways, they are widely used in patients with artificial tracheal airways—tracheostomy collar (Fig. 7) and T-tube (Fig. 8). When humidification is important they can be used in patient with intact airways—aerosol mask (Fig. 5) and face tent (Fig. 9).

As with all air entrainment devices, air entrainment nebulizers are able to deliver predictable FiO$_2$ concentrations of less than 35%. When higher FiO$_2$ is needed, most air-entrapment nebulizers have flow limits related to the jet nozzle size. To circumvent these limitations, several approaches have been used:
- Combining them with an increase in reservoir size by an open reservoir (T-tube) (Fig. 8)
- An inspiratory volume reservoir (2-5 L anesthesia bag) with one-way valve (Fig. 8)
- Connecting two or more devices through a Y connector to deliver up to 60% FiO$_2$
- Addition of oxygen into the delivery tubing of a lower FiO$_2$ delivery high flow device.

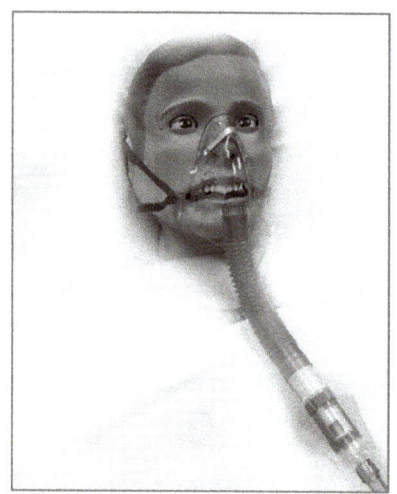

**Fig. 5:** Air entrainment mask (Venturi).

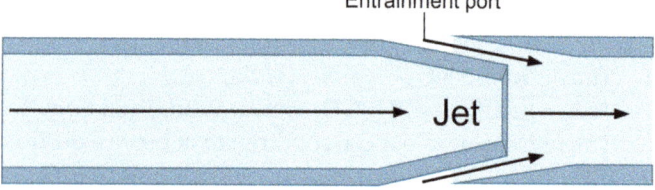

**Fig. 6:** Jet entrainment.

**Table 4:** Air entrainment device characteristics based on desired FiO$_2$ and the minimum flows to overcome dilutional entrainment of air for a patient with a respiratory rate of 30 and tidal volume of 600 mL.

| % Oxygen | Approximate air/oxygen ratio (using formula 2) | Total ratio parts | Minimum device flow to achieve desired FiO$_2$ (LPM) | Total output flow using 15 LPM O$_2$ (Formula 3) | Minimum O$_2$ flow to achieve desired FiO$_2$ |
|---|---|---|---|---|---|
| 100 | 0:1 | 1 | 60 | 15 | 60 |
| 80 | 0.3:1 | 1.3 | 60 | 20.1 | 46 |
| 70 | 0.6:1 | 1.6 | 60 | 24.2 | 37.5 |
| 60 | 1:1 | 2 | 60 | 30.4 | 30 |
| 50 | 1.7:1 | 2.7 | 60 | 40.9 | 22.2 |
| 45 | 2:1 | 3 | 60 | 49.4 | 20 |
| 40 | 3:1 | 4 | 60 | 62.3 | 15 |
| 35 | 5:1 | 6 | 60 | 84.6 | 10 |
| 30 | 8:1 | 9 | 60 | 131.7 | 6.6 |
| 28 | 10:1 | 11 | 60 | 169.3 | 5.5 |
| 24 | 25:1 | 26 | 60 | 395 | 2.3 |

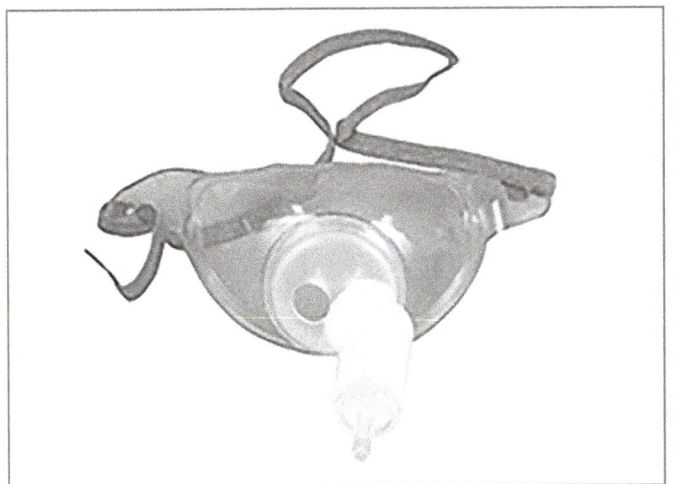

**Fig. 7:** Trach collar mask.

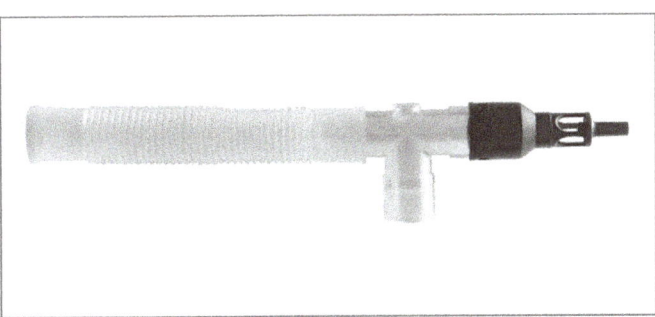

**Fig. 8:** T-tube.

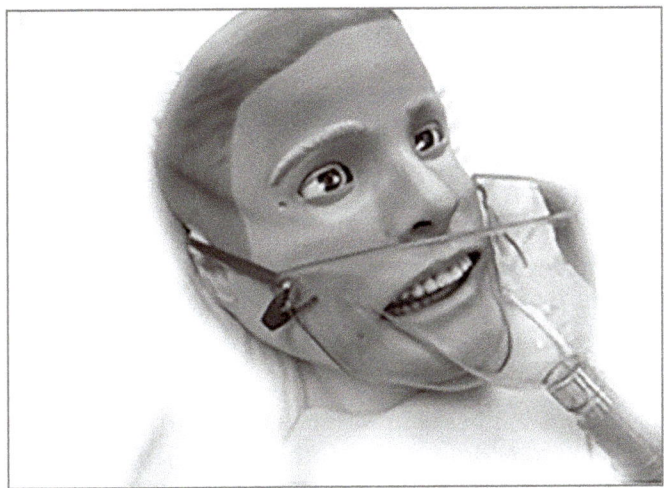

**Fig. 9:** Face tent aerosol mask.

## High Flow Nasal Cannula

High flow nasal cannula (HFNC) (Fig. 10) is a variation of the standard nasal cannula. It can provide both $FiO_2$ and humidity of greater than 90% at flows of 40 LPM (Vapotherm, Exeter, New Hampshire) or 50 LPM (Fisher and Paykel, Irvine, California).

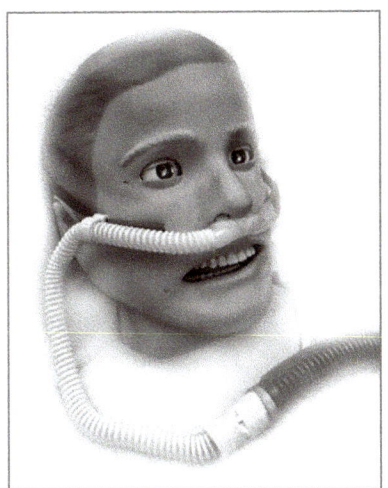

**Fig. 10:** High flow nasal cannula.

There is increasing evidence regarding usability and tolerability of HFNC.[23-26] Physiological data indicate that HFNC is associated with an increase of 1–8 $cmH_2O$ in oropharyngeal pressure[27] and an increased functional residual capacity. These positive pressures reduce airway resistance and improve oxygenation.[28] These effects are likely affected by mouth opening and fit of the cannula to the nares. One study in humans with congestive heart failure[29] indicates that pressures generated by HFNC may actually have an effect on right ventricular preload, a therapeutic target in acute pulmonary edema. Additionally, animal models have shown that gas flows tend to decrease physiological dead space by improving $CO_2$ washout and to decrease work of breathing.[30] Both of these properties could be relevant to the treatment of acute airway obstruction. Taken together, available physiologic observations provide support for using HFNC in various forms of hypoxic and hypercarbic respiratory failure.[28]

Two recent meta-analyses analyzed the effect of HFNO on intubation rate in studies of patients with acute hypoxemic respiratory failure. Ou and colleagues[31] determined from six randomized controlled trails that HFNC was associated with a lower intubation rate compared to standard oxygen therapy (RR 0.6, 95% CI 0.38–0.91), but there was no difference in the intubation rate when HFNC was compared with noninvasive positive pressure ventilation (NIPPV). Same observation of no significant difference in the rate of intubation between HFNC and NIPPV was noted by Ni and colleagues[32] looking at 18 trials with 3,881 patients.

As a result the use of HFNC has been increasing in recent years[33] in populations that have acute respiratory failure with moderate hypoxemia. While best indications for use are still probed, it remains an area for fruitful future research endeavors.

High flow nasal cannula's main advantages stem from delivering reliable FiO$_2$ and humidity at high flows supporting the ventilatory needs of patients with significant work of breathing and respiratory distress. It is usually much better tolerated than noninvasive ventilation as patients can speak, eat, and are less claustrophobic. It has been used in all populations—neonates, infants, children, and adults.

### Bag Mask Devices

Bag mask devices (Fig. 11) are widely used in critical care and the hospital and prehospital setting for life-threatening or emergency life support as a temporary way to deliver oxygen and ventilation. Bag mask devices use a self-inflating bag with one way non-rebreathing valve. With proper seal over the mouth and nose they can provide 100% FiO$_2$. During advanced cardiac life support (ACLS) one rescuer or two rescuer techniques can be employed to assure oxygenation and ventilation.

The use of *noninvasive positive pressure ventilation* and *invasive mechanical ventilation* is discussed in separate chapters in this book.

## Enclosure Oxygen Devices

### Oxygen Hoods and Tents

Enclosure devices, such as oxygen hoods and tents, are usually used in infants and children, although they are becoming much less used due to wide variation in FiO$_2$ due to leakage.

### Hyperbaric Oxygen (HBO) Therapy

HBO therapy can be considered a special enclosure device which uses 100% oxygen at pressures greater than 1 atmosphere. Most HBO therapies are performed between 2 to 3 ATA (atmospheric pressure absolute), but in cases of decompression sickness or air embolism can go up to 6 ATA or more. Figure 12 illustrates the effect of HBO therapy on bubble size as the pressure increases.

Hyperbaric oxygen therapy can be provided in either a monoplace (single person) chamber with compressed oxygen or a multiplace chamber (multiple persons) compressed with air where oxygen is delivered by either a hood or mask. The benefits of treatment are the result of both primary and secondary effects. Boxes 1 and 2 list the physiologic effects and indications[34] of HBO therapy.

Primary effects are the result of increased pressure and hyperoxia. Indeed, PaO$_2$ can increase from less than 100 mm Hg at 1 atmospheres absolute (ATA) room air to more than 2,000 mm Hg at 3 ATA. This also translates into

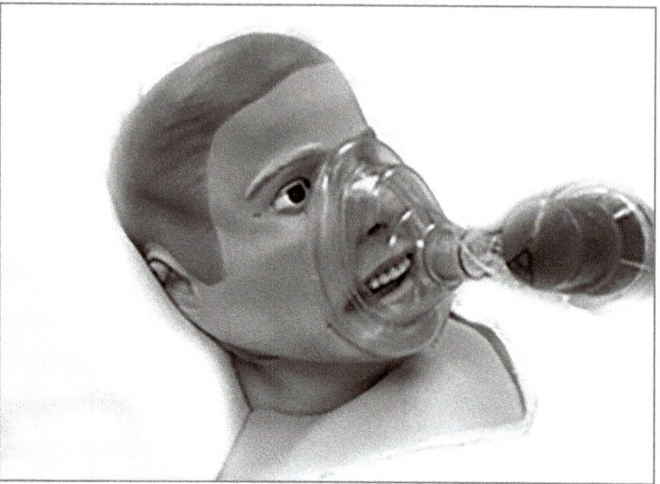

**Fig. 11:** Bag mask device.

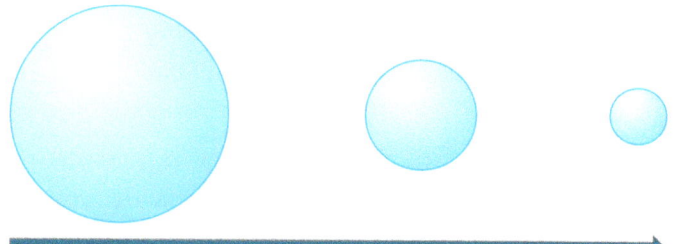

**Fig. 12:** Effect of hyperbaric oxygen therapy on bubble size as the pressure increases.

**Box 1:** Physiologic effects of hyperbaric oxygen (HBO) therapy.

*Physiologic effects of HBO therapy*
- Bubble reduction (Boyle's law)
- Hyper oxygenation
- Vasoconstriction
- Enhanced host immune function
- Neovascularization

significant increases in tissue oxygen partial pressures (200–400 mm Hg).[35] This can be used as an advantage in anaerobic infections or in cases of severe anemia in patients that cannot receive blood transfusions (Jehovah's Witness). Secondary effects are the result of a controlled oxidative stress, through reactive oxygen species (ROS) and reactive nitrogen species, resulting in improved leukocyte function, amelioration of ischemia–reperfusion injury, and neovascularization as a result of increased local growth factors and release of autologous progenitor stem cells.[15]

> **Box 2:** Current indications and therapeutic uses of hyperbaric oxygen (HBO) therapy.
>
> *Current indications and therapeutic uses of hyperbaric oxygen*
>
> - Strong scientific evidence
>   - Main treatment
>     - Decompression sickness
>     - Arterial gas embolism
>     - Severe carbon monoxide poisoning and smoke inhalation
>   - Adjunctive treatment
>     - Prevention and treatment of osteoradionecrosis
>     - Improved skin graft and flap healing
>     - Clostridial myonecrosis
> - Suggestive scientific evidence
>   - Adjunctive treatment
>     - Refractory osteomyelitis
>     - Radiation induced injury
>     - Acute traumatic ischemic injury
>     - Prolonged failure of wound healing
>     - Exceptional anemia from blood loss

> **Box 3:** Side effects of hyperbaric oxygen (HBO) therapy.
>
> *Side effects of HBO therapy*
>
> - Effects of pressure
>   - Middle ear barotrauma
>   - Rupture of tympanic membrane
>   - Sinus/paranasal trauma
>   - Dental barotrauma and pain
>   - Pulmonary barotrauma and pneumothorax
>   - Arterial gas embolism
> - Effects of hyperoxia/radical oxygen species
>   - Central nervous system toxicity/seizures
>   - Pulmonary oxygen toxicity
>     - Interstitial/alveolar edema
>     - Intra-alveolar hemorrhage
>     - Fibrinous exudate
>     - Capillary endothelium destruction
>   - Ocular side effects/vision changes
>     - Hyperoxic myopia
>     - Cataract
>     - Retrolental fibroplasia
>   - Other side effects
>     - Claustrophobia
>     - Blood pressure increase (increased systemic vascular resistance)
>     - Pulmonary edema (in patients with low left ventricular function)
>     - Hypoglycemia in diabetics (increases insulin and utilization of glucose in brain)

These same therapeutic effects that are used to patient's advantage can be the cause of side effects[36] of HBO therapy (Box 3).

## SALIENT POINTS

- The therapeutic use of oxygen is ubiquitous in today's medicine.
- It is important to understand that as with any therapy, oxygen prescription should have written in: the indication, the dose, the rate, the target oxygen saturation, and the method of delivery.
- The indication for oxygen therapy should always be hypoxemia and not breathlessness. Monitoring via pulse oximetry should be available in all clinical situations in which oxygen is used.
- Side effects are relatively rare, but not always immediately observable. There is increased evidence that inappropriate use of oxygen can be harmful, so guidelines have been published to avoid overuse and inappropriate delivery.
- Understanding the benefits and limitations of the available oxygen delivery devices along with understanding of the underlying physiology of hypoxemia can be helpful in selecting the appropriate method of oxygen delivery.
- Patient factors should be taken into consideration when selecting an oxygen delivery device.
- With technological advances the devices used to deliver oxygen have improved, but always remains the clinician's task to adjust the delivery of oxygen to the lowest $FiO_2$ possible to achieve the desired therapeutic effects.

## REFERENCES

1. Grainge C. Breath of life: the evolution of oxygen therapy. J R Soc Med. 2004;97(10):489-93.
2. Priestley J. Experiments and Observations on Different Kinds of Air. Birmingham: Thomas Pearson; 1775.
3. Blodgett AN. The continuous inhalation of oxygen in cases of pneumonia otherwise fatal, and in other diseases. Boston Med Surg J. 1890;123(21):481-5.
4. Sekhar KC, Rao SSCC. John Scott Haldane: The father of oxygen therapy. Indian J Anaesth. 2014;58(3):350-2.
5. Haldane JS. The therapeutic administration of oxygen. Br Med J. 1917;1(2928):181-3.
6. Haldane JS. Respiration. London: Oxford University Press; 1922.
7. Massaro DJ, Katz S, Luchsinger PC. Effect of various modes of oxygen administration on the arterial gas values in patients with respiratory acidosis. Br Med J. 1962;2(5305):627-9.
8. Petty TL, Finigan MM. Clinical evaluation of prolonged ambulatory oxygen therapy in chronic airway obstruction. Am J Med. 1968;45(2):242-52.
9. Roffe C, Nevatte T, Crome P, et al. The Stroke Oxygen Study (SO2S) - a multi-center, study to assess whether routine

oxygen treatment in the first 72 hours after a stroke improves long-term outcome: study protocol for a randomized controlled trial. Trials. 2014;15:99.
10. Ronning OM, Guldvog B. Should stroke victims routinely receive supplemental oxygen? A quasi-randomized controlled trial. Stroke. 1999;30(10):2033-7.
11. Rawles JM, Kenmure AC. Controlled trial of oxygen in uncomplicated myocardial infarction. Br Med J. 1976;1(6018):1121-3.
12. Stub D, Smith K, Bernard S, et al. Air versus oxygen in ST-segment elevation myocardial infarction. Circulation. 2015;131(24):2143-50.
13. Jackson RM. Pulmonary oxygen toxicity. Chest. 1985;88(6):900-5.
14. Askie LM, Darlow BA, Davis PG, et al. Effects of targeting lower versus higher arterial oxygen saturations on death or disability in preterm infants. Cochrane Database Syst Rev. 2017;4:CD011190.
15. Heyboer M, Jennings S, Grant WD, et al. Seizure incidence by treatment pressure in patients undergoing hyperbaric oxygen therapy. Undersea Hyperb Med. 2014;41(5):379-85.
16. Siemieniuk RAC, Chu DK, Kim LH, et al. Oxygen therapy for acutely ill medical patients: a clinical practice guideline. BMJ. 2018;363:k4169.
17. Shapiro BA HR, Trout CA. Clinical applications of respiratory care, 4th edition. Chicago: Mosby; 1991.
18. Marti S, Pajares V, Morante F, et al. Are oxygen-conserving devices effective for correcting exercise hypoxemia? Respir Care. 2013;58(10):1606-13.
19. Lee GJ, Lee SW, Oh YM, et al. A pilot study comparing 2 oxygen delivery methods for patients' comfort and administration of oxygen. Respir Care. 2014;59(8):1191-8.
20. Dobson MB. Use of jet mixing devices with an oxygen concentrator. Thorax. 1992;47(12):1060-2.
21. Cox D, Gillbe C. Fixed performance oxygen masks. Hypoxic hazard of low-capacity drugs. Anaesthesia. 1981;36(10):958-64.
22. Hui DS, Chow BK, Chu LCY, et al. Exhaled air and aerosolized droplet dispersion during application of a jet nebulizer. Chest. 2009;135(3):648-54.
23. Cuquemelle E, Pham T, Papon JF, et al. Heated and humidified high-flow oxygen therapy reduces discomfort during hypoxemic respiratory failure. Respir Care. 2012;57(10):1571-7.
24. Rittayamai N, Tscheikuna J, Rujiwit P. High-flow nasal cannula versus conventional oxygen therapy after endotracheal extubation: a randomized crossover physiologic study. Respir Care. 2014;59(4):485-90.
25. Roca O, Riera J, Torres F, et al. High-flow oxygen therapy in acute respiratory failure. Respir Care. 2010;55(4):408-13.
26. Sztrymf B, Messika J, Bertrand F, et al. Beneficial effects of humidified high flow nasal oxygen in critical care patients: a prospective pilot study. Intensive Care Med. 2011;37(11):1780-6.
27. Frizzola M, Miller TL, Rodriguez ME, et al. High-flow nasal cannula: impact on oxygenation and ventilation in an acute lung injury model. Pediatric Pulmonol. 2011;46(1):67-74.
28. Lee JH, Rehder KJ, Williford L, et al. Use of high flow nasal cannula in critically ill infants, children, and adults: a critical review of the literature. Intensive Care Med. 2013;39(2):247-57.
29. Carratala Perales JM, Llorens P, Brouzet B, et al. High-flow therapy via nasal cannula in acute heart failure. Revista Espanola De cardiologia. 2011;64(8):723-5.
30. Lampland AL, Plumm B, Meyers PA, et al. Observational study of humidified high-flow nasal cannula compared with nasal continuous positive airway pressure. J Pediatr. 2009;154(2):177-82.
31. Ou X, Hua Y, Liu J, et al. Effect of high-flow nasal cannula oxygen therapy in adults with acute hypoxemic respiratory failure: a meta-analysis of randomized controlled trials. CMAJ. 2017;189(7):E260-e267.
32. Ni YN, Luo J, Yu H, et al. Can high-flow nasal cannula reduce the rate of endotracheal intubation in adult patients with acute respiratory failure compared with conventional oxygen therapy and noninvasive positive pressure ventilation?: a systematic review and meta-analysis. Chest. 2017;151(4):764-75.
33. Stefan MS, Eckert P, Tiru B, et al. High flow nasal oxygen therapy utilization: 7-year experience at a community teaching hospital. Hosp Prac (1995). 2018;46(2):73-6.
34. Leach RM, Rees PJ, Wilmshurst P. Hyperbaric oxygen therapy. British Med J. 1998;317(7166):1140-3.
35. Thom SR. Hyperbaric oxygen: its mechanisms and efficacy. Plast Reconstr Surg. 2011; 127(Suppl 1):131S-141S.
36. Heyboer M, Sharma D, Santiago W, et al. Hyperbaric oxygen therapy: side effects defined and quantified. Adv Wound Care. 2017;6(6):210-24.

# CHAPTER 3

# Approach to the Patient with Hypoxemia

*Aaron Lim*

## CASE

You are called to assess a 64-year-old male in respiratory distress on postoperative day 1 from an exploratory laparotomy and bowel resection. He is on 2 liters of nasal cannula with pulse oximetry reading 84% and arterial blood gas of pH 7.30, $PaCO_2$ 50, and $PaO_2$ 50. He is hemodynamically stable with a heart rate of 105/min and blood pressure of 137/85 mm Hg.

What is your differential diagnosis? How will you manage this patient?

## HYPOXIA AND HYPOXEMIA

While often used interchangeably, the terms hypoxia and hypoxemia are not synonymous. Hypoxia refers to an inadequate oxygen supply or utilization in the tissues.[1-3] Hypoxemia is an abnormally low partial pressure of oxygen in the arterial blood ($PaO_2$).[1-3] Indeed, hypoxemia and hypoxia often co-exist, however, they can be present independently of one another.

A normal $PaO_2$ for a patient breathing room air is 80–100 mm Hg and decreases with age.[2] The expected $PaO_2$ can be calculated with the following equation:

$$PaO_2 = 100 - 0.3 \text{ (Age)}$$

For example, a 40-year-old would be expected to have a $PaO_2$ of about 88 mmHg. Though age should be taken into account, a patient is generally considered hypoxemic if the $PaO_2 < 60$ mm Hg, which corresponds to a hemoglobin oxygen saturation of 90%.[1,3,4]

## OXYGENATION: NORMAL PHYSIOLOGY

Oxygen is vital to normal physiologic function serving as the final acceptor in the electric transport chain of aerobic respiration.[1] During inspiration, the majority of oxygen that passively diffuses into the pulmonary capillaries is bound to hemoglobin while a relatively small fraction remains dissolved in the plasma.[2] Together, this comprises the arterial oxygen content ($CaO_2$).

Arterial $O_2$ Content
$$CaO_2 = 1.39(Hgb)(SaO_2) + 0.003(PaO_2)$$
1.39 mL $O_2$/g of Hgb = capacity of Hgb for $O_2$
0.003 mL $O_2$/dL/mm = solubility of oxygen

The adequacy of tissue oxygenation depends on both oxygen delivery and consumption. Oxygen delivery ($DO_2$) is the product of arterial oxygen content ($CaO_2$) and cardiac output (CO). The amount of hemoglobin-bound oxygen is directly related to the hemoglobin concentration (Hgb) and the arterial oxygen saturation ($SaO_2$). Oxygen uptake or consumption ($VO_2$) reflects the amount of oxygen taken up by the tissues.

Oxygen Delivery
$$DO_2 = CaO_2 \times CO$$

Oxygen Consumption
$$VO_2 = (CaO_2 - CvO_2) \times CO$$
$CvO_2$ = mixed venous oxygen content.

The fraction of delivered oxygen that is taken up by the tissues is the oxygen extraction ratio ($O_2ER$) which under normal conditions is approximately 0.25.

Oxygen Extraction Ratio
$$O_2ER = VO_2/DO_2$$

During times of decreased oxygen supply or increased demand, the $O_2ER$ can increase to up to 0.5–0.6 to maintain adequate oxygenation.[5] However, beyond this point the $O_2ER$ becomes fixed, $VO_2$ becomes supply-dependent, and further decreases in $DO_2$ will result in dysoxia.[1] It is at this critical $DO_2$ tissues begin to switch to anaerobic respiration to make high-energy phosphates while forming lactate as a byproduct.[1,2] Lactate can serve as an oxidative fuel in several vital organs including the brain, heart, liver, and skeletal muscle during limited periods of tissue hypoxia, but if not corrected can lead to intracellular acidosis, impaired cellular function, and ultimately cell death.[1]

The relationships described above demonstrate that tissue dysoxia can be caused by a number of abnormalities including anemia, low oxygen saturation, hypoxemia, low cardiac output, or increased oxygen consumption. Because hypoxemia can potentially lead to end-organ dysfunction, and most significantly anoxic brain injury after only 4–6 minutes of hypoxic stress, it is a serious matter that should be immediately addressed when encountered.[2]

### *Monitoring*

Most commonly, the oxygenation status of patients in the intensive care unit (ICU) is monitored with pulse oximetry. Pulse oximetry provides the peripheral capillary oxygen saturation ($SpO_2$) which closely reflects the $SaO_2$ of blood at clinically acceptable levels.[1,4] Technically speaking, one must have a low $PaO_2$ by way of arterial blood gas (ABG) to make the diagnosis of hypoxemia. However, several clinical studies have shown continuous pulse oximetry to be superior to periodic blood gas sampling in detecting significant hypoxemia and therefore *$SpO_2$ is used as an acceptable surrogate for $PaO_2$ in the ICU setting*.[1] It is a low saturation via pulse oximetry that often prompts the clinician to obtain an ABG to diagnose hypoxemia.

## Pulmonary Gas Exchange

The basic purpose of pulmonary gas exchange is to oxygenate blood and remove carbon dioxide from blood passing through the lungs.[5] The lungs are composed of approximately 300 million alveoli surrounded by a network of billions of capillaries.[4,5] During inspiration, the alveoli expand and are filled with $O_2$-rich and $CO_2$-poor fresh gas. At the alveolar-capillary membrane, oxygen passively diffuses from the alveolus into the blood and $CO_2$ diffuses from the blood into the alveoli until both sides are in equilibrium. The newly oxygenated blood flows to the pulmonary veins and into the left heart from where it is pumped to the rest of the body. During expiration, the alveoli collapse and the $CO_2$-rich gas is exhaled.[5]

### *V/Q matching*

The adequacy of gas exchange depends on the balance of ventilation (V) and perfusion (Q) throughout the lung. An idealistic lung model would be homogeneous with perfectly matched ventilation and perfusion throughout resulting in a V/Q ratio of 1.[5] In reality, the normal lung is heterogeneous with varying V/Q ratios across different lung units. The distribution of ventilation and perfusion is not uniform. The right lung receives more ventilation than the left lung (~53% vs. 47%) and there is greater blood flow in the hilar regions than the periphery in both lungs.[4] Since both ventilation and perfusion are gravity-dependent, both individually increase from the lung apices to the bases. However, because the flow of blood is more gravity-dependent, perfusion increases at a greater rate than ventilation resulting in a decrease in V/Q ratios from top to bottom.[6] This explains why normal V/Q ratios in West zones 1, 2, and 3 are 3.4, 0.8, and 0.6, respectively.[2] Thus, there is an inherent component of clinically insignificant V/Q inequality in the normal lung. In the diseased lung, such mismatch can cause hypoxemia.

V/Q mismatch throughout the lung can be placed on a spectrum with the extremes being dead space and shunt.[1] When there is ventilation in excess of perfusion (V/Q > 1), this is called alveolar dead space. Anatomic dead space refers to the conducting airways that do not participate in gas exchange (i.e. pharynx, larynx, trachea, bronchi, and bronchioles). Together, anatomic and alveolar dead spaces comprise physiologic dead space.

When there is perfusion in excess of ventilation (V/Q < 1), this is called a shunt or venous admixture.[3] When there is no ventilation at all to a perfused lung segment (V/Q = 0), this is a total shunt and the physiology mimics that of an intracardiac right-to-left shunt. An example of this is a right endobronchial intubation, where the left lung is not ventilated but continues to be perfused. The blood that flows through the left lung is not oxygenated and goes on to mix in with the pulmonary venous return from the ventilated right lung.

Many pulmonary diseases result in varying degrees of both dead space and shunt physiology, but they are rarely absolute, meaning at least some perfusion or ventilation persists in affected lung units.[6] When lung units have decreased ventilation with resultant hypoxia, the blood vessels in these regions get vasoconstricted, a normal physiologic mechanism known as hypoxic pulmonary vasoconstriction (HPV). HPV curbs the effect of shunt in areas of low V/Q by diverting blood to better ventilated lung regions. In response to areas of low perfusion, the bronchioles reflexively constrict thereby decreasing the degree of intrapulmonary shunt. V/Q mismatch will be discussed in more detail later in this chapter.

## Alveolar Gas Equation

The alveolar gas equation describes the transfer of oxygen from the environment into the alveoli and can be used to calculate the partial pressure of oxygen in the alveolus ($P_AO_2$).[7] In its most simplistic form it is expressed as:

Alveolar Gas Equation
$$P_AO_2 = PiO_2 - PaCO_2/R$$
After substituting $PiO_2 = FiO_2 (P_{atm} - P_{H_2O})$,
$$P_AO_2 = FiO_2 (P_{atm} - P_{H_2O}) - PaCO_2/R$$

The $PiO_2$ is the partial pressure of inspired oxygen and is directly related to the fraction of inspired oxygen ($FiO_2$) and the gradient between atmospheric pressure (760 mm Hg at sea level) and the barometric pressure of water ($P_{H_2O}$ = 47 mm Hg). The $PaCO_2$ is the partial pressure of carbon dioxide and R is the respiratory quotient which under normal conditions is 0.8.

## Alveolar-arterial (A-a) Gradient

The alveolar-arterial (A-a) gradient is the difference between the partial pressure of oxygen in the alveolus ($P_AO_2$) and the partial pressure of oxygen in the arterial blood ($PaO_2$). It is useful in determining the mechanism of hypoxemia and reflects the integrity of the alveolar-capillary unit.

$$\text{A-a gradient} = P_AO_2 - PaO_2$$

After substituting the alveolar gas equation for $P_AO_2$,

$$\text{A-a gradient} = [FiO_2 (P_{atm} - P_{H_2O}) - PaCO_2/R] - PaO_2$$

Under normal conditions, there is an A-a gradient of 5–10 mm Hg explained by the bronchial and thebesian veins draining directly into the left atrium without participating in gas exchange (physiologic shunt).[4] Of note, the normal A-a gradient increases with age.

$$\text{Normal A-a gradient} = (\text{Age}/4) + 4$$

An increased A-a gradient suggests V/Q mismatch, right-to-left shunt, or diffusion impairment in the alveolar-capillary membrane preventing normal gas exchange.

Below is an example of the calculated A-a gradient in a normal patient breathing room air ($FiO_2$ 0.21) at sea level with normal $PaO_2$, $PaCO_2$, and R values.

$$\begin{aligned}\text{A-a gradient} &= [FiO_2 (P_{atm} - P_{H_2O}) - PaCO_2/R] - PaO_2 \\ &= [0.21 (760 - 47) - 40/0.8] - 90 \\ &= 100 - 90 \\ &= 10 \text{ mm Hg}\end{aligned}$$

## MECHANISM OF HYPOXEMIA

There are five main mechanisms of hypoxemia—V/Q mismatch, shunt, hypoventilation, low $PiO_2$, and diffusion impairment.[1-5,8] V/Q mismatch is the most common mechanism of hypoxemia, though multiple can overlap.

## V/Q Mismatch

V/Q mismatch is the most common cause of hypoxemia and refers to an imbalance of blood flow and ventilation causing variation in the composition of gasses throughout lung regions.[1] As discussed earlier in this chapter, V/Q mismatch is a spectrum that can include areas of excess ventilation, such as dead space, or areas of excess perfusion, such as intrapulmonary shunt or venous admixture.[2] There can also be areas where both ventilation as well as perfusion is absent, known as silent units or silent spaces. There is an increase in the A-a gradient and hypoxemia caused by V/Q mismatch will improve with supplemental oxygen.

In areas where there is excess ventilation, increasing the amount of inspired oxygen ($PiO_2$) will increase the $P_AO_2$ and therefore the amount of oxygen that diffuses into the arterial blood ($PaO_2$). In ventilated areas where perfusion exceeds ventilation (1 > V/Q > 0), increasing the amount of oxygen will still increase the $PaO_2$ of blood that leaves the capillary beds, therefore decreasing the severity of the resultant venous admixture. In areas of total shunt where there is no ventilation (V/Q = 0), supplemental oxygen will have no effect on the blood that passes through the capillary bed and the affected segments will physiologically mimic a right-to-left shunt.[1]

A classic example of hypoxemia caused by V/Q mismatch is a pulmonary embolus (PE). Lung units downstream from the obstruction continue to be ventilated with decreased or no perfusion and therefore have high V/Q ratios. Meanwhile, the "extra" blood that would usually go to the obstructed areas flows to other lung regions resulting in lower V/Q ratios. When ventilation cannot keep up with excess perfusion in these areas, hypoxemia occurs. Supplemental oxygen increases the $P_AO_2$ in these ventilated areas of low V/Q and therefore the $PaO_2$ will also increase.[5]

## Shunt

Shunt occurs when blood from the right side of the heart enters the left side of the heart without taking part in any gas exchange.[4] The two types of shunts are intrapulmonary and intracardiac shunts. As previously mentioned, intrapulmonary shunt occurs in unventilated areas and is an extreme form of V/Q mismatch (V/Q = 0).[4] Examples of intrapulmonary shunt include mainstem intubation, atelectasis, acute respiratory distress syndrome (ARDS), and unventilated areas distal to mucus plugs. In these areas, there is absolutely no ventilation so adding supplemental oxygen will have no discernible benefit to the affected segments.[5]

Intracardiac shunts occur when there is a communication from the right heart circuit to the left heart circuit (e.g. atrial septal defect, ventricular septal defect (VSD), patent foramen ovale) and a driving pressure to cause blood to flow from right to left.[1] For example, most patients with a VSD will have left-to-right shunting unless over time, right ventricular pressure increases to the point that it exceeds left ventricular pressure and there is a reversal of the shunt to right-to-left (i.e. Eisenmenger's syndrome).

Like in V/Q mismatch, there is an increased A-a gradient in shunt. The distinguishing feature of hypoxemia caused by shunt is no improvement with supplemental or 100% oxygen.

### Shunt Fraction

The shunt fraction is the percentage of total blood flow that is not exposed to inhaled gas and can be calculated using the shunt equation.[2]

Shunt Equation

$$Q_s/Q_t = (C_{C'O_2} - C_{aO_2}) / (C_{C'O_2} - C_{vO_2})$$

$Q_s$ = shunt blood flow
$Q_t$ = total cardiac output
$C_{C'O_2}$ = alveolar oxygen content
$C_{aO_2}$ = arterial oxygen content
$C_{vO_2}$ = mixed venous oxygen content

The greater the shunt fraction, the more severe the hypoxemia will be. While $PaO_2$ continues to decrease as shunt fraction increases, $PaCO_2$ stays constant until the shunt fraction exceeds 50%. Many patients with shunt physiology will still have normal or decreased $PaCO_2$ secondary to hyperventilation triggered by hypoxemia and/or the disease process.[2] In general, in regions of low V/Q ratio (e.g. shunt), oxygen is the more affected gas while in regions of high V/Q ratio (e.g. dead space), $CO_2$ is more affected.

### a-A Oxygen Tension Ratio

The arterial/alveolar oxygen tension ratio ($PaO_2/P_AO_2$) can be used to assess the severity of gas exchange abnormalities. Unlike the A-a gradient, it is *less affected by $FiO_2$ or barometric pressure*. A ratio <0.75 is abnormal and may be due to either V/Q mismatch, diffusion impairment, or an increase in the oxygen extraction ratio. Normal ratio ranges from 0.75 to 1.0 and in a hypoxic patient suggests a mechanism of either alveolar hypoventilation or low atmospheric pressure. The a-A oxygen tension ratio can be used to determine the change in $FiO_2$ necessary to achieve a certain $PaO_2$.

*An example:* A patient has a $PaO_2$ 50 and $PaCO_2$ 50 on 30% $FiO_2$. What $FiO_2$ will be required to increase $PaO_2$ to 60?

$$(PaO_2/P_AO_2)_{initial} = (PaO_2 / P_AO_2)_{final}$$

Using the alveolar gas equation to solve for $P_AO_{2\,initial}$ gives us:

$$(50/150) = (60 / P_AO_2)_{final}$$
$$P_AO_{2\,final} = 180$$

Again, use the alveolar gas equation and this time solve for $FiO_2$:

$P_AO_2$ = $FiO_2 (P_{atm} - P_{H_2O}) - PaCO_2/R$
180 = $FiO_2 (760 - 47) - 50/0.8$
$FiO_2$ = 0.34

Therefore, in order to increase the $PaO_2$ from 50 to 60, you would need to increase the $FiO_2$ from 0.30 to 0.34.

### $PaO_2/FiO_2$ Ratio

The $PaO_2/FiO_2$ ratio or "P/F ratio" is useful to estimate the degree of shunt and can be quickly calculated at the bedside. A normal P/F ratio is greater than 300. P/F < 300 indicates abnormal gas exchange and P/F < 200 indicates severe hypoxemia, as in moderate ARDS. For example, a normal healthy person breathing room air has a P/F ratio of 100/0.21 or approximately 500, while a patient with a $PaO_2$ of 90 on 50% $FiO_2$ would have a P/F ratio of 90/0.5 = 180 indicating severe hypoxemia secondary to shunt.

### Effect of Cardiac Output on Shunting

Generally speaking, an increase in cardiac output will cause an increase in shunting in both normal and diseased lungs, however, hypoxemia may be more pronounced in the latter due to the presence of increased heterogeneity.[9] This is because increased CO results in increased blood flow to all lung units in the heterogeneous lung and in low V/Q lung units (i.e. V/Q < 1) this increased flow will further decrease the V/Q ratio. This decrease in regional V/Q ratio will increase venous admixture and shunt.

## Hypoventilation

Alveolar hypoventilation is another cause of hypoxemia and usually comes in the form of shallow breathing, hypopnea or apnea, or airway obstruction.[2] The major distinguishing feature of hypoxemia secondary to hypoventilation is accompanying hypercapnia (increased $PaCO_2$) which can cause respiratory acidosis.[2,4,10] Because the alveolus is a space comprised of only gasses, the sum of the partial pressures of gasses remains constant (Dalton's Law). Therefore, as $P_ACO_2$ increases during hypoventilation, $P_AO_2$ decreases leading to an increased $PaCO_2$ and decreased $PaO_2$ once the partial pressures equilibrate at the alveolar-capillary membrane.[2]

In hypoxemia secondary to pure hypoventilation, there is no compromise at the level of gas exchange at the alveolar-capillary membrane and the V/Q ratios are normal. Therefore, there is no increase in the A-a gradient and PaO$_2$ improves with supplemental oxygen. However, hypoventilation is commonly accompanied by other causes of hypoxemia like V/Q mismatch.[5]

Most hypoventilation in ICU patients can be attributed to either central respiratory depression or respiratory muscle weakness. Examples of central respiratory depression include opiate-induced narcosis, structural, or ischemic central nervous system lesions that affect the respiratory center, and obesity-hypoventilation syndrome (Pickwickian syndrome).[1,2] Conditions leading to respiratory muscle weakness include those impairing neural conduction (e.g. amyotrophic lateral sclerosis, Guillain–Barre syndrome, high cervical spine injuries), or causing skeletal muscle weakness (e.g. myasthenia gravis, muscular dystrophy).[1] Hypoventilation can occur in mechanically-ventilated patients if minute ventilation (tidal volume × respiratory rate) is inadequate for gas exchange.

## Low PiO$_2$

While the initial step in management of a patient with hypoxia or hypoxemia is typically providing supplemental oxygen and thereby increasing FiO$_2$, a low PiO$_2$ or FiO$_2$ is rarely the true cause of hypoxemia except in unusual circumstances. The classic example of low PiO$_2$ causing hypoxemia is at high altitude where atmospheric pressure is decreased.[5] Although the FiO$_2$ at altitude remains unchanged, the PiO$_2$ is decreased because it is directly related to atmospheric pressure as PiO$_2$ = FiO$_2$ (P$_{atm}$ – P$_{H_2O}$).[5] Below is an example comparing the P$_A$O$_2$ of a person at sea level versus one climbing Mount Everest at 18,000 feet where the atmospheric pressure is approximately 400 mm Hg.[11]

At sea level
P$_A$O$_2$ = FiO$_2$ (P$_{atm}$ – P$_{H_2O}$) – PaCO$_2$/R
= 0.21 (760 – 47) – 40/0.8
= 100 mm Hg

At Mount Everest
P$_A$O$_2$ = FiO$_2$ (P$_{atm}$ – P$_{H_2O}$) – PaCO$_2$/R
= 0.21 (400 – 47) – 40/0.8
= 24 mm Hg

As you can see, at high altitude though the FiO$_2$ remains 0.21 the PiO$_2$ decreases because atmospheric pressure decreases as one ascends. This leads to decreased P$_A$O$_2$ and therefore decreased PaO$_2$ and hypoxemia. The example above also shows the benefit of supplemental oxygen (increased FiO$_2$) and compensatory hyperventilation (decreases PaCO$_2$) to correct hypoxemia at altitude.[5,6]

In the ICU, hypoxemia due to low PiO$_2$ can be caused by faulty connections between the oxygen source and ventilator or bag-mask-ventilation devices. For example, an intubated patient being transported from the ICU to the operating room while being ventilated by hand with a self-inflating bag connected to an empty oxygen tank will become hypoxemic if the PiO$_2$ is inadequate for their current condition.

Hypoxemia secondary to inadequate PiO$_2$ will improve with 100% oxygen. However, it is important to remember that improvement with supplemental oxygen does not rule out other causes of hypoxemia like hypoventilation, V/Q mismatch, or diffusion impairment. The A-a gradient will be normal as there is no disruption of gas exchange at the alveolar-capillary membrane.

## Diffusion Impairment

The final cause of hypoxemia, diffusion impairment, results from disruption of the alveolar-capillary membrane. The most common example of this is in a patient with interstitial lung disease during exertion.[10] In a normal patient at rest, a red blood cell (RBC) travels through the pulmonary capillaries in 0.75 second. It takes 0.25 second for diffusion equilibrium of O$_2$ and CO$_2$ to occur, so there is some allowance for circumstances such as exercise when blood flow rates increase and RBC transit times decrease.[7] Pulmonary fibrosis increases the distance gasses must diffuse to reach RBCs and during exertion, this in combination with faster blood flow rates may lead to hypoxemia.[5] Still, diffusion impairment-induced hypoxemia is rarely seen at rest unless there is greater than 50% lung damage and is a less common mechanism of hypoxemia in ICU patients.[5] Because there is damage to the alveolar-capillary membrane, there will be an increased A-a gradient and PaO$_2$ should improve with supplemental oxygen.

## MANAGEMENT

The approach to a patient with hypoxemia should include initial assessment and stabilization in addition to workup and definitive treatment of the underlying cause(s). A patient with hypoxemia is at risk for clinical deterioration, so it is important to quickly address the ABC's (airway, breathing, and circulation) and rule out hemodynamic instability. One should ensure a patent and secure airway, adequate breathing—whether spontaneous, assisted, or controlled (mechanical) ventilation, and adequate circulation to perfuse vital organs. If any of these are abnormal, the patient should be supported immediately. If the patient does not have a pulse or is having any type of malignant arrhythmia—such as ventricular fibrillation—advanced cardiac life support (ACLS) should be initiated.

Once the patient has been deemed stable from a cardiovascular standpoint and a patent airway confirmed, a systematic approach should be used to determine the cause of hypoxemia (Flowchart 1), provide supportive measures, and address the underlying etiology. A simplified approach to a patient with hypoxemia is shown in Flowchart 1.

## Physically Assess the Patient

Often overlooked and sometimes abandoned in the modern era of medicine is the physical examination of patients, especially in the ICU where data such as vital signs, fluid balances, laboratory values, medications, and imaging studies are readily and remotely accessible via electronic medical records. While physical exam findings alone might not be diagnostic, they can provide important clues to a diagnosis and help rule out other possible causes of hypoxemia.

In the setting of hypoxemia, a focused physical exam should include at the least, an assessment of cardiovascular, respiratory, and neurologic systems. Auscultation of the lungs can reveal shallow breathing in the setting of hypoventilation, diminished or absent lung sounds if there is upper airway obstruction, mucus plugging, or endobronchial intubation, crackles or rales in the setting of fluid overload, wheezing or rhonchi in obstructive lung disease, etc. Cardiovascular physical exam can hint towards conditions such as heart failure, valvulopathy, or cardiac tamponade. It is important to assess neurologic status as conditions such as neuromuscular weakness or altered mentation can lead to respiratory compromise as well as an unprotected airway.

## Analysis of the Arterial Blood Gas

Evaluate the pH, $PaO_2$, and $PaCO_2$ and identify any acid-base abnormalities (more detailed analysis of ABG discussed in other chapters). If the patient has a primary respiratory acidosis—low pH and high $PaCO_2$—in the setting of hypoxemia, hypoventilation should be high on your differential as the cause.

## Calculate the A-a Gradient

As previously discussed, this can be determined using the alveolar gas equation to obtain the $P_AO_2$ and the $PaO_2$ from the ABG.

If the A-a gradient is normal, the most likely cause of hypoxemia is hypoventilation, though low $PiO_2$ is also possible. To distinguish between the two, look at the $PaCO_2$ which will be high in hypoventilation, but normal or low if there is insufficient $PiO_2$. Both conditions will improve with supplemental oxygen.

If the A-a gradient is abnormally high, the differential includes V/Q mismatch, shunt, or diffusion impairment, with the latter being the least likely cause in ICU patients. At this point, administration of supplemental oxygen can help distinguish between V/Q mismatch and shunt. Hypoxemia caused by V/Q mismatch will improve with supplemental oxygen whereas shunt-induced hypoxemia is less likely to improve. With shunt, the A-a gradient will actually become greater with supplemental oxygen. For completion, hypoxemia due to diffusion impairment would also improve with 100% $O_2$, but again it is less likely to be the primary culprit in this setting.

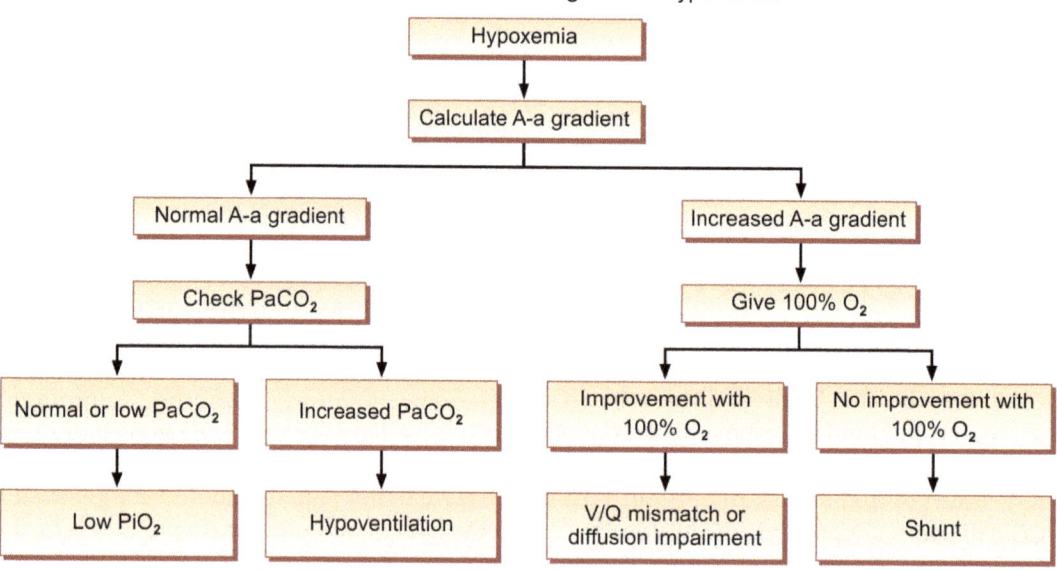

**Flowchart 1:** Differential diagnosis of hypoxemia.

## Administration of 100% Oxygen

The most common initial intervention in the management of a hypoxemic patient is the administration of 100% oxygen to ideally achieve a goal $PaO_2 > 60$ mm Hg and/or $SpO_2 > 92\%$.[12] This is a reasonable intervention, particularly if the patient is severely hypoxemic and in extremis, but it is important to understand the implications. If an initial arterial blood gas has been obtained, an A-a gradient and P/F ratio can still be retrospectively calculated. However, if a gas (and therefore $PaO_2$) is not obtained prior to giving oxygen, you will not be able to calculate the initial A-a gradient or P/F ratio to aid in diagnosis. Four of the five mechanisms of hypoxemia will respond to 100% oxygen with the exception being shunt. Therefore, if there is no improvement with supplemental oxygen, one should consider shunt as a mechanism. However, if there is improvement prior to calculation of an A-a gradient, it is now more difficult to distinguish among the other four possible causes. In the grand scheme of things, this exercise and limitation is probably more academic than practical because there will be more information available to aid in diagnosis and the presence of more than one mechanism of hypoxemia is not uncommon. It is also important to keep in mind that prolonged administration with 100% $FiO_2$ can lead to absorption atelectasis as oxygen replaces nitrogen in the lungs and this can further worsen hypoxemia.[12,13]

## Temporizing and Supportive Measures

In addition to administration of 100% oxygen typically by nonrebreathing mask in nonintubated patients, other maneuvers should be considered to stabilize hypoxemic patients while working to initiate definitive treatment. For example, narcotic-induced hypoventilation may require escalation of airway management, such as a jaw thrust or chin lift, insertion of a nasal trumpet, noninvasive positive pressure ventilation, or even endotracheal intubation prior to and during careful administration of naloxone. If the patient is apneic, bag-mask ventilation or mechanical ventilation will be needed until spontaneous breathing is restored.

## Further Workup and Treatment of Underlying Cause(s)

Once the mechanism(s) of hypoxemia has been determined and the patient stabilized, the underlying cause needs to be diagnosed and addressed. Appropriate labs such as a complete metabolic panel, complete blood count, liver function tests, and cultures may provide important diagnostic information. An electrocardiogram is quickly obtained and can be used to evaluate for arrhythmias, ischemia, infarction, etc. Imaging studies like chest X-ray and computerized tomography (CT) scan can help identify causes such as pneumonia, ARDS, mainstem intubation, atelectasis, pleural effusion, pulmonary edema, mucus plugging, and pneumothorax. CT angiogram, V/Q scans, and transesophageal echocardiogram can help diagnose PE.

As with any medical condition, treatment should be appropriately initiated. For example, pneumonia should be treated with appropriate antibiotics. ARDS ought to be managed with lung-protective ventilation strategies which include low tidal volume ventilation, avoidance of high plateau pressures, and addition of positive end-expiratory pressure (PEEP) to prevent alveolar collapse. Albuterol and ipratropium nebulizers could be beneficial in the setting of asthma or COPD exacerbation. Hypoxemia due to pulmonary edema from congestive heart failure may benefit from diuretics and inotropic support, mucus plugging might require therapeutic bronchoscopy, and severe atelectasis may benefit from recruitment maneuvers, etc.[8]

## Case Revisit

The broad differential diagnosis for hypoxemia in this patient includes V/Q mismatch, shunt, hypoventilation, low $PiO_2$, and diffusion impairment. For the reasons previously discussed, low $PiO_2$ and diffusion impairment would be low on the differential for this particular patient leaving hypoventilation, V/Q mismatch, and shunt. In addition to an abnormally low $PaO_2$, the ABG is significant for respiratory acidosis (low pH, high $PaCO_2$) which might suggest hypoventilation (e.g. narcotic overdose, rapid shallow breathing from pain) as a possible mechanism, however, because the A-a gradient is elevated (~94 mm Hg), V/Q mismatch in the form of deadspace and/or shunt (e.g. atelectasis, pneumonia) is likely present.

A reasonable approach to the initial management of this hemodynamically stable patient includes focused physical examination to assess neurologic status, airway patency, adequacy and depth of respirations, and presence and quality of bilateral breath sounds while simultaneously administering supplemental oxygen, for example 100% $FiO_2$ via a nonrebreathing mask. In most instances, supplemental oxygen will "temporize" the patient by acutely improving hypoxemia and preventing further deterioration and will buy some time while further workup is performed and more definitive measures taken. Should the patient not improve with supplemental oxygen, further escalation of airway management such as intubation should be considered and total intrapulmonary shunt (e.g. mucus plugging, pneumothorax) or intracardiac shunt rises on the differential. This case demonstrates that the mechanisms/causes of hypoxemia often overlap and management should take into consideration the entire clinical picture including history, physical exam, laboratory findings, and imaging studies.

## SALIENT POINTS

- Hypoxia refers to abnormally low oxygen content in the tissues. Hypoxemia refers to abnormally low dissolved oxygen in the blood and is clinically significant if $PaO_2$ < 60 mm Hg.
- Adequacy of pulmonary gas exchange is affected by the balance of ventilation and perfusion in the lung. V/Q mismatch occurs when there is loss of this equality and can result in hypoxemia.
- The five main mechanisms of hypoxemia are V/Q mismatch, shunt, hypoventilation, low $PiO_2$, and diffusion impairment. In the ICU, low $PiO_2$ and diffusion impairment fall lower on the differential.
- Arterial blood gas analysis, calculation of the A-a gradient, and response to supplemental oxygen aid determining the mechanism of hypoxemia, though often more than one is present.
- V/Q mismatch is a spectrum with the extremes being deadspace and shunt. Hypoxemia due to V/Q mismatch is characterized by an increased A-a gradient and improvement with supplemental oxygen.
- Shunt can be intrapulmonary or intracardiac. Hypoxemia due to shunt is characterized by an increased A-a gradient and little to no improvement with supplemental oxygen.
- Hypoventilation-induced hypoxemia is characterized by an increased $PaCO_2$, a normal A-a gradient, and improvement with supplemental oxygen.
- Inadequate $PiO_2$-induced hypoxemia is characterized by a normal A-a gradient and improvement with supplemental oxygen.
- Management of the patient with hypoxemia should begin with immediate assessment and stabilization of airway, breathing, and circulation followed by more definitive workup, diagnosis, and treatment.

## REFERENCES

1. Marino PL. Marino's the ICU Book, 4th edition. Philadelphia: Wolters Kluwer Health/Lippincott Williams & Wilkins; 2014.
2. Theodore AC. (2017). Oxygenation and Mechanisms of Hypoxemia. UpToDate. [online] Available from: https://www.uptodate.com/contents/oxygenation-and-mechanisms-of-hypoxemia. [Accessed Jan., 2019].
3. Yao FF, Fontes ML, Malhotra V (Eds). Yao & Artusio's Anesthesiology: Problem-Oriented Patient Management, 7th edition. Philadelphia: Wolters Kluwer Health/Lippincott Williams & Wilkins; 2012.
4. Wasnick J, Butterworth J, Mackey D. Morgan and Mikhail's Clinical Anesthesiology, 5th edition. New York, NY: McGraw-Hill Education LLC.; 2013.
5. Wagner PD. The physiological basis of pulmonary gas exchange: Implications for clinical interpretation of arterial blood gases. Eur Respir J. 2015;45(1):227-43.
6. Barash PG. Clinical Anesthesia, 7th edition. Philadelphia, PA: Lippincott Williams & Wilkins; 2013.
7. Miller RD, Eriksson LI, Fleisher L, Wiener-kronish JP, Cohen NH. Miller's Anesthesia, 8th edition. Philadelphia, PA: Elsevier; 2015.
8. Department of Medicine. Washington University, School of Medicine. In: Hemant G, Hirbe A, Nassif M, Otepka H, Rosenstock A (Eds). The Washington Manual of Medical Therapeutics, 34th edition. Philadelphia, Baltimore, New York, London, Buenos Aires, Hong Kong, Sydney, Tokyo: Wolters Kluwer Health, Lippincott Williams & Wilkins; 2014.
9. Tsang JY. Mechanism for worsening gas exchange at increased cardiac output: It's time for an Occam's razor. J Pulm Respir Med. 2014;4:217.
10. Sarkar M, Niranjan N, Banyal PK. Mechanisms of hypoxemia. Lung India. 2017;34(1):47-60.
11. West JB, Lahiri S, Maret KH, et al. Barometric pressures at extreme altitudes on Mt. Everest: physiological significance. J Appl Physiol Respir Environ Exerc Physiol. 1983;54(5):1188-94.
12. Duarte AG, Bidani A. Evaluating hypoxemia in the critically ill. J Respir Dis. 2005;5:209-21.
13. Rodríguez-Roisin R, Roca J. Mechanisms of hypoxemia. Intensive Care Med. 2005;31(8):1017-9.

# CHAPTER 4

# Approach to the Patient with Hypercapnia

*Malvika Sagar, Char Ogborn, Shekhar Ghamande*

## CASE

A 38-year-old morbidly obese male was admitted to the hospital with acute respiratory illness including cough, fever and dyspnea over 3 days. The patient denied history of smoking or any chronic lung disease. His body mass index (BMI) was 50. Despite a diagnosis of obstructive sleep apnea, he was not adherent with his continuous positive airway pressure machine. Due to hypoxemia with oxygen saturation ($SpO_2$) of 82% on room air, a respiratory rate of 36/minute, pulse of 102/minute and a blood pressure of 108/60 mm Hg, he was placed on oxygen ($O_2$) at 3L/minute. He had diminished breath sounds in both lung fields and faint heart sounds. He had pedal edema with dark discoloration of his skin on his feet.

Laboratory indicated white blood cell (WBC) of 16,000/µL, blood urea nitrogen (BUN) of 22 mg/dL and creatinine of 1.5 mg/dL. The arterial blood gas (ABG) showed partially compensated respiratory acidosis with pH 7.23, $pCO_2$ 76, $pO_2$ 52, $HCO_3$ of 32 and $SaO_2$ of 86% on 3 liters/minute through nasal cannula. Bilevel positive airway pressure (BiPAP) therapy with an inspiratory pressure of 16 cm and expiratory pressure of 12 cm with fraction of inspired oxygen ($FiO_2$) of 0.4 was applied. The chest radiograph revealed prominent interstitial infiltrates with cardiomegaly (Fig. 1). His electrocardiogram (ECG) showed sinus tachycardia. Subsequently, the patient became somnolent and his ABG value changed to pH 7.16, $pCO_2$ 83, $pO_2$ 72, $HCO_3$ 30 and $SaO_2$ 93% despite being on BiPAP. At this point, he was managed with invasive mechanical ventilation (IMV) on volume assist-control.

A review of his prior records indicated that he was seen about 8 months ago in clinic and his pulmonary function tests (PFTs) revealed a restrictive pattern with forced expiratory volume in first second (FEV1) 70% predicted, forced vital capacity (FVC) of 72% predicted with a FEV1/FVC ratio of 80. His total lung capacity was 76% of predicted. His diffusing capacity was 68% of predicted.

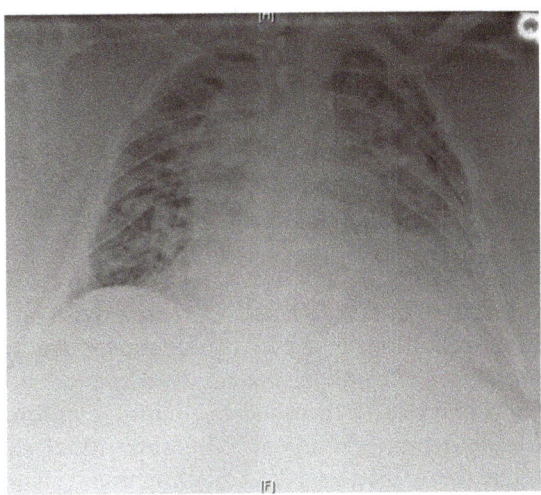

**Fig. 1:** Chest radiograph of the case showing prominent interstitial infiltrates with cardiomegaly.

What should be the approach to this patient's hypercapnia? This case has been revisited at the end.

## INTRODUCTION

Hypercapnia is an elevation in the partial pressure of carbon dioxide ($CO_2$) in the artery. It is easy to miss this diagnosis in neuromuscular patients. If not treated in time, acute hypercapnic respiratory failure (AHRF) could become life threatening. Clinical scenario, definition, pathophysiology, causes, clinical features, advantages and disadvantages, evaluation, management and prognosis of hypercapnia are discussed in this chapter.

## DEFINITION

Hypercapnia is defined as an elevation in the partial pressure of $CO_2$ in the artery ($PaCO_2$) greater than 45 mm Hg.[1]

## PATHOPHYSIOLOGY

The level of $CO_2$ in arterial blood ($PaCO_2$) is directly proportional to the rate of $CO_2$ production ($VCO_2$) and inversely related to the rate of $CO_2$ elimination, i.e. alveolar ventilation. However, alveolar ventilation ($V_A$) is determined by minute ventilation ($V_E$) and the ratio of dead space ($V_D$) to tidal volume ($V_T$).[2]

$$V_A = V_E \times (1 - V_D/V_T)$$

### Dead Space

Dead space refers to the space in which there is no exchange of $O_2$ and $CO_2$ gasses across the alveolar membrane in the respiratory tract. More specifically, anatomic dead space refers to the volume of air found in the sections of the respiratory tract that conduct air to the alveoli and respiratory bronchioles but do not participate in gas exchange. The alveolar dead space refers to the volume of air in the alveoli that are ventilated but not perfused indicating no gas exchange. True alveolar dead space is the space where no perfusion exists [ventilation-perfusion (V/Q) ratio is equal to infinity]. Relative alveolar dead space is when there is excessive ventilation and V/Q ratio is greater than 1.[3] Usually alveolar dead space is zero in normal lungs and hence, anatomical dead space is synonymous with physiological dead space. The only air which reaches to terminal bronchioles and alveoli is available for gas exchange.[4] Therefore, tidal volume must exceed the dead space, so that functional alveoli get ventilated by inhaled air.

Mechanical dead space refers to cavity in within an apparatus where the gas flows in both directions as the user breathes in and out. This increases the needed respiratory effort to get the required amount of usable air with the risk of shallow breaths causing an accumulation of $CO_2$. In effect, it is an external extension of the physiological dead space.[3]

With acute respiratory distress syndrome (ARDS), disturbances are created in the pulmonary microvasculature, increasing the dead space. However, it is not clear if these portions are ventilated enough to be considered dead space.[5]

### Minute Ventilation versus Alveolar Ventilation

Minute ventilation is the product of tidal volume and the respiratory rate. The alveolar ventilation is lesser than the minute ventilation as dead space is subtracted while calculating alveolar ventilation.

Alveolar ventilation = (Tidal volume – Dead space) × Respiratory rate

For example if tidal volume is 500 mL, respiratory rate 12 breaths/minute, anatomic dead space 150 mL; then minute ventilation will be 500 mL × 12 breaths/minute = 6 L/minute; while alveolar ventilation will be (500 mL – 150 mL) × 12 breaths/minute = 4.2 L/minute.

Another equation for alveolar ventilation is:

$$V'_A = (V'CO_2/PaCO_2) \times K$$

Where $V'_A$ = Alveolar ventilation, $V'CO_2$ = Rate of carbon dioxide exhalation, $PaCO_2$ = Partial pressure of arterial carbon dioxide, and K = Unit correction factor.[6]

According to the alveolar ventilation equation, $PaCO_2$ is inversely proportional to the alveolar ventilation.

If the tidal volume is doubled and the rate is halved or vice versa, the minute ventilation would not change but the alveolar ventilation as well as $PaCO_2$ changes significantly. Alveolar ventilation can be more effectively increased by increasing tidal volume instead by increasing respiratory rate.

### Role of Peripheral and Central Chemoreceptors in Maintaining $CO_2$ Balance

Arterial $pCO_2$ is tightly regulated by feedback mechanism through peripheral and central chemoreceptors. Peripheral chemoreceptors are located in the carotid and aortic bodies. They respond quickly to decreased arterial partial pressure of $O_2$ ($PO_2$), increased $PCO_2$ and hydrogen ion ($H^+$) concentration, but the effect is less as compared to central chemoreceptors. However, the central chemoreceptors respond to high $PCO_2$ and not $PO_2$ or $H^+$.[7]

### Mechanism of Hypercapnia in Chronic Obstructive Pulmonary Disease

- Increased dead space ventilation in areas with high V/Q ratio is the major mechanism for hypercapnia in chronic obstructive pulmonary disease (COPD) patients. Increased dead space is due to low tidal volume, high respiratory rate, loss of capillaries and overinflation.
  - Pink puffers are those who can compensate by increasing minute ventilation and hence perfusion
  - Blue bloaters are those who cannot compensate.[2]
- Mechanism of hypercapnia with supplemental $O_2$:
  - Worsening of V/Q mismatch leading to increased dead space[2,8]
  - Decreased binding affinity of hemoglobin for $CO_2$ (Haldane effect) in the presence of $O_2$.[2]
  - The administration of $O_2$ reduces hypoxic drive, but its contribution to hypercapnia is minor.

## CAUSES

Common causes of hypercapnia include reduced minute ventilation and increased dead space. Increase in $CO_2$ production rarely results in clinically important hypercapnia unless a patient has limited pulmonary reserve. In critically ill patients, the weakness of the respiratory muscles is responsible for a large number of alveolar hypoventilation cases. Metabolic disturbances like hypokalemia, hypocalcemia, hypophosphatemia, and hypomagnesemia can also cause weakness of respiratory muscles.[9]

It is important to determine whether the hypercapnia is due to V/Q mismatch or hypoventilation. A neurological event can lead to central hypoventilation which would result in hypoxemia with hypercapnia without an increase in alveolar-arterial gradient. Computed tomography of the head and basic laboratory tests include screening for drug toxicity would be a useful quick screen.

The presentation can be subacute in cases of amyotrophic lateral sclerosis (ALS) and Duchenne muscular dystrophy (DMD). Guillain-Barré syndrome (GBS) is the most common neuropathy leading to acute paralysis worldwide[10] and respiratory involvement occurs in 25% of cases.[11] By the end of the second week of presentation, Albuminocytologic dissociation in cerebrospinal fluid (CSF) (increased protein with normal CSF leukocytes) in GBS occurs in more than 90% of patients.[11] Nerve conduction studies (NCSs) provide valuable diagnostic information on demyelination but may be normal early in the course of disease.[11] Myasthenia gravis is the most common neuromuscular disease (NMD) with fluctuation of weakness and involvement of bulbar and ocular muscles.[12] A myasthenic crisis occurs in 20% of patients, usually within the first year of presentation. Diagnosis can be made with repetitive nerve stimulation and single fiber electromyographic testing. They have a sensitivity of 75% and 95% respectively.[13] A positive edrophonium test[14] has a high sensitivity of 85–90% but low specificity. Antibodies directed against acetylcholine receptor (positive in 85% cases) can aid in the diagnosis. In the patients with negative acetylcholine receptor antibodies, antibodies against specific muscle tyrosine kinase occur in 38–50% of generalized myasthenia gravis.[15]

In patients with COPD, hypercapnia develops with progressively worsening lung function. During COPD acute exacerbations, high expiratory resistance with flow limitation can lead to dynamic hyperinflation and development of intrinsic positive end-expiratory pressures (iPEEP).[16] The elastic work needed to overcome the iPEEP requires extra work in breathing.[17] Gas exchange impairment (V/Q mismatch) leads to higher dead space which increases the need to maintain higher minute ventilation.[18] Failure inability to keep up with the ventilation needs, and increased work of breathing can result in hypercapnic respiratory failure.[19]

The asthmatics do not develop hypercapnia until they develop respiratory failure with an exacerbation. Hypoxia and hypercapnia which result from poorly ventilated areas contribute to the regional perfusion redistribution of blood flow in these patients.[20]

### Permissive Hypercapnia

The permissive hypercapnia refers to the purposeful hypoventilation of mechanically ventilated patients to reduce ventilator-associated lung injury in disease states like bronchopulmonary dysplasia, ARDS and status asthmaticus.[1]

## CLINICAL FEATURES

Patients with mild to moderate hypercapnia may be anxious, or complain of mild dyspnea, daytime headaches and excessive daytime sleepiness. Those with higher levels of $CO_2$ develop central nervous system (CNS) side effects and papilledema. Clinical features are enlisted below in detail based on the organ systems involved (Table 1).[21]

### Neurologic Symptoms

Acute hypercapnia is often associated with headaches, breathlessness, anxiety, confusion, disorientation,

**Table 1:** Significant effects of hypercapnia on different organ systems.

| Organ system | Effects |
|---|---|
| Cardiovascular | • Improved cardiac output and oxygen delivery to tissues |
| Respiratory | • Increased pulmonary vascular resistance and hence acute hypercapnia can worsen pulmonary hypertension<br>• Improved lung compliance and improved V/Q matching |
| Central nervous system | • Increased intracranial pressure<br>• Increased cerebral blood flow and improved oxygenation and hence potential benefit in ischemic states |
| Inflammation | • Increased inflammation and hence potential to prolong the sepsis |
| Metabolism | • Decreased metabolic demand and hence potential benefit in ischemic states |

incoherence, and combativeness. In patients with chronic hypercapnia, a narcotic-like effect may be seen. Motor disturbances, including myoclonic jerks, tremor, and asterixis are observed with both acute and chronic hypercapnia. Signs and symptoms of increased intracranial pressure (ICP) related to the vasodilating effects of $CO_2$ on cerebral blood vessels can be observed occasionally in acute or chronic hypercapnia. Sustained myoclonus and seizure activity may also develop. When hypercapnia is severe, papilledema may be found. Hypercapnic coma usually occurs in patients with acute exacerbations of chronic respiratory insufficiency who are treated with excessive $O_2$.

## Cardiovascular Symptoms

Acute hypercapnia is usually characterized by warm and flushed skin, sweating, bounding pulse, increased cardiac output, and normal or increased blood pressure. However, severe hypercapnia might be associated with a decrease in both cardiac output and blood pressure. Cardiac arrhythmias are frequently observed in patients with either acute or chronic hypercapnia, especially those receiving digoxin.

## Renal Symptoms

Mild to moderate hypercapnia causes renal vasodilation, but acute rise in $PaCO_2$ above 70 mm Hg can induce renal vasoconstriction and hypoperfusion. Salt and water retention typically are associated with sustained hypercapnia, especially in the presence of cor pulmonale. Multiple other factors might play a role, including the stimulation of the sympathetic nervous system and the renin-angiotensin-aldosterone axis and the elevated levels of antidiuretic hormone and cortisol.

## Clinical Features due to an Underlying Cause[1]

The presence of an underlying disorder or risk factor should raise the suspicion for hypercapnia and prompt ABG analysis. Clinicians should look for a history of common risk factors, including sedative use, the clinical features of chronic lung disease and central or peripheral NMDs (e.g. hemiplegia, obesity, snoring, and neuromuscular weakness). It is common to miss the presentation of acute hypercapnia in a postanesthetic patient who becomes hypoxemic. Usually giving supplemental $O_2$ treats hypoxemia, but that may worsen the hypercapnia by reducing the respiratory drive and hence lead to more hypoxemia and finally respiratory failure.

## ADVANTAGES AND DISADVANTAGES OF HYPERCAPNIA

Hypercapnia has both beneficial and detrimental effects on various organ systems in the body (Table 1). While, it reduces systemic vascular resistance and increases cardiac output, it increases pulmonary vascular resistance and hence worsens pulmonary hypertension. Hypoxia is a more potent pulmonary vasoconstrictor as compared to hypercapnia.[21]

### Advantages

In a multicenter trial, hypercapnia was associated with good outcomes in patients resuscitated from out-of-hospital cardiac arrest after 1 year.[22] During the early postresuscitation period, cardiac arrest patients, who were on ventilators and had mild hypercapnia had higher cerebral oxygenation than those in whom hypercapnia was not present.[23] A study which recruited fourteen competitive divers who could breath-hold in the Croatian national team, revealed that hypercapnia may protect the brain against severe $O_2$ deprivation associated with prolonged apnea.[24] Additionally, permissive hypercapnia plays a role in vasodilating cerebral vessels and increasing cerebral blood flow.[25]

### Disadvantages

Increased risk of atrial fibrillation has been noted in hypercapnia associated with COPD.[26] Exposure to both hypocapnia and hypercapnia within a day of coronary artery bypass grafting was associated with increased risk of 30-day mortality and delayed extubation.[27] A study found that hypercapnia, but not hypoxia caused electroencephalogram (EEG) slowing, implying that hypercapnia may be more significant in neurobiological impairments in patients with sleep-disordered breathing.[28] Children with obstructive sleep apnea and snorers have reduced response to hypercapnia when awake as compared to controls.[29] Compensated respiratory acidosis may increase delta wave activity in preterm babies born before 32-week gestation.[30] Hypercapnia and sleepiness may be mediated by reduced neuroelectrical brain activity.[31] Severe hypercapnia can cause intracranial hemorrhage in neonates.[25] Dysfunction of brainstem regions responsible for central $CO_2$ chemoreception has been proposed as one of the pathophysiologies of sudden infant death syndrome.[32] Infants of mothers who smoke and substance abuse exhibited a blunted ventilatory response to hypercapnia.[33] Maintenance of normal $PaCO_2$ may prevent morbidity. Hypercapnia may increase cerebral blood flow and the risk of developing intraventricular hemorrhage.[25]

## EVALUATION OF HYPERCAPNIA

### Differential Diagnosis of the Symptoms of Hypercapnia

Since hypercapnia most frequently presents with dyspnea and altered sensorium, many of the additional etiologies associated with both symptoms (e.g. pulmonary embolus, heart failure, encephalopathy, and sepsis) need to be differentiated by a thorough history and examination.

### Differential Diagnosis of Hypercapnic Respiratory Failure

Flowcharts 1 and 2 show the broad differential of hypercapnia.

### Diagnostic Workup

#### Arterial Blood Gas Analysis

- *Acute versus chronic respiratory acidosis:* If pH is below 7.35 then it is either acute or acute on chronic respiratory acidosis. In acute respiratory acidosis, pH would be same as predicted, while in acute on chronic respiratory acidosis, pH would be higher than predicted. On the other hand, in chronic respiratory acidosis, pH is near normal.[1]

- *Alveolar-arterial oxygen gradient (A-a gradient):* Hypercapnia may not occur initially in the conditions in which the A-a gradient is increased. This is because, when the gas exchange is impaired, the total minute ventilation may actually increase due to increased dead space. This will cause hypocapnia instead of hypercapnia.

There is an invaluable role of alveolar-arterial gradient to distinguish patients with hypercapnia due to global hypoventilation and from hypercapnia due to intrinsic pulmonary disease which is displayed in Flowchart 1.

**Calculation of alveolar-arterial $O_2$ gradient**

$PaO_2$ is the partial pressure of arterial $O_2$ obtained from the ABG and $PAO_2$ is the alveolar $O_2$ tension that can be estimated from the alveolar gas equation:

$$PAO_2 = FiO_2 (P_B - PH_2O) - PaCO_2/R$$

Where $FiO_2$ = Fractional concentration of inspired $O_2$ (0.21 when breathing room air), $P_B$ = Barometric pressure (760 mm Hg at sea level), $PH_2O$ = Water vapor pressure (47 mm Hg at 37°C), and R = Respiratory exchange ratio.

#### Other Laboratory Tests

They can assist in determining the presence of hypercapnia and identify the etiology of hypercapnic respiratory failure.

- *Serum chemistry:* An elevated bicarbonate level may suggest underlying chronic hypercapnia at the baseline, although this is nonspecific as diuretics can increase the

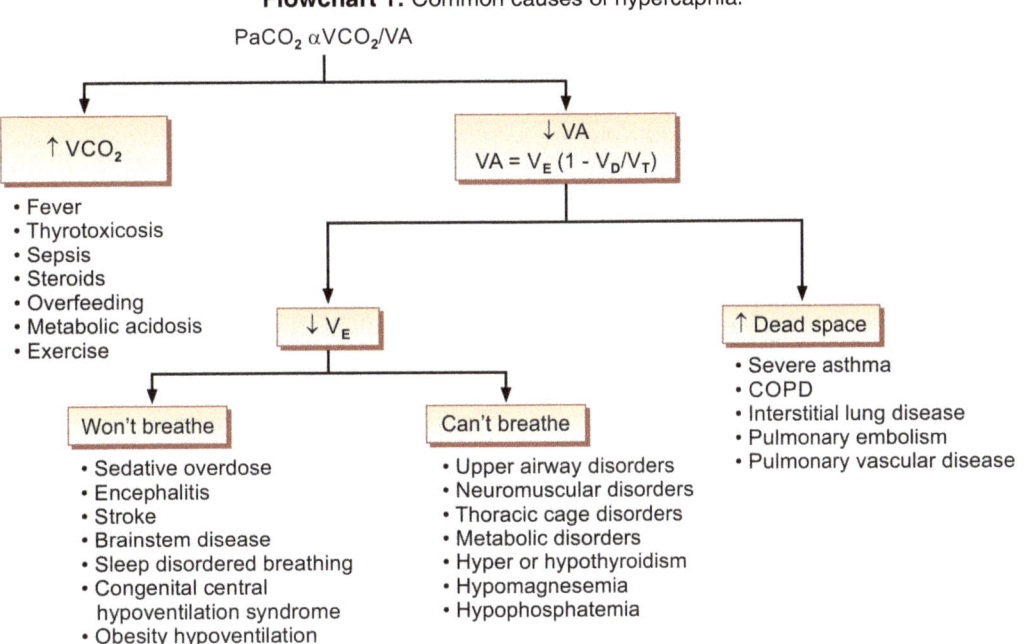

**Flowchart 1:** Common causes of hypercapnia.[2]

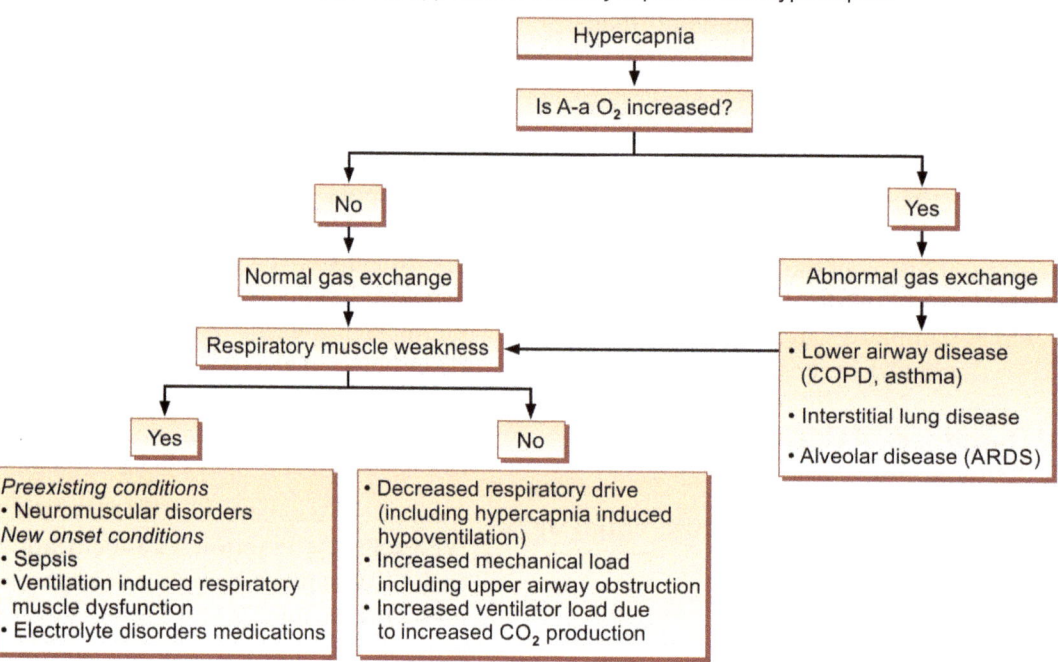

Flowchart 2: Diagnostic approach to critically ill patient with hypercapnia.[9]

bicarbonate concentration without causing high $PCO_2$. Low phosphate and magnesium levels may suggest the etiology for hypercapnia.

- *Complete blood count:* Chronic hypoxemia from lung disease may be associated with polycythemia.[1]
- *Toxicology screen:* A toxicology screen should be considered when an overdose is suspected and drug history unavailable.
- *Thyroid function tests:* Hypothyroidism can cause hypercapnia.
- *Creatine phosphokinase (CPK):* Elevated CPK may suggest infectious or autoimmune polymyositis, hypothyroidism, rhabdomyolysis secondary to colchicine or chloroquine toxicity, or procainamide myopathy.[1]

## Imaging Assessment

Imaging abnormalities are not sensitive or specific for the diagnosis of hypercapnia. A chest radiograph should be performed with acute hypercapnia to look for pulmonary pathology.

- *Chest imaging:* A chest radiograph or computed tomography of the chest may reveal underlying COPD (e.g. hyperinflation, flattened diaphragms) and interstitial lung disease (reticular nodular pattern shadows), as well as rib cage abnormalities (kyphoscoliosis, pectus excavatum or diaphragmatic paralysis (unilateral or bilateral elevation of diaphragm). The latter may also be diagnosed with ultrasound.[1]
- *Brain and spinal cord imaging:* Computed tomography or magnetic resonance imaging of the neck or brain may reveal central (especially brainstem) or peripheral nervous system etiologies for hypercapnia (stroke, tumor, traumatic transection of the spinal cord).[1]

## Physiologic Assessment

Measurement of vital capacity and negative inspiratory force in monitoring hypercapnic respiratory failure in patients with muscular weakness is instrumental. A vital capacity less than 1 L in a patient with NMD warrants admission to an intensive care unit (ICU) because of the due to risk of acute respiratory failure.[1]

Previous PFTs, sleep studies, NCSs, or electromyography (EMG), including phrenic NCS and diaphragmatic EMG may suggest underlying lung disease, sleep apnea or neuromyopathy, respectively.[1] During sleep studies, nocturnal capnometry helps with diagnosing hypercapnia.[34]

## Carbon Dioxide Monitoring

Besides an ABG analysis, other methods for determining $CO_2$ include end-tidal $CO_2$ ($ETCO_2$) and transcutaneous $CO_2$ ($PtcCO_2$) monitoring. Continuous $ETCO_2$ detectors or capnometers measure exhaled $CO_2$ tension. Continuous $ETCO_2$ monitoring is widely accepted and used in both adult and pediatric patients.[35] There have been several studies comparing the different modalities for $CO_2$ monitoring with conflicting results. A retrospective study involving 39 adults showed that $PtcCO_2$ was significantly greater than $ETCO_2$.[36] Additionally, a prospective study on 81 adults comparing $PtcCO_2$ and ABG showed an acceptable agreement of $PtcCO_2$ monitoring with ABG analysis. However, $PtcCO_2$ underestimates $PaCO_2$ levels when they are high. Hence, this method may not be ideal for patients with severe hypercapnia.[37] $PtcCO_2$ can be used to monitor $CO_2$ overnight during noninvasive ventilation (NIV).[38]

## MANAGEMENT

### First-Line Therapy

Assess and stabilize the airway, breathing, and circulation. Perform a brief clinical bedside assessment with continuous monitoring.

Draw an ABG. ABG analysis is preferred over venous blood gas (VBG) as it is more accurate. VBGs typically tend to have a slightly higher $PaCO_2$ and bicarbonate level, and a lower pH, but can be used if ABGs cannot be obtained.[1]

### Antidotes

Naloxone could be used for opioid-induced hypercapnic encephalopathy.

Flumazenil is used to reverse acute benzodiazepine toxicity.

For oral sedative overdoses, gastric emptying and activated charcoal administration is not recommended due to the increased risk of aspiration, but could be used in those patients with protected airways (e.g. intubated patients).

Sedatives should be avoided in patients with hypercapnic respiratory failure as they can worsen the respiratory acidosis and may result in respiratory arrest.[1]

### Role of Bronchodilators

In patients undergoing mechanical ventilation, albuterol nebulization is commonly prescribed. This β2-agonist does bronchodilatation as well as improves mucociliary clearance and alveoli fluid clearance.[39] Recently, Festic et al.[40] did a "Lung Injury Prevention Study with Budesonide and Beta agonist (LIPS-B)". The study revealed a significant improvement in oxygenation in the group treated with inhaled budesonide/formoterol that became evident on days 2 and 4 of the study as compared with formoterol alone or placebo.

Ipratropium bromide, an anticholinergic bronchodilator, is another drug commonly administered in mechanically ventilated patients by nebulization.

Acute respiratory distress syndrome survivors frequently present a decrease in expiration flow rate with airway hyperreactivity and air trapping due to small airways disease, supporting a need to maintain bronchodilator treatment for 6 months after hospital discharge.[39]

Nebulized drugs should normally be administered during breaks from NIV. However, if the patient is dependent on NIV, bronchodilators can be given via a nebulizer inserted into the ventilator tubing.[25]

### Respiratory Support

#### Noninvasive Ventilation

Many patients with acute respiratory failure improve on NIV; however, others need intubation and full respiratory support.

- *Patients suitable for noninvasive ventilation:* In general, patients with acute respiratory acidosis (e.g. pH <7.3) who are in moderate to severe respiratory distress, with tachypnea (respiratory rate >25) and an increased work of breathing are frequently suitable candidates for NIV. Management of patients with mild to moderate $CO_2$-induced somnolence from sleep apnea or sedatives (will not breathe), and patients with NMDs (cannot breathe) can include NIV.[1] Advanced age alone should not deter a trial of NIV.[41] An ABG must be performed within 2 hours of being on NIV along with clinical assessment while on NIV. Based upon data derived from patients with COPD, those who respond are likely to do so in the first 2 hours.[1]
- *Mode:* The optimal mode and initial settings vary depending upon the underlying disease and patient comfort. While most patients are started on pressure-controlled NIV (e.g. BiPAP), some patients may demonstrate improved tolerance on volume-controlled NIV (e.g. patients with NMD).[1]
- *Settings:* The optimal initial settings vary depending upon the mode of NIV chosen. Usually patients are started on lower settings and titrated up based on tolerability and response to it.[1]
- *Administration of oxygen:* Patients who present with acute hypercapnic acidosis frequently (but not always) have hypoxemia as well that necessitates supplemental $O_2$ therapy. NIV settings should be optimized before increasing the $FiO_2$. The flow rate of supplemental $O_2$ may need to be increased when ventilatory pressure is

increased to maintain the same target for oxygenation. Mask leak and delayed triggering may occur when $O_2$ flow rates greater than 4 L/minute, which risks patient-ventilator asynchrony. Hence, the requirement for high-flow rates should prompt a check for patient-ventilator asynchrony. A ventilator with an integral $O_2$ blender is recommended if $O_2$ at 4 L/minute fails to maintain $SaO_2$ greater than 88%.[41]

The major concern with the delivery of $O_2$ is the development of worsening hypercapnia and consequently acidosis by reducing the respiratory drive. However, it is essential to administer $O_2$ to patients who have significant hypoxemia to prevent the life-threatening complications of a low arterial oxygen tension ($PaO_2$). Thus, the primary goal of $O_2$ therapy in patients with hypoxemic hypercapnic respiratory failure is the adequate treatment of hypoxemia while avoiding significant worsening of hypercapnia, The target pulse oxygen saturation ($SpO_2$) should be 90–93% or a $PaO_2$ of 60–70 mm Hg.[1]

For those who require small amounts of supplemental $O_2$, starting with low flow (e.g. 1–2 L/minute or 0.24–0.28 $FiO_2$) to achieve an $SpO_2$ at or close to this goal is appropriate. Gradual increases in increments of 1 L/minute (via nasal cannula) or 4–7% (via Venturi mask) with close monitoring of both $PaO_2$ and $PaCO_2$ may be required. Once the target goal is achieved, supplemental $O_2$ can be maintained at this level and then weaned as tolerated.[1]

While high-flow nasal $O_2$ has a proven role in the treatment of hypoxemic respiratory failure, it has no proven role in the treatment of hypercapnic respiratory failure and should not be used.[1]

- *Weaning noninvasive ventilation:* Clinical reassessments and ABG are used to wean NIV. A regimen or decreasing hours of usage such as 4 hours on, 4 hours off followed by 2 hours on, 4 hours off can be implemented to transition over to a nasal cannula alone. Mild to moderate upper airway compromise due to laryngitis, may be treated by a mixture of helium and $O_2$ (heliox) in order to reduce turbulent flow.[1]
- *Sedation with noninvasive ventilation:* Sedation should be sparingly used and only with close monitoring in an ICU setting. If needed, intravenous morphine (± benzodiazepine) or dexmedetomidine may provide symptom relief and may improve tolerance to NIV.
- *Special considerations:* Previous episodes of ventilator-associated pneumothorax may lead to a low threshold for admission to ICU and use of NIV at lower than normal inspiratory pressures.[1]

Carbonic anhydrase inhibitors should not be routinely used in AHRF.[41]

In patients with NMD, mechanical insufflation and exsufflation should be used, in addition to standard physiotherapy techniques, when cough is weak and the patient retains secretions.[1]

In obesity hypoventilation, weight loss could potentially reverse hypercapnia without any significant improvement in apnea-hypopnea index. In addition, this also improves oxygenation (both during sleep and while awake) and minimizing hypoxia-induced organ dysfunction.[42]

### Intensive Care Unit Admission

Admission for severe hypercapnic respiratory failure is typically due to COPD or obesity hypoventilation syndrome (OHS). Criteria for ICU admission are:
- Need for intubation and mechanical ventilation
- Patients with NMD with vital capacity at or less than 15 mL/kg.

### Invasive Mechanical Ventilation

Worsening physiological parameters, particularly pH and respiratory rate, indicate the need to change the management strategy and endotracheal intubation.[41]

Controlled IMV may need to be continued in some patients with severe airflow obstruction, weak muscles or for chronic hypercapnia. In obstructive diseases, controlled IMV should be continued until airway resistance falls.[41]

In IMV, mechanical dead space is added because of artificial airway, circuits like tubing, HME filter, etc.[3]

In mechanically ventilated patients, both cough and mucociliary clearances are reduced. N-acetylcysteine is the most widely used mucolytic, but evidence for its efficacy is not enough. However, strong evidence for the efficacy of nebulized hypertonic (3–14%) saline has been reported. Animal studies of nebulized hypertonic saline suggest that the administration of hypertonic saline reduces the severity of lung injury.[39]

- *Invasive ventilation strategy:* The ventilator management is dictated by the underlying disease process rather than the hypercapnia itself. During controlled ventilation, dynamic hyperinflation should be minimized by prolonging expiratory time [inspiratory-to-expiratory (I:E) ratio of 1:3 or greater] and setting a low rate (10–15 breaths/minute). Permissive hypercapnia (aiming for pH 7.2–7.25) may be required to avoid high airway pressures when there is severe airflow obstruction. Positive end-expiratory pressure (PEEP) should not usually exceed 12 cm.

> **Box 1:** Risk factors for extubation failure.[41]
> - Previous failed extubation
> - Bulbar dysfunction
> - Fluid overload
> - Tachypnea
> - Underlying pneumonia or pulmonary disease requiring invasive mechanical ventilation (IMV)
> - Older patients
> - Prolonged duration of IMV
> - Anemia
> - Increased severity of illness
> - Low albumin

- *Sedation in invasive mechanical ventilation:* Patient-ventilator asynchrony should be considered in all agitated patients.

### Tracheostomy

For those who fail extubation, tracheostomy should be considered. The risk factors for extubation are shown in Box 1. Performing routine tracheostomy within a week of initiating IMV is not recommended based on two large multicenter studies and meta-analysis. The need and timing of a tracheostomy should be individualized. Tracheostomy procedure has its own risk at the time of insertion and subsequently. This is particularly the case in progressive NMD and chest wall disease when tracheostomy may be difficult to reverse. In COPD, NMD or OHS, NIV-supported extubation should be employed in preference to inserting a tracheostomy. The decision to perform tracheostomy should be multidisciplinary.[41]

### Other Therapies

#### Extracorporeal $CO_2$ Removal

Patients with severe ARDS with poor compliance can develop hypercapnia with worsening dead space fraction. At that point, extracorporeal membrane oxygenation (ECMO) could facilitate $CO_2$ removal in addition to maintaining oxygenation. Extracorporeal $CO_2$ removal ($ECCO_2R$) is being investigated for targeting lower $CO_2$ while the tidal volume is reduced as part of a lung-protective strategy for management of ARDS. Indication for $ECCO_2R$ are:
- Despite optimizing IMV using lung-protective strategies, severe hypercapnic acidosis (pH <7.15) persists
- When "lung-protective ventilation" is needed but hypercapnia is contraindicated like patient with brain injury
- For patients on IMV awaiting a lung transplant
- If expertise exists, $ECCO_2R$ might be considered.[41]

Extracorporeal $CO_2$ removal can serve as a bridge to lung transplant. A study on 20 patients with life-threatening hypercapnia who received $ECCO_2R$ by interventional lung-assist (iLA; Novalung) as bridge to lung transplant showed that the common underlying diagnoses were bronchiolitis obliterans syndrome, cystic fibrosis, and idiopathic pulmonary fibrosis.[43] The technique is still experimental as no randomized trial is available. However, it is associated with frequent and potentially severe complications.

#### High-Frequency Oscillation Ventilation

High-frequency oscillation ventilation (HFOV) could be a useful alternative in patients with ARDS with hypercapnic failure if conventional ventilation fails.[44]

#### Modafinil

Modafinil is a respiratory stimulant and routinely used for narcolepsy, but is not commonly used for hypercapnia. In a case series of six patients with hypercapnic respiratory failure, the use of modafinil was beneficial.[8] These patients were at risk of death due to refusal of nasal ventilation or its failure. Hence, modafinil may have a role in shortening hospital stay, improving outcome and quality of life, and reducing deaths and readmissions in selected patients.[8]

## IMPACT OF HYPERCAPNIA ON OUTCOME

Hypercapnia is detrimental in majority of respiratory conditions.

### Acute Respiratory Distress Syndrome

The effects of hypercapnia on alveolar fluid clearance are well studied. Hypercapnia leads to endocytosis of sodium potassium ATPase and thereby therefore reduction in alveolar fluid clearance.[45] Additionally, it has been shown to impair alveolar epithelial cell proliferation and repair which is detrimental in lung injury.[46] Recently, severe hypercapnia ($paCO_2$ >50) in the first 2 days was shown to be associated with higher mortality in a large study of patients with ARDS on mechanical ventilation.[47]

### Pneumonia

Hypercapnia has been associated with impaired host defense mechanisms including reduced levels of tumor necrosis factor-α and interleukin-6.[48] It has been linked to increased mortality[49] and increased length of hospital stay[50] in patients with community-acquired pneumonia.

### Chronic Obstructive Pulmonary Disease

Hypercapnic patients with COPD treated with home NIV experience improved quality of life[51] and mortality.[52,53]

A large, multicenter retrospective study in Australia and New Zealand revealed that uncompensated hypercapnia in the first 24 hours in mechanically ventilated patients was associated with increased mortality.[54]

## FUTURE IMPLICATIONS

The link between obesity and hypercapnia is intriguing. Kikuchi et al.[51] recently showed that hypercapnia might be associated with adipogenesis and thus contribute to the obesity. In their study, human preadipocytes were induced to differentiate into adipocytes under different concentrations of $CO_2$ and $O_2$. They found hypercapnia led to faster adipogenesis but not adipocyte hypertrophy and this was independent of $O_2$ concentration. This effect was mediated via cyclic adenosine monophosphate (AMP). There was activation of protein kinase A which stimulated proadipogenic transcription factors including cyclic AMP response element-binding protein and peroxisome proliferator-activated receptor-γ. This could set up a feedback where OHS worsens hypercapnia which perpetuates accelerated adipogenesis and obesity.

The role of nonconventional ventilatory techniques with ultra-low tidal volume ventilation in ARDS with $ECCO_2R$ is currently under study. This technology can be used to reduce plateau pressures further with lower tidal volumes and yet allow adequate $CO_2$ removal. A pilot multicenter study demonstrated the feasibility and safety of this approach in ARDS.[55]

Mesenchymal stem cells are being pursued to treat patients with severe ARDS. They have been shown to be safe in early trials.[56,57] The paracrine factors carried by these cells are thought to be responsible for beneficial effects in the acute lung injury.

### Case Revisit

This patient had OHS as a cause of hypoventilation.

As the prevalence of obesity rises worldwide, OHS is being recognized as a more common cause of hypercapnic respiratory failure. It is recognized as the presence of obesity (BMI >30 kg/m²), daytime hypercapnia $PaCO_2$ greater than or equal to 45 mm Hg while awake after ruling out other causes, accompanied by obstructive sleep apnea or sleep-related hypoventilation.[58] The PFTs are characterized by restrictive lung defect. The case discussed fulfills the criteria for OHS. It is not uncommon to identify these patients on presentation to the hospital. As many as 30% of OHS patients are first diagnosed at the time of respiratory failure[59] in the hospital. OHS is the second most common reason for use of NIV in AHRF. In this patient with OHS, NIV was used initially but he had to be intubated for failure of NIV likely from his pneumonia and poorly resolved hypercapnia.

## SALIENT POINTS

- Hypercapnia is an elevation in the arterial $CO_2$.
- Neuromuscular weakness and pulmonary disorders are the common causes of hypercapnia.
- Permissive hypercapnia is the approach used for ventilator strategies in conditions like ARDS, asthma and bronchopulmonary dysplasia to minimize ventilator-induced lung injury.
- Clinical features are mainly neurological and may range from headaches to seizures and coma.
- Respiratory support in the form of noninvasive or invasive ventilation is the mainstay of therapy. NIV is preferred whenever feasible. However, invasive ventilation may be inevitable in cases of worsening clinical status.
- Prognosis depends on the underlying etiology.
- It is very important to identify hypercapnia and manage it promptly as it can be life threatening.

## REFERENCES

1. Feller-Kopman DJ, Schwartzstein RM. (2019). The evaluation, diagnosis, and treatment of the adult patient with acute hypercapnic respiratory failure. [online] Available from: https://www.uptodate.com/contents/the-evaluation-diagnosis-and-treatment-of-the-adult-patient-with-acute-hypercapnic-respiratory-failure. [Last accessed April, 2019].
2. Feller-Kopman DJ, Schwartzstein RM. (2019). Mechanisms, causes, and effects of hypercapnia. [online] Available from: https://www.uptodate.com/contents/mechanisms-causes-and-effects-of-hypercapnia. [Last accessed April, 2019].
3. Malley WJ. Clinical Blood Gases: Assessment and Intervention, 2nd edition. St. Louis: Elsevier Health Sciences; 2013. pp. 150-1.
4. Respiratory minute volume: an overview. (2019). [online] Available from: https://www.sciencedirect.com/topics/agricultural-and-biological-sciences/respiratory-minute-volume. [Last accessed April, 2019].
5. Quinn M, Rizzo A. Anatomy, anatomic dead space. (2018). [online] Available from: http://www.ncbi.nlm.nih.gov/books/NBK442016/. [Last accessed April, 2019].
6. Alveolar ventilation. (2017). [online] Available from: http://www.pathwaymedicine.org/alveolar-ventilation. [Last accessed April, 2019].

7. West JB. Respiratory Physiology: The Essentials, 9th edition. Philadelphia: Wolters Kluwer Health/Lippincott Williams and Wilkins; 2011.
8. Parnell H, Quirke G, Farmer S, et al. The successful treatment of hypercapnic respiratory failure with oral modafinil. Int J Chron Obstruct Pulmon Dis. 2014;9:413-9.
9. Laghi F. Hypoventilation and respiratory muscle dysfunction. In: Parrillo JE, Dellinger RP (Eds). Critical Care Medicine: Principles of Diagnosis and Management in the Adult, 4th edition. Philadelphia: Saunders; 2014. pp. 674-91.
10. Chio A, Cocito D, Leone M, et al. Guillain-Barre syndrome: a prospective, population-based incidence and outcome survey. Neurology. 2003;60(7):1146-50.
11. Willison HJ, Jacobs BC, van Doorn PA. Guillain-Barre syndrome. Lancet. 2016;388(10045):717-27.
12. Juel VC. Myasthenia gravis: management of myasthenic crisis and perioperative care. Semin Neurol. 2004;24(1):75-81.
13. Literature review of the usefulness of repetitive nerve stimulation and single fiber EMG in the electrodiagnostic evaluation of patients with suspected myasthenia gravis or Lambert-Eaton myasthenic syndrome. Muscle Nerve. 2001;24(9):1239-47.
14. Meriggioli MN, Sanders DB. Autoimmune myasthenia gravis: emerging clinical and biological heterogeneity. Lancet Neurol. 2009;8(5):475-90.
15. Ohta K, Shigemoto K, Kubo S, et al. MuSK antibodies in AChR Ab-seropositive MG vs AChR Ab-seronegative MG. Neurology. 2004;62(11):2132-3.
16. Rodarte J, Rehder K. Dynamics of respiration. In: Macklem PT, Mead J (Eds). Handbook of Physiology: The Respiratory System, Mechanics of Breathing. Bethesda, MD: American Physiological Society; 1986. pp. 131-44.
17. Sliwinski P, Kaminski D, Zielinski J, et al. Partitioning of the elastic work of inspiration in patients with COPD during exercise. Eur Respir J. 1998;11(2):416-21.
18. Scano G, Grazzini M, Stendardi L, et al. Respiratory muscle energetics during exercise in healthy subjects and patients with COPD. Respir Med. 2006;100(11):1896-906.
19. Ohar JA, Sadeghnejad A, Meyers DA, et al. Do symptoms predict COPD in smokers? Chest. 2010;137(6):1345-53.
20. Dorrington KL, Balanos GM, Talbot NP, et al. Extent to which pulmonary vascular responses to $PCO_2$ and $PO_2$ play a functional role within the healthy human lung. J Appl Physiol (1985). 2010;108(5):1084-96.
21. Curley GF, Kavanagh BP, Laffey JG. Hypocapnia and hypercapnia. In: Broaddus VC, Mason RJ, Gotway MB (Eds). Murray and Nadel's Textbook of Respiratory Medicine, 6th edition. Philadelphia: Saunders; 2016. pp. 1527-46.
22. Vaahersalo J, Bendel S, Reinikainen M, et al. Arterial blood gas tensions after resuscitation from out-of-hospital cardiac arrest: associations with long-term neurologic outcome. Crit Care Med. 2014;42(6):1463-70.
23. Eastwood GM, Tanaka A, Bellomo R. Cerebral oxygenation in mechanically ventilated early cardiac arrest survivors: the impact of hypercapnia. Resuscitation. 2016;102:11-6.
24. Bain AR, Ainslie PN, Hoiland RL, et al. Cerebral oxidative metabolism is decreased with extreme apnoea in humans; impact of hypercapnia. J Physiol. 2016;594(18):5317-28.
25. Zhou W, Liu W. Hypercapnia and hypocapnia in neonates. World J Pediatr. 2008;4(3):192-6.
26. Terzano C, Romani S, Conti V, et al. Atrial fibrillation in the acute, hypercapnic exacerbations of COPD. Eur Rev Med Pharmacol Sci. 2014;18(19):2908-17.
27. Choi JH, Lee EH, Jang MS, et al. Association between arterial carbon dioxide tension and outcome in patients admitted to the intensive care unit after coronary artery bypass surgery. J Cardiothorac Vasc Anesth. 2017;31(1):61-8.
28. Wang D, Yee BJ, Wong KK, et al. Comparing the effect of hypercapnia and hypoxia on the electroencephalogram during wakefulness. Clin Neurophysiol. 2015;126(1):103-9.
29. Busch DR, Lynch JM, Winters ME, et al. Cerebral blood flow response to hypercapnia in children with obstructive sleep apnea syndrome. Sleep. 2016;39(1):209-16.
30. Victor S, McKeering CM, Roberts SA, et al. Effect of permissive hypercapnia on background cerebral electrical activity in premature babies. Pediatr Res. 2014;76(2):184-9.
31. Wang D, Piper AJ, Yee BJ, et al. Hypercapnia is a key correlate of EEG activation and daytime sleepiness in hypercapnic sleep disordered breathing patients. J Clin Sleep Med. 2014;10(5):517-22.
32. Ravindran CR, Bayne JN, Bravo SC, et al. Intracellular acidosis and pH regulation in central respiratory chemoreceptors. J Health Care Poor Underserved. 2011;22(4 Suppl):174-86.
33. Ali K, Wolff K, Peacock JL, et al. Ventilatory response to hypercarbia in newborns of smoking and substance-misusing mothers. Ann Am Thorac Soc. 2014;11(6):933-8.
34. Jaimchariyatam N, Dweik RA, Kaw R, et al. Polysomnographic determinants of nocturnal hypercapnia in patients with sleep apnea. J Clin Sleep Med. 2013;9(3):209-15.
35. Lin YJ. Is capnometry monitoring useful in nonintubated neonates? Pediatr Neonatol. 2010;51(6):309-10.
36. Won YH, Choi WA, Lee JW, et al. Sleep transcutaneous vs. end-tidal $CO_2$ monitoring for patients with neuromuscular disease. Am J Phys Med Rehabil. 2016;95(2):91-5.
37. Ruiz Y, Farrero E, Cordoba A, et al. Transcutaneous carbon dioxide monitoring in subjects with acute respiratory failure and severe hypercapnia. Respir Care. 2016;61(4):428-33.
38. Aarrestad S, Tollefsen E, Kleiven AL, et al. Validity of transcutaneous $PCO_2$ in monitoring chronic hypoventilation treated with non-invasive ventilation. Respir Med. 2016;112:112-8.
39. Artigas A, Camprubi-Rimblas M, Tantinya N, et al. Inhalation therapies in acute respiratory distress syndrome. Ann Transl Med. 2017;5(14):293.
40. Festic E, Carr GE, Cartin-Ceba R, et al. Randomized clinical trial of a combination of an inhaled corticosteroid and beta-agonist in patients at risk of developing the acute respiratory distress syndrome. Crit Care Med. 2017;45(5):798-805.
41. Davidson AC, Banham S, Elliott M, et al. BTS/ICS guideline for the ventilatory management of acute hypercapnic respiratory failure in adults. Thorax. 2016;71 Suppl 2:ii1-35.
42. Javaheri S, Simbartl LA. Respiratory determinants of diurnal hypercapnia in obesity hypoventilation syndrome. What does weight have to do with it? Ann Am Thorac Soc. 2014;11(6):945-50.

43. Schellongowski P, Riss K, Staudinger T, et al. Extracorporeal $CO_2$ removal as bridge to lung transplantation in life-threatening hypercapnia. Transpl Int. 2015;28(3):297-304.
44. Friesecke S, Stecher SS, Abel P. High-frequency oscillation ventilation for hypercapnic failure of conventional ventilation in pulmonary acute respiratory distress syndrome. Crit Care. 2015;19:201.
45. Vadasz I, Hubmayr RD, Nin N, et al. Hypercapnia: a nonpermissive environment for the lung. Am J Respir Cell Mol Biol. 2012;46(4):417-21.
46. O'Toole D, Hassett P, Contreras M, et al. Hypercapnic acidosis attenuates pulmonary epithelial wound repair by an NF-kappaB-dependent mechanism. Thorax. 2009;64(11):976-82.
47. Nin N, Muriel A, Penuelas O, et al. Severe hypercapnia and outcome of mechanically ventilated patients with moderate or severe acute respiratory distress syndrome. Intensive Care Med. 2017;43(2):200-8.
48. Gates KL, Howell HA, Nair A, et al. Hypercapnia impairs lung neutrophil function and increases mortality in murine pseudomonas pneumonia. Am J Respir Cell Mol Biol. 2013;49(5):821-8.
49. Laserna E, Sibila O, Aguilar PR, et al. Hypocapnia and hypercapnia are predictors for ICU admission and mortality in hospitalized patients with community-acquired pneumonia. Chest. 2012;142(5):1193-9.
50. Iqbal N, Irfan M, Khan JA, et al. Hypercapnia as a marker of ICU admission and prolonged hospitalization in patients with community-acquired pneumonia. Eur Respir J. 2015;46(Suppl 59):OA3261.
51. Liao H, Pei W, Li H, et al. Efficacy of long-term noninvasive positive pressure ventilation in stable hypercapnic COPD patients with respiratory failure: a meta-analysis of randomized controlled trials. Int J Chron Obstruct Pulmon Dis. 2017;12:2977-85.
52. Kohnlein T, Windisch W, Kohler D, et al. Non-invasive positive pressure ventilation for the treatment of severe stable chronic obstructive pulmonary disease: a prospective, multicentre, randomised, controlled clinical trial. Lancet Respir Med. 2014;2(9):698-705.
53. Murphy PB, Rehal S, Arbane G, et al. Effect of home noninvasive ventilation with oxygen therapy vs oxygen therapy alone on hospital readmission or death after an acute COPD exacerbation: a randomized clinical trial. JAMA. 2017;317(21):2177-86.
54. Tiruvoipati R, Pilcher D, Buscher H, et al. Effects of hypercapnia and hypercapnic acidosis on hospital mortality in mechanically ventilated patients. Crit Care Med. 2017;45(7):e649-56.
55. Peperstraete H, Eloot S, Depuydt P, et al. Low flow extracorporeal $CO_2$ removal in ARDS patients: a prospective short-term crossover pilot study. BMC Anesthesiol. 2017;17(1):155.
56. Zheng G, Huang L, Tong H, et al. Treatment of acute respiratory distress syndrome with allogeneic adipose-derived mesenchymal stem cells: a randomized, placebo-controlled pilot study. Respir Res. 2014;15:39.
57. Wilson JG, Liu KD, Zhuo H, et al. Mesenchymal stem (stromal) cells for treatment of ARDS: a phase 1 clinical trial. Lancet Respir Med. 2015;3(1):24-32.
58. Berger KI, Ayappa I, Chatr-Amontri B, et al. Obesity hypoventilation syndrome as a spectrum of respiratory disturbances during sleep. Chest. 2001;120(4):1231-8.
59. Nowbar S, Burkart KM, Gonzales R, et al. Obesity-associated hypoventilation in hospitalized patients: prevalence, effects, and outcome. Am J Med. 2004;116(1):1-7.

# CHAPTER 5

# Noninvasive Ventilation

*Zbigniew Szkulmowski, Antonio M Esquinas*

## INTRODUCTION

Noninvasive ventilation (NIV), i.e. a set of mechanical ventilation techniques not using artificial airways, such as intubation or tracheotomy, is currently becoming standard therapy in the treatment of respiratory failure.[1,2] Currently, the most frequently applied NIV techniques include positive pressure ventilation with the use of various nasal masks, face masks, mouthpieces, and recently also helmets.

Noninvasive ventilation owes its increasing popularity to its efficiency in achieving the desired physiological effects of mechanical ventilation, i.e. reduction of atelectasis under positive pressure, reduction of work of breathing, improvement of oxygenation, increase of carbon dioxide ($CO_2$) elimination, at the same time avoiding adverse effects related to intubation and invasive ventilation, mainly infections.[3] This is particularly important for the patients with particularly high risk of infection with hospital species, i.e. patients who can be potentially difficult to wean from ventilator, or with immunodeficiency.[4,5]

In the countries where NIV is a long-established treatment method, the NIV techniques are usually applied to patients with deterioration of chronic obstructive lung disease and to patients with cardiogenic lung edema, not only in intensive care units (ICUs), but also in emergency units or medical treatment wards.[6,7] The application of NIV to patients with acute lung damage or as part of weaning from ventilator is limited to ICUs.[8] The frequency of application of NIV in ICUs, as compared to nationwide application frequency in Poland, is surprisingly high. It is estimated that NIV is applied, on various stages of treatment, to 35% of patients treated in ICUs; in some medical centers specializing in ventilation treatment, NIV may be applied to as many as 60% of patients.[9-11]

## BASIC PRINCIPLE FOR NONINVASIVE VENTILATION USE

Respiratory failure is caused by two main factors: deterioration of the pulmonary gas exchange, which results in hypoxemia, and/or the failure of the pumping function of the respiratory system, which in turn leads to hypercapnia.[12-14]

Pulmonary gas exchange disruption are caused by ventilation to perfusion mismatching, increased pulmonary shunt, alveolar derecruitment, or atelectatic lesions.[15]

Hypercapnic respiratory failure can be caused by respiratory center depression, increased work of breathing (due to increased airway resistance, reduced chest wall or pulmonary compliance, or dynamic hyperinflation), or fatigue of ventilatory muscles (due to labored breathing or the weakness of respiratory muscles caused by either acute or chronic factors).[12] Alveolar hypoventilation leads to $CO_2$ retention caused by disproportion between the production of this gas and the capability of the ventilatory system to exhale it. Patients with $CO_2$ retention breathe more rapidly, have shorter inspiration time ($T_i$) and lower tidal volumes ($V_t$) than patients with normal $CO_2$ levels.[12] Positive pressure mechanical ventilation should have the following effects:
- Improvement of pulmonary gas exchange resulting from the application of positive pressure, the alveolar recruitment capability, the increase of $V_t$, the reduction of atelectatic areas, and
- Reduction of respiratory load due to the facilitation of respiratory muscles with positive pressure synchronized with the patient's inspiratory effort that results in reduction of work of breathing.

Periodical reduction of ventilatory load allows the ventilatory muscles to rest. As a result, between the NIV sessions the respiratory muscles can provide more efficient ventilation or coughing with secretion elimination.

By assisting patient's ventilation in sessions lasting several hours, NIV also enables temporary improvement of pulmonary gas exchange by applying positive pressure and reducing the load on the respiratory muscles. This has been confirmed many times by showing lower pressures during NIV than in the case of breathing.[12]

## NONINVASIVE VENTILATION USE IN CLINICAL CONDITIONS

The clinical use of NIV arises from the ability to apply positive pressure to the airways, reduce the load on ventilatory muscles, avoid complications related to artificial airways required for invasive ventilation, and the possibility to provide "preventive" positive pressure ventilation in the developing ventilatory failure, in order to avoid the need for intubation and invasive ventilation. A number of reports has shown that, compared to invasive ventilation, NIV is related with a lower risk of nosocomial infections, reduced need for antibiotic therapy, shorter treatment in the ICU, and lower mortality rate.[16] Furthermore, the patient's comfort is improved and the need for sedatives and analgesics is reduced,[17] which independently affect the weaning time and the length of treatment in the ICU.[18]

Noninvasive ventilation should be applied when a rapid improvement of the patient's clinical condition and respiratory function can be expected as a result of etiological treatment of the underlying disease. The main indications for NIV include acute ventilatory failure in patients in whom invasive ventilation is related to particularly high risk of infections (e.g. patients with immunodeficiency), significant difficulties with weaning from the ventilator [patients with severe chronic obstructive pulmonary disease (COPD)], or in patients in whom the respiro-circulatory failure can improve rapidly with treatment, e.g. in patients with lung edema[19] (Box 1).

Low invasiveness of the method makes it suitable not only for fully developed respiratory failure, as it is with invasive ventilation, but also as a preventive measure against the aggravation of the respiratory function. Thus, NIV can be used preventively in conditions which, if not managed, will result in the onset of ventilatory failure symptoms.[12,20,21] The impact of positive pressure ventilation techniques on the ventilatory system, with the reduction of atelectatic lesions, increasing the vital capacity and, consequently, the work of breathing, and reducing the load on ventilatory muscles with support ventilation makes it possible to apply NIV in a noncontinuous manner.[22]

**Box 1:** Indications for noninvasive ventilation in intensive care.

*Clinical signs/symptoms*
- Dyspnea: Moderate to severe
- Tachypnea: >24/min in patients with obstructive lung disease, >30/min in patients with restrictive lung disease
- Symptoms of increased work of breathing, using additional respiratory muscles, paradoxical respiration

*Arterial blood gases*
- $PaCO_2$ >45 mm Hg, pH <7.35 in severe or exacerbated chronic ventilatory failure
- Hypoxemia $PaO_2/FiO_2$ <200

($FiO_2$: fraction of inspired oxygen; $PaCO_2$: partial pressure carbon dioxide; $PaO_2$: partial pressure arterial oxygen)

This is one of the key features differentiating NIV from invasive ventilation techniques. The patient undergoes NIV in 1–2 hour sessions (the time required for ventilatory muscles to rest and for glycogen in the muscles to be replenished); between the sessions, the patient is able to breathe spontaneously, under passive oxygen therapy, communicating with his/her surroundings and undergoing intensive physiotherapy. In the meantime, the patient is able to breathe with less effort (higher pulmonary compliance and less fatigued respiratory muscles), and produce more efficient cough to eliminate secretions from the airways. The patient should restart the session of NIV when is not yet fatigued with spontaneous breathing.[23] On the initial stages of treatment, NIV sessions can last several hours and spontaneous breathing periods can extend from several dozen minutes to 1 hour, depending on the patient's tolerance. With the improvement of the patient's general condition, the periods between subsequent ventilation sessions are extended. An NIV session should always last 1–2 hours. The longest session is the night time ventilation, which should take approximately 4–6 hours, to avoid nocturnal hypoventilation and desaturation episodes and thus to ensure efficient, restful sleep. In particularly severe conditions, the NIV sessions can be extended in the initial stages of treatment to improve the patient's comfort of breathing for the period required for the etiological treatment which improves the condition of the respiratory system (e.g. antibiotics, diuretics or continuous renal replacement therapy, medications improving the performance of the circulatory system). Long-term, uninterrupted, and comfortable NIV sessions, which may last up to several dozen hours, can be enabled by helmets, which are attached more comfortably than face or nasal masks.

The efficacy of NIV in acute ventilatory failure has been proven for a number of clinical conditions. Depending on the underlying cause of ventilatory failure, the treatment

**Table 1:** Recommendations for noninvasive ventilation (NIV) in treating acute ventilatory failure.

| Level of recommendation | Medical conditions |
|---|---|
| Review of randomized controlled trials (RCTs) and individual RCTs | • COPD exacerbation<br>• Weaning the COPD patient from the ventilator<br>• Cardiogenic lung edema<br>• Patients with immunosuppression |
| Review of cohort trials, individual cohort trials | • Patients not qualifying for intubation<br>• As palliative care of terminal patients<br>• Extubation failures (in particular for COPD and circulatory failure)<br>• Out-of-hospital pneumonia in COPD patients<br>• Postoperative ventilatory failure (treatment, prevention)<br>• Acute ventilatory failure prevention in asthma<br>• Acute out-of-hospital pneumonia<br>• Weaning from the ventilator |
| Review of controlled clinical trials, individual controlled clinical trials | • Neuromuscular disorders, kyphoscoliosis<br>• Partial upper airway obstruction<br>• Chest trauma<br>• Acute ventilatory failure in asthma<br>• ARDS |
| Series of cases and low-quality individual controlled clinical trials | • Very old patients<br>• Cystic fibrosis<br>• Obesity hypoventilation syndrome<br>• Idiopathic pulmonary fibrosis |

(ARDS: acute respiratory distress syndrome; COPD: chronic obstructive pulmonary disease)

effects may vary.[24] Thus far, the best effects have been observed in patients undergoing NIV for exacerbation of COPD and in cardiogenic lung edema[25,26] (Table 1).

## Chronic Obstructive Pulmonary Disease Exacerbation

A number of randomized trials and meta-analyses have confirmed the efficacy of NIV in improving the effects of treatment of COPD exacerbation complicated with hypercapnic acidosis.[27-29]

In a 2004 meta-analysis, covering 14 randomized controlled trials (RCTs) and 758 COPD patients with hypercapnia more than 45 mm Hg, it was determined that the treatment using NIV reduced mortality rate from 21% to 11%, and the need for intubation from 33% to 16%; also, the hospitalization time was reduced.[30,31] Patients treated with NIV would also require intubation and invasive ventilation less frequently than patients treated conventionally.[30,32] Patients with severe exacerbation of COPD respond to NIV better than patients with moderate exacerbation of the disease. In patients with moderate COPD, the outcomes of standard therapy did not differ from NIV treatment.[28,33]

The efficacy of NIV in treating COPD exacerbation has become the basis for making the technique a standard treatment procedure.[34-36]

Some researchers also consider severe COPD resistant to standard therapy an indication for long-term, home-based treatment with NIV; however, thus far no mortality rate reduction has been shown, but only a reduction in the hospitalization incidence and improvement of the quality of life of the patients.[37]

## Cardiogenic Pulmonary Edema

Similarly to COPD exacerbation, the efficacy of NIV in treating cardiogenic pulmonary edema has been confirmed a number of times. This treatment method improves the ventilation parameters, facilitates treatment and normalization of arterial blood gases parameters,[38] and reduces the need for intubation,[39-42] in particular in patients with co-occurring hypercapnia.[20] The mechanism of clinical condition improvement depends on reducing not only the work of breathing, but also the myocardial afterload. The efficacy of continuous positive airway pressure (CPAP) and NIV in terms of improving the vital parameters and reducing intubation incidence is similar; both therapies are well-tolerated and are not related to severe complications risk.[20,43]

## Patients with Immunodeficiency

Administering NIV to patients with immunodeficiency may not produce such spectacular outcomes as with COPD or cardiogenic lung edema due to the underlying disease of the ventilatory failure, which may not be as easily reversible. For this reason, the indications for NIV should be carefully considered in order to avoid starting the treatment in patients with high risk of failure. This might apply to patients with severe forms of underlying disease, as classified according to the Simplified Acute Physiology Score (SAPS) system; patients with tachypnea during NIV;

patients in whom NIV was initiated late after admission to the ICU; patients requiring catecholamines, renal replacement therapy; or patients with severe hypoxemic respiratory failure.[44-46] NIV is recommended as the first-line therapy in patients with immunodeficiency in the case of mild or moderate form of acute respiratory failure.[45-48]

In patients correctly qualified for NIV treatment, positive effect of NIV has been shown frequently in patients after organ transplantation, the observed positive outcomes included oxygenation improvement, reduction of intubation incidence, reduction of treatment time, and reduction of mortality in the ICU, with no impact on mortality on later stages; in another trial including patients with immunodeficiency originating from various diseases, NIV has reduced the incidence of severe pulmonary complications, the incidence of intubations, and mortality rate, both in the ICU and in the hospital care.[15,46,49]

## Weaning from Mechanical Ventilation

Noninvasive ventilation has been mentioned in reports on various forms of weaning the patient from invasive ventilation. NIV techniques are particularly efficient in patients with COPD, but have also been shown to work for respiratory failure of different origin.[46,50]

### Protection against Development of Ventilatory Failure after Extubation

Noninvasive ventilation efficacy may be higher, if NIV is initiated immediately after extubation, rather than only after the onset of respiratory failure.[23,51,52] This applies in particular to patients with higher reintubation risk. Such risk is higher in patients with hypercapnia more than 45 mm Hg, circulatory failure, after previous extubation failures, with COPD, bronchiectasis, obesity hypoventilation syndrome, chest deformations, asthma or muscle weakness, and cough of various origins.[51,52]

### Postextubation Ventilatory Failure Treatment

In patients with developed ventilatory failure, the outcomes of NIV treatment are much poorer. The ventilatory capacity in those patients is considerably lower due to the spreading atelectatic pulmonary lesions, increased work of breathing, and weakening of the ventilatory muscles in the time between extubation and the onset of acute ventilatory failure. Those patients often become ineligible for NIV techniques. In such cases, NIV only delays the inevitable intubation and efficient ventilatory treatment with invasive techniques. Such delay may deteriorate prognosis and increase the mortality rate.[53]

Randomized trials have shown that applying NIV to patients with developed acute ventilatory failure extends the time to intubation, but has no impact on reintubation incidence, the time of treatment in the ICU, and sometimes even increases mortality.[53,54]

### Facilitating Weaning from the Ventilator

Noninvasive ventilation makes it possible to remove the intubation tube earlier in patients who do not yet meet the extubation criteria.[55,56] This applies in particular to patients with COPD.[57] In those patients, administering NIV immediately after extubation reduces the time of treatment in the ICU, the ventilator-associated pneumonia (VAP) incidence, the mortality rate, and reduces the total mechanical ventilation time by as much as 7.3 days.[57]

## Acute Respiratory Distress Syndrome

A number of reports suggest that NIV may be useful in treating patients with acute hypoxemic lung injury caused by underlying disease other than cardiogenic lung edema.[58,59] NIV is reported to reduce mortality rate (by 17% of absolute risk), intubation incidence (by 23% of absolute risk), and the treatment time in the ICU (by 2 days).[60,61] The efficacy of NIV in patients with ARDS has not yet been fully confirmed.[62] The method may be helpful on earlier stages of the disease. The patients should be carefully screened and monitored. This treatment method must not be applied to patients with severely impaired pulmonary gas exchange, as in the group of patients, in which NIV proved inefficient, the mortality rate was significantly higher than in the group receiving standard treatment with invasive ventilation.[63,64] In patients eligible for treatment, NIV is able to improve the pulmonary gas exchange parameters, help avoid intubation for 54% of patients, and reduce the incidence of VAP, multiple organ failure, and mortality in the ICU.[11,65] However, the patients treated with NIV must be carefully monitored, especially in the case of increased risk of failure (SAPS > 34, severe hypoxemia $PaO_2/FiO_2$ < 175, shock, acidosis), so that intubation is not unnecessarily delayed if noninvasive techniques fail.[47,66]

## Long-term Ventilation

Noninvasive ventilation can also be administered in out of hospital scenario. One of the possible NIV applications is long-term ventilation of patients with chronic ventilatory failure of various origins. The patients undergo NIV, usually with the use of nasal masks, face masks or mouthpieces, and special ventilators designed for home applications.

Ventilation for several or several dozen hours a day relieves the ventilatory muscles and allows them to work more efficiently during periods of spontaneous ventilation. It also reduces the work of breathing and sensation of dyspnea, and enables more efficient cough and secretions elimination from the airways.[67-72] It is crucial to improve the efficiency of $CO_2$ elimination and minimize the symptoms of chronic hypercapnia, which often significantly restricts the patients' activities.[67,72]

## EQUIPMENT USED IN NONINVASIVE VENTILATION

### Masks

The mask types include nasal masks, face masks, and total face masks. Mouthpieces, mouth masks, and helmets are also used (Figs. 1A to F).

*Nasal Masks*

It is used mainly by patients with obstructive sleep apnea (OSA). It is intended mainly for patients without disturbance of consciousness, cooperative, and able to keep their mouth closed during positive pressure ventilation. The advantages of nasal masks include small dead space under the mask and lower risk of claustrophobic episodes. Also, in the case of vomiting, the risk of aspiration is negligible. A modified version of the nasal mask is the so-called "nasal pillow masks", with two soft tubes ("pillows") inserted into the nostrils. The ends of the tubes are slightly wider to ensure that there are no air leaks. The advantages of nasal pillow masks include convenience, small size, and weight, and elimination of pressure on the bridge of the nose, where pressure ulcers most frequently occur if nasal or half masks are used.

*Face Masks*

Face masks are the most frequently used type of masks in the ICUs or emergency units.[25] They cover both nose and mouth, and provide better tightness than nasal masks. In most cases, the masks maintain tightness event if the patient opens their mouth, e.g. after falling asleep, or when the patient is agitated. The disadvantage of face masks is that the size of the mask must fit perfectly (which means the patient must have several masks). The pressure on the bridge of the nose may damage the skin. The dead space under the mask is larger, which makes synchrony of the ventilator with the patient more difficult (trigger issues) and that in turn causes the risk of $CO_2$ rebreathing. Some total face masks appear to be free of the majority of issues of face masks. The total face masks are supported on the

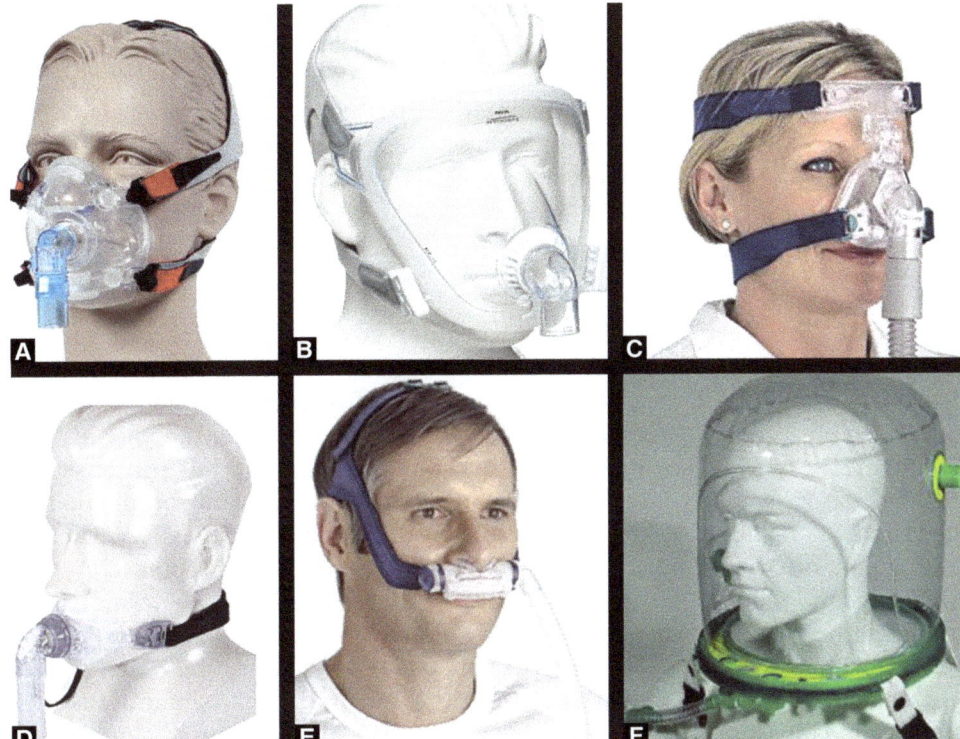

**Figs. 1A to F:** Different types of masks and a helmet used in noninvasive ventilation, from the top left corner: (A) Hans Rudolph half mask; (B) Philips Respironics face mask; (C) ResMed nasal mask; (D) Fischer and Paykel Healthcare mouth mash; (E) ResMed nasal pillows mask; (F) Harol helmet. *Source:* Advertising materials of mask producers.

forehead, chin, and face sides. Therefore, there is no risk of pressure ulcers on the nose or pressure on the eyes. Total face masks are particularly useful for patients with nontypical face shapes (very thin or obese patients), for patients with nose injuries, patients in whom the gastric tube cannot be removed, or agitated patients (who speak and open their mouths). The disadvantages, similarly to half masks, include large dead space and the risk of $CO_2$ rebreathing. Nevertheless, face masks are well tolerated and particularly useful for patients treated in the ICU.[73-75]

### Helmets

Unlike the masks, a helmet is attached with straps under the patient's arms, and sealed with a soft flange on the neck and shoulders. This solution ensures proper tightness and makes it possible to apply slightly higher pressure values than in typical masks. Because there is no pressure on the face, the ventilation session may be much longer, if necessary, from several to several dozen hours at a time; on the initial stage of treatment, ventilation may even be continuous. The helmet also makes it possible to use NIV in difficult anatomical situations (orofacial injuries, gastric tubes, thick facial hair), and can improve the patient's comfort, as it allows free talking, reading, etc. The disadvantages of helmets are mainly related to their large volume and the associated considerable dead space, which makes it difficult to choose an appropriate trigger and properly synchronize the patient with the ventilator; also, it requires high gas flow rates through the helmet to reduce the risk of $CO_2$ rebreathing.[76-78] The minimum required flow rates reach 40–60 L/min,[79] which in turn might cause significant noise (up to 100 dB) originating from the turbulent gas flow at the inlet of the helmet. The noise level can be reduced by installing a filter or a heat and moisture exchanger (HME) on the helmet inlet port.[64]

## Ventilator Breathing Circuits

In the ICU setting, reusable breathing circuits are usually used. Reusable circuits are cheaper, but usually made from thick rubber and heavier than disposable circuits. Consequently, reusable circuits may pull the mask down and unseal the breathing system. For this reason, lighter disposable circuits are preferable. The ventilator breathing systems can be traditional with double patient circuit: inspiration and expiration tubes. In this system, there is practically no contact between the inspiratory and the expiratory air. The disadvantage of the traditional system is larger weight and less convenient use; however, the ability to measure the volume of expired air and thus more accurate monitoring of ventilation make this system a standard in ICUs. An alternative is the single patient circuit system, either with external expiratory valve or without expiratory valve and with a leak port. The advantages of the single circuit system include simplicity and low weight. The single patient circuit systems always include a section of the system, between the patient and the expiration valve or leak port, which is common for both inspiration and expiration. Leakage systems are becoming increasingly popular in NIV, especially for long-term home-based therapy, but also in hospital settings. The pros of leak systems include simplicity of the system, resistance to dirt, and very low weight compared to traditional systems. The entire system consists of a straight tube coming from the ventilator to the NIV mask and the leak port with precisely specified area, located on the mask or from a few to a dozen or so cm from it. The leak port can have different shapes, e.g. can resemble gills, or could be formed by a number of smaller holes, but its total surface area is always identical. During inspiration and expiration, the air from the breathing circuits continues to "leak" through the leak port. The leak has a precisely specified flow rate and depends on the pressure in the breathing circuits; if the pressure is higher, the leak flow rate is higher during inspiration; if the pressure is lower, the leak flow rate is lower during expiration. The presence of a continuous leak is accounted for by the control algorithm of the ventilator which produces the pressure and flow necessary to achieve the set ventilation parameters [inspiratory positive airway pressure (IPAP), $V_t$] during inspiration, and constant expiratory positive airway pressure (EPAP). If this type of breathing circuit is used, maintaining EPAP at constant level (and the related expiration air leak) is necessary, as it protects the patient from $CO_2$ rebreathing.

## Ventilators

Having only an older ventilator model without the special functions designed for NIV should not prevent the healthcare personnel from attempting to apply that method. In such cases, synchronizing the patient with the ventilator can be more difficult, but still possible. Currently, most new ventilators available on the market have the necessary features for performing NIV. The key features include: the NIV mode with acceptance of leaks around the mask, which prevents the ventilator from constantly raising alarms and switching into emergency mode, and the leak compensation feature, which adjusts the ventilator's basic flow to the current volume of air leaks, thus maintaining the trigger at a constant level regardless of the air-tightness of the mask. The leak compensation feature greatly facilitates the ventilator-patient synchrony and reduces the work of breathing.[10,80,81]

## VENTILATION MODES USED IN NONINVASIVE VENTILATION

When administering NIV, similarly to invasive ventilation, the ventilator can operate in either volume-targeted ventilation (VTV) mode or pressure-targeted ventilation (PTV) mode. The PTV mode is much more frequently applied, both in acute settings and for long-term ventilation. Due to variable inspiratory flow and, consequently, improved leak compensation, the PTV is better tolerated than VTV where the inspiratory flow is fixed. In PTV mode, the patient adapts to NIV more quickly and tolerates ventilation better, the work of breathing is reduced, and there are fewer complications related to aerophagia.[82,83]

The VTV mode is still applied, particularly in long-term ventilation of patients with neuromuscular disorders. In such cases, the cough efficiency can be improved by applying the technique of air stacking (i.e. double $V_t$ intake). The patient does not exhale after inspiring the first $V_t$ and generates a subsequent assisted inspiration immediately after completing the first one. A double tidal volume improves the expiration efficiency (often with assistance of a second person), as well as cough efficiency and phlegm elimination from the airways.[84] The technique is most frequently used in patients ventilated with a mouthpiece and cannot be used in pressure-targeted ventilation. The specified peak airway pressure allows the patient to inspire one $V_t$ in this ventilation mode. Additional pulmonary volume without increasing the peak pressure can only be achieved with the patient's active inspiration at high $V_t$, which is not possible in patients with severely weakened muscles suffering from neuromuscular disorders. Mastering the air stacking technique and the assistance of an experience healthcare team makes it possible to achieve a long-term NIV period without the need for artificial airways.[85-88] A number of authors have reported long-term survival and reduced incidence of complications related to artificial airways; however, one disadvantage of the method is its limited availability due to the small number of healthcare centers with the relevant know-how and experience to apply it.[84-86,89]

For some new respirators, special software has been developed which enables achieving the same outcomes with PTV, as with air stacking in VTV.[88] One of those software developments is called LIAM (Lung Insufflation Assist Maneuver).

## IMPLEMENTATION TECHNIQUE

The moment of initiation of the NIV in the patient may determine the patient's acceptance of the method and further course of treatment. Positive pressure created by the ventilator may be surprising to the patient and for some patients, the sensation after attaching the mask might be unpleasant. For this reason, in each case, the NIV must be preceded by a conversation with the patient in order to explain to him/her the principle of the method, its purpose, and procedure[19] (Box 2). It is important to make the patient aware that the method is a noncontinuous one and after a ventilation session is complete, the patient will be able to breathe spontaneously for some time. Before attaching the mask to the patient's face with straps, it should be first held to the patient's face in order to demonstrate that the inconvenience for the patient will be minor. It should be emphasized that the efficacy of the method largely depends on the patient's cooperation with the healthcare team and any steps increasing the patient's acceptance of the mask and the ventilator are fully justified. The patient should be placed in half-sitting position. Ventilation begins with low IPAP and EPAP. IPAP should be set at 8–10 cmH$_2$O and EPAP at 0 cmH$_2$O. The trigger sensitivity should be set at the lowest level preventing autotriggering, in order to reduce the work of breathing related to initiating inspiration, and to improve

---

**Box 2:** Noninvasive ventilation implementation technique.

- Explaining the technique to the patient
- Select appropriate size and type of the interface/mask
- Setting inspiratory and expiratory pressure at low levels (e.g. IPAP 8 cmH$_2$O, EPAP 3–5 cmH$_2$O)
- Lifting the patient to sitting position (if possible)
- Attaching the mask gently, starting ventilation
- Tightening mask straps, if there are leaks and the patient is not complaining
- Setting FiO$_2$ at a level making it possible to achieve SpO$_2$ >90%
- Setting alarms—low pressure above EPAP
- Observation of the patient and taking the necessary steps to improve the patient's comfort and synchrony with the ventilator
- Modifying the inspiration pressure levels to achieve $V_t$ of 6 mL/kg/breath or higher, in order to achieve SpO$_2$ >90%
- Skin protection against pressure ulcers (artificial skin, dressings, periodical mask replacement)
- Mild sedation should be considered if the patient is agitated
- Monitoring the patient's comfort, respiratory rate, SpO$_2$, and dyspnea every 30 minutes for the first 6–12 hours, then every hour
- Measuring the baseline blood pressure, then repeating BP measurement after 1 hour from starting the ventilation
- Consider humidification, if prolonged use is planned (over 6 hours)

(BP: blood pressure; EPAP: expiratory positive airway pressure; FiO$_2$: fraction of inspired oxygen; IPAP: inspiratory positive airway pressure; SpO$_2$: peripheral capillary oxygen saturation)

the ventilator-patient synchrony. Usually, the sensitivity level is set at 0.3–0.5 cmH$_2$O. The O$_2$ concentration level in the breathing gas should be set at the appropriate level to maintain SpO$_2$ within the range of 92–95%. Excessive SpO$_2$ levels may cause breathing regulation disturbances, particularly in patients with chronic CO$_2$ retention. The inspiration time T$_i$ must be limited, particularly if pressure ventilation mode is used. Otherwise, while the leak around the mask intensifies, the ventilator may not be able to reach the set pressure value and will extend the inspiration time, often significantly, which will considerably affect the patient synchrony. Once the patient has accepted ventilation with low IPAP and EPAP values, the pressure level should be gradually increased until positive clinical effect is achieved, or significant leak around the mask occurs than cannot be compensated with reasonable tightening of the straps. It should be borne in mind that NIV sessions take several hours at a time and excessive mask pressure will be uncomfortable for the patient, and may lead to pressure ulcers and rejection of the mask and the NIV technique by the patient. The need for excessive pressure is a signal that the mask does not fit properly and that another mask size or type should be used. To test if the mask fits properly, the healthcare professional should be able to put 1–2 fingers between the straps and the patient's head, without causing air leaks or complaints from the patient.

## MONITORING

The primary efficacy endpoint for the applied NIV techniques will be the achieved clinical outcomes. The patient's breathing slows down, the V$_t$ increases, the patient calms down and the ventilator-patient synchrony improves. Over the course of several to ten-odd minutes, SpO$_2$ increase is observed. Gasometric analysis indicates a rapid increase of PaO$_2$, while partial pressure carbon dioxide (PaCO$_2$) decreases slowly, sometimes not until the next session. After fully calming their breath, the patient often falls asleep, especially if he/she has previously breathed with substantial effort for a prolonged period of time.

Monitoring the efficacy of NIV is mainly based on clinical monitoring and, to a smaller extent, gasometric analysis or monitoring the parameters of breathing mechanics. The monitored parameters are listed in Table 2.

The efficiency of monitoring largely depends on the experience of the healthcare team, especially the midlevel personnel. On the initial stage of NIV of the patient, the nurses' labor input related to attaching and adjusting the masks, and regular, careful monitoring, is larger than in the case of patients undergoing invasive ventilation. This

**Table 2:** Objective and subjective signs of noninvasive ventilation efficacy.

| Objective parameters | Subjective parameters |
|---|---|
| • State of consciousness<br>• Respiratory rate<br>• Heart rate<br>• Blood pressure<br>• Using additional respiratory muscles<br>• Volume of phlegm in airways<br>• Leakages around the mask<br>• Skin damage<br>• SpO$_2$, EtCO$_2$, Vt, P$_{imax}$, curves: P, V, P$_{di}$ | • Dyspnea<br>• Discomfort<br>• Symptom of claustrophobia<br>• Pain at the pressure site of the mask, straps |

(EtCO$_2$: end-tidal CO$_2$; P: pressure; P$_{di}$: transdiaphragmatic pressure; P$_{imax}$: maximal inspiratory pressure; SpO$_2$: peripheral capillary oxygen saturation; V: volume; Vt: tidal volume)

should be taken into account in planning the staffing in the wards applying NIV. When the patient has adapted to ventilation and his/her condition has improved in subsequent NIV sessions, the labor input related to patient care is reduced.

## CAUSES OF NONINVASIVE VENTILATION FAILURE

Around 10–15% of patients do not tolerate NIV.[12] In each case, it is the operator who should be investigated first for reasons of rejection. The patient may reject NIV for various reasons, including, but not limited to, equipment-related issues, ventilator-patient asynchrony, or incorrect qualification of the patient for NIV.

### Equipment-related Issues

It is usually due to improper adjustment of the mask. The type of the applied mask plays a crucial role. In the ICU settings, face masks are more frequently used than nasal masks. Using face masks, it is easier to achieve air-tightness in patients who are unconscious, agitated, or talking. It is also easier to maintain air-tightness in sleeping patients. Efficient NIV quickly improves gas exchange, reduces the work of breathing, and improves respiratory comfort. The patient, tired from prolonged and deteriorating respiratory malady, often falls asleep within minutes from starting ventilation. Sometimes, the sleeping patient opens his/her mouth and, if nasal mask is used, leaks might occur. Mask leaks also require frequent adjustments or tightening of the straps, which reduces the comfort of ventilation and may prompt the patient to reject ventilation. It is recommended to apply NIV with a number of masks available on place that can be replaced quickly, if necessary, in order to set up the most appropriate arrangement. Rapid respiratory support and improvement of respiratory comfort will increase the patient's confidence in the treatment method. Quick and efficient initiation of noninvasive respiratory support is of particular importance in patients with limited respiratory reserve. This is the case, for instance, when NIV is initiated in patients weaned from invasive ventilation. After extubation, the patient may experience rapid deterioration of ventilation comfort due to doubled anatomical dead space (intubation decreases anatomical dead space from about 150 mL to 70 mL by omitting upper airways) and the need to eliminate secretions from the airways.

Another reason of failure may be the lack of appropriate ventilator-patient synchrony. The asynchrony degree may vary, from complete misalignment between the ventilator operation and the patient's spontaneous breathing (and consequently, the patient's "fight" against the apparatus), to more subtle asynchrony, such as maladjustment of the peak flow increases time from the apparatus, or overextension of inspiration. However, each type of asynchrony increases the work of breathing and deteriorates the gas exchange; therefore, the operator should always attempt to eliminate the issue. The efficacy of NIV is reduced, which is reflected in the increased $CO_2$ retention. Also, the efficacy of humidification of inspiratory air deteriorates, as humidifier is released into the environment through the leak. Asynchrony disrupts the patient's sleep; a number of researchers have reported sleep fragmentation and frequent waking up caused by leaks. The ventilation comfort can also be affected by different procedures administered by the healthcare team to manage the leaks. These include tightening the mask straps, or other efforts to minimize leak through open mouth. As these procedures can create unnecessary risks for patients, due to the increased risk of aspiration to the airways, it should be avoided.

However, the aspect distinguishing NIV from invasive ventilation is the presence of air leak around the mask and its impact on synchronization.

The leak is an inherent element of NIV; the leak rate may reach up to several dozen liters per minute. The leak between the mask and the patient's face significantly disrupts the pressure transfer from the patient's respiratory system to the pressure and flow sensors in the ventilator, and affects the ventilator-patient synchrony on each stage of the breathing cycle, mainly: the positive end-expiratory pressure (PEEP) level, the inspiratory triggering, the pressurization phase, and inspiration to expiration cycling.[90]

The leak compensation capability will usually depend on the applied ventilation mode and the quality of the leak compensation function of the ventilator.

The leak compensation ratio will also depend on whether the PTV or VTV is applied. In the traditional VTV, the target parameter of each inspiration is achieving the set $V_t$. In this mode, the inspiratory flow is constant. Of course, the inspiratory flow can have different waveforms: square, decelerating, accelerating, or sine, but cannot exceed the predefined value based on the $V_t$ and inspiratory time. In the PTV, the target parameter is the inspiratory pressure; in order to maintain the pressure at a specified level, the flow is adjusted according to the compliance and resistance in the respiratory system. Morphologically, the flow changes in this ventilation mode are similar to the changes occurring during spontaneous breathing. Therefore, by definition, the PTV is better suited to compensate the leaks (Figs. 2A and B).

### Leakage Compensation in Volume-targeted Ventilation

Despite the rising interest in pressure-targeted ventilator, caused mainly by the lower manufacturing costs, the ventilators with volume-targeted capabilities are still widely applied, in particular in patients undergoing long-term ventilation for respiratory failure arising from neuromuscular disorders.[91] The advantages of VTV in those patients include higher comfort and efficient correction of daytime and nocturnal hypoventilation, and lower risk of hypoventilation in the case of a reduction of the respiratory system compliance (e.g. secretions accumulation in the airways.[68,92]

The main disadvantage of volume-targeted ventilators and ventilation modes is the inability to maintain the set ventilation parameters, in particular the $V_t$, in case of leak.[93,94]

The leak is usually unstable and its rate is sometimes much higher than the inspiratory flow.[95] As a result, efficient compensation of the leak and achieving the set $V_t$ is not possible in volume ventilation. Sabil assessed the $V_t$ achieved during VTV of patients with neuromuscular disorders who received NIV during nocturnal sleep. He determined that when the active ventilation was reduced after the patient had fallen asleep, the real $V_t$ decreased due to leakage to values lower than 50% of the initial $V_t$.[96]

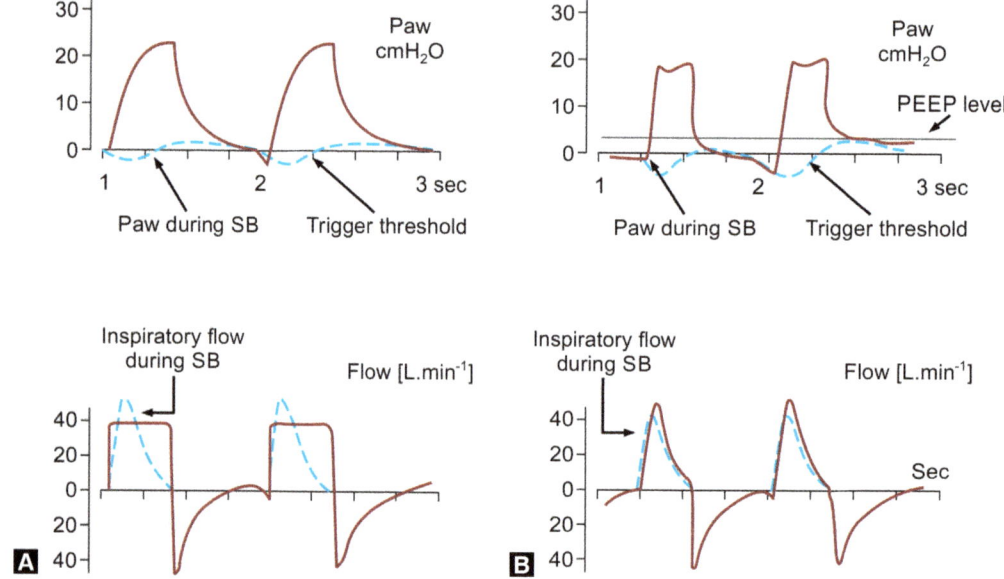

**Figs. 2A and B:** Correlation of pressure and flow during—(A) Volume-targeted ventilation; (B) Pressure-targeted ventilation. (Paw: airway pressure; PEEP: positive end-expiratory pressure; SB: spontaneous breathing)

### Leakage Compensation during Pressure-targeted Ventilation

In the PTV, leak compensation is by default more efficient than in volume-targeted modes. However, the efficiency of the compensation largely depends on the mechanical and software solutions applied by the equipment manufacturers, and is not uniform for different ventilators. Numerous studies comparing different ventilators have been made and the majority of them had similar outcomes. In 2001, Mehta compared six ventilators for NIV, working in pressure-targeted mode, with three volume-targeted ventilators, including one ventilator used in the ICU.[97] The comparison included the ventilation parameters in three settings: without leak, with small leak (25% of the baseline $V_t$), and with large leak (50% of baseline $V_t$). In the setting without leak, the differences in tidal volume between the ventilators were already significant—the achieved Vt ranged from 800 mL to 1200 mL at identical inspiratory pressure (peak inspiratory pressure was 18 cm $H_2O$ for pressure-targeted ventilators), and the target volume of 1 L for volume-targeted ventilators. The presence of even a small leak caused a deficiency of the supplied tidal volume that differed significantly between the ventilators. It was considerably higher for volume-targeted ventilators, particularly with a large leak. The ICU ventilator was unable to supply any tidal volume at all with large leak.

Furthermore, in some pressure-targeted ventilators, a large leak caused rapid $V_t$ drop. This was caused by the appearance of an autotrigger, i.e. quick initiation of subsequent inspirations from the ventilator which were unrelated to the patient's respiratory effort. This phenomenon would subside only after reducing the trigger sensitivity; however, this in turn affects the ventilator-patient synchrony and the comfort of ventilation. In the case of VTV with a large leak, the $V_t$ loss cannot be compensated even by increasing the $V_t$ substantially. Even significant increase of the supplied $V_t$ from 0.5 L to as much as 2 L would not even partially compensate the $V_t$ lost through the leak.[97]

The difficulties with leak compensation, as described herein, prompt the equipment manufacturers to develop systems that would neutralize, to the maximum extent possible, the negative consequences of the leak. These systems are usually based on software controlling the flow in the ventilator's breathing circuits and adjusting it in order to maintain the set pressure level in the system. As a result, the pressure value which the patient must generate in order to activate change in the respiratory cycle (mainly related to the inspiratory and expiratory trigger) is maintained at a constant level.

The leak compensation control algorithms can be very complicated. Examples include AutoTrak,[98] based on seven algorithms applied simultaneously during each respiratory cycle, or the modification of the ventilator's factory algorithm which improved the trigger sensitivity for NIV of children, as reported by Khiriani[99] (Fig. 3).

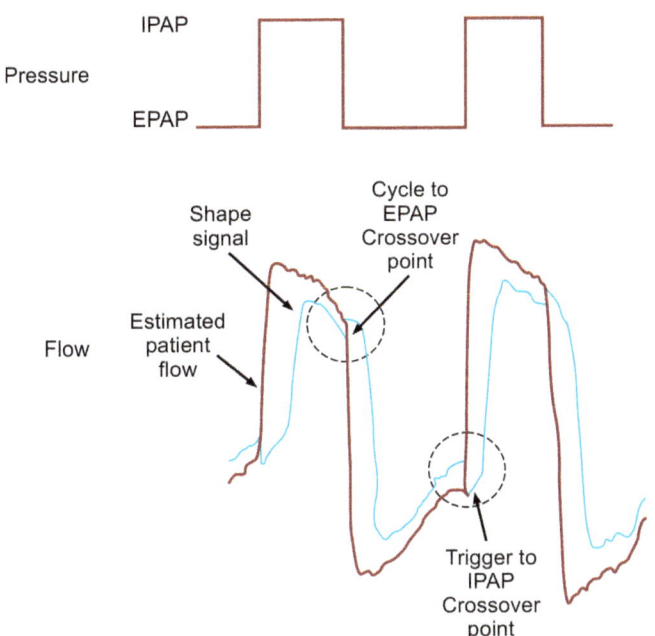

**Fig. 3:** Leakage compensation: Left side—in the AutoTrak system, the flow rate is modified according to the flow and pressure signal level, on the basis of the algorithms: Leak estimation: Average and parabolic, volume trigger, shape signal, spontaneous expiratory threshold (SET), flow reversal, maximum IPAP time, volume control cycle.
(EPAP: expiratory positive airway pressure; IPAP: inspiratory positive airway pressure)
*Source:* Advertising materials of Phillips Respironics.[98]

> **Box 3:** Factors which can influence synchronization during noninvasive ventilaton.
>
> *Patient related:*
> - Proper selection of patients
> - Accepting the method by the patient
> - Body position
>
> *Equipment related:*
> - A suitable respirator
> - The right interface
> - A proper ventilation mode
> - Control of $CO_2$ rebreathing
> - Humidification
> - Adjustment of ventilation parameters (pressure, flow) to the patient's needs
>
> *Others* (sedation, oxygen therapy)

## Ventilator-patient Asynchrony

Synchronization of the mechanical work of the ventilator with the neuromuscular respiratory effort of the patient is one of the most important elements in the treatment by mechanical ventilation. Synchronization should include all components of each respiratory cycle, including respiration rate, inspiration (trigger), inspiratory phase (pressure, inspiration time, inspiratory flows, tidal volumes) and transition from inspiration to exhalation. The lack of synchronization or respiratory-patient desynchronization has a significant impact on the patient's course of treatment not only because of the lack of comfort of the patient who "fights with the ventilator" but also the deterioration of the efficiency of gas exchange, increased respiratory muscle load, increased respiration and fatigue in the respiratory muscles and often the need for deeper sedation of the patient.[80,100,101] The consequence is the extension of the time of weaning from the ventilator, the time of mechanical ventilation, the time of treatment at the ICU and, as a result, the risk of complications related to mechanical ventilation, which may have a significant impact on the patient's prognosis.[102,103] In the case of NIV noninvasive ventilation, synchronization may be particularly difficult due to the fact that the NIV is a "semi-open" system due to the presence of air leaks around the mask that give the unsealing effect of the respirator-patient system. Leaks are inherently associated with noninvasive ventilation and most often occur in the initial phase of ventilation, when the patient adapts to a new mode of breathing and at a later stage of prolonged ventilation. In addition to the leakage itself, the patient will be influenced by the type of mask used, the emotional state of the patient and our efforts and changes in ventilation parameters to correct the problem.[101] This may cause the respirator-patient synchronization to be more difficult during NIV use than during invasive ventilation.

Synchronization does not only depend on the adjustment of the ventilator's parameters but is a complex and multifactorial process. It is important to take care of all the elements that determine the acceptance of the method by the patient. They are listed in Box 3.

## Proper Qualification for Noninvasive Ventilation

In this case, the failure of the applied NIV usually occurs due to the fact that the patient's condition is too severe, i.e. the breathing gas must have high oxygen levels, the inspiratory or expiratory pressure must be high as well; the patient may be agitated and thus uncooperative and refusing to accept ventilation, the patient may experience disturbance of consciousness; also, the patient may be suffering from excessive secretion quantity which is difficult to eliminate, the respiratory effort might be too high, or the patient might be hemodynamically unstable. Insufficient experience of the healthcare team could also be a factor.

When it becomes clear that the method has failed, i.e. within 1–2 hours from initiating NIV, the patient's respiratory rate and effort do not drop, the $V_t$ does not increase, hemodynamic instability occurs, and the patient's gasometry parameters do not improve, the NIV should be discontinued and the patient should be intubated.[101,104] If the signs of failure become apparent, NIV should be discontinued immediately, as prolonging the ventilation might lead to the patient's exhaustion and extreme fatigue of respiratory muscles, which will extend the recuperation time of the muscles and delay another attempt to administer NIV.

## HUMIDIFICATION OF INSPIRATORY AIR

Insufficient humidification of inspiratory air during NIV causes drying of the mucus membranes of the oral cavity and throat, as well as structural changes and swelling, which in turn increases airways resistance even by 30%. This phenomenon is referred to as increased nasal airway resistance (NAWR), and may be one of crucial, though underestimated factors leading to the rejection of NIV by the patients. Besides, during NIV, despite maintaining the natural airway and the possibility of heating up and humidifying the inspiratory air in the nasal cavity, efficient humidification is required, since patients who need respiratory support often breathe rapidly and deeply, generating high air flow rates and affecting the humidification efficiency in the nasal cavity. The patients frequently breathe through their mouths, bypassing the nasal cavity due to the presence of feeding tubes or catheters in the nostrils, or because of the sensation of dyspnea (breathing through the mouth causes less resistance for the airflow). During NIV, the usually applied humidification techniques might prove inefficient, due mainly to the unidirectional leak of the inspiratory (humidified) air from the ventilator to the patient, caused by either intentional (systems operating in leak mode) or unintentional (leaks between the mask and the patient's face) inspiratory air leaks. The inspiratory air can be humidified with the use of HMEs (widely used filters), or heated humidifiers (HHs). The HMEs work efficiently if the entire volume of expiratory air, heated and maximally saturated with water vapor, returns to the exchangers to heat it up and saturate it with vapor. In the case of NIV, the leaks between the mask and the patient's face, or intentional leaks (breathing circuits operating in leak mode, especially those where the leak port is located between the HME and the patient's face, e.g. on the mask) cause some of the humidified air expired by the patient to be released into the environment and be lost for the humidification process. As a result, the expiratory air only partially returns to the HME. Consequently, the HME's saturation and heating is insufficient, thus reducing the filter's performance in the next inspiration. Furthermore, in patients with borderline respiratory stability and the related low $V_t$, the high volume of the extension and HME (up to 130 mL) may prevent a significant portion of the $V_t$ and the humidified expiratory air from reaching the filter, thus reducing HME performance. In the case of invasive ventilation, large dead space of the apparatus is not a major issue, as it can be easily compensated by increasing the inspiratory volume or pressure. In patients undergoing NIV, the issue is far more serious, as increasing either volume or pressure would only feed the leaks and cause further loss of humidified expiratory air. Such inconveniences are eliminated if HH is used, which is why the HHs should be the standard for inspiratory air humidification during NIV.

## REBREATHING DURING NONINVASIVE VENTILATION

During NIV, all types of patient circuits can be used, i.e. traditional double circuits or single circuits. However, the single patient circuits are becoming increasingly popular, especially for long-term ventilation, as they are lighter and do not pull the mask off the patient's face, thus making the ventilation process more comfortable. The simplified ventilator structure and the elimination of the expiratory valve are also important factors.

The single patient circuit systems can come in two types: with valves or without valves. The valve systems have an external expiratory valve at the distal end, controlled by the pressure in the ventilator system. During inspiration, the valve membrane extending under inspiratory pressure covers the end of the T-tube in the valve, and the entire inspiration is directed to the patient. During expiration, the pressure in the entire system, including above the expiratory valve membrane, drops exposing the end of the T-tube and enabling the patient to expire (Fig. 4).

In both the double and the single patient circuit systems with expiratory valve, the issue of rebreathing is virtually nonexistent. The patient inspires only the expiratory air rich with $CO_2$ that is found between the mask and the branching of the Y-connector in the double patient circuit, or is present to the expiratory valve level in the single patient circuit system. Potential problems might arise only if the connectors or filters which are used between the mask and the Y-connector or the valve, are too long and do not match the patient's ventilation parameters. It should be borne in mind that the typical connectors and filters

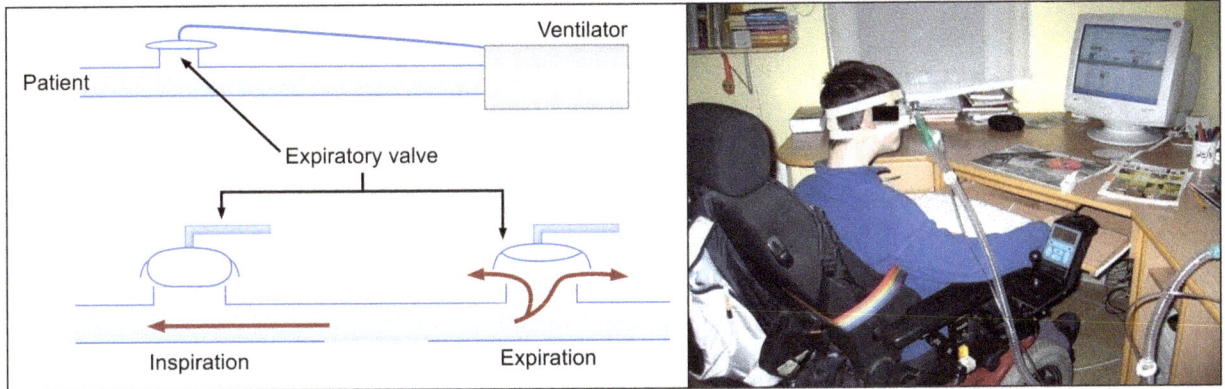

**Fig. 4:** Principle of operation of external expiratory valve. To the right: Patient undergoing noninvasive ventilation with the use of a single patient circuit with expiratory valve, as part of a long-term ventilation program (published with the patient's consent).

used in adult patients have the internal capacity of 40 mL and 90 mL, respectively. Hence, they might affect the $CO_2$ rebreathing in patients with low $V_t$s.

The problem of $CO_2$ rebreathing may occur in a single leak circuit. Such systems are becoming increasingly popular due to their simplicity, light weight, and resistance to dirt. The ventilator is connected to the mask via a straight tube. In the system, the so-called "leak" is installed near the mask. The leak might take the form of a mushroom with openings (Whisper-Swivel connector), or a connector with several openings or cuts. In each case, the total surface area of the hole is equal to the area of the circle with a diameter of 4 mm. In modern masks, the leak openings are located in the mask itself in order to simplify the system and minimize the issue of rebreathing (Figs. 5A to D). The leak through the leak openings is referred to as intentional, unlike the unintentional leak caused, e.g. by the mask failure.

During ventilation with intentional leak, this is usually the bilevel positive airway pressure (BiPAP) mode, where the ventilator generates two pressure levels: higher inspiratory pressure and lower expiratory pressure. The controlling algorithms adjust the inspiratory and expiratory flow rates to compensate the expiration leak, and generate the appropriate IPAP and maintain the constant expiratory positive airway pressure (EPAP or PEEP).

The crucial factors for the rebreathing issue are the expiration and the PEEP level. If expiration is too rapid (high expiratory flow rate), too short (expiratory time), or the PEEP level is too low (higher PEEP means higher rate of the flow flushing the system toward the leak), it may happen during the expiration that not all air will be expired through the intentional leak openings and some of the expiratory air will move into the section of the tube between the leak openings and the ventilator (Fig. 6). This happens in particular with rapid expiration when, in order to maintain

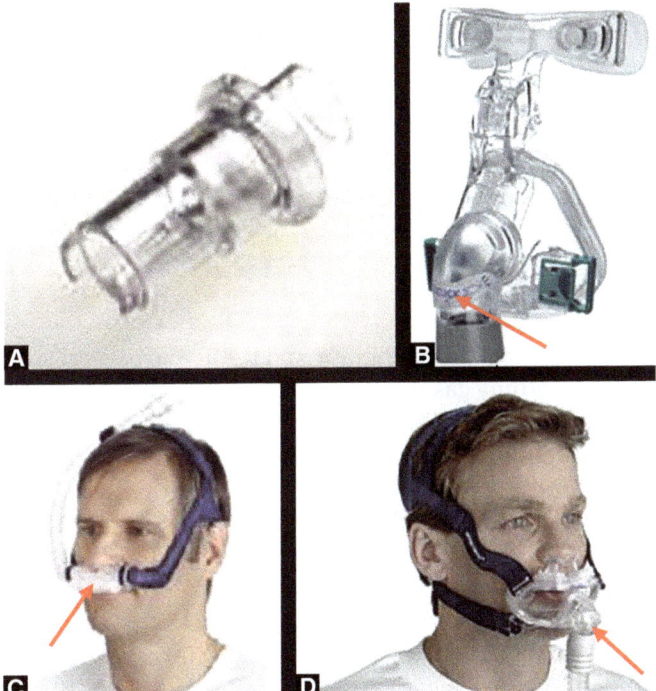

**Figs. 5A to D:** Elements of a system operating in leak mode: Whisper-Swivel connector (A), masks with leak openings (marked by arrows) (B to D).
*Source:* From commercial materials of mask producers.

the constant PEEP level, the pressure valve on the ventilator opens. In such cases, the expiratory air, rich in $CO_2$, may fill a substantial portion of the tube connecting the patient to the ventilator, and the patient might subsequently inspire the $CO_2$.[105]

On average, the issue of rebreathing may affect 10–20% of respiratory cycles of NIV, particularly in patients breathing rapidly and with low levels of specified PEEP.[105,106] For this reason, in the ventilators operating in the leak mode, it is not possible to set the PEEP below 4 cmH$_2$O.

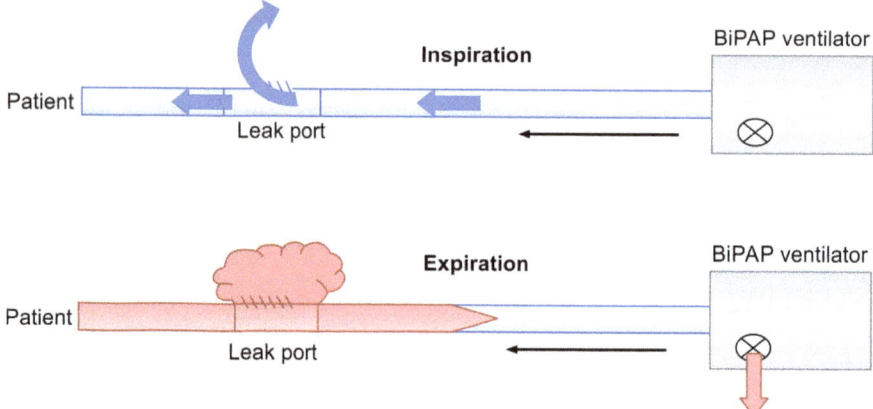

Fig. 6: Ventilation with intentional leak.
(BiPAP: bilevel positive airway pressure)

The volume of inspired $CO_2$ is usually relatively low and is not a significant clinical issue; however, in certain cases the issue might become serious and cause substantial increase of the work of breathing by stimulating the respiratory center with $CO_2$, resulting in NIV intolerance.

## OXYGEN THERAPY DURING NONINVASIVE VENTILATION

The efficacy of oxygen therapy and the actual oxygen level in the breathing gas may largely depend on the type of the ventilator's breathing circuit and the method of oxygen administration, but also on the volume of the unintentional leak.

The issue might occur if oxygen is administered in a low-flow system, i.e. when oxygen is added to the system with fixed flow rate, from an oxygen concentrator, oxygen tank, or by the flow meter in the hospital system. In that case, the flow rate usually is set within the range of 2–10 L $O_2$/min; the oxygen flow is fixed, regardless of the momentary flow rate in the ventilator's breathing circuit (Fig. 7). The differences occur depending on whether we use the volume or pressure variable mode. In volumetric mode, regardless of the size of the leak, the proportions: oxygen and inspiratory flow will always be constant and the percentage of oxygen in the breathing mixture will also be constant, regardless of the amount of inspiratory air that eventually reaches the patient. It is different in the course of pressure-variable ventilation. The inspiratory flow is variable to maintain a constant inspiratory pressure, and in principle the oxygen in the constant flow will have a different share in the variable inspiratory flow. In the case of leaks, often significantly exceeding the normal inspiratory flow, this problem will increase. As a result, when using

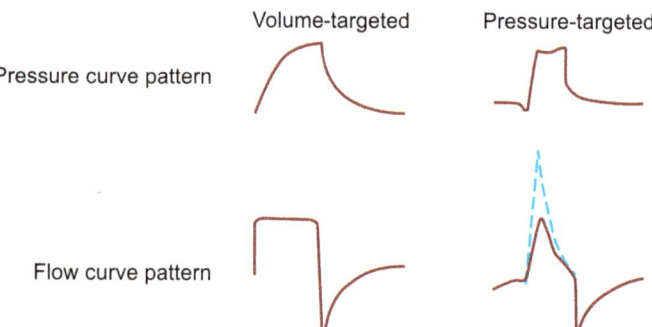

Fig. 7: Pressure and flow curves during volume-targeted and pressure-targeted ventilation. Gray band—fixed $O_2$ flow, the air/$O_2$ proportion is fixed during volume-targeted ventilation (fixed gas flow rate), but change in the pressure-targeted ventilation if leaks are present—dotted line.

variable pressure ventilation, in the presence of leaks or significantly increased respiration with large inspiratory flows, the actual oxygen concentration in the breathing mixture can be significantly lower than we expected.[107]

This issue does not occur if a high flow system is used, for instance a hospital ventilator connected to the hospital gas network, where the air/oxygen proportion is maintained regardless of the gas flow rate.

The issue also does not occur if VTV is used, as it is characterized with fixed flow independent from the leak ratio.

## CONTRAINDICATIONS FOR NONINVASIVE VENTILATION

An absolute contraindication for NIV is, first of all, the patient's condition requiring immediate intubation and the application of ventilation techniques enabling full control of ventilation parameters and effect, and to protect the patient's airways. Furthermore, there are relative contraindications for NIV, as listed in Box 4.[108]

The exception from the contraindications listed above may be the disturbance of consciousness resulting from hypercapnia in the course of the underlying disease. In such cases, NIV may be attempted provided that the patient is carefully monitored. If the patient's state of consciousness and condition does not improve within 1–2 hours from initiating NIV, the patient should be intubated and ventilation should continue in invasive mode.[109,110] The higher the hypercapnia level, the lower the probability of improvement with NIV.[111]

## SALIENT POINTS

- Noninvasive ventilation is a recognized and effective method of treatment of respiratory failure. For NIV, there is no need to intubate the patient (that increase the risk of complications, mainly infectious) or the use of sedation that may extend the duration of mechanical ventilation.
- In contrast to invasive ventilation, this method can be used not only therapeutically, in developed respiratory failure, but also prophylactically, in borderline respiratory function, which often allow to avoid intubation.
- Noninvasive ventilation improves respiratory efficiency not only through the effects of positive inspiratory pressures but mainly by relieving the respiratory muscles through the pressure support of the patient's inspiration. For this reason, there is no need to use it continuously as it is necessary while applying invasive ventilation.
- Most often, we use NIV sessions lasting up to several hours between which the patient is able to, having refreshed respiratory muscles, breathe with less work of breathing and more efficiently eliminate airway secretions.

**Box 4:** Relative contraindications for noninvasive ventilation.
- Circulatory arrest
- Obstruction of the airways
- Uncooperative patient
- Protection of the airways is impossible
- High risk of choking
- Ineffective cough
- Severe disturbance of consciousness
- Status postsurgical procedures or trauma of the facial skeleton
- Anticipated long term of mechanical ventilation
- Fresh fixations in the esophageal region

- The most important conditions for the success of NIV are correct: (1) qualification for NIV and (2) respirator-patient synchronization.
- Proper synchronization is crucial for effective relief of the patient's respiratory muscles and depends on many factors, including, but not limited to, proper interface, leak control, selection of a proper ventilation mode, and adjustment of ventilation parameters to the patient's breathing pattern.

## REFERENCES

1. Demoule A, Girou E, Richard JC, et al. Increased use of noninvasive ventilation in French intensive care units. Intensive Care Med. 2006;32:1747-55.
2. Maheshwari V, Paioli D, Rothaar R, et al. Utilization of noninvasive ventilation in acute care hospitals: a regional survey. Chest. 2006;129:1226-33.
3. Bersten AD. Best practices for noninvasive ventilation. CMAJ. 2011;183:293-4.
4. Ambrosino N, Vagheggini G. Noninvasive positive pressure ventilation in the acute care setting: where are we? Eur Respir J. 2008;31:874-86.
5. Carrey Z, Gottfried SB, Levy RD. Ventilatory muscle support in respiratory failure with nasal positive pressure ventilation. Chest. 1990;97:150-8.
6. Vanpee D, el-Khawand C, Rousseau L, et al. Influence of respiratory behavior on ventilation, respiratory work and intrinsic PEEP during noninvasive nasal pressure support ventilation in normal subjects. Respiration. 2002;69:297-302.
7. Esquinas AM, Groff P, Cosentini R. Noninvasive ventilation in the emergency department: are protocols the key? Eur J Emerg Med. 2014;21:240.
8. Hill NS, Brennan J, Garpestad E, et al. Noninvasive ventilation in acute respiratory failure. Crit Care Med. 2007;35:2402-7.
9. Crimi C, Noto A, Princi P, et al. Survey of non-invasive ventilation practices: a snapshot of Italian practice. Minerva Anestesiol. 2011;77:971-8.
10. Crimi C, Noto A, Princi P, et al. A European survey of noninvasive ventilation practices. Eur Respir J. 2010;36:362-9.
11. Antonelli M, Conti G, Esquinas A, et al. A multiple-center survey on the use in clinical practice of noninvasive ventilation as a first-line intervention for acute respiratory distress syndrome. Crit Care Med. 2007;35:18-25.
12. Esquinas AM. Noninvasive mechanical ventilation: theory, equipment, and clinical applications. Berlin, London: Springer; 2010.
13. Esquinas AM, Egbert PS, Scala R, et al. Noninvasive mechanical ventilation in high-risk pulmonary infections: a clinical review. Eur Respir Rev. 2014;23:427-38.
14. Tobin MJ. Principles and practice of mechanical ventilation. New York: McGraw-Hill, Medical Pub. Division; 2006.
15. Antonelli M, Conti G, Bufi M, et al. Noninvasive ventilation for treatment of acute respiratory failure in patients undergoing solid organ transplantation: a randomized trial. JAMA. 2000;283:235-41.

16. Girou E, Schortgen F, Delclaux C, et al. Association of noninvasive ventilation with nosocomial infections and survival in critically ill patients. JAMA. 2000;284:2361-7.
17. Devlin JW, Nava S, Fong JJ, et al. Survey of sedation practices during noninvasive positive-pressure ventilation to treat acute respiratory failure. Crit Care Med. 2007;35:2298-302.
18. Girard TD, Kress JP, Fuchs BD, et al. Efficacy and safety of a paired sedation and ventilator weaning protocol for mechanically ventilated patients in intensive care (Awakening and Breathing Controlled trial): a randomised controlled trial. Lancet. 2008;371:126-34.
19. Nava S, Hill N. Non-invasive ventilation in acute respiratory failure. Lancet. 2009;374:250-9.
20. Nava S, Carbone G, DiBattista N, et al. Noninvasive ventilation in cardiogenic pulmonary edema: a multicenter randomized trial. Am J Respir Crit Care Med. 2003;168:1432-7.
21. Carlucci A, Delmastro M, Rubini F, et al. Changes in the practice of non-invasive ventilation in treating COPD patients over 8 years. Intensive Care Med. 2003;29:419-25.
22. Brochard L, Harf A, Lorino H, et al. Inspiratory pressure support prevents diaphragmatic fatigue during weaning from mechanical ventilation. Am Rev Respir Dis. 1989;139: 513-21.
23. Ferrer M, Valencia M, Nicolas JM, et al. Early noninvasive ventilation averts extubation failure in patients at risk: a randomized trial. Am J Respir Crit Care Med. 2006;173:164-70.
24. Mehta S, Hill NS. Noninvasive ventilation. Am J Respir Crit Care Med. 2001;163:540-77.
25. Liesching T, Kwok H, Hill NS. Acute applications of noninvasive positive pressure ventilation. Chest. 2003;124:699-713.
26. Keenan SP, Sinuff T, Burns KE, et al., Group CCCTGCCCSNVG. Clinical practice guidelines for the use of noninvasive positive-pressure ventilation and noninvasive continuous positive airway pressure in the acute care setting. CMAJ. 2011;183:E195-214.
27. Ram FS, Wellington S, Rowe BH, et al. Non-invasive positive pressure ventilation for treatment of respiratory failure due to severe acute exacerbations of asthma. Cochrane Database Syst Rev. 2005:CD004360.
28. Keenan SP, Sinuff T, Cook DJ, et al. Which patients with acute exacerbation of chronic obstructive pulmonary disease benefit from noninvasive positive-pressure ventilation? A systematic review of the literature. Ann Intern Med. 2003;138:861-70.
29. Williams TL. Effect of non-invasive ventilation on survival, quality of life, respiratory function and cognition: a review of the literature. Amyotroph Lateral Scler. 2007;8:317; author reply 317-318.
30. Ram FS, Picot J, Lightowler J, et al. Non-invasive positive pressure ventilation for treatment of respiratory failure due to exacerbations of chronic obstructive pulmonary disease. Cochrane Database Syst Rev. 2004:CD004104.
31. Chandra D, Stamm JA, Taylor B, et al. Outcomes of noninvasive ventilation for acute exacerbations of chronic obstructive pulmonary disease in the United States, 1998-2008. Am J Respir Crit Care Med. 2012;185:152-9.
32. Collaborative Research Group of Noninvasive Mechanical Ventilation for Chronic Obstructive Pulmonary Disease. Early use of non-invasive positive pressure ventilation for acute exacerbations of chronic obstructive pulmonary disease: a multicentre randomized controlled trial. Chin Med J (Engl). 2005;118:2034-40.
33. Keenan SP, Powers CE, McCormack DG. Noninvasive positive-pressure ventilation in patients with milder chronic obstructive pulmonary disease exacerbations: a randomized controlled trial. Respir Care. 2005;50:610-16.
34. Sliwinski P, Gorecka D, Jassem E, et al. [Polish respiratory society guidelines for chronic obstructive pulmonary disease]. Pneumonol Alergol Pol. 2014;82:227-63.
35. Celli BR, MacNee W, Force AET. Standards for the diagnosis and treatment of patients with COPD: a summary of the ATS/ERS position paper. Eur Respir J. 2004;23:932-46.
36. British Thoracic Society Standards of Care C. Non-invasive ventilation in acute respiratory failure. Thorax. 2002;57:192-211.
37. Conti G, Antonelli M, Navalesi P, et al. Noninvasive vs. conventional mechanical ventilation in patients with chronic obstructive pulmonary disease after failure of medical treatment in the ward: a randomized trial. Intensive Care Med. 2002;28:1701-7.
38. Peter JV, Moran JL, Phillips-Hughes J, et al. Effect of non-invasive positive pressure ventilation (NIPPV) on mortality in patients with acute cardiogenic pulmonary oedema: a meta-analysis. Lancet. 2006;367:1155-63.
39. Masip J. Noninvasive ventilation in acute cardiogenic pulmonary edema. Curr Opin Crit Care. 2008;14:531-5.
40. Masip J, Roque M, Sánchez B, et al. Noninvasive ventilation in acute cardiogenic pulmonary edema: systematic review and meta-analysis. JAMA. 2005;294:3124-30.
41. Filippatos G, Mebazaa A, Masip J. Noninvasive ventilation improved dyspnea but did not reduce short-term mortality in acute cardiogenic pulmonary edema. ACP J Club. 2008;149:9.
42. Weng CL, Zhao YT, Liu QH, et al. Meta-analysis: Noninvasive ventilation in acute cardiogenic pulmonary edema. Ann Intern Med. 2010;152:590-600.
43. Mehta S, Al-Hashim AH, Keenan SP. Noninvasive ventilation in patients with acute cardiogenic pulmonary edema. Respir Care. 2009;54:186-95.
44. Adda M, Coquet I, Darmon M, et al. Predictors of noninvasive ventilation failure in patients with hematologic malignancy and acute respiratory failure. Crit Care Med. 2008;36:2766-72.
45. Bello G, De Pascale G, Antonelli M. Noninvasive ventilation for the immunocompromised patient: always appropriate? Curr Opin Crit Care. 2012;18:54-60.
46. Aboussouan LS M-CE. Noninvasive Positive Pressure Support. Center for Continuing Education, Cleveland Clinic Foundation. 2014. [online] Available from http://www.clevelandclinicmeded.com/ [Last Accessed May 2019].]
47. Gristina GR, Antonelli M, Conti G, et al. Noninvasive versus invasive ventilation for acute respiratory failure in patients with hematologic malignancies: a 5-year multicenter observational survey. Crit Care Med. 2011;39:2232-9.

48. Aboussouan LS, Ricaurte B. Noninvasive positive pressure ventilation: Increasing use in acute care. Cleve Clin J Med. 2010;77:307-16.
49. Hilbert G, Gruson D, Vargas F, et al. Noninvasive ventilation in immunosuppressed patients with pulmonary infiltrates, fever, and acute respiratory failure. N Engl J Med. 2001;344:481-7.
50. Boles JM, Bion J, Connors A, et al. Weaning from mechanical ventilation. Eur Respir J. 2007;29:1033-56.
51. Ferrer M, Sellares J, Valencia M, et al. Non-invasive ventilation after extubation in hypercapnic patients with chronic respiratory disorders: randomised controlled trial. Lancet. 2009;374:1082-8.
52. Nava S, Gregoretti C, Fanfulla F, et al. Noninvasive ventilation to prevent respiratory failure after extubation in high-risk patients. Crit Care Med. 2005;33:2465-70.
53. Esteban A, Frutos-Vivar F, Ferguson ND, et al. Noninvasive positive-pressure ventilation for respiratory failure after extubation. N Engl J Med. 2004;350:2452-60.
54. Keenan SP, Powers C, McCormack DG, et al. Noninvasive positive-pressure ventilation for postextubation respiratory distress: a randomized controlled trial. JAMA. 2002;287:3238-44.
55. Ferrer M, Esquinas A, Leon M, et al. Noninvasive ventilation in severe hypoxemic respiratory failure: a randomized clinical trial. Am J Respir Crit Care Med. 2003;168:1438-44.
56. Trevisan CE, Vieira SR, Research Group in Mechanical Ventilation W. Noninvasive mechanical ventilation may be useful in treating patients who fail weaning from invasive mechanical ventilation: a randomized clinical trial. Crit Care. 2008;12:R51.
57. Burns KE, Adhikari NK, Meade MO. A meta-analysis of noninvasive weaning to facilitate liberation from mechanical ventilation. Can J Anaesth. 2006;53:305-15.
58. Martin TJ, Hovis JD, Costantino JP, et al. A randomized, prospective evaluation of noninvasive ventilation for acute respiratory failure. Am J Respir Crit Care Med. 2000;161:807-13.
59. Wysocki M, Tric L, Wolff MA, et al. Noninvasive pressure support ventilation in patients with acute respiratory failure. A randomized comparison with conventional therapy. Chest. 1995;107:761-8.
60. Hernandez G, Fernandez R, Lopez-Reina P, et al. Noninvasive ventilation reduces intubation in chest trauma-related hypoxemia: a randomized clinical trial. Chest. 2010;137:74-80.
61. Keenan SP, Sinuff T, Cook DJ, et al. Does noninvasive positive pressure ventilation improve outcome in acute hypoxemic respiratory failure? A systematic review. Crit Care Med. 2004;32:2516-23.
62. Agarwal R, Reddy C, Aggarwal AN, et al. Is there a role for noninvasive ventilation in acute respiratory distress syndrome? A meta-analysis. Respir Med. 2006;100:2235-8.
63. Nava S, Schreiber A, Domenighetti G. Noninvasive ventilation for patients with acute lung injury or acute respiratory distress syndrome. Respir Care. 2011;56:1583-8.
64. Agarwal R, Aggarwal AN, Gupta D. Role of noninvasive ventilation in acute lung injury/acute respiratory distress syndrome: a proportion meta-analysis. Respir Care. 2010;55:1653-60.
65. Zhan Q, Sun B, Liang L, et al. Early use of noninvasive positive pressure ventilation for acute lung injury: a multicenter randomized controlled trial. Crit Care Med. 2012;40:455-60.
66. Rana S, Jenad H, Gay PC, et al. Failure of non-invasive ventilation in patients with acute lung injury: observational cohort study. Crit Care. 2006;10:R79.
67. Robert D, Argaud L. Clinical review: long-term noninvasive ventilation. Crit Care. 2007;11:210.
68. Leger P, Bedicam JM, Cornette A, et al. Nasal intermittent positive pressure ventilation. Long-term follow-up in patients with severe chronic respiratory insufficiency. Chest. 1994;105:100-5.
69. Bach JR, Robert D, Leger P, et al. Sleep fragmentation in kyphoscoliotic individuals with alveolar hypoventilation treated by NIPPV. Chest. 1995;107:1552-8.
70. Robert D, Argaud L. Noninvasive positive ventilation in the treatment of sleep-related breathing disorders. Handb Clin Neurol. 2011;98:459-69.
71. Nicolini A, Banfi P, Grecchi B, et al. Non-invasive ventilation in the treatment of sleep-related breathing disorders: A review and update. Rev Port Pneumol. 2014;20:324-35.
72. Make BJ, Hill NS, Goldberg AI, et al. Mechanical ventilation beyond the intensive care unit. Report of a consensus conference of the American College of Chest Physicians. Chest. 1998;113:289S-344S.
73. Girault C, Briel A, Benichou J, et al. Interface strategy during noninvasive positive pressure ventilation for hypercapnic acute respiratory failure. Crit Care Med. 2009;37:124-31.
74. Cuvelier A, Pujol W, Pramil S, et al. Cephalic versus oronasal mask for noninvasive ventilation in acute hypercapnic respiratory failure. Intensive Care Med. 2009;35:519-26.
75. Conti G, Cavaliere F, Costa R, et al. Noninvasive positive-pressure ventilation with different interfaces in patients with respiratory failure after abdominal surgery: a matched-control study. Respir Care. 2007;52:1463-71.
76. Navalesi P. Internal space of interfaces for noninvasive ventilation: dead, but not deadly. Crit Care Med. 2009;37:1146-7.
77. Nava S, Navalesi P, Gregoretti C. Interfaces and humidification for noninvasive mechanical ventilation. Respir Care. 2009;54:71-84.
78. Nava S, Navalesi P. Helmet to deliver noninvasive ventilation: "Handle with care". Crit Care Med. 2009;37:2111-3.
79. Rocco M, Dell'Utri D, Morelli A, et al. Noninvasive ventilation by helmet or face mask in immunocompromised patients: a case-control study. Chest. 2004;126:1508-15.
80. Vignaux L, Vargas F, Roeseler J, et al. Patient-ventilator asynchrony during non-invasive ventilation for acute respiratory failure: a multicenter study. Intensive Care Med. 2009;35:840-6.
81. Fanfulla F, Taurino AE, Lupo ND, et al. Effect of sleep on patient/ventilator asynchrony in patients undergoing chronic non-invasive mechanical ventilation. Respir Med. 2007;101:1702-7.

82. Aboussouan LS, Khan SU, Meeker DP, et al. Effect of noninvasive positive-pressure ventilation on survival in amyotrophic lateral sclerosis. Ann Intern Med. 1997;127: 450-3.
83. Windisch W, Storre JH, Sorichter S, et al. Comparison of volume- and pressure-limited NPPV at night: a prospective randomized cross-over trial. Respir Med. 2005;99:52-9.
84. Nicolini AR, Barlascini CO, Sclifò F, et al. Mouthpiece ventilation in patients with neuromuscular disease. A brief clinical review. Phys Med Rehabil Int. 2014;1(3):1-4.
85. Bach JR. Amyotrophic lateral sclerosis: prolongation of life by noninvasive respiratory AIDS. Chest. 2002;122:92-8.
86. Bach JR, Alba AS, Saporito LR. Intermittent positive pressure ventilation via the mouth as an alternative to tracheostomy for 257 ventilator users. Chest. 1993;103:174-82.
87. Mellies U, Goebel C. Optimum insufflation capacity and peak cough flow in neuromuscular disorders. Ann Am Thorac Soc. 2014;11:1560-8.
88. Khirani S, Ramirez A, Delord V, et al. Evaluation of ventilators for mouthpiece ventilation in neuromuscular disease. Respir Care. 2014;59:1329-37.
89. Bach JR GM, Hon A, Ishikawa Y, et al. Changing trends in the management of end-stage neuromuscular respiratory muscle failure. Am J Phys Med Rehab. 2012;91:1.
90. Rabec C, Rodenstein D, Leger P, et al. Ventilator modes and settings during non-invasive ventilation: effects on respiratory events and implications for their identification. Thorax. 2011;66:170-8.
91. Janssens JP, Derivaz S, Breitenstein E, et al. Changing patterns in long-term noninvasive ventilation: a 7-year prospective study in the Geneva Lake area. Chest. 2003;123:67-79.
92. Schonhofer B, Sortor-Leger S. Equipment needs for noninvasive mechanical ventilation. Eur Respir J. 2002;20: 1029-36.
93. Gonzalez J, Sharshar T, Hart N, et al. Air leaks during mechanical ventilation as a cause of persistent hypercapnia in neuromuscular disorders. Intensive Care Med. 2003;29: 596-602.
94. Lofaso F, Fodil R, Lorino H, et al. Inaccuracy of tidal volume delivered by home mechanical ventilators. Eur Respir J. 2000;15:338-41.
95. Oscroft NS, Smith IE. A bench test to confirm the core features of volume-assured non-invasive ventilation. Respirology. 2010;15:361-4.
96. Sabil A MG, Prignet H, Orlikowski D, et al. Air leakage during nocurnal mechanical ventilation in patients with neuromuscular diseases. ITBM-RBM. 2006;27:227-32.
97. Mehta S, McCool FD, Hill NS. Leak compensation in positive pressure ventilators: a lung model study. Eur Respir J. 2001; 17:259-67.
98. Phillips-Respironics. Trilogy workshop. Koninklijke Philips Electronics NV: 2010:1-23.
99. Khirani S, Louis B, Leroux K, et al. Improvement of the trigger of a ventilator for non-invasive ventilation in children: bench and clinical study. Clin Resp J. 2014;10:559-66.
100. Thille AW, Contou D, Cordoba-Izquierdo A. Noninvasive ventilation for acute hypercapnic respiratory failure: is it the same as in hypercapnic coma?--reply. Respir Care. 2014; 59:e60-e61.
101. Nava S. Patient-ventilator interaction during noninvasive ventilation: practical assessment and theoretical basis. Breathe. 2009;5:323-33.
102. Williams JW, Cox CE, Hargett CW, Gilstrap DL, Castillo CE, Govert JA, et al. Noninvasive Positive-Pressure Ventilation (NPPV) for Acute Respiratory Failure, Rockville (MD); 2012.
103. Achour L, Letellier C, Cuvelier A, et al. Asynchrony and cyclic variability in pressure support noninvasive ventilation. Comput Biol Med. 2007;37:1308-20.
104. Nava S, Ceriana P. Causes of failure of noninvasive mechanical ventilation. Respir Care. 2004;49:295-303.
105. Lofaso F, Brochard L, Touchard D, et al. Evaluation of carbon dioxide rebreathing during pressure support ventilation with airway management system (BiPAP) devices. Chest. 1995;108:772-8.
106. Szkulmowski Z, Belkhouja K, Le QH, et al. Bilevel positive airway pressure ventilation: factors influencing carbon dioxide rebreathing. Intensive Care Med. 2010;36:688-91.
107. Miyoshi E, Fujino Y, Uchiyama A, et al. Effects of gas leak on triggering function, humidification, and inspiratory oxygen fraction during noninvasive positive airway pressure ventilation. Chest. 2005;128:3691-8.
108. Organized jointly by the American Thoracic Society tERS, the European Society of Intensive Care Medicine, and the Société de Réanimation de Langue Française, and approved by ATS Board of Directors, December 2000, International Consensus Conferences in Intensive Care Medicine: noninvasive positive pressure ventilation in acute Respiratory failure. Am J Respir Crit Care Med. 2001;163:283-91.
109. Díaz GG, Alcaraz AC, Talavera JC, et al. Noninvasive positive-pressure ventilation to treat hypercapnic coma secondary to respiratory failure. Chest. 2005;127:952-60.
110. Scala R, Naldi M, Archinucci I, et al. Noninvasive positive pressure ventilation in patients with acute exacerbations of COPD and varying levels of consciousness. Chest. 2005;128:1657-66.
111. Squadrone E, Frigerio P, Fogliati C, et al. Noninvasive vs invasive ventilation in COPD patients with severe acute respiratory failure deemed to require ventilatory assistance. Intensive Care Med. 2004;30:1303-10.

# CHAPTER 6

# Mechanical Ventilators

*Fabrice Galia, Samir Jaber, Audrey De Jong*

## BRIEF HISTORICAL RECALL OF VENTILATION

The concern for respiratory control and more particularly ventilation is very old. Major civilizations were already interested in ventilation 2,000 years ago. For example, the first tracheostomies were indirectly referenced in the *Rig Veda*, that is a group of written Indian texts of sciences between 1000 BC and 2000 BC.

The world continued being interested in breathing in the course of ages. In the 17th century, the first use of the bellows to insufflate air in the rib cage appeared, notably into the drowned men. However, its use was hanged by the academy of medicine of epoch because of undesirable effects it could cause (too big volumes or "Volotraumatismes" described by James Leroy d' Etiolles at the beginning of the 18th century).[1] This put a temporary end to the beginnings of positive pressure ventilation but opened the door to the concept of negative pressure ventilation with the patient inside the bellows generating overpressure and underpressure.

In the late 19th century, a first mechanical ventilator by external application of a variation in negative pressure was created by Alfred Jones; it was the "tank respirator" (1864), which worked with a super syringe.[2] A few years later, the French physician Eugène Woillez, following successful trials on its experimental model of porcine lung ventilated by applying an external negative pressure, created the spirophore, a device based on the principle of negative external pressure. The advent of mechanical ventilation was achieved through the "iron lung" by Drinker and Shaw, created in 1929, which operated by applying an external negative pressure on the chest wall to generate ventilation.[3] This type of ventilator was used for the treatment of poliomyelitis epidemics for the lengthy duration of ventilation in 1948 in the USA. In 1952 in Copenhagen, the high mortality rate (80%) due to the poliomyelitis epidemic and associated patients respiratory paralysis diminished only when the anesthesiologist Bjørn Ibsen decided to tracheostomize and ventilate patients with positive pressure breathing bag.[4] The first positive pressure ventilator was created in the early 20th century (Pulmotor by Henrich and Alexander Bernhard Dräger in 1907) and worked in pressure controlled ventilation mode at 20 mbar for inspiration while expiration was also facilitated by applying a negative pressure of −20 mbar.[5] From 1948 to 1993 many ventilators were developed (Table 1). Subsequently, in the years 1970–80, with electronic ventilators and the increase of ventilated patients, ventilators evolved (separation of the patient breathing circuit from machine, adjustable inspiratory time, pause time, cycling inspiration to expiration, triggering system to patient effort, and positive expiratory pressure).

Since the 80s, the evolution of ventilation in medical view followed the technological change, parallel with that of informatics.[6] Nowadays, the sensors became more precise (10 mL in volume and 0.1 mbar in pressure) and the ventilators integrate more powerful microprocessors. Many ventilatory modes appeared since 1990 but all did not consistently show an interest and a clinical effectiveness, and some even appeared to be noxious.[7-9]

## BASIC PRINCIPLE OF MECHANICAL VENTILATION

In medicine, mechanical ventilation[10] consists in compensating for or assisting spontaneous breathing with the help of a device named ventilator or artificial respirator. It is used in emergency context (emergency medicine, intensive care) or for general anesthesia, but can also be given at home to patients attained by chronic respiratory insufficiency.

A mechanical ventilator is a device which manages medical gases between the source of gases and the patient.

**Table 1:** Ventilators from 1948.

| Brand/Ventilator | Year | Brand/Ventilator | Year |
|---|---|---|---|
| Bennet TV-2P | 1948 | Engstrom Erica | 1980 |
| Engstrom 150 | 1950 | Siemens Servo 900C | 1982 |
| Dräger Poliomat | 1954 | Biomed IC-5 | 1983 |
| Thompson Portable Respirator | 1954 | Puritan Bennett 7200 | 1984 |
| Morch "Piston" | 1955 | Sechrist Adult 2200B | 1984 |
| Bird Mark 7 | 1955 | Dräger Evita | 1985 |
| Emerson High-Frequency Ventilator | 1955 | Bear Medical Bear 5 | 1985 |
| Emerson Assistor/Controller | 1958 | Ohmeda CPU | 1985 |
| Air-Shields 1000 | 1963 | Hamilton Veolar | 1986 |
| Puritan Bennett PR-2 | 1963 | Bird 6400 ST | 1986 |
| Emerson "Post-Op" 3-PV | 1964 | Infrasonics Infant Star | 1988 |
| Bourns LS-104-150 | 1964 | Bear 3 | 1988 |
| Puritan Bennett MA-1 | 1967 | Hamilton Amadeus | 1988 |
| Dräger Spiromat | 1968 | Siemens E | 1988 |
| Ohio/Monaghan 560 | 1968 | Bird 8400 ST | 1989 |
| Loos Co. Amsterdam | 1968 | Bunnel Life Pulse | 1989 |
| Engstrom 300 | 1968 | Dräger PPG IRISA | 1989 |
| Verifo CV 2000 | 1970 | Bird VIP | 1989 |
| Hamilton Standard PAD 1 | 1970 | Infrasonics Adult Star | 1989 |
| Monaghan 225 | 1972 | Siemens Servo 300 | 1991 |
| Bird Baby Bird | 1972 | Bear 100 | 1993 |
| Bird IMV Bird | 1972 | **Among many new** | |
| Siemens Servo 900/900B | 1972 | Dräger Evita (s) | **From 1993 to now** |
| Chemtron Gill 1 | 1973 | Hamilton Galileo(s) | |
| Emerson IMV | 1974 | Maquet Servo (x) | |
| Searle VVA | 1974 | Puritan Bennett PB 840 | |
| Ohio 550 | 1974 | General Electrics Engström | |
| Bourns Bear 1 | 1975 | Puritan Bennett 980 | |
| Forreger 21D | 1976 | Dräger V500 | |
| Puritan Bennett MA-2 | 1978 | Hamilton S1 | |

## GAS SUPPLY

### Air

To provide air to a mechanical ventilator there are two main types of gas supply. For the first type of gas supply, medical air is compressed at 3–6 bars, filtered, and dried by specific and dedicated air compressors within the hospital facilities.

For the second type of gas supply, turbines situated within the device take ambient air from the room to pressurize it within the ventilator.

### Other Medical Gases

Oxygen is supplied in the same manner like air or in pressurized cylinder. Other medical gases (e.g. NO, $N_2$) are often supplied in cylinders.

Then gases are mixed at the specific melange setting controlled by the anesthetist or automatically by the device.

Last, according to the settings ventilatory mode, a flow or pressure generator delivers the gas to the patient inspiratory limb.

## TURBINE OR WALL GAS

On the one hand, a turbine (Figs. 1A and B) is a rotary mechanism which extracts air from room to pressurize it into the ventilator. A turbine did not need compressed wall type gas.

On the other hand, compressed wall type gas are delivered at 3–6 bars to the ventilator and then to a servo-valve. A servo-valve is an electronic and hydraulic valve which receives a pressurized hydraulic fluid and pressurizes it to a cylinder proportionally to a received electrical signal.

Most of anesthesia ventilators and intensive care unit (ICU) ventilators are connected to wall type gas outlets. Transport ventilators are connected to oxygen cylinder and a turbine or air pressure driven by oxygen. Home ventilators are often equipped with turbine and sometimes with oxygen cylinder.

In a study made by Thille AW, et al.[11] on ICU ventilators in 2009, four turbine-based ventilators (Resmed/Elisée 350, Respironics/Esprit, Dräger Medical/Savina, Carefusion/Vela) were compared to nine servo-valve compressed gas-based ventilators (Carefusion/Avea, Newport Medical Instruments/E500, General Electric Healthcare/Engstöm and Centiva, Air Liquide/Extend, Dräger Medical/Evita XL, Hamilton Medical/Galileo, Tyco/PB840, Maquet/Servo-i) on a test lung model. On average, they found that turbine-based ventilators had a slightly shorter triggering at 51 ms vs. 62 ms delay in pressure support with a greater pressurization.

More recently, Delgado C, et al.[12] showed that pressure support ventilation (PSV) mode worked properly for each of their seven bench-tested turbine-based ventilators and triggering and pressurization in PSV were superior in the newest machines (Hamilton Medical/C2, Philips-Respironics/V60, Respironics/Trilogy, Philips-Respironics/

# Chapter 6
## Mechanical Ventilators

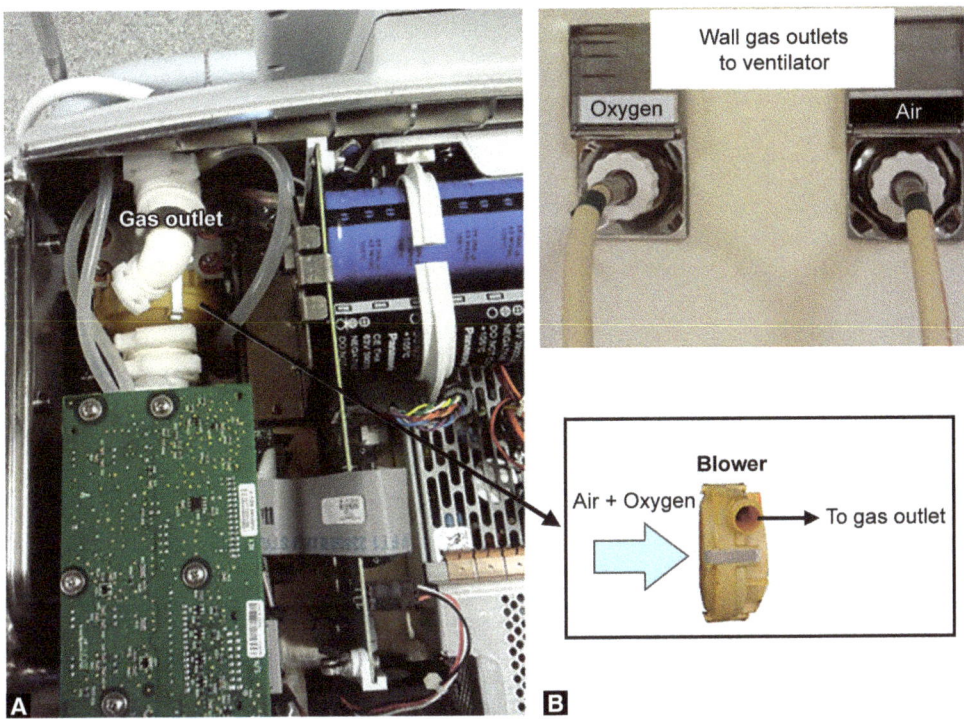

**Figs. 1A and B:** Wall and gas turbine. (A) Inside of ventilator with turbine (blower) to provide air supply. Air and oxygen are mixed and then pressurized with the blower; (B) Gas provided by wall gas outlets to the mixer of the ventilator and then to the servo-valve to provide breath according to the settings.

V680) to the oldest ones (Carefusion/Vela, Dräger Medical/Savina, Dräger Medical/Carina).

Turbine-based ventilators work properly and slightly better than conventional compressed gas-based ventilators. Such devices are found in area of home care, ICU or continuing care unit.

## TRIGGERING

In spontaneous or assisted controlled modes of ventilation, triggering is a major component. It is the detection by the device of the start of a breath by the patient. Then the ventilator triggers a cycle either in pressure or in volume. To achieve this triggering, muscles of the patient, diaphragm and/or accessory muscles have to generate a depression which produces a flow within the trachea. Then when, flow, volume or depression exceeds the triggering threshold, the mechanical ventilator triggers a cycle.

Basically, trigger types can be split between flow trigger and pressure trigger. For pressure triggering, patient effort has to overcome the pressure threshold set on the ventilator. For flow trigger, a continuous flow-by-flows within the circuit, and when there is a deviation of flow or measured volume that overcomes the flow threshold, the ventilator triggers. 20 years ago, Sassoon CS et al.[13] estimated that flow-triggering appears to offer measurable advantages over pressure-triggering, particularly during spontaneous breathing.

With modernization of devices, there are less and less differences between pressure triggering and flow triggering even though flow triggering showed a better efficiency with less workload of patient in the past[13-15] and that most of ICU ventilators propose this type of trigger. For some ICU ventilators, Thille et al.[11] found that a technological ceiling may have been reached when comparing ventilator generation between 2000 and 2006 in terms of pressurization and triggering. A similar result on recent ICU ventilators has been found in terms of triggering delay between 50 ms and 100 ms by Garnier et al. (Fig. 2).[16] When comparing one ICU ventilator to mid-level ICU ventilator Ferreira et al.[17] concludes that most mid-level ICU ventilators do not perform as well as the ICU one even though 6 ventilators on 11 had a triggering delay around 100 ms whatever the level of effort. Of note, one ventilator has based one part of its triggering on electrical activity of the diaphragm measured by a probe situated in the nasogastric tube.[18]

If the patient cannot trigger the ventilator, controlled or assisted controlled ventilation in pressure or volume is used. Respiratory rate (RR) is set by the physician and the

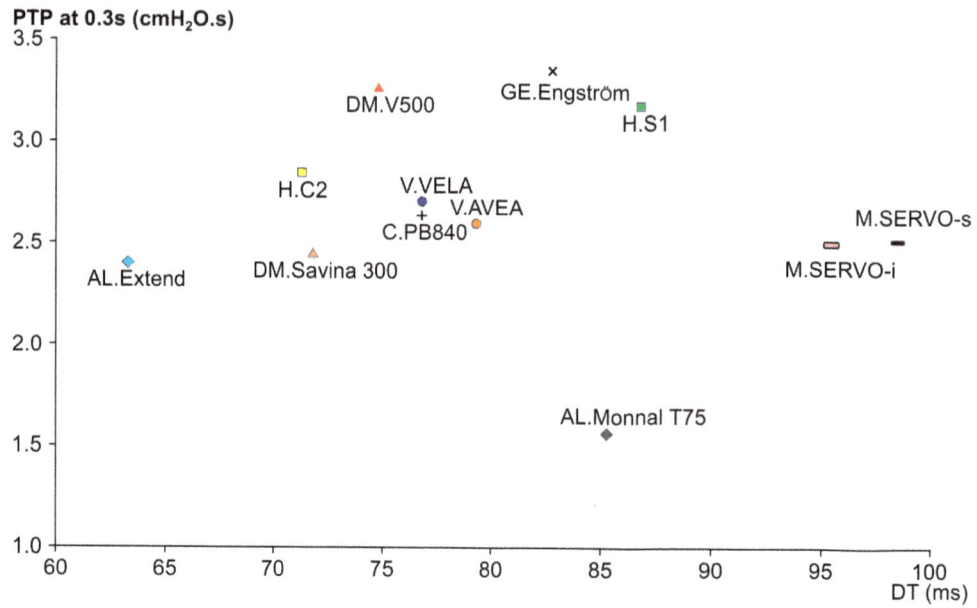

**Fig. 2:** Comparison of pressurization and triggering. Pressurization performance (PTP at 0.3 s) vs. triggering delay of recent ventilators studied on bench.[16] PTP at 0.3s: pressure time product at 0.3s from onset of effort, DT: trigger delay, AL: air liquide, C: covidien, DM: dräger medical, GE: general electics, H: hamilton, M: maquet, V: viasys.

ventilator provides a defined breath to the patient at the selected rate.

## CYCLING

When a cycle is triggered and the setting either volume or pressure is reached, then comes the cycling from inspiratory phase to expiratory phase.

In PSV, cycling depends on the maximum inspiratory flow. Thus the cycling threshold is a percentage of the maximum inspiratory flow or a flow value. During inspiration, after the maximum inspiratory flow has been reached, as soon as the flow decreases under the threshold, the ventilator stops insufflation and open exhalation valve until level of positive end-expiratory pressure (PEEP).

In continuous mandatory ventilation (CMV), cycling is set on time. Thus, as soon as inspiratory time (Ti) is reached, cycling is processed.

## CIRCUIT

For most of ICU ventilators, a dual limb circuit is used. This circuit is composed of one inspiratory limb by which fresh gas is provided to the Y-piece of the circuit at which are connected either an endotracheal tube or a tracheal cannula or a face mask if noninvasive ventilation (NIV) is used. Inspiratory sensors, inside the ventilators, allow the measure of inspiratory volume and flow.

At exhalation, the gas goes from the patient lungs to expiratory limb through the tube by mechanical retraction of chest and lungs. Sensors positioned at the end of expiratory limb within the ventilator measure inspiratory and expiratory pressures, and expiratory flow and volumes. PEEP is monitored and maintained through these sensors. A heat and moisture exchanger or a heated humidifier allows gas conditioning by heating and humidifying cold and dry medical gas.

For some ventilators (NIV, home), single limb circuit is sometimes used. This single inspiratory limb brings gas to the patient. It is provided at the distal end of the circuit either with intentional calibrated leaks (whisper swivel or mask with conditioned leaks) or with exhalation valve which opens at expiration to avoid $CO_2$ rebreathing. Whisper swivel valves are associated with $CO_2$ rebreathing; while nonrebreathing valves with more effort according to Lofaso et al.[19] However, in their study on nasal ventilation, Hill NS et al.[20] found no advantages in substituting plateau exhalation valve to whisper swivel. As compared to dual limb, single limb circuits are lighter and cheaper but with less advanced technology than dual limb ventilators.

## VENTILATION IN ICU

Schematically, the ventilation of a patient is a succession of stages (Table 2). Initially, if the clinician estimates that the patient will not manage to ensure suitably his/her own

## Chapter 6
## Mechanical Ventilators

**Table 2:** Ventilatory modes.

| Mode | Main setting | Type | Process | Settings | Monitoring | Interests | Limits |
|------|-------------|------|---------|----------|------------|-----------|--------|
| V-CMV | Flow/Volume | Controlled | Cycles set on ventilator | TV RR PEEP $FiO_2$ Ti Flow | Pplat PPeak | Control of VE | No spontaneous activity of the patient possible |
| P-CMV | Pressure | Controlled | Cycles set on ventilator | PINSP RR PEEP $FiO_2$ Ti Te | TV VE | Control of VE | No spontaneous activity of the patient possible |
| V-ACV | Flow/Volume | Assisted | V-CMV with possible triggering by patient | TV RR PEEP $FiO_2$ Ti Flow | Pplat PPeak VE | Control of minimum VE; Allow an increase of VE on patient will | Decrease of VE impossible even though patient wants |
| P-ACV | Pressure | Assisted | P-CMV with possible triggering by patient | PINSP RR PEEP $FiO_2$ Ti Te | TV VE | Theoretical control of minimum VE; Allow an increase of VE on patient will | Decrease of VE impossible even though patient wants |
| PSV | Pressure | Assisted | Pressure level set on ventilator with patient's triggering and cycling | Pinsp PEEP $FiO_2$ | TV VE | Allows spontaneous activity. Only mode for which patient chooses his Ti and so his TV | Set assistance while patient needs are variable with time |
| SIMV | Flow/Volume | Controlled | V-CMV with possible spontaneous breaths | TV RR PEEP $FiO_2$ Ti Flow | Pplat PPeak VE | Allows controlleds cycles with spontaneous breaths | Patient's muscles don't rest on controlled cycles |
| BIPAP | Pressure | Controlled | PCV with possible spontaneous breaths | Pinsp RR PEEP $FiO_2$ Ti Te | TV VE | Theoretical control of minimum VE; Allows spontaneous breaths | Set assistance while patient needs are variable with time |

V-CMV: volume continuous mandatory ventilation; P-CMV: pressure continuous mandatory ventilation; V-ACV: volume assist control ventilation; P-ACV: pressure assist control ventilation; PSV: pressure support ventilation; SIMV: synchronized intermittent ventilation; BIPAP: bilevel positive airway pressure; TV: tidal volume; RR: respiratory rate; PEEP: positive end expiratory pressure; $FiO_2$: fraction of inspired oxygen; Ti: inspiratory time; Te: expiratory time; VE: minute ventilation (Vt × RR); Pplat: plateau pressure; Ppeak: inspiratory peak pressure; Pinsp: set inspiratory pressure.

ventilation efficiently, the patient is placed in volume- or pressure-continuous mandatory ventilation. When the respiratory state of the patient improves, the clinician can then place him in assist-control ventilation which is close to continuous mandatory ventilation except that the patient can start or trigger the ventilatory cycles. Spontaneous ventilation with inspiratory assistance also known as PSV, that is a mode for which the clinician sets the level of pressure brought by the ventilator to the patient, is then used followed by the weaning of mechanical ventilation and the return to spontaneous breathing without assistance. These stages correspond to conventional ventilation.[21]

## Continuous Mandatory Ventilation or Assist-Control Ventilation

Continuous mandatory ventilation (CMV) or controlled ventilation (Fig. 3) is a mode for which, because of sedation (and curarization) or by incapacity of the patient, ventilation is fully controlled by the ventilator, according to the settings made by the clinician. The clinician sets most of the ventilatory settings for the patient. In assist-control ventilation (ACV), the possibility exists for the patient to trigger the respiratory cycles with a minimum value of RR, set by the clinician. Triggering depends on the value of the threshold set in flow or pressure as well as sedation of the patient, of patient muscular force, and his/her pulmonary hyperinflation.

### CMV/ACV in Volume

Volumetric CMV mode is more used than the barometric one in ICU.[22] The clinician sets the tidal volume (Vt), RR, the inspiratory flow (often of square waveform), PEEP (pressure higher than the atmospheric pressure in airways during expiration), and the time of inspiration with the inspiratory pause time. The pressures must be monitored.

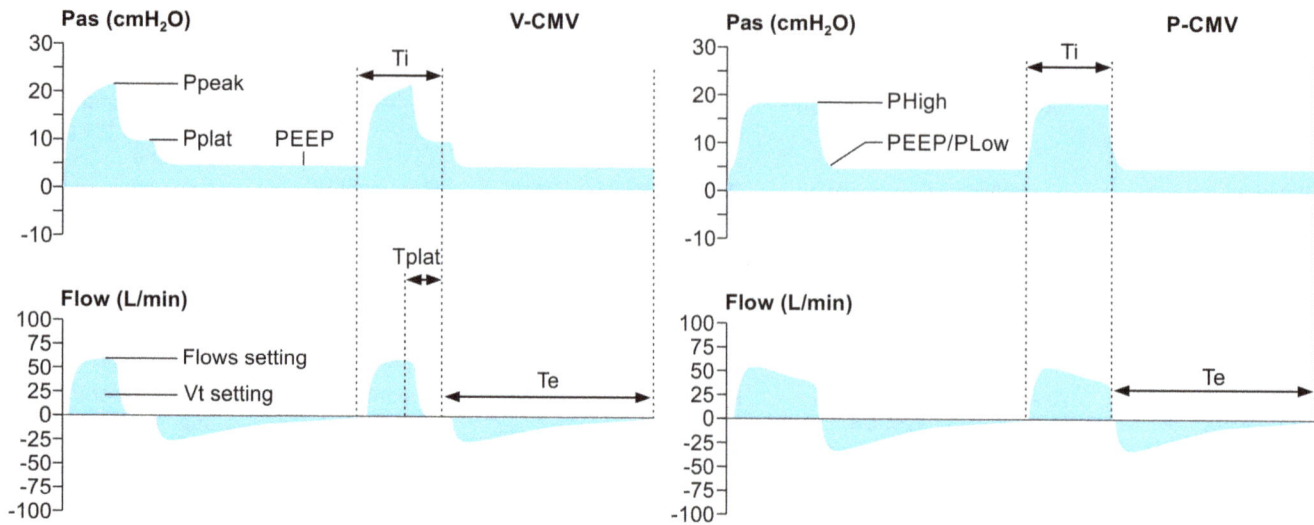

**Fig. 3:** Ventilatory modes P-CMV and V-CMV. Presentation of main ventilatory parameters of continuous mandatory ventilation in volume (V-CMV) and pressure (P-CMV) waveforms. Paw: pressure airway; PHigh: high pressure setting; Ppeak: maximum peak pressure within a breath; Pplat: plateau pressure; PEEP/PLow: positive end expiratory pressure; Vt: tidal volume; Ti: inspiratory time; Te: expiratory time; Tplat: plateau time (no flow).

A minimum minute ventilation is always assured (RR.Vt). To avoid the risks of barotraumatism or volotraumatism, many recommendations exist for the use, the monitoring, and the settings of this mode. In particular, the value of plateau pressure (pressure at end of inspiration with zero flow, which represents the maximum alveolar pressure at end of inspiration) must be lower than 30 mbar. Some clinical studies showed that a higher Vt (>12 mL per kilo of predicted body weight) could cause volotraumatism and that for some restrictive pathologies such as the acute respiratory distress syndrome, 6 mL/kg of Vt or less was recommended and was associated with decreased mortality.[23] The main reason to use this mode is the discharge of the respiratory workload for the patient, the improvement of blood gases and ventilatory function. The limitation of CMV/ACV in volume is its setting of a certain number of constraints on the ventilation of the patient[24] (flow, volume, frequency).

### CMV/ACV in Pressure

In barometric CMV mode, the clinician sets the settings of pressure to be reached, RR, PEEP, and inspiratory time per cycle with this pressure. The waveform of the inspiratory flow is decelerating due to the flow decrease when it has reached the pressure target. In this ventilatory mode, it is important to monitor volume as it is not controlled by the ventilator. Ventilation minute is not controlled either and depends on the respiratory mechanics of the patient which can change during ventilation. In clinical practice, any increase in resistances of the airways (obstruction, clogged tube, bronchospasm) results in a reduction of the inspiratory flow and Vt.[25]

### Volume versus Pressure

Choosing the best appropriate ventilation mode to the patients' lung conditions is a very important question. Recent reviews[22,26] of randomized controlled trials showed no superiority of one mode to another in patients suffering of acute lung injury or acute respiratory distress syndrome. Current recommendations are to use the ventilation mode that allows the clinician to reach the objectives individually adapted to the clinical condition of the patient in the most effective way possible.[22]

ACV/CMV is not a mode adapted for ventilatory weaning because of many ventilatory constraints imposed to the patient, of possible associated sedation, and patient's impossibility to carry out a spontaneous respiratory activity. Ventilatory weaning is usually carried out via pressure support ventilation (PSV).[27]

## Pressure Support Ventilation

Pressure support ventilation (Fig. 4) is a mode in pressure known as of ventilatory assistance to the patient. The patient triggers all his/her breathing cycles, and the ventilator assists him during inspiration by generating a pressure (Fig. 2) set by the clinician.[28] When the inspiratory flow decreases up to the threshold value of flow stopping (expiratory trigger, by default set at 25% of peak flow for most ventilators), the ventilator ends the inspiratory phase

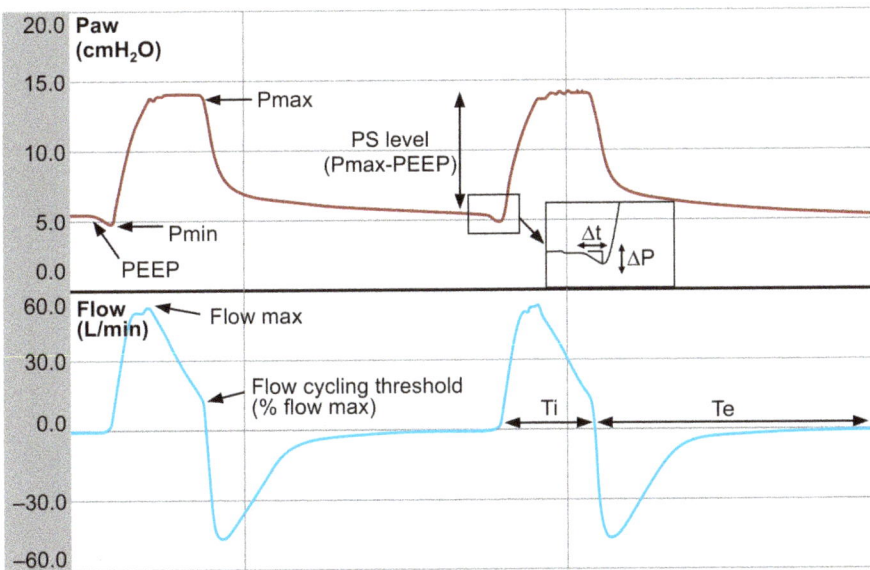

**Fig. 4:** Pressure support ventilation mode. Presentation of main ventilatory parameters including triggering and cycling of pressure support ventilation. Paw: airway pressure; Pmax: maximum airway pressure within a breath; PEEP: positive end expiratory pressure; PS level: pressure support level above PEEP; Pmin: minimum pressure during trigger phase; $\Delta t$: trigger delay from onset of effort to ventilator start of pressurization; $\Delta P$: pressure drop during trigger phase (PEEP-Pmin); Ti: inspiratory time; Te: expiratory time.

and turns in expiratory phase (inspiration-expiration transition or cycling). In this barometric mode, the clinician will set the pressure level of inspiratory assistance (pressure support, PS), the level of PEEP, the value of the inspiratory triggering threshold, and the slope of pressure rise. The clinician sets the ventilatory parameters according to the patient response in terms of RR, Vt, and clinical tolerance.[25] Consequently, as a barometric mode of assistance, the data to be monitored will be RR (spontaneous) as well as patient's Vt. This more physiological mode can be used in a ventilatory context of weaning associated with low level pressure (<10 mbar); then it is very close to spontaneous breathing. Moreover, this mode can also be used in an acuter phase with little sedation for which synchronization between patient and ventilator will be better than in controlled volume or pressure modes.

## VENTILATION APART ICU

Mechanical ventilators are used at home for sleep troubles or chronic disease, in anesthesia, for transport within hospital or outside for emergency medical services (EMS), for adults or children.

### Anesthesia Ventilators

The anesthesia ventilator has different objectives:[29]
- Managing ventilation that is removing carbon dioxide ($CO_2$) from alveoli and bringing oxygen.
- Gas conditioning that is heating and humidifying gas.
- Managing halogenated anesthetic agents by bringing them to alveoli.

Different types of ventilator systems exist depending upon flow generator type (ascending or descending bellow, volume reflector) and recycling of halogenated anesthetic agents with $CO_2$ elimination.

The main specific parts of an anesthesia ventilator are:
- A gas mixer which can blend oxygen with air and possibly with nitrous oxide.
- A flow generator which can both pressurize and mix gas (expiratory ascending bellows, volume reflector) or pressurizes them only (turbine, piston, expiratory descending bellows).
- A circled breathing system with unidirectional inspiratory and expiratory valves ideally with a heating system to avoid condensation inside the breathing system.
- A soda lime canister which allows $CO_2$ absorption and rebreathing of exhaled halogenic agents.
- A reservoir bag to receive and mix fresh continuous flow gas and intermittent expired gas.
- A servo valve which drives exceeding gas to scavenging interface.
- A scavenging system which evacuates anesthetic gases outside of the operating room.
- A system for spontaneous and manual ventilation which requires a reservoir bag and an adjustable pressure limiting valve (APL valve).

- A gas analyzer system for measuring inspiratory and expiratory gas concentration.
- A fast oxygen delivery (oxygen flush) which can deliver oxygen high flow to manage hypoxemia or sudden leaks on the breathing system.
- An emergency oxygen supply and its breathing system to manually ventilate the patient in case of ventilator failure.

There are different types of anesthesia ventilators according to their flow generator type. The oldest have descending (hanging) bellows during expiratory phase while most of newest have ascending (standing) bellows at expiration and could be safer.[30] Among ascending bellows ventilators there are Kion (Siemens), Felix (Air Liquide), Avance (General Electric Healthcare) and among descending bellows anesthesia ventilators are Leon plus (Heinen und Loewenstein), Julian (Dräger Medical). Some ventilators use other techniques: Zeus and Perseus (Dräger Medical) ventilators use turbine, Primus (Dräger Medical) use cylinder with piston, Flow-i (Maquet) use Volume reflector.™

Concerning performances of anesthesia ventilators, in a bench test study made 10 years ago, Jaber S et al.[31] have shown that recent anesthesia ventilators of this time showed comparable results to some ICU ventilators in terms of triggering, below 100 ms, and pressurization in PSV mode.

In a recent bench test study, Wallon G et al.[32] showed that alteration of respiratory mechanisms or fresh gas flow may impair accuracy of Vt delivery of most recent anesthesia ventilators (General Electric/Aisys, Maquet/Flow-i, Dräger Medical/Primus, Dräger Medical/Zeus) even though not clinically significant. In his PhD report on mechanical ventilation,[33] Coisel Y showed (Fig. 5) that accuracy of measure of delivered Vt is in the expected range with less than 10% difference but worth than that of ICU ventilators.

Another main characteristic of the anesthesia ventilator is the closed or opened breathing circuit. With opened circuit ventilators (e.g. ICU ventilators), there is no rebreathing of $CO_2$ or halogenated agents, a higher fresh gas flow than minute ventilation allows a cleaning of the circuit. The main disadvantage in the opened circuit is the loss of anesthetic agents during each patient exhalation resulting in higher costs.

With semi-closed circuit, fresh gas flow is higher than patient minute volume, and there is rebreathing with soda canister to remove $CO_2$. An exhausting valve allows evacuation of gas excess.

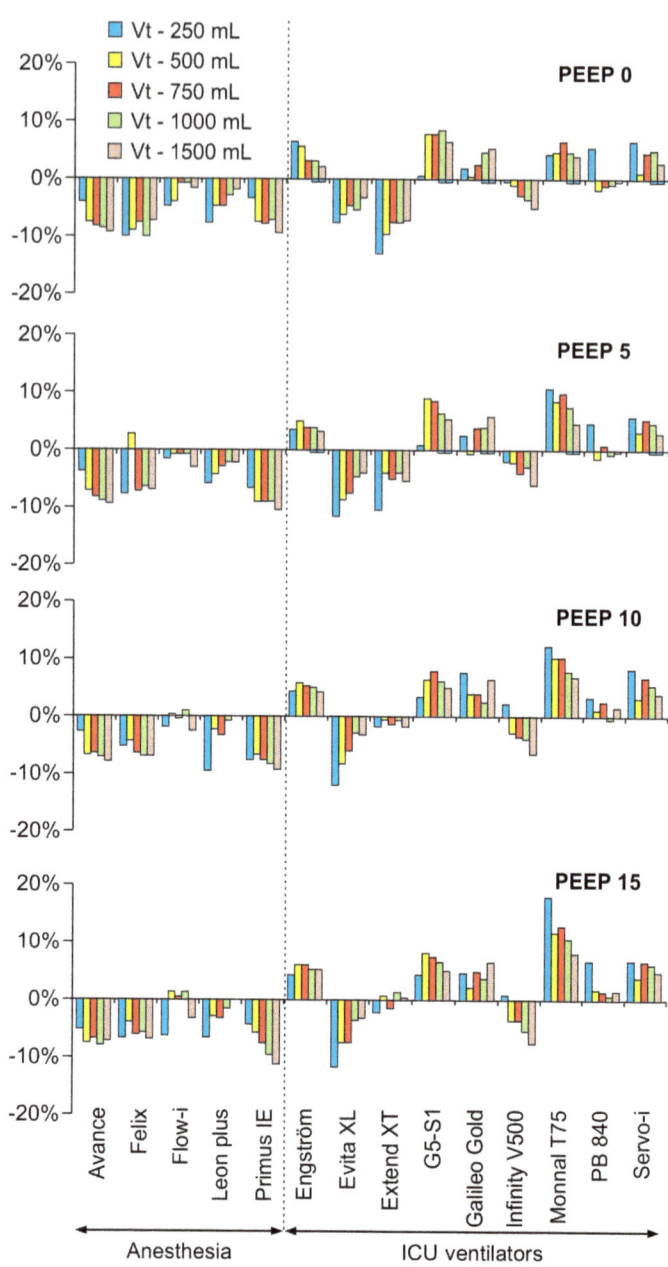

**Fig. 5:** Accuracy of expired tidal volume measurement. Measurement on bench[33] of accuracy of ICU and Anesthesia ventilators. Measures are made without end-inspiratory pause.
*Source:* With permission from Dr. Coisel Yannael.

With closed circuits, fresh gas flow equals minute volume, there is a full rebreathing of expired gas through soda canister and reuse of expired halogenated agents.

Some closed circuits ventilators (Dräger Medical Zeus, Air Liquide Felix, General Electric Healthcare Aisys) allow closed-loop target-controlled anesthesia[34] for volatile anesthetics management. These ventilators use feedback gas measurements to control direct injection of gas in the breathing circuit. For example, expired fraction of oxygen gives information on patient preoxygenation[35] and allows to adapt fraction of inspired oxygen ($FiO_2$) level. Feedback gas allows an adapted administration of anesthetics agents.

## Emergency Medical Services and Transport Ventilators

Transport ventilators are frequently used in daily practice, although transport of ventilated patients remains potentially dangerous. The ventilator should be adapted to the type of transport. Recovery room ventilators do not need the same specifications than prehospital or ICU patients transport ones.

For critically ill patients, ventilators should have adjustable $FiO_2$, reliable PEEP, continuous monitoring of pressure, flow, and end tidal $CO_2$ waves.

Ideal transport ventilator[36] should be solid and resistant, with moderate size and weight. Its electrical autonomy should be sufficient. With user-friendly human-machine interface, it should monitor main ventilatory settings among which RR, Vt, PEEP, peak pressure, plateau pressure, possibly end-tidal $CO_2$ and delivered $FiO_2$.

In terms of performances, L'Her E et al.[37] made an exhaustive bench study on 26 emergency and transport ventilators. They found heterogeneity in terms of characteristics and performances of ventilators and that some of them may be influenced by lung mechanics or leaks. Sophisticated transport ventilators, with waves display and NIV mode, tend to have better results than simple ones, even though probably more expensive. All sophisticated ones have acceptable accuracy in Vt with less than 10% difference at setting whatever the resistance.

In terms of triggering, among sophisticated devices, LTV 1200 (Viasys Carefusion), T1 (Hamilton Medical) and T60 (Air Liquide) have inspiratory delay, which is the time during triggering before return to PEEP level after triggering at start of pressurization, below 200 ms and 3 others, Crossvent 3 (Bio-Med Devices), Elisée 350 (Resmed) and iVent 201 (General Electric Healthcare) have inspiratory delay below 300 ms among 10 evaluated ventilators. Last in terms of pressurization accuracy with leaks, among sophisticated ventilators, Elisée 350 (Resmed), M. Transport (Weinmann), Oxylog 3000 (Dräger Medical), and T1 (Hamilton Medical) have less than 5% difference as compared to settings. Newport™ HT70 (Medtronic) and T60 (Air Liquide) have less than 10%.

## EVOLUTION OF MECHANICAL VENTILATION

Modern mechanical ventilation started more than 50 years ago. In 2002, Richard JC, et al.[38] found in a bench test study on 22 ventilators that, in terms of triggering and pressurization in PSV, new generation ventilators post 1993 outperformed most of previous generation ones. A few years later, Thille et al.[11] performed a similar study on 13 ICU ventilators and concluded that ICU ventilators seemed to have reached a technical ceiling. In this way, industrialists tend to center ventilators development on more user-friendly human-machine interface such as interactive-touch screen setting availability and new advanced ventilatory modes.

With technological advance, new modern modes[39,40] using more powerful sensors were developed by the industrialists sometimes in collaboration with the clinicians. The principle of these modes is to be more physiological and/or to reduce the load of the clinician in terms of control and handling of the ventilator. Main ventilator parameters are automatically set as a function of one or more ventilatory data, while being based on more or less complex physiological models and by introducing rules of clinical guidelines. The base of these modes of ventilation is the closed-loop operation. These modes self-set their control according to the measured ventilatory data, by adjusting their parameters according to clinical algorithms. The current closed-loop modes are the Neurally Adjusted Ventilatory Assist (NAVA®, Maquet) and Proportional Assist Ventilation Plus (PAV+®, Medtronic-Covidien) as well as Intellivent-Adaptive Support Ventilation (Intellivent-ASV®, Hamilton Medical) and SmartCare® (Dräger Medical).

## NAVA® AND PAV+®

The two first modes, NAVA and PAV+, in pressure, base their closed-loop on the evaluation of the patient's inspiratory effort. They reply with a pressure proportional to the effort of the patient and require an adjustment of the ventilatory assistance's gain.

### NAVA®[18]

In NAVA®, the assistance signal of control corresponds to the electric activity of the diaphragm (EAdi) collected by a esophageal catheter equipped with electrodes. The algorithm filters and calculates the signal amplitude. Then the ventilator provides a pressure proportional to the Eadi signal times a set gain constant. The greater the constant, the greater assistance the patient will receive.

### PAV Plus®[41]

In PAV Plus®, the pressure produced by the ventilator is proportional to the ventilatory demand; the more effort the patient exerts, the more the machine assists and, conversely, if the demand diminishes, the less the machine assists. Ventilator continuously measures the pulmonary characteristics of the patient's lung, resistance, and compliance. The system instantaneously measures flow and volume, and knowing resistance and compliance, provides a pressure proportional to patient effort determined by the algorithm breath by breath. The clinician sets a percentage of assistance corresponding to the part of work of breathing assisted by the ventilator.

## INTELLIVENT-ASV® AND SMARTCARE®

Intellivent-ASV® and SmartCare® are adaptive modes respectively cycle-by-cycle and on 2–5 minutes which adapt their level of assistance according to the ventilatory data of the previous periods and of safety clinical instructions as well as of patient's effort optimization or weaning. These modes can be used from the acute phase of the patient disease until weaning.

### Intellivent-ASV[42,43]

Adaptive support ventilation is a ventilatory mode which, according to RR and Vt, will regulate cycle-by-cycle its level of inspiratory support according to an algorithm. ASV proposes to maintain a preset minute ventilation by taking into account the spontaneous respiratory cycles, adding some pressure-controlled ventilatory cycles if necessary and adapting pressure level to provide the desired Vt. Intellivent is based on ASV but minute ventilation objective is automatically adjusted to maintain end-tidal $CO_2$ within expert-defined ranges. Furthermore, it adjusts automatically PEEP and $FiO_2$ settings function of pulsatil oxygen saturation ($SpO_2$) and based on acute respiratory distress syndrome (ARDS) network PEEP-$FiO_2$ table.

### SmartCare[44,45]

The system functions with the ventilatory mode clinically used which is PSV. Its operation is based on three essential principles:
a. Maintaining the patient in a respiratory comfort zone by adapting the level of pressure support
b. Progressive decrease of the level of pressure support in the event of patient stability
c. Automated attempt of weaning tests with a minimum level of pressure support followed by the posting of a message if these tests are positive.

The algorithm used by SmartCare is based on RR, Vt, and expired $CO_2$ ($etCO_2$) of the patient, obtained from the ventilator data each 2 or 5 minutes, and on data thresholds set by ventilation experts.

Interests of these adaptive servo-controlled modes are various. These modes are more physiological and in constant harmony with the patient's ventilation. Moreover, clinicians cannot monitor patients as frequently as an adaptative servo-controlled mode, which does it cycle-by-cycle or every 2 or 5 minutes. The ventilator could therefore be better adapted to the patient, potentially reducing sedation requirement and associated length of mechanical ventilation,[46,47] stay, and associated morbidity and mortality. However, in particular situations, these modes could not be as efficient as the individualized setting of ventilation by the experimented physician[48] and some settings are still remained to be made for proportional modes.

## USABILITY

As noticed in the study by Marjanovic NS et al.,[49] recent ventilators are very close in terms of technical efficiency; the difference being now based on usability which may be related to safety.[50]

Morita PP and Marjanovic NS,[49,50] studies are different in terms of place (USA and France ICUs), recruitment (48 respiratory therapists and 20 senior physicians), used simulators (dedicated simulator and test lung) but compared almost the same recent modern ventilators G5-S1 (Hamilton Medical), PB980 (Medtronic-Covidien), Servo-U (Maquet), V500 (Dräger Medical), plus V680 (Philips), and R860 (General Electric Healthcare) in Marjanovic NS study. They have both strong methodologies, and advanced statistical analysis but have opposite results. In North American study by Morita PP, SERVO-U tends to be the more usable and V500 the least while, in French study, V500 tends to be the more usable and G5-S1 the least. These differences are probably caused by different ventilators' experience from subjects and subjectivity of usability by itself. A combination of their evaluation criteria (Table 3) could be used when ventilator usability has to be assessed.

To conclude, having a very performing ventilator is nothing without knowledge on how to use it, its capacities, and when using it.

## SALIENT POINTS

From the first tracheostomies 2000 BC to present days with automated ventilation modes and more physiological

**Table 3:** Criteria for evaluation of usability.

| Type | Criteria |
|---|---|
| Set | Power on ventilator |
| Watch | Change ventilatory mode and recognize it |
| Set-Watch | Identifying and modifying humidification system from the screen |
| Set | Set ventilatory parameters among which trigger and inspiratory flow and cycling to predefined values |
| Set | Start Ventilation |
| Set-Watch | Alarms control (setting, identifying reason, shutdown) |
| Watch | Read ventilatory settings and monitored data. Read data not directly available from the screen. |
| Set | Performing inspiratory and expiratory pause in V-CMV |
| Set | Performing a leak test |
| Set | Change to NIV mode |
| Set | Standing by ventilator |
| Set | Switch off ventilator |

modes, ventilators, and mechanical ventilation have greatly evolved.

Understanding ventilation means understanding differences between gas supply types, and between circuit types, and understanding triggering, cycling, and setting of main pressure or volume ventilation modes.

Different but close to ICU ventilators, anesthesia, and transport ones are also to be known and understood because their ventilation modes and ventilators are similar to ICU ventilators but different on certain points such as working principle or leaks. Different studies compare performances of these ventilators.

Having one of the most technically advanced mechanical ventilators is nothing if you cannot use it; usability of mechanical ventilator interfaces is a key point.

## REFERENCES

1. Leroy d'Etiolles JJ. Second mémoire sur l'asphyxie. J Physiol Exp Pathol. 1828;8:97-135.
2. Colice GL. Historical perspective on the development of mechanical ventilation. In: Tobin MJ (Ed). Principles and Practice of Mechanical Ventilation, 3rd edition. New York: McGraw-Hill; 1994. pp. 1-35.
3. Drinker P, Shaw LA. An apparatus for the prolonged administration of artificial respiration: I. A design for adults and children. J Clin Invest. 1929;7(2):229-47.
4. Ibsen B. The anaesthetist's viewpoint on the treatment of respiratory complications in poliomyelitis during the epidemic in Copenhagen, 1952. Proc R Soc Med. 1954;47(1):2-4.
5. Alluaume R. Pulmotor; apparatus for assisted or controlled respiration. Anesth Anal. 1951;8(1):42-6.
6. Lellouche F. Modes asservis complexes. In: Brochard L, Mercat A, Richard J (Eds). Ventilation Artificielle: De La Physiologie À La Pratique. 2008. pp. 35-42.
7. Jaber S, Delay JM, Matecki S, et al. Volume-guaranteed pressure-support ventilation facing acute changes in ventilatory demand. Intensive Care Med. 2005;31(9):1181-8.
8. Branson RD. Dual control modes, closed loop ventilation, handguns, and tequila. Respir Care. 2001;46(3):232-3.
9. Branson RD, Johannigman JA. What is the evidence base for the newer ventilation modes? Respir Care. 2004;49(7):742-60.
10. Tobin MJ. Mechanical ventilation. N Engl J Med. 1994;330(15):1056-61.
11. Thille AW, Lyazidi A, Richard JC, et al. A bench study of intensive-care-unit ventilators: New versus old and turbine-based versus compressed gas-based ventilators. Intensive Care Med. 2009;35(8):1368-76.
12. Delgado C, Romero JE, Puig J, et al. Performance of the new turbine mid-level critical care ventilators. Respir Care. 2017;62(1):34-41.
13. Sassoon CS. Mechanical ventilator design and function: The trigger variable. Respir Care. 1992;37(9):1056-69.
14. Aslanian P, El Atrous S, Isabey D, et al. Effects of flow triggering on breathing effort during partial ventilatory support. Am J Respir Crit Care Med. 1998;157(1):135-43.
15. Nava S, Ambrosino N, Bruschi C, et al. Physiological effects of flow and pressure triggering during non-invasive mechanical ventilation in patients with chronic obstructive pulmonary disease. Thorax. 1997;52(3):249-54.
16. Garnier M, Quesnel C, Fulgencio JP, et al. Multifaceted bench comparative evaluation of latest intensive care unit ventilators. Br J Anaesth. 2015;115(1):89-98.
17. Ferreira JC, Chipman DW, Kacmarek RM. Trigger performance of mid-level ICU mechanical ventilators during assisted ventilation: A bench study. Intensive Care Med. 2008;34(9):1669-75.
18. Sinderby C. Neurally adjusted ventilatory assist (NAVA). Minerva Anestesiol. 2002;68(5):378-80.
19. Lofaso F, Brochard L, Touchard D, et al. Evaluation of carbon dioxide rebreathing during pressure support ventilation with airway management system (BiPAP) devices. Chest. 1995;108(3):772-8.
20. Hill NS, Carlisle C, Kramer NR. Effect of a nonrebreathing exhalation valve on long-term nasal ventilation using a bilevel device. Chest. 2002;122(1):84-91.
21. Chatburn RL. Classification of mechanical ventilators. In: Tobin MJ (Ed). Principles and Practice of Mechanical Ventilation, 3rd edition. New York: McGraw-Hill; 1994. pp. 37-64.
22. Garnero AJ, Abbona H, Gordo-Vidal F, et al. Pressure versus volume controlled modes in invasive mechanical ventilation. Med Intensiva. 2013;37(4):292-8.
23. Brower RG, Matthay MA, Morris A, et al. Acute Respiratory Distress Syndrome Network. Ventilation with lower tidal volumes as compared with traditional tidal volumes for acute lung injury and the acute respiratory distress syndrome. N Engl J Med. 2000;342(18):1301-8.

24. Mancebo J. Assist-control ventilation. In: Tobin MJ (Ed). Principles and Practice of Mechanical Ventilation. New York: McGraw-Hill, Inc; 2006. pp. 183-200.
25. Mercat A. Les modes ventilatoires conventionnels et mixtes. In: Brochard L, Mercat A, Richard J (Eds). Ventilation Artificielle: De La Physiologie À La Pratique. 2008. pp. 23-35.
26. Chacko B, Peter JV, Tharyan P, et al. Pressure-controlled versus volume-controlled ventilation for acute respiratory failure due to acute lung injury (ALI) or acute respiratory distress syndrome (ARDS). Cochrane Database Syst Rev. 2015;1:CD008807.
27. Burns KE, Raptis S, Nisenbaum R, et al. International practice variation in weaning critically ill adults from invasive mechanical ventilation. Ann Am Thorac Soc. 2018;15(4):494-502.
28. Brochard L, Lellouche F. Pressure support ventilation. In: Tobin MJ (Ed). Principles and Practice of Mechanical Ventilation. New York: McGraw-Hill, Inc; 2006. pp. 221-50.
29. Coisel Y, Millot A, Carr J, et al. How to choose an anesthesia ventilator? Ann Fr Anesth Reanim. 2014;33(7-8):462-5.
30. Jain RK, Swaminathan S. Anaesthesia ventilators. Indian J Anaesth. 2013;57(5):525-32.
31. Jaber S, Tassaux D, Sebbane M, et al. Performance characteristics of five new anesthesia ventilators and four intensive care ventilators in pressure-support mode: A comparative bench study. Anesthesiology. 2006;105:944-52.
32. Wallon G, Bonnet A, Guérin C. Delivery of tidal volume from four anaesthesia ventilators during volume-controlled ventilation: A bench study. Br J Anaesth. 2013;110:1045-51.
33. Coisel Y. Ventilation Mécanique En Anesthésie-Réanimation: Évaluation Des Nouveaux Modes Ventilatoires En Médecine Péri-Opérative. 48 - Anesthésie Réanimation. Montpellier, France: Universite Montpellier 1; 2014. p. 319.
34. Hendrickx JF, De Wolf AM. The anesthesia workstation: Quo vadis? Anesth Analg. 2018;127(3):671-5.
35. Bouroche G, Bourgain JL. Preoxygenation and general anesthesia: A review. Minerva Anestesiol. 2015;81(8):910-20.
36. Coisel Y, Conseil M, Galia F, et al. Ventilateurs de transport (cahier des charges, fonctionnalités, etc.). Le Praticien en Anesthésie Réanimation. 2012;16(1):54-62.
37. L'Her E, Roy A, Marjanovic N. Bench-test comparison of 26 emergency and transport ventilators. Crit Care. 2014;18(5):506.
38. Richard JC, Carlucci A, Breton L, et al. Bench testing of pressure support ventilation with three different generations of ventilators. Intensive Care Med. 2002;28(8):1049-57.
39. Lellouche F, Brochard L. Advanced closed loops during mechanical ventilation (PAV, NAVA, ASV, Smartcare). Best Pract Res Clin Anaesthesiol. 2009;23(1):81-93.
40. Navalesi P, Costa R. New modes of mechanical ventilation: Proportional assist ventilation, neurally adjusted ventilatory assist, and fractal ventilation. Curr Opin Crit Care. 2003;9(1):51-8.
41. Mancebo J. Proportional assist ventilation. Minerva Anestesiol. 1999;65(5 Suppl 1):12-5.
42. Brunner JX, Iotti GA. Adaptive support ventilation (ASV). Minerva Anestesiol. 2002;68(5):365-8.
43. Clavieras N, Wysocki M, Coisel Y, et al. Prospective randomized crossover study of a new closed-loop control system versus pressure support during weaning from mechanical ventilation. Anesthesiology. 2013;119(3):631-41.
44. Dojat M, Pachet F, Guessoum Z, et al. NéoGanesh: A working system for the automated control of assisted ventilation in ICUs. Artif Intell Med. 1997;11(2):97-117.
45. Lellouche F, Mancebo J, Jolliet P, et al. A multicenter randomized trial of computer-driven protocolized weaning from mechanical ventilation. Am J Respir Crit Care Med. 2006;174(8):894-900.
46. Rose L, Schultz MJ, Cardwell CR, et al. Automated versus non-automated weaning for reducing the duration of mechanical ventilation for critically ill adults and children: A cochrane systematic review and meta-analysis. Crit Care. 2015;19:48.
47. Chanques G, Conseil M, Roger C, et al. Immediate interruption of sedation compared with usual sedation care in critically ill postoperative patients (SOS-ventilation): A randomized, parallel-group clinical trial. Lancet Respir Med. 2017;5:795-805.
48. Morato JB, Sakuma MT, Ferreira JC, et al. Comparison of 3 modes of automated weaning from mechanical ventilation: A bench study. J Crit Care. 2012;27(6):741.e1-8.
49. Marjanovic NS, De Simone A, Jegou G, et al. A new global and comprehensive model for ICU ventilator performances evaluation. Ann Intensive Care. 2017;7(1):68.
50. Morita PP, Weinstein PB, Flewwelling CJ, et al. The usability of ventilators: A comparative evaluation of use safety and user experience. Crit Care. 2016;20:263.

# CHAPTER 7

# Mechanical Ventilation in Specific Clinical Scenarios

*Afzal Azim*

## INTRODUCTION

Respiratory failure is one of the most common indications for admission to the emergency department and specialist wards, and the need for respiratory system support represents the most common indication for admission to intensive care unit (ICU). Approach to patients with respiratory failure based on the principles of noninvasive and invasive respiratory support is essential for all healthcare professionals involved in patient management.

Clinical application of mechanical ventilation requires strategy modulation according to disease pathophysiology. Physiologically, hindrances to lung movement during respiration can be grouped into elastic resistance and nonelastic resistance.[1,2]

- Elastic resistance includes resistance due to lung tissue and chest wall. It also includes resistance from surface tension at the alveolar gas liquid interface. It is measured when no air flows in the respiratory system. Increased elastic resistance is seen in acute respiratory distress syndrome (ARDS) and restrictive lung diseases.
- Nonelastic resistance includes the influence of friction to gas flow through the airway, friction resistance from thoracic tissue deformation, and a small contribution due to inertia of gas and movement of tissues. It is measured when air is flowing through the respiratory system. Nonelastic resistance is increased in obstructive airway disease.

Work of breathing consists of overcoming these resistances. Increase in one or other forms of resistance leads to increased work of breathing.

Two classic examples of fundamentally different approaches of mechanical ventilation are chronic airflow obstruction and adult respiratory distress syndrome. The current chapter deals with managing mechanical ventilation in patient having obstructive airway disease, bronchopleural fistula, severe metabolic acidosis and ARDS.

## OBSTRUCTIVE AIRWAY DISEASES

Airflow limitation is the hallmark feature of obstructive airway diseases, which mainly comprise of asthma and chronic obstructive pulmonary disease (COPD).[3] Traditionally asthma is characterized by a childhood or early adulthood onset disease with reversible airflow limitation while COPD frequently manifests at a later stage in life and has irreversible or partially reversible airflow limitation. Some patients have features of both COPD and asthma and are termed as overlap syndrome. Airway inflammation is neutrophil predominant in COPD, eosinophil predominant in asthma, and mixed in overlap syndrome.

## BRONCHIAL ASTHMA[4,5]

Indications for intubation include:
- Progressive fatigue and exhaustion
- Depressed level of consciousness
- Respiratory arrest.

### Physiological Concepts

Before discussing ventilator strategy, some basic physiological concepts are discussed below.

### Concept of Time Constant

Time constant is the product of airway resistance and compliance. Expiratory time is a function of time constant. It takes approximately three times the time constants for complete exhalation of given volume of gas. At higher lung volumes lung compliance decreases and shortens the time constant. Patients with increased airway resistance increase their lung volume and thus reduce their time constants and expiratory time.

$$\text{Time Constant} = \text{Resistance} \times \text{Compliance}.$$

At higher lung volumes lung compliance decreases (you cannot inflate an already inflated balloon).

In patients with increased airway resistance, decrease in lung compliance finally results in decreased time constant and decreased expiratory time. Thus, a new steady state is achieved where end-expiratory lung volume (EELV) is higher than resting functional residual capacity (FRC), but permits expiration of the entire tidal volume.

### Concept of Functional Residual Capacity or End Expiratory Lung Volume

During the embryonic development of the fetus, the chest wall grows faster than the lung. As a result of this differential growth, a negative pressure develops in the intrapleural space, which is responsible for the inward recoil of the lungs and the opposite recoil of the chest wall. FRC or EELV represents the point of respiratory system where inward recoil of lungs is equal to the outward recoil of chest wall with respiratory muscles at rest. This state is achieved at the end of expiration after normal tidal breathing.

### Static and Dynamic Hyperinflation

Pulmonary hyperinflation is term used for increase in lung volume above its resting FRC.[6] Static hyperinflation is term used for increased lung volume due to loss of elastic recoil of the lung tissue as seen in patients of emphysema and old age. The resting point of the respiratory system is now shifted at higher FRC and the tendency of lung to recoil reduces. Dynamic hyperinflation (DH) is the term used when time between two inspiratory efforts is insufficient to completely decompress the lung to its resting state.

*Pulmonary hyperinflation is the key deciding factor for initial ventilator settings in severe asthma.*[7,8]

### Mechanism of Hyperinflation

Patients with acute severe asthma breathe near their total lung capacity and with mechanical ventilation, lung volumes are likely to increase further. DH is triggered when there is insufficient time during expiration for complete exhalation of delivered tidal volume. This results in an increase in EELV leading to generation of auto-positive end-expiratory pressure (auto-PEEP). Subsequent breaths lead to progressive increase in lung volume which ultimately leads to improved expiratory gas flow due to increase in elastic recoil pressure and an increase in airways diameter, thereby permitting the entire tidal volume to be exhaled.

Although DH may be an adaptive process that enhances expiratory flow, it can result in severe hypotension and barotraumas. Several terms are used inconsistently as synonyms as listed below (Table 1):
- Dynamic hyperinflation
- Auto-PEEP (AP)
- Intrinsic PEEP (PEEPi)
- Gas trapping
- Occult PEEP
- Breath stacking.

Dynamic hyperinflation is not always the same as air trapping. DH can also occur without physically entrapping the air in certain conditions (Dependent gas trapping observed in obesity, recumbent position in ARDS patients). DH can also be better understood by the statements given below:
- Persistent inspiratory muscle activity during early part of expiration
- Beginning of inhalation before the respiratory system has returned to Vrel (resting lung volume).

### Factors Contributing to Dynamic Hyperinflation or PEEPi

- Bronchospasm
- Mucosal edema
- Inspissated mucus plugs
- Tachypnea
- Anxiety leading to increased ventilatory demands.

Dynamic hyperinflation decreases the effectiveness of the respiratory system predisposing to respiratory fatigue and exhaustion which is attributed to the following points:
- Increased inspiratory effort to generate negative pressure equal in magnitude to PEEPi (resulting in loss of 20–30% of inspiratory muscle effort)

**Table 1:** Various terminologies related to PEEP (Positive end-expiratory pressure).

| | |
|---|---|
| PEEP | Refers to extrinsic PEEP, which is preselected |
| Intrinsic PEEP | Refers to total PEEP (PEEPtot) |
| Intrinsic PEEP/total PEEP | Extrinsic PEEP + Auto-PEEP |
| Auto-PEEP (AP) | Intrinsic PEEP – Extrinsic PEEP |
| Auto-PEEP | Total PEEP – Extrinsic PEEP |
| Auto-PEEP | Equals to intrinsic PEEP when extrinsic PEEP is 0 |
| PEEPi | Abbreviation for both AP and intrinsic PEEP |

# Chapter 7
## Mechanical Ventilation in Specific Clinical Scenarios

- It decreases length tension relationship of muscles characterized by:
  - Decreased zone of apposition of diaphragm
  - Decreasing perfusion
- Increases end inspiratory lung volume reducing compliance and cause alveolar overdistension.

### Hemodynamic Consequences of Dynamic Hyperinflation

This should always be kept in mind. These include:
- Reduced preload to right ventricular
- Increased right ventricular afterload
- Increased right ventricular end-diastolic volume (EDV)
- Shift of interventricular septum toward left
- Increased left ventricular afterload as a result of increased negative intrapleural pressure during inspiration.

### Identification of Air Trapping and Auto-Positive End-expiratory Pressure in Flow-Time Scalar and Flow-Volume Loop

See Figures 1 and 2.

### Initial Ventilator Settings

In severe asthma, the most important factors that determine the degree to which VEE (lung volume at end-expiration) increases during mechanical ventilation are:
- Expiratory resistance
- Tidal volume
- Expiratory time.

The ventilator settings that influence the severity of hyperinflation are tidal volume, respiratory rate, and inspiratory flow rate. In initial management, these variables must have optimal settings (Table 2); while subsequent ventilator adjustment should be based on pH and/or $P_{plat}$ levels (Table 3).

The following therapies have to be used in conjunction with the ventilator therapy:
- Sedation with or without paralysis
- Therapies for airflow obstruction which include bronchodilator therapy and steroids as a part of bronchial hygiene therapy.

### Monitoring during Ventilation

Pulmonary hyperinflation is the key deciding factor for ventilator settings in severe asthma: The degree of hyperinflation varies from patient to patient. Monitoring trends of hyperinflation is essential to bring changes in ventilator settings.[9,10]

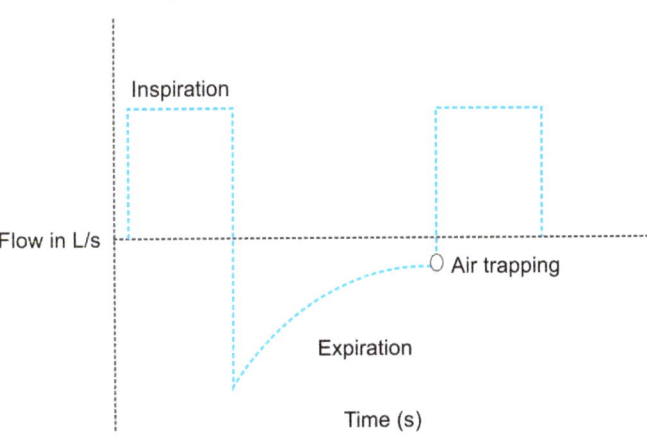

**Fig. 1:** The diagram represents the flow time scalar of patient on volume control mode and square wave pattern of flow. The graph does not touch the baseline at the end of expiration, thus representing air tapping.

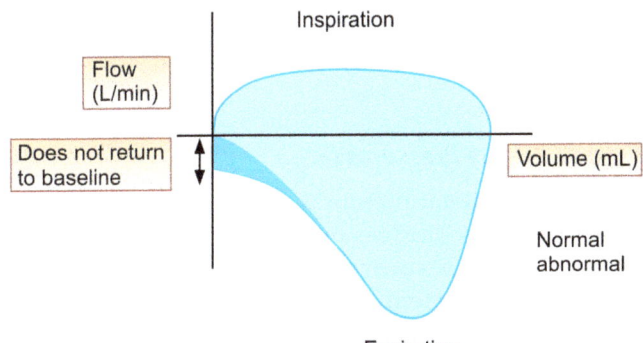

**Fig. 2:** Flow volume loop showing air trapping.

| Table 2: Initial ventilator settings in severe asthma. | |
|---|---|
| *Initial ventilator settings* | |
| Mode | Assist control |
| Tidal volume | 6–8 mL/kg |
| Respiratory rate | 12–14 breaths/min |
| Inspiratory flow | 60–70 liters per minute |
| Waveform | Decelerating or constant |
| PEEP | <5 cmH$_2$O |
| FiO$_2$ | Target a saturation of >90% |
| PEEP: positive end-expiratory pressure | |

### Peak Airway Pressures ($P_{peak}$)

Monitoring peak airway pressures are routinely done and easy to monitor. However, we need to understand its limitations with such patients.
- Peak airway pressures depend upon the resistive properties of the airway to inspiratory flow and may not be true representative of actual hyperinflation.

**Table 3:** Ventilatory adjustments based on pH and/or $P_{plat}$.
*Subsequent ventilatory targets*

| Parameters | Ventilator adjustment |
|---|---|
| $P_{plat}$ > 30 cmH$_2$O | Decrease minute ventilation (decrease rate) |
| If blood pH < 7.2 and $P_{plat}$ < 25 cmH$_2$O | Increase minute ventilation (increase rate) |
| If blood pH < 7.2 and $P_{plat}$ 25–30 cmH$_2$O | Consider to add buffers to counter effects of acidosis |

- There is very limited evidence to suggest a direct relationship between peak airway pressures and barotrauma.
- Initial peak airway pressure in asthmatic patients may be ≥50 cmH$_2$O. A factor which may be contributing to high-peak airway pressures is the high inspiratory flow which is used in these patients.
- Moreover, decrement in $P_{peak}$ may not even represent the decrease in DH with prolonged expiratory time due to increased airway resistance and decreased lung volume.

### Plateau Airway Pressures ($P_{plat}$)

Monitoring plateau pressures may be better than peak airway pressures. The reasons are explained below:
- Patients with severe asthma have near-normal respiratory system compliance and an increase in $P_{plat}$ may represent DH. Hence, if the patient is being ventilated at constant tidal volume, changes in the amount of DH in response to bronchodilator therapy or manipulation of I:E ratio can be due to changes in $P_{plat}$.
- No safe limit of $P_{plat}$ has been described in literature but the usual practice is to keep it between 25 cmH$_2$O and 30 cmH$_2$O (Lung protective ventilation).
- One should be aware that $P_{plat}$ measured on the ventilator is representative of average of all alveolar pressures. It is possible that some alveolar units may have higher alveolar pressures than the average.
- Measuring auto-PEEP in a mechanically ventilated patient may provide just an estimate of end-expiratory alveolar pressures, thereby representing plateau pressures.

### Measurement of Auto-Positive End-expiratory Alveolar Pressure[11,12]

There is no ideal technique to measure auto-PEEP in a ventilated patient. The method of estimation of auto-PEEP varies from an actively breathing patient to a passively ventilated patient. PEEPi depends on factors other than respiratory mechanics of the patient which includes respiratory rate, tidal volume, position of the patient, and it keeps on changing in response to the adjunct therapies and also during the course of the disease. Still no consensus exists on the optimal method for its measurement. We will be discussing the common techniques practiced for its measurement.

### Measurement of Static Auto-Positive End-expiratory Alveolar Pressure

*End-expiratory occlusion technique (EEOT):* This technique requires the occlusion of the airways at the end of exhalation. The difference between end-of-occlusion Paw and pre-occlusion Paw is known as static PEEP (Fig. 3) and represents the average auto-PEEP of a nonhomogeneous lung with different time constants of different lung units.

Timing of occlusion is important and it should begin just before the next inspiratory flow of the ventilator is about to begin. If it is applied too early then there is a chance of overestimation of auto-PEEP. Since occlusion at exhalation port compresses the gas within the ventilator tubings and the humidifier it can give falsely low values of auto-PEEP. As a rule shorter tubings should be used and the humidifier should be removed during measurement of auto-PEEP with this technique.

### Measurement of Dynamic Auto-Positive End-expiratory Alveolar Pressure

It is measured as the increase in Paw from end-exhalation to the point corresponding to the beginning of inspiratory flow. The concept is that rise in Paw preceding inspiratory flow is equal the pressure required to counter the elastic recoil of the respiratory system. Theoretically this measurement should represent the lung units with the shortest time constants, meaning thereby the lung units which empty at the earliest. *Hence, there is a possibility that this technique can underestimate auto-PEEP.*

Measurement of both static and dynamic auto-PEEP can give an estimate about the severity of time constant inequalities existing in the respiratory system of the patient.

### Measurement of Auto-Positive End-expiratory Alveolar Pressure by Esophageal Pressure (Pes) Change Predicting the Inspiratory Flow (Also Known as Counter-Balance Method)

This technique requires inserting an esophageal balloon catheter system and it estimates the changes in pleural pressure. It is invasive technique with limitations and

# Chapter 7
## Mechanical Ventilation in Specific Clinical Scenarios

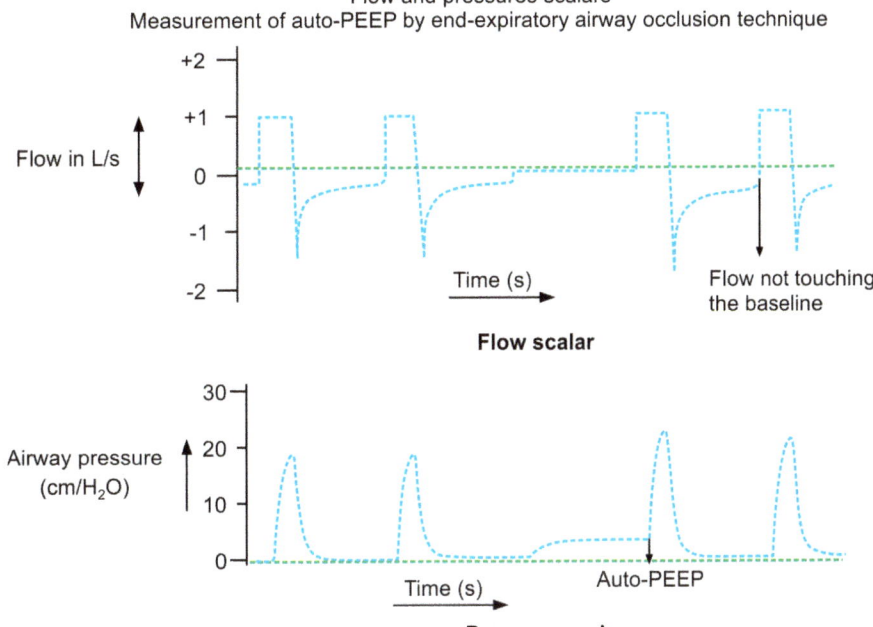

**Fig. 3:** Flow and pressures scalars. Measurement of auto-PEEP by end-expiratory airway occlusion technique.

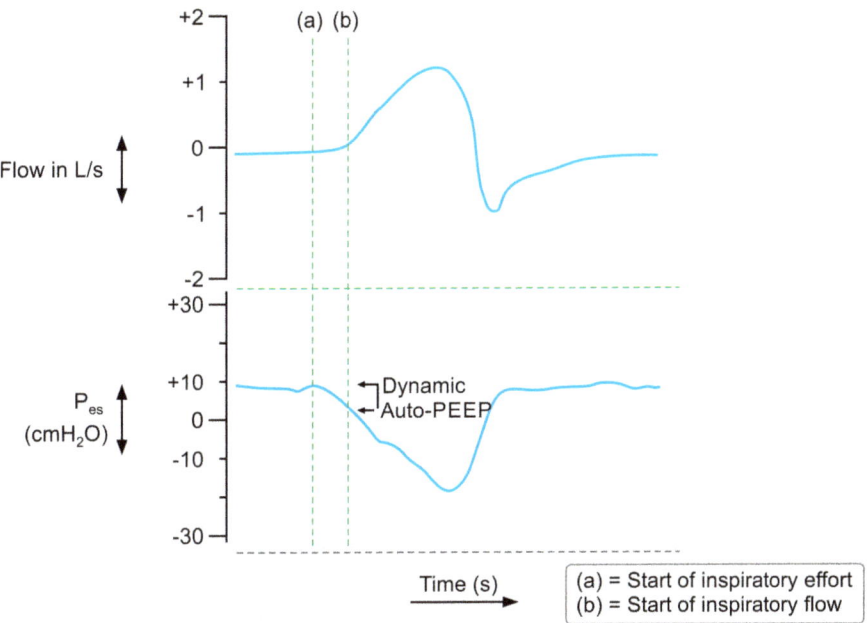

**Fig. 4:** Method of measuring dynamic auto-PEEP (difference between start of inspiratory effort as measured by esophageal pressure, an indirect measure of pleural pressure and start of inspiratory flow).

also not readily available in most of the ICUs and has not become the standard practice for measuring auto-PEEP.

It measures the dynamic auto-PEEP as change in esophageal pressure from the initiation of patient's inspiratory effort to the beginning of inspiratory flow (Fig. 4). It measures the inspiratory muscle pressure which is required to offset the end-expiratory recoil of the respiratory system. This technique is based on certain *assumptions* which add to the limitations of this technique.

- End-expiratory alveolar pressure represents the elastic recoil pressure when the respiratory system is relaxed.

- Changes in esophageal pressure from the beginning of inspiratory effort to start of inspiratory flow reflects the inspiratory muscle pressure which is required to counter the elastic recoil of respiratory system at the end of exhalation.
- Time constant inequalities do exist.
- It means that PEEPi represents the pressure to start inspiratory flow in alveolar units with short time constants.
- Exhalation is passive.
- It assumes that at the end of exhalation there is absent expiratory muscle contraction.

### Selection of Positive End-expiratory Pressure

The optimal PEEP should be the PEEP that does not harm the patient and at the same time it is able to balance the auto-PEEP. The waterfall theory explains that increasing the pressure away from the small airway closure or collapse should not cause any decrement in expiratory flow until the downstream water (external positive end-expiratory pressure) reaches the critical pressure (Fig. 5). Hence, it is advisable that the external PEEP should be kept below 75–85% of auto-PEEP. It would lessen DH and avoid circulatory compromise.

## CHRONIC OBSTRUCTIVE PULMONARY DISEASE

The pathophysiology of COPD patients is similar to asthmatic patients with some extra considerations which are described below.[13,14]

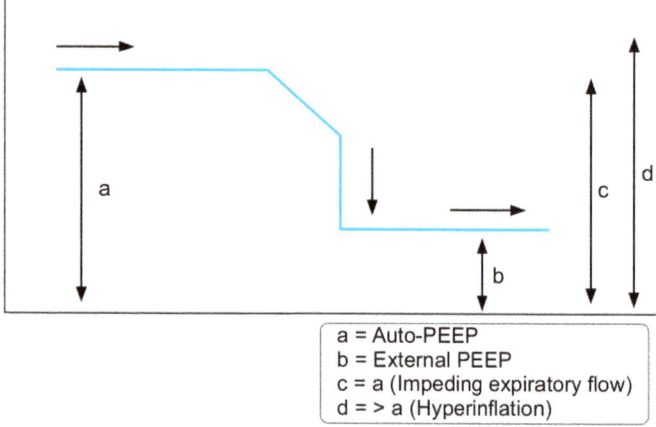

**Fig. 5:** Represents the water fall concept for determination of PEEP requirement during mechanical ventilation.

Some features associated with respiratory mechanics with these patients include:
- Increased inspiratory airway resistance
- Increased expiratory airway resistance
- Respiratory muscle weakness
- Respiratory muscle fatigue.

Chronic obstructive pulmonary disease patients have greatly increased expiratory resistance. The mechanisms are listed below:
- Resistance is more at low lung volume due to dynamic narrowing of small airways during exhalation
- "Wave speed limitation"—tracheobronchial tree cannot adjust to airflow resulting in expiratory flow limitation (EFL)
- Small airway collapse at critical closing pressures
- EFL exists in as many as 60% of stable patients even during resting breathing
- The consequences of EFL include
- EFL → Air trapping → Activation of expiratory muscles → Increases alveolar pressure
- Expiratory flow limitation seen in these patients is a condition that occurs because gas flow cannot be increased any more by:
  - Raising alveolar pressures
  - Reducing the airway opening pressure.

### Consequences of Expiratory Flow Limitation[15,16]

- Expiratory muscle contraction—do not achieve storage of elastic energy at end of exhalation
- Relaxed expiratory muscles at the onset of inhalation do not assist inspiratory muscles in expanding the respiratory system during inhalation
- Entire burden of breathing is borne by inspiratory muscles
- Expiratory muscle recruitment dissipates precious energy substrate.

Breathing at low respiratory rates is recommended for hyperinflated lungs to improve their gas exchange. Hence, it is recommended that for these patients the most effective combination of respiratory rate and the ratio of inspiratory time divided by the total respiratory cycle (IT/TRC) should be used.

The ability of the respiratory muscles to sustain an increased inspiratory load in these patients depends on two ratios:
1. Respiratory duty cycle, which is equal to inspiratory time divided by the time of a total respiratory cycle (IT/TRC) and

2. Mean transdiaphragmatic pressure per breath divided by the maximum static transdiaphragmatic pressure (MTDP/Mx STDP).

When we combine the above two ratios we get tension time index (TTI) which give us an idea regarding mechanical load, utilization of energy during the process of breathing, blood flow, and susceptibility of muscles to get fatigued.

IT/TRC × MTDP/Mx STDP = tension–time index (TTI)
TTI > 0.15 = Task failure (Healthy subjects TTI = 0.02)
Stable COPD patients have TTI = 0.05 which extrapolates to more than 2 times the phrenic motor neuron discharge and almost 5 times greater diaphragmatic recruitment at resting breathing.

The main goal of mechanical ventilation in patients with obstructive airway disease is to facilitate pulmonary gas exchange and allowing sufficient rest to compromised respiratory muscles. Ventilating a COPD patient is often difficult because the disease may not have a reversible component. However, adequate planning of ventilation strategy with modifications based on response to adjunct therapies can influence the overall outcome of these patients.

## BRONCHOPLEURAL FISTULA

Bronchopleural fistula (BPF) in patients who have not undergone thoracic surgery is an infrequently encountered complication in intensive care units.[17,18] Ventilatory management of such patients is a challenge for the intensivist. The reported mortality in patients with BPF can be anywhere between 18% and 50%, with tension pneumothorax and aspiration pneumonia as leading causes of death. A patient of BPF developing ARDS becomes all the more difficult case to manage on ventilator.

### Definition and Classification

Bronchopleural fistula is defined as leakage of inspired air from the airways into the pleural cavity persisting for more than 24 hours. Classification according to timing
- Early (1–7 days)
- Intermediate (8–30 days)
- Late fistulas (more than 30 days)
- PAL (persistent air leak)—if ≥5–7 days.

### Pathophysiology

*"Patients do not die because of BPF/they die with BPF."*

Anatomically BPF is a sinus tract between the main bronchi, lobar bronchi, or segmental bronchus, and the pleural space. Acute BPF can be life-threatening due to clinical manifestations of tension pneumothorax or asphyxiation from pulmonary flooding of secretions. Clinical features may include sudden onset of dyspnea, hypotension, subcutaneous emphysema, expectoration of purulent fluid, tracheal or mediastinal shift, persistent air leak, and a reduction or disappearance of pleural effusion on the chest radiograph. The mechanisms for BPF in nonsurgical patients are enumerated below (Table 4).

In routine clinical practice, the severity of the air leak can be classified into three categories (from least to most severe):
- Air bubbling present during inspiration only
- Air bubbling present during both inspiration and expiration
- Air bubbling present during both inspiration and expiration with a measurable difference in the inspired and expired tidal volumes.

### Diagnosis

Diagnosis of BPF can be based on:
- Clinical (pneumothorax with chest tube)
- Fiberoptic bronchoscopy
- Selective bronchography
- CT-scan to diagnose the site/size/etiology of BPF
- Methylene blue test
- Ventilation scintigraphy (postsurgical cases).

The harmful effects of BPF should be first understood which aid in optimizing the ventilatory strategy for these patients (Table 5).

**Table 4:** Etiologies of bronchopleural fistula (BPF) in ICU settings.

| Mechanisms for BPF in ICU settings | |
|---|---|
| Spontaneous rupture | Direct injury |
| Volutrauma | Chest trauma |
| High PEEP therapy/High plateau pressures | Difficult airway with multiple intubation attempts |
| Severe ARDS | Central line placement |
| Necrotizing pneumonia | Thoracocentesis |
| Right main bronchus intubation | Chest tube placement |
| Pneumonectomy | Transbronchial biopsy |
| Manual ventilation | |

(ARDS: acute respiratory distress syndrome; PEEP: positive end-expiratory pressure)

**Table 5:** Harmful effects of bronchopleural fistula.

| Effect | Problem |
| --- | --- |
| Incomplete lung expansion | Atelectasis and V/Q mismatch |
| Loss of tidal volume | Decreased minute ventilation/respiratory acidosis |
| Loss of PEEP | Hypoxemia |
| Secretions seep into pleural space | Pleural space infections |
| Factitious triggering | Asynchrony/inadequate ventilation |

(PEEP: positive end-expiratory pressure)

## General Management Principles

*In general, management of the patient with a bronchopleural fistula is the same as if the fistula were not there.*

- Use the lowest number of mechanical breaths (it helps to decrease both mean airway pressure and number of high pressure breaths).
- Partial ventilatory support is preferred to total ventilatory support [pressure support ventilation/assist control mode of ventilation/synchronized intermittent mandatory ventilation-pressure support (PSV/ACV/SIMV-PS)].
- Limit the effective tidal volume based on permissive $CO_2$ levels.
- Minimize the inspiratory time by keeping low inspiration to expiration ratio (1:2).
- Use high inspiratory flow.
- Avoid pause at the end of inspiration.
- Avoid inverse ratio ventilation.
- Use low compressible-volume ventilator circuit to minimize the delivered tidal volume.
- Minimize PEEP (Best PEEP for acceptable oxygenation).
- Monitor auto-PEEP (Take measures to reduce auto-PEEP).
- Explore positional differences in BPF leak. Use the position with least leak.
- Treat other causes of expiratory flow obstruction.

## Specific Strategies for Management of Bronchopleural Fistula

Bronchopleural fistula can usually be managed by conventional ventilation. The need for special ventilation techniques is uncommon.

- Chest tube manipulation (Theoretical with few anecdotal reports)
  - Intermittent inspiratory chest tube occlusion
  - Application of intrapleural pressure at expiration
- One lung ventilation
- High frequency ventilation
- Extracorporeal oxygenation.

### Chest Tube Management

A short wide-bore chest tube should be used to achieve the best results when a large air leak is present.

- Small negative pressures can be applied (up to 10 $cmH_2O$) but we should be aware that it
  - Can increase fistula
  - Can lead to autotriggering
- A specialized pleural drainage unit (PDU) should be used to provide suction and a water seal to prevent backflow of air into the pleural cavity
  - The traditional PDUs regulate suction pressures by the height of the water column (keep a watch on Ht. of column)
- Newer-generation "dry" suction units are also available now.

### Preventive Strategies for Bronchopleural Fistula

- Use lung protective ventilation (low tidal volume strategy)
- Monitor for auto-PEEP
- Monitor the static respiratory system compliance (tidal volume/plateau airway pressure-PEEP)
  - Decrease applied PEEP if the static compliance decreases when the applied PEEP is increased.
- Separate the patient from mechanical ventilation as soon as possible
- Extreme care when inserting a subclavian or internal jugular central venous catheter, or performing thoracentesis.

## SEVERE METABOLIC ACIDOSIS

Critically ill patients are prone to encounter disturbances of acid–base equilibrium. Acidosis can be either respiratory due to increases in arterial partial carbon dioxide tension ($PCO_2$: respiratory acidosis) or metabolic due to accumulation of a variety of organic or inorganic, fixed acids. Understanding the pathophysiology is crucial for proper management. Though metabolic acidosis is not uncommon in patients admitted in intensive care unit, the precise incidence and prevalence of metabolic acidosis has not been established. Often acid–base disorders are diagnostic markers of some underlying pathology. The true cause–effect relationship between acidosis and adverse clinical outcomes remains uncertain for critically ill patients. Clinical manifestations of severe acidemia can include cerebral edema, seizures, diaphragm dysfunction, poor cardiac function, increased pulmonary vasoconstriction, and decreased systemic vascular resistance manifesting as hypotension.

Metabolic acidosis is defined as an arterial blood pH of less than 7.35 with plasma bicarbonate levels of less than 22 mmol/L. Respiratory compensation is the first to occur and normally starts immediately. Compensation can be partial (very early in time course) or full compensation bringing back the pH to normal. Winter's formula can be helpful to calculate the $CO_2$ compensation for the existing metabolic acidosis—(the formula allows calculation of the expected compensating $pCO_2$). If the measured $pCO_2$ is more than what is expected for that metabolic acidosis then coexisting respiratory acidosis may also be present in the same patient. Clinically the patients experience dyspnea due to stimulation of the respiratory center in an attempt to "blow off" $CO_2$ and thereby increasing the blood pH. Sometimes they may not have significant tachypnea but instead they hyperventilate (large tidal volumes) to compensate for their pH (Kussmaul's breathing).

### Physiological Effects of Hyperventilation may Influence Ventilator Settings

- Hemodynamic disturbances
- Asynchrony
- Dyssynchrony
- Increased work of breathing (WOB)
- Predisposes to barotrauma
- Interferes with respiratory mechanics
- Dynamic hyperinflation.

Intubation and ventilation can lead to decompensation of physiological compensations and hence caution is advised at initiation of mechanical ventilation.[19] Patients with a metabolic acidosis rely on their hyperventilation to maintain their pH. Hence, it is advised to *maintain hyperventilation in such patients* till we provide therapy or the etiology of acidosis.

If ventilation is set to some standard value and the $pCO_2$ is allowed to rise toward 40 mm Hg, then this represents further worsening of acute respiratory acidosis and pH can fall rapidly. Anesthetic agents and initial ventilator settings to a normal respiratory rate may lead to further decompensation. The target of mechanical ventilation is to keep the pH in the normal range (7.35–7.45). Initiation of mechanical ventilation in these patients should be with adequate precautions and knowledge about heart–lung interactions which can occur after initiation of positive pressure ventilation.

### Factors that may Worsen the Hemodynamic Effects of MV in Acidotic Patients

- Decrease in venous return (in situations of hypovolemia, venodilation)
- Increase in mean intrathoracic pressure (e.g. the use of large tidal volume or use of high PEEP)
- Blunting of compensatory sympathetic reflexes (e.g. sedatives).

## ACUTE RESPIRATORY DISTRESS SYNDROME

Acute respiratory distress syndrome is a disease in which the lungs suffer severe heterogeneous injury, interfering with their ability to take up oxygen. It is the final common pathway of lung damage caused of a variety of insults ranging from direct causes like aspiration pneumonia, inhalational injury, etc. to indirect causes like cardiopulmonary bypass and disseminated infection of extrapulmonary origin.

### Definition

Acute respiratory distress syndrome was first defined in 1994 during the American-European Consensus Conference (AECC) as:[20]

- A condition with acute respiratory failure
- Bilateral infiltrates on chest radiology
- $PaO_2/FiO_2$ ratio ≤200 mm Hg
- No evidence of left atrial hypertension or a pulmonary capillary pressure <18 mm Hg (if measured).

Acute lung injury (ALI) was less severe form of ARDS with $PaO_2/FiO_2 \leq 300$ mm Hg.[19] During the year 2011, a revised definition of ARDS was given by European Society of Intensive Care Medicine with endorsement from the American Thoracic Society (ATS) and the Society of Critical Care Medicine (SCCM) to address the limitations of the above definition.[21] The term acute lung injury was dropped and ARDS was classified on the basis of $PaO_2/FiO_2$ as mild (200 mm Hg to 300 mm Hg), moderate (100 mm Hg to 200 mm Hg), and severe ($PaO_2/FIO_2 \leq 100$ mm Hg). Other salient features of Berlin definition included acute onset respiratory distress as new worsening within 1 week, bilateral chest infiltrates NOT fully explained by lung pathologies like effusion, nodule or collapse and pulmonary edema, fluid overload or heart failure.

### Pathophysiology of ARDS

The affected areas in ARDS are the alveoli (air sacs). The thin wall between the blood and air (alveolar-capillary membrane—less than 0.5 micrometers in width) is at its thinnest segment where the gas exchange takes place. ARDS pathology involves both the capillary and alveolar cells are injured. This injury results in fluid spillage into the alveolar units, thus hindering or preventing gas exchange.[22] Regardless of the triggering event, an inflammatory chain reaction is set off. Molecules released by infected or injured cells attract white cells from the blood to enter the affected area. The incoming white blood cells combine with resident lung cells to produce more chemicals (called cytokines and chemokines), thereby exaggerating the inflammatory process. The inflammatory exudates decrease the surfactant function leading to collapse/consolidation of distal airspaces subsequently leading to loss of gas exchange. This would normally be compensated for by hypoxic pulmonary vasoconstriction, if the inflammatory process did not also effectively paralyze the vascular tone thereby allowing deoxygenated blood to flow through unventilated lung units. The combination of these two processes initially causes hypoxemia but if allowed to persist eventually leads to type 2 respiratory failure with $CO_2$ retention.

From mechanical ventilation point of view, ARDS comprises of heterogeneous lung with different ventilatory requirements in different zones of lungs. These patients have some normal alveoli, some consolidated while some alveoli recruitable with ventilatory strategies.

## Ventilatory Management of ARDS

Management of these patients consists of appropriate treatment of the underlying or causative illness, supportive care, and prevention of complications associated with mechanical ventilation. Appropriate treatment of an underlying infection consists of identifying the causative organism as best as possible and treated with appropriate/sensitive antibiotics. Mechanical ventilation is a key component of holistic supportive care and in this chapter we highlight the important principles of mechanical ventilation in patients with ARDS.

Last few decades have highlighted the injurious effects of mechanical ventilation. In the 1970s, ventilator settings were titrated to normalize blood gas values. Clinicians used tidal volume of 12-15 mL/kg of body weight. Barotrauma in the form of pneumothorax, pneumomediastinum, and pneumoperitoneum were common, and mortality in severe ARDS was as high as 90%. In order to reduce mortality associated with ARDS and design optimal management strategy, the National Heart, Lung, and Blood Institute (NHLBI), National Institutes of Health (NIH), conducted multiple multicenter clinical trials from 1994 to 2014. Over this period of two decades almost 10 randomized controlled trials and one observational study were conducted. Out of these 11 studies showed that lung protective ventilation strategy was associated with improved outcome and decreased mortality.

### Lung Protective Mechanical Ventilation

Work by Amato and colleagues and later the landmark ARDSNet (Acute Respiratory Distress Syndrome Network) trial in 2000 showed improved outcomes with low tidal volume (TV) ventilation strategies [4-6 mL/kg of ideal body weight (IBW)] versus higher traditional TV (10-12 mL/kg IBW).[23,24] A better understanding of ventilator-induced lung injury (VILI) in recent years has created a renewed interest on practicing lung protective ventilation strategy. Recent data favor low tidal volume ventilation not only in ARDS but in patients without ARDS also.

It incorporates two major components:
1. Low tidal volume ventilation (4-6 mL/kg of predicted body weight)
2. Limiting the plateau pressures to less than 30 cmH$_2$O.

The recommendation to use lower tidal volume (less than or equal to 6 mL/kg predicted body weight) ventilation with a plateau pressure less than or equal to 30 cmH$_2$O is strong despite moderate quality of evidence for hospital mortality and barotrauma, and low quality of evidence for 60 day mortality. Additional studies and meta-analysis have showed large tidal volume ventilation and high pressures are harmful.[25-27] However, lack of adverse effects, strong mechanistic and physiologic rationale for its use and supportive data from ARDS prevention studies have resulted in *its universal acceptance as a gold standard of care.*

There is no safe plateau pressure in ARDS. However, the recommendations are to keep them less than 30 cmH$_2$O. Some experts believe it should be kept as low as 20 cmH$_2$O. It has been chosen as a surrogate for transpulmonary pressures because measuring transpulmonary pressures is not clinically possible. Methods to reduce plateau pressures are to work on low tidal volumes but one should be cautious regarding PaCO$_2$ and pH (try keeping these parameters in acceptable range). This is one more reason to choose high respiratory rates in ARDS patients to maintain minute ventilation.

### PEEP Selection in ARDS

The treatment for hypoxemia in ARDS is to recruit collapsed lung alveolar units by recruiting them through use of external PEEP. The optimal PEEP settings, or even the best method to go about choosing PEEP, are controversial.

The ARDSnet trial also provides algorithms for bedside selection of PEEP based on $FiO_2$ but still it is best left to the treating clinician to choose the right PEEP for each individual patient.

The use of relatively higher PEEP in patients with moderate or severe ARDS did not get support from high-quality evidences, as there is inconsistency among studies for strategy to set the level of PEEP. The evidences favoring use of higher PEEP in patients with at least moderate ARDS is based on subgroup and individual patient data, rather than the evidence based on a randomized controlled trial investigating higher PEEP in this group of patients. Also, the risk of barotrauma with the use of higher PEEP in moderate or severe ARDS is not quantified very well in studies. The quality of evidence to quantify risks' of high PEEP is also limited by inconsistency as the meta-analysis has included trials of high PEEP with different tidal volume strategies. There is no universal consensus as of now regarding the methodology used to optimize PEEP or to manage the respiratory acidosis that can be frequent accompaniment of lung protective ventilation. However, the suggestions for clinical practice are to use of high PEEP strategies for patients with moderate/severe ARDS.[28]

Default PEEP setting in ARDS can be kept at 10 $cmH_2O$. Patients likely to benefit from PEEP above 10 cm are the ones with reduced chest wall compliance and those with airway and alveolar edema that can be easily redistributed. It should be noted that edema fluid can be more easily redistributed only in early phase of inflammation as in latter stages it gets converted to gel state. With further progression of ARDS there is remodeling and fibrosis.

Plateau airway pressure is useful only when it is able to recruit more lung units otherwise it can cause harmful effects like decreased venous return, increased intrathoracic pressure, decreased cardiac output, and ventilation perfusion mismatch.

## Prone Ventilation

Prone ventilation is one of the strategies to improve oxygenation in ARDS patients. Edema fluid redistribution and recruitment of alveoli are most easily achievable in early phase of the disease and that is why prone ventilation works best in initial phase.

Current evidence regarding prone ventilation favors survival outcome when combined with lung-protective ventilation and when delivered for minimum 12 hours to patients with moderate/severe ARDS.[29,30] The most recent and well-conducted randomized study (PROSEVA trial) focused on severe ARDS, and involved a multimodal intervention comprising lung-protective ventilation with prolonged-duration prone positioning resulting in significant reduction in short as well as long-term mortality.[31] This study provides the strong rationale for practicing prone ventilation.

The possibility for substantial patient benefit must be considered despite possibilities of prone position-related adverse events (facial edema, potential dislodgement of invasive lines, pressure sores, and ocular complications); as prevalence of these adverse events are either low or very low. However, it should be ensured that sufficient skilled personnel should deliver this intervention.

Recent data by the PROSEVA group examined prone positioning in severe ARDS ($PaO_2/FiO_2$ ratio < 150 mm Hg) and found an overall reduction in 28-day mortality (16.0% vs 32.8%) without any increase in complications in the prone group.[31] Though the investigators who participated in this trial had significant experience with prone positioning that could have minimized complications (airway and central line dislodgment, pressure ulcers).

The recommendations for clinical practice are to use prone positioning for at least 12 hours per day in patients with moderate/severe ARDS.

## Recruitment Maneuvers

Increased lung weight due to interstitial and alveolar edema can cause collapse of dependent alveolar units.[32,33] Recruitment maneuvers (RMs) are used to achieve recruitment of collapsed alveolar units by transiently increasing applied airway pressure and driving pressure (Plateau airway pressure—PEEP). Various RMs have been described in literature including progressive incremental PEEP at constant driving pressure, continuous positive airway pressure (30–40 $cmH_2O$ for 40 seconds), etc. RMs cause transient improvement in oxygenation and lung compliance in patients with recruitable alveolar units. These maneuvers are potentially dangerous in patients with shock and fluid deficit as they can worsen hemodynamic compromise. Current guidelines suggest use of RMs in ARDS patients. There are no recommendations for the best RM in ARDS. The clinicians can practice the maneuver they are best versed with.

## Extracorporeal Membrane Oxygenation

Extracorporeal membrane oxygenation (ECMO) is a modality of oxygenating the blood via an extracorporeal circuit. Blood is drawn from the patient via large bore catheter placed in artery or vein, passed through an oxygenator, and returned back into a large central vein.

| Table 6: Outline for management of ARDS. | | |
|---|---|---|
| Mild ARDS | Moderate ARDS | Severe ARDS |
| 200 mm Hg < $PaO_2/FIO_2$ < 300 mm Hg<br>PEEP or CPAP ≥ 5 $cmH_2O$ | 100 mm Hg < $PaO_2/FIO_2$ < 200 mm PEEP ≥ 5 $cmH_2O$ | $PaO_2/FIO_2$ < 100 mm Hg<br>PEEP ≥ 5 $cmH_2O$ |
| Conservative fluid strategy for all grades of ARDS | | |
| Low tidal volume ventilation with Plateau pressures less than 30 $cmH_2O$ for all grades of ARDS | | |
| | Prone ventilation for >12 hours/day | |
| | PEEP optimization/recruitment (Preferred high PEEP ≥ 10 $cmH_2O$) | |
| | | Referral to ECMO center |

(ARDS: acute respiratory distress syndrome; ECMO: extracorporeal membrane oxygenation; PEEP: positive end-expiratory pressure)

Extracorporeal support techniques were extensively used in 2009 H1N1 pandemic with promising results.[34] However, current evidence in this field is limited. More robust data is needed before strong recommendations can be made regarding ECMO use in ARDS. Current recommendation for ECMO is that patients with severe ARDS to be referred to ECMO center with trained staff (also see chapter on ECMO).

## Extracorporeal Carbon Dioxide Removal

It is still at research level and should be the subject of a suitably powered multicenter randomized controlled trial (RCT) with long-term follow up and economic analysis, that focuses on both potential benefits and harms (also see chapter on $ECCO_2R$).

## High Frequency Oscillatory Ventilation

The use of HFOV for the management of ARDS has a poor recommendation based on moderate quality evidence. Current evidence from multiple RCTs demonstrated no benefit from HFOV and one RCT even demonstrated an increase in mortality with HFOV (also see Chapter on HFOV).

Our knowledge regarding mechanical ventilation for ARDS has evolved significantly over last few decades. Lung protective ventilation, prone ventilation, restrictive fluid strategy, optimal PEEP and RM are the cornerstone of ventilating ARDS patients (Table 6).

## SALIENT POINTS

- Lung protective ventilation is the key in any form of ventilator strategy, following the principle of "do no harm".
- Low tidal volume ventilation (VT: 6–8 mL/kg) targeting $P_{plat}$ < 30 $cmH_2O$ should be the target in all patients.
- Full support ventilation is initially provided targeting adequate minute ventilation and avoiding hyperoxia (Target: $SpO_2$: 88–92%; $PaO_2$: 70–100 mm Hg).
- Analgosedation is to be provided to maintain patient's synchrony with the ventilator. Daily sedation vacation should be practiced after initial stabilization.
- Neuromuscular blockade should be considered in select cases but should be withdrawn early.
- After initial management, subsequent changes in mechanical ventilation settings should be based on clinical condition and regular monitoring of arterial blood gases.

## REFERENCES

1. Banner MJ, Kirby RR, Blanch PB. Differentiating total work of breathing into its component parts. Essential for appropriate interpretation. Chest. 1996;109(5):1141-3.
2. Banner MJ, Downs JB, Kirby RR, et al. Effects of expiratory flow resistance on inspiratory work of breathing. Chest.1988;93(4):795-9.
3. Dima E, Rovina N, Gerassimou C, et al. Pulmonary function tests, sputum induction, and bronchial provocation tests: diagnostic tools in the challenge of distinguishing asthma and COPD phenotypes in clinical practice. Int J Chron Obstruct Pulmon Dis. 2010;5:287-9.
4. Mims JW. Asthma: definitions and pathophysiology. Int Forum Allergy Rhinol. 2015;5(1Suppl):S2-6.
5. Afzal M, Tharratt RS. Mechanical ventilation in severe asthma. Clin Rev Allergy Immunol. 2001;20(3):385-97.
6. Ferguson GT. Why does the lung hyperinflate? Proc Am Thorac Soc. 2006;3(2):176-9.
7. Ahmed SM, Athar M. Mechanical ventilation in patients with chronic obstructive pulmonary disease and bronchial asthma. Indian J Anaesth. 2015;59(9):589-98.
8. Stather DR, Stewart TE. Clinical review: Mechanical ventilation in severe asthma. Crit Care. 2005;9(6):581-7.
9. Brochard L, Martin GS, Blanch L, et al. Clinical review: Respiratory monitoring in the ICU – a consensus of 16. Crit Care. 2012;16(2):219.

10. Theerawit P, Sutherasan Y, Ball L, et al. Respiratory monitoring in adult intensive care unit. Expert Rev Respir Med. 2017;11(6):453-68.
11. Blanch L, Bernabé F, Lucangelo U. Measurement of air trapping, intrinsic positive end-expiratory pressure, and dynamic hyperinflation in mechanically ventilated patients. Respir Care. 2005;50(1):110-23.
12. Laghi F, Goyal A. Auto-PEEP in respiratory failure. Minerva Anestesiol. 2012;78(2):201-21.
13. Scano G, Grazzini M, Stendardi L, et al. Respiratory muscle energetics during exercise in healthy subjects and patients with COPD. Respir Med. 2006;100(11):1896-906.
14. Gagnon P, Guenette JA, Langer D, et al. Pathogenesis of hyperinflation in chronic obstructive pulmonary disease. Int J Chron Obstruct Pulmon Dis. 2014;9:187-201.
15. Koutsoukou A, Pecchiari M. Expiratory flow-limitation in mechanically ventilated patients: A risk for ventilator-induced lung injury? World J Crit Care Med. 2019;8(1):1-8.
16. Pedersen OF, Butler JP. Expiratory flow limitation. Compr Physiol. 2011;1(4):1861-82.
17. Shekar K, Foot C, Fraser J, et al. Bronchopleural fistula: an update for intensivists. J Crit Care. 2010;25(1):47-55.
18. Alohali AF, Abu-Daff S, Alao K, et al. Ventilator Management of Bronchopleural Fistula Secondary to Methicillin-Resistant *Staphylococcus aureus* Necrotizing Pneumonia in a Pregnant Patient with Systemic Lupus Erythematosus. Case Rep Med. 2017;2017:1492910.
19. Ahmed A, Azim A. Difficult tracheal intubation in critically ill. J Intensive Care. 2018;6:49.
20. Bernard GR, Artigas A, Brigham KL, et al. Report of the American-European consensus conference on ARDS: definitions, mechanisms, relevant outcomes and clinical trial coordination. The Consensus Committee. Intensive Care Med. 1994;20(3):225-3.
21. ARDS Definition Task Force, Ranieri VM, Rubenfeld GD, Thompson BT, et al. Acute respiratory distress syndrome: the Berlin Definition. JAMA. 2012;307(23):2526-33.
22. Fujishima S. Pathophysiology and biomarkers of acute respiratory distress syndrome. J Intensive Care. 2014;2(1):32.
23. Amato MB, Barbas CS, Medeiros DM, et al. Effect of a protective-ventilation strategy on mortality in the acute respiratory distress syndrome. N Engl J Med. 1998;338(6):347-54.
24. Acute Respiratory Distress Syndrome Network, Brower RG, Matthay MA, Morris A, et al. Ventilation with lower tidal volumes as compared with traditional tidal volumes for acute lung injury and the acute respiratory distress syndrome. N Engl J Med. 2000;342(18):1301-8.
25. Putensen C, Theuerkauf N, Zinserling J, et al. Meta-analysis: ventilation strategies and outcomes of the acute respiratory distress syndrome and acute lung injury. Ann Intern Med. 2009;151(8):566-76.
26. Slutsky AS, Ranieri VM. Ventilator-induced lung injury. N Engl J Med. 2013;369:2126-36.
27. Hager DN, Krishnan JA, Hayden DL, et al. ARDS clinical trials network. Tidal volume reduction in patients with acute lung injury when plateau pressures are not high. Am J Respir Crit Care Med. 2005;172(10):1241.
28. Fan E, Del Sorbo L, Goligher EC, et al. American Thoracic Society, European Society of Intensive Care Medicine, and Society of Critical Care Medicine. An Official American Thoracic Society/European Society of Intensive Care Medicine/Society of Critical Care Medicine Clinical Practice Guideline: Mechanical ventilation in adult patients with acute respiratory distress syndrome. Am J Respir Crit Care Med. 2017;195(9):1253-63.
29. Scholten EL, Beitler JR, Prisk GK, et al. Treatment of ARDS with prone positioning. Chest. 2017;151(1):215-24.
30. Taccone P, Pesenti A, Latini R, et al. Prone positioning in patients with moderate and severe acute respiratory distress syndrome: A randomized controlled trial. JAMA. 2009;302:1977-84.
31. Guerin C, Reignier J, Richard JC, et al. Prone positioning in severe acute respiratory distress syndrome. N Engl J Med. 2013;368(23):2159-68.
32. Valente Barbas CS. Lung recruitment maneuvers in acute respiratory distress syndrome and facilitating resolution. Crit Care Med. 2003;31(4 Suppl):S265-71.
33. Esan A, Hess DR, Raoof S, et al. Severe hypoxemic respiratory failure part 1–ventilatory strategies. Chest. 2010;137(5):1203-16.
34. Australia and New Zealand Extracorporeal Membrane Oxygenation (ANZ ECMO) Influenza Investigators, Davies A, Jones D, Bailey M, et al. Extracorporeal Membrane Oxygenation for 2009 Influenza A (H1N1) Acute Respiratory Distress Syndrome. JAMA. 2009;302(17):1888-95.

# CHAPTER 8

# Graphic Analysis of Mechanical Ventilation

Daniel Arellano Sepúlveda

## INTRODUCTION

In the past few years, the mechanical ventilation development has been remarkable, allowing the incorporation of important innovations for the ventilation to patients with respiratory insufficiency. Within this novelty we can include the systems to improve the oxygen and other gasses supply, advanced ventilatory modalities and the graphic monitoring of mechanical ventilation. This monitoring through graphic screens has given the possibility to implement the physiological elements of breathing, the primary ventilatory evaluation and the optimization of mechanical ventilation and the respiratory care.[1] Although most mechanical ventilators (MVs) of latest technology bring in this technology to the graphic analysis of the ventilation and the capacity to assess parameters of pulmonary mechanics. This information is not completely incorporated to the intensive care professionals' daily practice. Many times, technology has surpassed the capacity of the specialists to be able to understand and use this information.

Despite these factors, the ventilatory graphics have begun to be a usual item in the environment of the critical patient and require proper interpretation, in the same way a musician reads the chords on a staff. This same capacity of symbol analysis is needed to adequately read the graphed curves in the MV. The use of the ventilatory graphics to enhance the care of our patients requires the understanding of the clinical context under which this information is taken, the factors that influence them and can interfere in their correct understanding.[2]

## BASIC CONCEPTS

Usually, the mechanical ventilation is typified by three traditional variables—(1) the volume (capacity), (2) pressure, and (3) flow (and the time in which these variables are implemented), which will have specific performances facing certain factors and physiopathological conditions.[3] To the research of the pulmonary graphic, these variables interact and can be analyzed through the graphic curves (one variable in relation to time) or loops (more than one variable).[4]

## CURVES

The most used curves correspond to pressure/time curve (P/t), flow/time curve (F/t) and volume/time curve (V/t).

### Pressure/Time Curve

This curve shows the incremental changes of the air route pressure in relation to time. The pressure is expressed in centimeters of water ($cmH_2O$) and the time in seconds.

### Flow/Time Curve

In this case, the curve shows the changes of the air route (both inspiratory and expiratory) in relation to time. We must recall that flow corresponds to a speed concept and it is expressed in liters per minute (L/minute). Therefore, the changes in speed that a gas volume suffers during the input and output of the respiratory system will be shown in this graphic.

### Volume/Time Curve

It shows the relation between the input and output of an amount of gas applied to a respiratory system (flow volume) in a defined period. The volume can be shown in milliliters (mL) or liters (L) and its performance is related to the behavior of the flow curve.

## LOOPS

The loops are characterized by the relation of two variables, and not by comparing a variable in relation to time, with the intention to provide information of certain changes in the pulmonary function.[5] The most used loops are volume/pressure (V/P) and flow/volume (F/V).

### Volume/Pressure

It provides dynamic information of the respiratory system distensibility. It can be measured in quasi-static conditions, which improves the reliance in the information measured. It is of great help to evaluate the pulmonary overstretching in controlled mood by volume with constant flow.

### Flow/Volume

It relates the mobilized volume and the speed that the flow is provided. This loop expresses the airway resistance (Raw) and it is important when the bronchodilator's response is evaluated, or in case of leaks in the patient-ventilator system.

## NOMENCLATURE

The interpretation of the curves will depend on the ventilatory mode used and the preset parameters. For a correct reading of the alterations in these curves, it is necessary to know the standard components that must be evaluated in the ventilatory graphic as shown here.

### Pressure/Time Curve

This curve shows the behavior of the pressure in time (Fig. 1). The pressure applied in the airway can be of two types:
- The *positive pressure* which is externally blown to the respiratory system from a high-pressure system (usually an MV) and it is drawn above the horizontal (X-axis or abscissa) of the P/t curve.
- The *negative pressure* is drawn under the X-axis (abscissa) of the P/t curve.

The time during which the positive pressure is applied, corresponds to the inspiratory time.

When the patient has an expiratory pressure preset [positive end-expiratory pressure (PEEP) or continuous positive airway pressure (CPAP)], the P/t curve appears with an established positive pressure over its zero value (Fig. 2). When the PEEP is not used, all the generated pressure of this basal pressure (abscissa) corresponds to negative pressure generated by the patient's effort (Fig. 1).

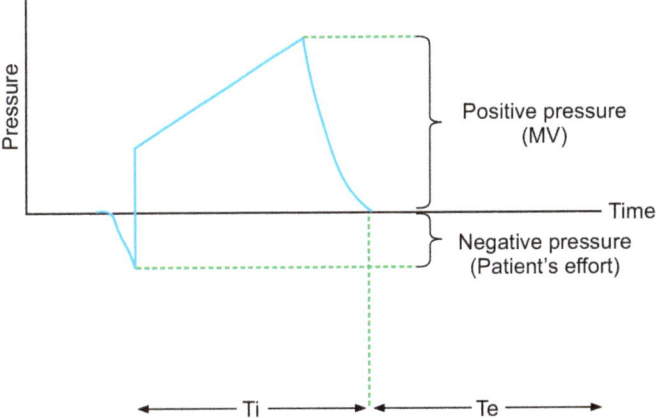

**Fig. 1:** Pressure/time (P/t) curve. All pressure generated over the abscissa (X-axis) is positive pressure blown to the airway by the mechanical ventilator. All the pressure generated under the abscissa (X-axis) is negative pressure generated by the patient's effort (Ti: inspiratory time; Te: expiratory time).

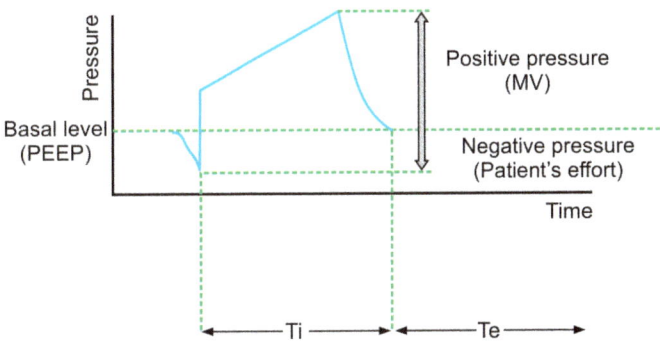

**Fig. 2:** Pressure/time (P/t) curve with positive end-expiratory pressure (PEEP) (basal level of pressure) (Ti: inspiratory time; Te: expiratory time).

When the patient is ventilated with PEEP or CPAP, the pressure generated by patient is graphed under the basal level of pressure (PEEP or CPAP) (Fig. 2).[4]

### Flow/Time Curve

This curve shows the flow pattern used or generated, it means, the speed the gas moves through the airway. It is considered inspiratory flow every plotted value for over the basal zero (abscissa or X-axis) and the expiratory flow corresponds to the plotted value under zero level. Since the expiratory flow has an opposite direction with respect to the inspiratory flow, it is represented as a negative value, under the x-axis (Fig. 3).

The morphology of the inspiratory flow curve will depend on the mode and the type of ventilatory control used.[4]

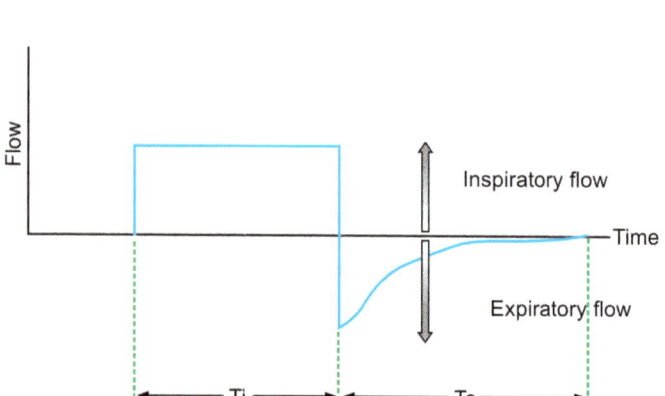

**Fig. 3:** Flow/time (F/t) curve in controlled mode by volume with constant flow. All plotted flow over the X-axis is inspiratory flow and the one generated under this axis is expiratory flow. The morphology of the inspiratory curve can vary according to the control mode used. The expiratory curve depends on the pulmonary mechanics (Ti: inspiratory time; Te: expiratory time).

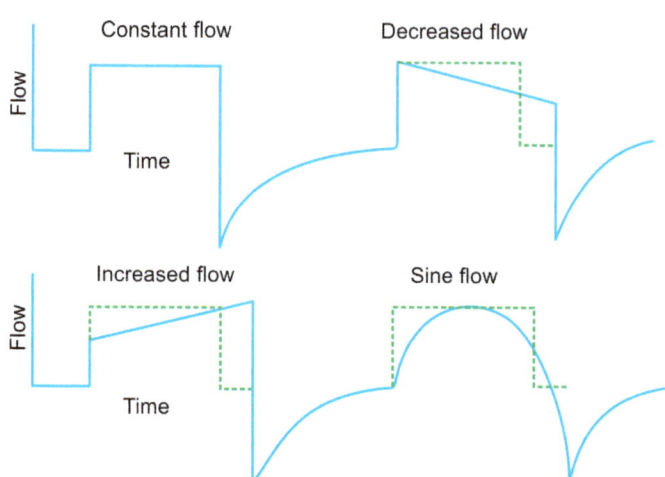

**Fig. 4:** Inspiratory flow patterns in volume control mode. The constant flow curve stands out for being the one which moves the gas volume in shorter time. The other types of flow patterns allow best adjustment under certain conditions and kinds of ventilated patients.

In modes controlled by pressure [pressure-controlled ventilation (PCV), pressure support (PS)], the inspiratory flow will behave according to:[5]
- Inspiratory pressure programed by the operator
- Preset inspiratory time
- The patient's thoracopulmonary mechanics (distensibility and stamina)
- The patient's ventilatory effort.

On the other hand, in modes controlled by volume, the inspiratory flow can be fixed and preset by the operator, and the waveform pattern flow can be programed according to the availability in different models of MVs: increased, decreased, constant or sine[6] (Fig. 4).

### Constant or Square Flow

It is one of the flow patterns most used in patients who require the entry of the tidal volume in the shortest time possible, with the intention of optimizing the expiratory time and the lung deflation (e.g. obstructive patients, chronic obstructive pulmonary disease, etc.). It is characterized because the gas always enters to the airway at the same speed (or flow), this will generate a rising pressure curve.

### Increasing Flow

In this pattern, the flow starts from zero and gets a maximum inspiratory flow (peak flow) preset. It is also used in patients who require high flows (obstructive and with a high ventilatory demand).

### Decreasing Flow

In this case, the flow starts at a maximum set value and usually goes down to zero at the end of the inspiration. This type of flow is used in restrictive patients because it generates less pressure in the airway and is better tolerated by the patient.

### Sinusoidal Flow

This flow pattern has an increasing flow phase followed by a decreasing flow phase. This pattern is most physiological and it is better tolerated by the patient.

In standard modalities, the MV functions only to input the gas volume in the lung, being the passive exhalation; for this reason, the expiratory flow depends on the elastic recoil of the lung, as well as the Raw. The normal morphology of the expiratory flow curve is similar in all ventilatory modes or inspiratory flow patterns. The expiratory flow can also be influenced or modified by patient's active expiratory effort, or by external maneuvers that compress the thorax [chest physiotherapy, cardiopulmonary resuscitation (CPR), etc.].

It should be noted that the area under the flow curve (both inspiratory and expiratory) corresponds to the gas volume moved in inspiratory phase: tidal volume (Fig. 5).

## Volume/Time Curve

This curve shows the behavior of the volume moved in time, and under standard conditions, both the inspired and exhaled tidal volume should be exemplified over the X-axis (Fig. 6). The inspiratory volume curve increases up

# Chapter 8
## Graphic Analysis of Mechanical Ventilation

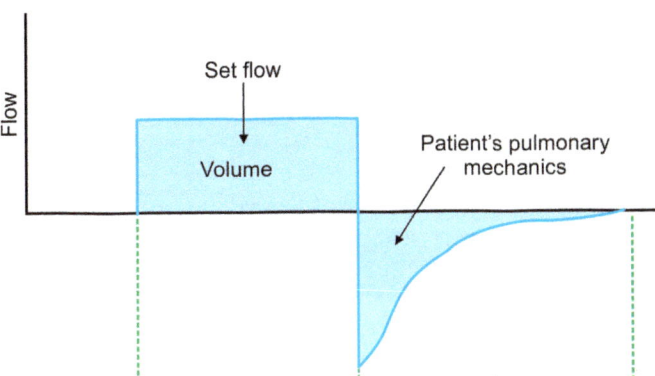

**Fig. 5:** Flow/time (F/t) curve. In volume-control modes, the inspiratory flow is programed, and the expiratory flow depends of respiratory mechanics. The area under the flow curve corresponds to the tidal volume (curve for mode volume control with constant flow) (Ti: inspiratory time; Te: expiratory time).

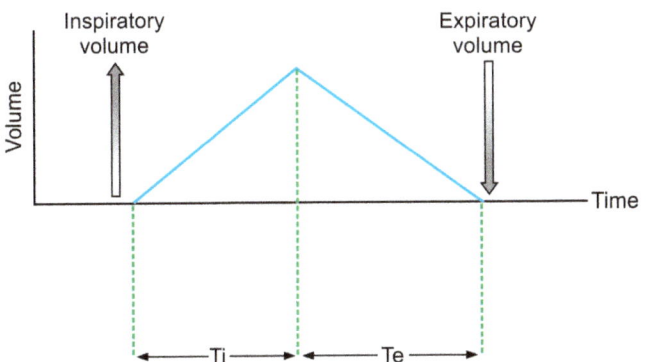

**Fig. 6:** Volume/time (V/t) curve. In this curve, the volume is expressed in the axis Y. The inclination of the volume curve determines the time used to provide volume (flow).

to the programed value (it is expressed in the Y-axis). The inclination of this part of the curve determines the used time to input the volume and it is related to inspiratory flow:
- If it is more inclined, indicate a lower inspiratory flow and therefore it will require more time to reach to the programed volume.[7]
- When this inspiratory volume curve is more vertical, indicate less inspiratory time and higher flow.

The decreasing part of this curve corresponds to the expiratory phase and therefore, to the gas output from the respiratory system. The morphology of the V/t curve depends on the behavior of the inspiratory and expiratory flow curves.

It should be noted that the beginning of the curve of volume must start and end in zero (in the X-axis). If the volume does not reach zero, it indicates leakage or air escapes. If the curve of expiratory volume surpasses under the X-axis shows the patient's active exhalation.

## CURVES INTERPRETATION

To read the pulmonary graphic and the different curves, the ventilatory mode and the flow patterns must be considered. For this reason, we will analyze the different types of curves in the two main control modes [pressure control (PC) and volume control (VC)][8] and in the most used programed flow patterns (constant and decreasing flow).

### Volume Control versus Pressure Control

#### Pressure Control

The ventilation pressure controlled (weather in mandatory or spontaneous modes) is characterized by generating curves of square pressure associated to a decreasing inspiratory flow (Fig. 7B). As the pressure is fixed and remains constant during the inspiratory time, the inspiratory flow decreases as the pressure gradient declines.[9]

It should be underlined that when "the inspiratory flow decreases" means that the gas enters to the lung increasingly slower. As it will be explained later, the morphology of the inspiratory flow curve will depend on the thoracopulmonary mechanic. Since the flow is increasingly slower (remind that flow = speed), the entry volume is higher at the beginning of the inspiratory time (upright curve) and then it begins to decrease as time passes (horizontal curve).

The expiratory flow, since exhalation is passive, it always depends on the elastic recoil of the lung and the Raw, consequently it is decelerating: at the beginning there is an expiratory peak flow that decreases its output speed up to zero.[10]

#### Volume Control

In this pattern, the flow is programed by the clinicians, for this reason, it can have several settings[6,10] (Fig. 4). The volume curve will behave according to the gas entry preset (flow). The pressure curve will vary in relation to the pulmonary mechanic and the programed flow pattern. If constant flow is used (square flow curve, Fig. 7A), the increase of the pressure will be exponential as the resistance increases the respiratory system, the MV must perform more work to keep a constant inspiratory flow which generates more pressure. If a decelerating flow is used, the morphology of the pressure curve is more "rectangular", since the programed drop of the inspiratory flow match with the increase of the elastic charge, which generates in the airways a kind of constant pressure.

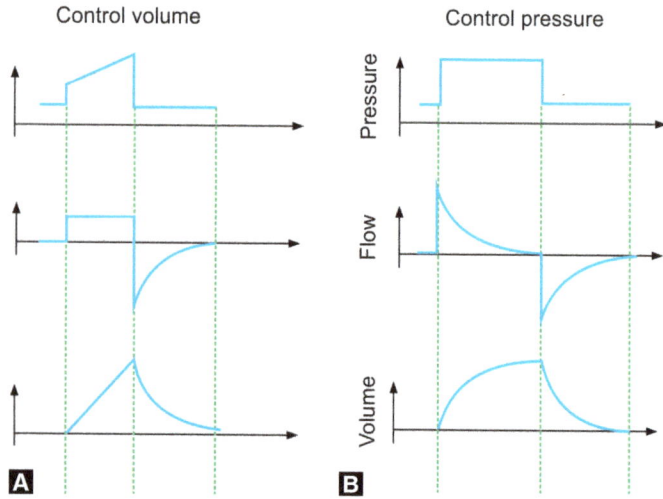

**Figs. 7A and B:** Volume control versus pressure control. Differences among P/t, F/t and V/t on modes controlled by volume (A) or pressure (B).

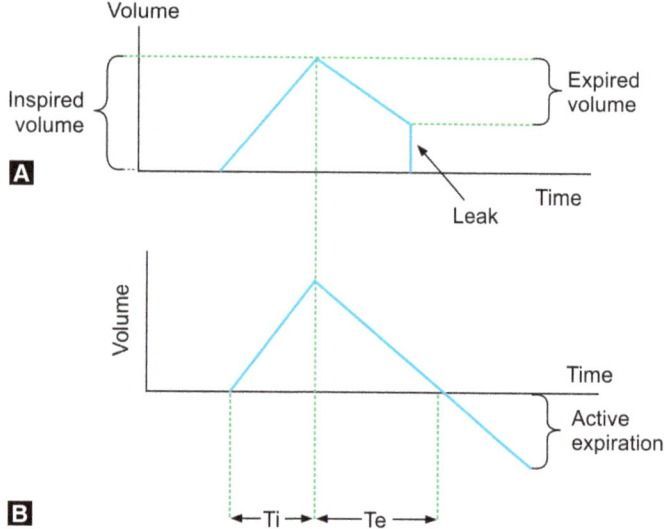

**Figs. 8A and B:** Volume/time curve. (A) Leakage. It shows the exhaled volume curve that does not get zero (the exhale volume is less than the inspired volume). (B) Active exhalation: the active exhalation occurs when the patient produces a higher expiratory volume than the inspired volume. In this case, the exhaled volume surpasses the baseline (zero volume).

## Interpretation of Volume/Time Curve

As it was mentioned previously, the V/t curve usually begins in zero and increases up to get the preset volume.[7] During the exhalation, while the exhaled volume leaves the lung, the curve volume should descend until zero. If the expired volume curve did not get zero, it would imply that possibly there is a gas leak in the patient-ventilator system (Fig. 8A). This signal could be showing an air leakage[11] at the ventilator circuit level (circuit connectors incorrectly set, etc.), at the artificial airways level [endotracheal tube (ETT) cuff flat], or at a patient's level (bronchopleural fistula, pneumothorax, etc.). When a V/t curve alteration is discovered, the hermeticism of the ventilator, the ETT or ventilator circuit, and the patient must be evaluated.

When the expiratory curve surpasses zero, under the abscissa (axis X or time line), indicates that the patient is exhaling a higher volume than the inspired one, it means, that the patient is producing an active exhalation (Fig. 8B). This phenomenon can also happen when there is active expiration or the patient coughs.

It should be noted that when patient produces an active exhalation, he eliminates a gas volume which is part of his functional residual capacity (FRC), which will be restored in sometime. For this reason, it is not rare that the expiratory volume curve does not get zero when a patient has active exhalation during some further respiratory phases. Therefore, to be sure of leakage presence, this ventilatory alteration must be present in all cycles (Fig. 9).

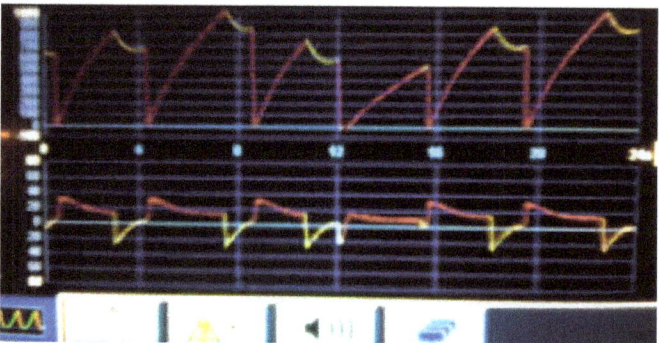

**Fig. 9:** Leak in volume/time (V/t) curve. A great leakage is shown in support pressure ventilation (PSV). It should be noted that in the V/t curve (up) the exhaled volume is little (yellow) and the curve does not reach zero, showing a great leakage.

## Interpretation of Pressure/Time Curve

The P/t curve will vary according to the control mode of the ventilatory phase (VC or PC) and the flow pattern used (when ventilation is controlled by volume). For this reason, the P/t curve will be evaluated under these following circumstances as shown here.

### Pressure/Time Curve in Pressure Control

As it was previously mentioned, the modalities controlled by pressure (PC) are characterized by being limited by pressure, which generates a square pressure curve (constant pressure) and a decelerating flow curve. In this case, the pressure curve can be considered constant and immutable; however, it is important to mention that in MV of newest generation, the setting could vary using rise time (or Ramp). This command allows to generate a slower pressurization of the airway, which generates a pressure curve of "upward" aspect (or accelerating).[12] In this method of control, the P/t curve does not change; consequently its observation will not provide information.

### Pressure/Time Curve in Volume Control with Constant Flow

As it was previously mentioned, the VC ventilation, which uses constant flow, characterizes for generating a square flow curve and an exponential pressure curve (upward). In this case, the flow curve is invariable and set by the clinician, while the pressure curve will vary according to the mechanical conditions of the lung. The generated pressure in the airway (peak inspiratory pressure, $P_{IP}$) is the result of the work performed by the MV to defeat the resistive load (flow and the Raw) and the elastic load (pulmonary compliance and volume) (Fig. 10). If the Raw and/or the compliance worsen, the pressure in the airways will increase. In this case, it is not possible to discriminate if the increase of the $P_{IP}$ was because of compliance or resistance alteration.[13,14]

To discriminate between the pressure generated by elastic and frictional resistances, we can carry out a maneuver usually available in most ventilators, and it is easy to perform: a hold inspiratory pause (or pause time). The pause time is carried out at the end of the inspiration and consists in the closing of the inspiratory and expiratory valves of the MV, which holds the gas volume trapped inside the lung for a determined time. During the pause time the airflow is zero, because of this the airway pressure drops (when there is not airflow there is not resistive load).[15] In the absence of airflow, the only resistance to be defeated by the MV is the elastic recoil of the lung (elastic load, expressed by the pause pressure, also known as plateau pressure or plateau, $P_{pl}$) (Fig. 11).

The difference between the $P_{IP}$ and the $P_{pl}$, i.e. $P_{IP} - P_{pl}$ corresponds to the necessary pressure to beat the resistive load impost to the respiratory system (Raw and flow). This difference in pressure can also be known as resistance pressure. Meanwhile, the difference between the $P_{pl}$ and the PEEP corresponds to the necessary pressure to beat the elastic load, given by the elastic recoil of the lung (elastance) and the mobilized volume. This difference in pressure is known as compliance pressure or driving pressure (Fig. 12).

The measurement of the pause pressure allows discriminating qualitatively between disturbances in the compliance or the Raw, which directs the therapeutic management to follow (Figs. 13A and B). An increase on the

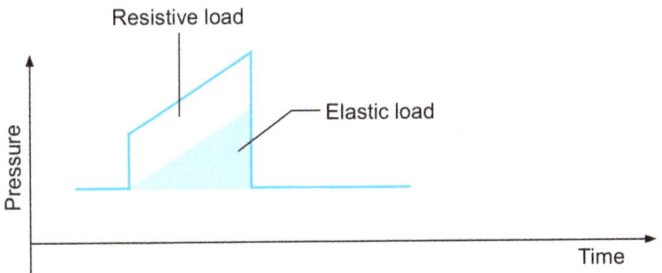

**Fig. 10:** Pressure/time curve in constant flow of volume control ventilation. The maximum pressure generated in the airway ($P_{IP}$) is necessary to defeat the elastic and resistive load. An increase of these loads will produce an upward of the $P_{IP}$, without discriminating which of the two resistances produced the raise in the pressure.

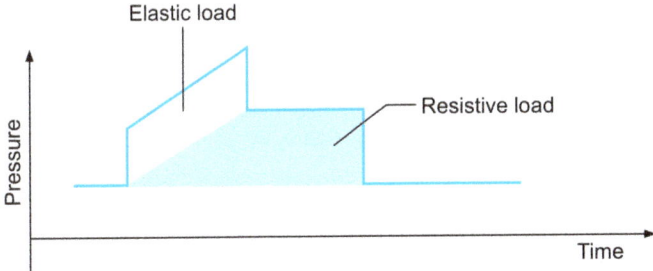

**Fig. 11:** Pressure/time curve in constant flow in volume control (VC) mode with pause time. In implementing an inspiratory pause (or pause time), the airway resistance is isolated since there is not flow. In this case, the only resistance which generates pressure is the elastic pulmonary load (elastance and volume) which is expressed as the pause pressure or plateau.

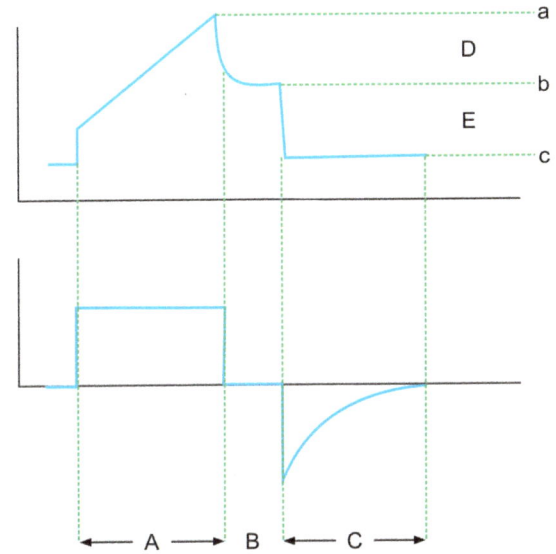

**Fig. 12:** Elements of a P/t curve in control volume ventilation, with pause time and constant flow. A: inspiratory time; B: pause time; C: expiratory time; D: resistance pressure ($P_{IP}$-$P_{plat}$, associated to resistive load); E: compliance pressure or driving pressure ($P_{plat}$-PEEP, associated to elastic load); a: peak inspiratory pressure ($P_{IP}$); b: plateau pressure ($P_{plat}$); c: PEEP.

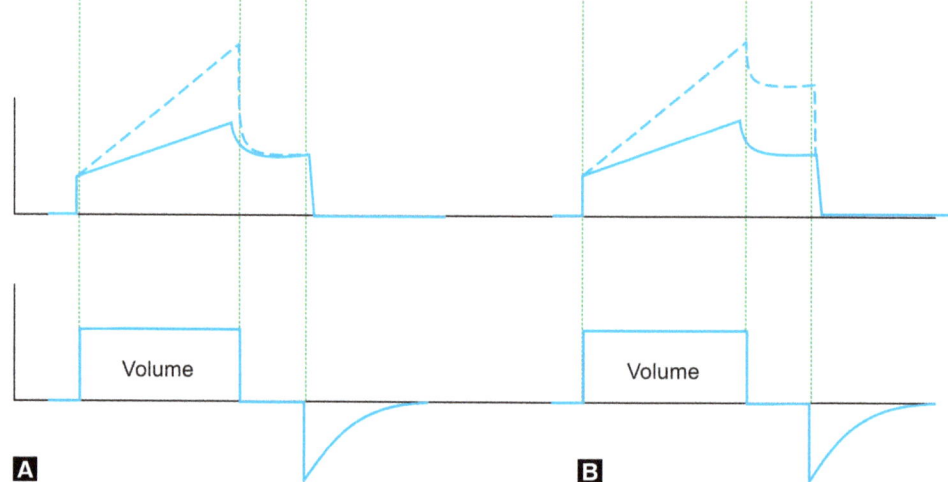

**Figs. 13A and B:** Variation of the P/t curve in the control volume ventilation, with pause time and constant flow. (A) An increase in the resistance of the airway (Raw) will produce an increase on the PIP, without varying the plateau pressure ($P_{plat}$). (B) A decrease in the compliance will produce an increase in the Pplat, with an increase associated to the $P_{IP}$. It should be noted that the difference between the PIP and the Pplat stays the same, which means that the Raw does not change.

Raw will produce an increase in the maximum inspiratory pressure ($P_{IP}$) without varying the $P_{pl}$. On the other hand, a decrease in the thoracopulmonary distensibility (consequently, an increase in the elastance or elastic recoil of the lung) will emerge by an increase on the $P_{IP}$ and the $P_{pl}$. If there is not a disturbance in the Raw, the difference between the $P_{IP}$ and the $P_{pl}$ should stay unaffected.

Under these same conditions, and if we know the numerical values of the ventilatory parameters, the static compliance (Cst)[16] and the Raw[17] can be quantitatively evaluated through the use of the following formula:

$$Cst = \frac{\text{Expired Tidal Volume}\,(mL)}{P_{pl} - PEEP\,(cmH_2O)}$$

$$Raw = \frac{P_{IP} - P_{pl}\,(cmH_2O)}{\text{Inspiratory flow}\,(L/sec)}$$

It should be noticed that to measure the Raw it is necessary a constant flow. To measure the Cst, it is necessary apply an inspiratory pause which generates the $P_{pl}$. In lots of MV, it is needed to perform this maneuver in modalities controlled by volume, although the newest MV also allows its measurement in modes controlled by pressure.

### Volume Control Ventilation with Decelerating Flow

The VC ventilation with decelerating flow is characterized by generating a flow pattern where the gas enters to the respiratory system at the beginning at a great speed, and then gradually decreases its speed until it reaches zero.

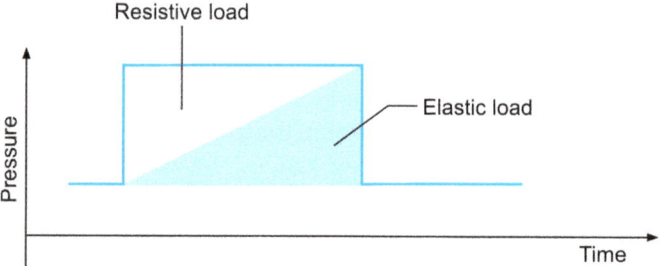

**Fig. 14:** Pressure/time (P/t) curve in volume control ventilation with decelerating flow. In the same way as the mode with constant flow, the generated pressure is necessary to defeat the elastic and resistive loads.

When this flow pattern is programed, the pressure curve tends to be square. In the same way as the constant flow, the flow curve is invariable, and the pressure curve will vary according to the mechanical conditions of the respiratory system[14] (Fig. 14). If there is an increment in the resistive load (Raw), the P/t curve shows an increase in the pressure generated to defeat these resistive forces, therefore, the P/t curve tends to take the appearance of a "decelerating curve", with a raise in the pressure at the beginning of the inspiratory phase (Fig. 15A). When the disturbance of the pulmonary mechanics is caused by the increase in the elastic load (increment of elastance and therefore, the drop of the compliance), the P/t curve has an appearance of "upward curve" (Fig. 15B), with an increase in pressure at the end of the inspiration.

To understand the behavior of P/t curve is of great help, since it allows them to evaluate the disturbances in the respiratory system mechanics. For example, the clearance

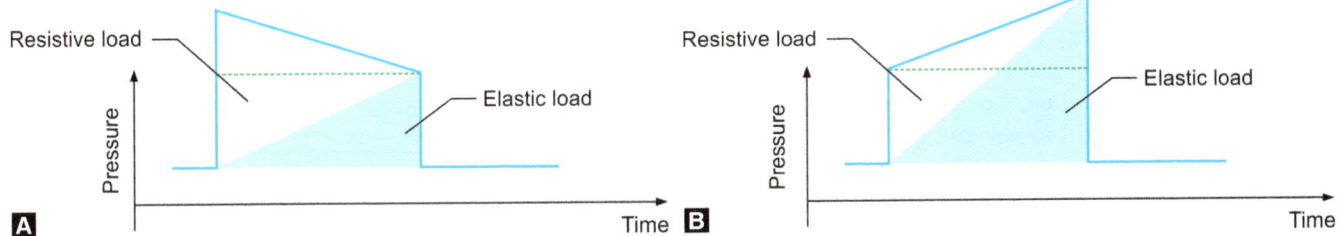

**Figs. 15A and B:** Variation of the P/t curve in volume control ventilation with decelerating flow. (A) Increase in the resistive work by the increment in the resistance of the airway (Raw). (B) Increase in the elastic work caused by fall in the respiratory system compliance.

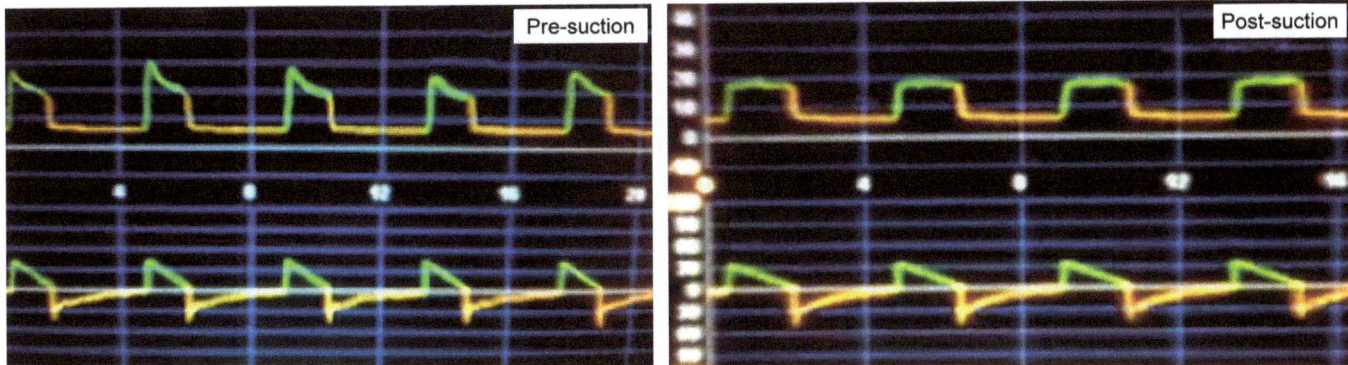

**Fig. 16:** Changes in the P/t (VC and decelerating flow) pre- and post-endotracheal suction (ETS). Note that the increment in the pressure at the beginning of the inhalation (curve P/t) prior to the ETS, which shows an increase in the Raw. Posterior to the ETS the configuration of the P/t curve is recovered, this shows a reduction in the Raw after clearing the airway.

of the airway would reduce the Raw, as well as the rescission of an atelectasis would improve the compliance[18] (Fig. 16).

## Interpretation of Flow/Time Curve

The behavior of the inspiratory flow will depend on the mode used, in VC modes it will be unchangeable, while in PC ventilation, the curve F/t will change and will depend on the behavior of the respiratory system compliance (Crs) and the Raw. Besides, we must remember that in mechanical ventilation the exhalation is passive, so the morphology of the expiratory flow curve will depend on the respiratory system mechanics. Since exhalation is similar in all modalities, the F/t curve in this phase will always provide important information.

### Curve Flow/Time: Inspiratory Flow

This curve must be studied in PC ventilation, where it is modified and depends on the respiratory mechanics. It is necessary to remember that the area under the flow curve corresponds to the mobilized volume (tidal volume). The tidal volume will depend on the preset inspiratory pressure, on the time applied and on the Crs of the patient (Fig. 17). At larger Crs, the greater tidal volume. It is also important to have in mind that the inspiratory flow will reach zero at the end of the final inspiration; in modes limited by pressure

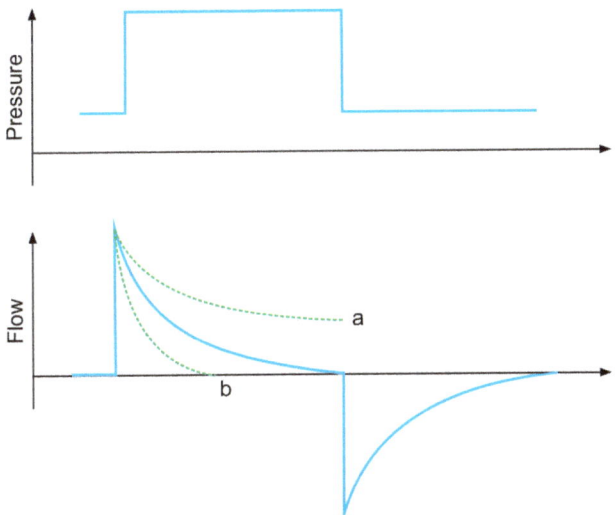

**Fig. 17:** Flow/time (F/t) curve in pressure control ventilation. The area under the flow curve corresponds to the tidal volume. According to the patient's static compliance (Cst), the mobilized volume will vary: if the Cst increases, the mobilized volume will be higher (a), if the opposite occurs, the tidal volume will be lower and the flow curve might quickly reach zero (b).

or cycled by time (PC), if the inspiratory time is short, the inspiratory flow will probably not reach zero, which shows that the patient, in relation to preset pressure and his/her Crs, might lead to higher volume. In other cases, the inspiratory time will be longer or the Crs will be shorter; therefore, the inspiratory flow will reach zero before the inspiratory time ends.[19]

Based on the information, the inspiratory flow curve can provide qualitative information on Crs. Variations on this curve would indicate disturbances in the elastic capacity of the lung, for example, pneumonia, acute respiratory distress syndrome (ARDS), atelectasis, pneumothorax, etc., which is revealed by the reduction in the tidal volume moved in PC ventilation, with a premature fall in the inspiratory flow curve to zero (Fig. 18). This curve can also be disturbed in cases of important disturbances in the artificial airway, as it will be discuss later.

### Curve Flow/Time: Expiratory Flow

In mechanical ventilation, the exhalation is passive and the gas outlet from the respiratory system depends directly from the Crs and the Raw, so that the evaluation of the expiratory flow (through the F/t curve) is of vital importance when you are doing the analysis of the respiratory system mechanics status and a specific pathology which affects it. As previously mentioned, the main factor that establishes the output of the gas is given by the lung elastance. The elastance of the lung [or lung elastic recoil (LER)], it can be defined as the mechanical property that certain elements have to suffer reversible deflections when they are submitted to the action of external forces and, recover their original form when these external forces stop their action.[20] These "external forces" would correspond to the inspiratory muscle action which help to generate the intrapulmonary volume changes and the "deformation" of the parenchyma during the insufflation. Under physical terms, a lung to be more elastic is going to need more energy to distort it (insufflate) and the exhalation is going to return more rapidly to its initial position. When it recovers the initial position faster, it implies that it will quickly empty itself, so that it will generate a higher expiratory flow. However, to a greater elastance, the higher energy is needed to insufflate, and a greater elastic recoil in the exhalation that generates a greater expiratory flow. It is important to remember that elastance corresponds to the reverse of compliance, as the compliance decreases the elastance increases, and vice versa. Based on these concepts, we can assume that a patient with low compliance will have a high elastance and, therefore, it will have great LER that will generate a higher expiratory flow (to a higher elastance, the higher expiratory flow. Remember, flow = speed).

When analyzing the exhalation in the F/t curve, it is possible to study the LER (through the peak expiratory flow, PEF) and the restriction to the airflow (Fig. 19).

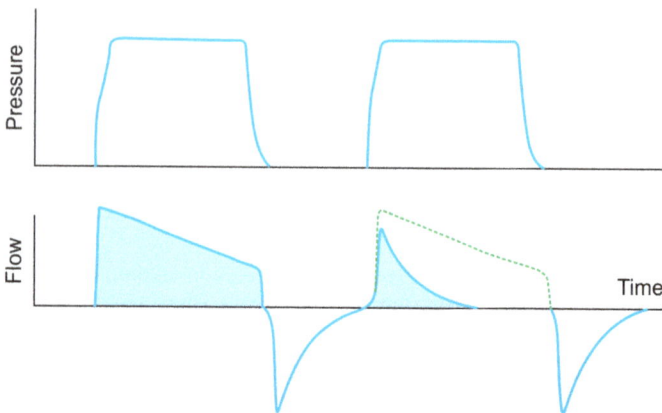

**Fig. 18:** The fall of the tidal volume by the reduction in the static compliance (Cst). It should be noted that the area under the curve F/t (tidal volume) decreases significantly, and the inspiratory flow reaches early zero.

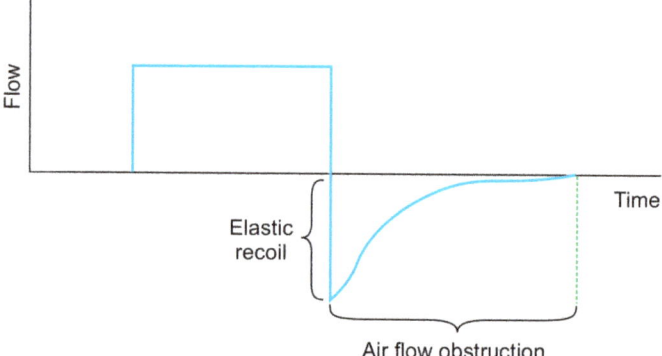

**Fig. 19:** Flow/time (F/t) curve. Analysis of the expiratory flow curve. The peak expiratory flow (PEF) is determined by the lung elastic recoil (LER): the higher the LER, the greater the PEF. The remainder of the curve allows the evaluation of the limitation in the airflow and the capacity of pulmonary emptying.

As it was commented, a patient with diminished compliance will have a high elastance, this increment of the LER will produce a high peak flow in the moment of the exhalation (Figs. 20A and B). Therefore, unlike the evaluation with spirometry, in MV the presence of a high maximum expiratory flow (peak) must be associated to patients with little distensible lung, with great LER.

The obstruction in the airway and the restriction of the airflow can be evaluated through the F/t curve, watching the behavior of the expiratory flow (Fig. 21). In standard conditions, the LER produces a high expiratory flow at the beginning (PEF), subsequently the expired gas starts to come out increasingly slower from the respiratory system until it reaches zero[21] (Fig. 19). In patients with obstruction in the airway, the gas will take more time to be exhaled, which increases the necessary time to empty the lung (Fig. 21). The expiratory flow must always reach

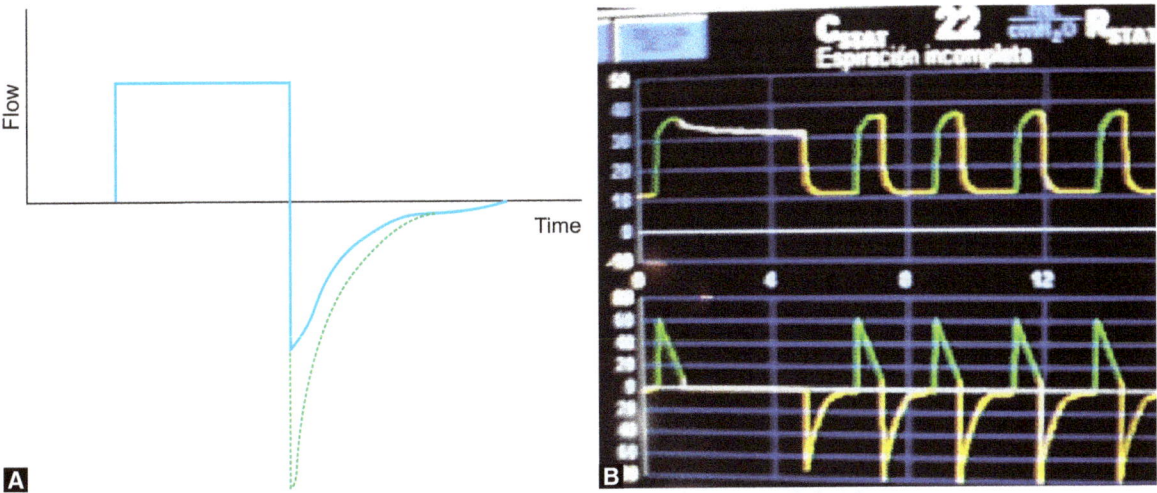

**Figs. 20A and B:** Peak expiratory flow (PEF) and the lung elastic recoil (LER). The elastance (LER) is inversely proportional to the compliance, so the PEF will be proportional to the elastance. Therefore, low compliance will generate an increment of the elastance and a high expiratory flow (shown as broken line in Figure 20A). (B) P/t and F/t curves in a patient with low compliance (22 mL/cmH$_2$O). Note a high P$_{plat}$ and high expiratory flows (even higher than inspiratory flows).

zero, which indicates the complete output of the standard volume that had been inspired.[22] When the expiratory flow does not reach zero before the beginning of a new ventilatory cycle would indicate that the volume of inspired air was not exhaled completely, showing air entrapment and a possible generation of auto-PEEP[23] (Fig. 22). The auto-PEEP (also known as intrinsic PEEP) corresponds to the generated pressure in the respiratory system by the air entrapment, which is neither programed nor desired and it can only be seen evaluated in the ventilator using an extended expiratory pause. The auto-PEEP can disturb the ventilatory mechanics, increase the respiratory work and promote the pulmonary overstretching. This air entrapment and the subsequent auto-PEEP can also appear when the MV setting is not well adjusted, especially if the preset respiratory frequency is too high or the expiratory time is too short.[22,23]

### Signs of Obstruction in the Flow/Time Curve

The expiratory flow curve can also highlight obstruction in the artificial airway caused by secretions or by the humidifier filters. It was previously mentioned that the PEF is influenced by the LER. It should be underlined that in cases where there is an important resistance to the expiratory flow (by bronchospasm or secretions) this PEF will be limited and will suddenly restrict the gas output, this phenomenon will trigger a change in the setting of the expiratory flow curve, producing a "spike" shape. The presence of this spike always denotes resistance of the gas output, which can suggest secretions in the artificial airway or important obstruction in the airway (Figs. 23A to C).

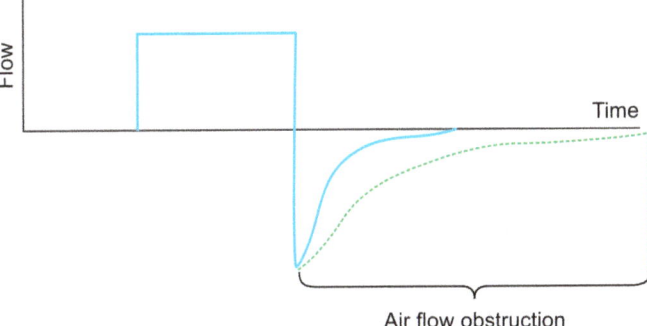

**Fig. 21:** Expiratory flow limitation. The bronchial obstruction can be detected in the pulmonary graphic. When there is a decrease in the diameter of the airway, the gas comes out slowly from the lung, increasing the necessary time to produce the exhalation (shown as broken line).

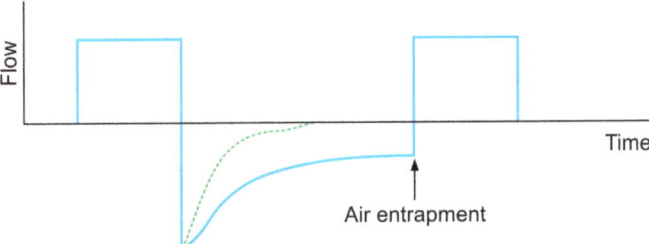

**Fig. 22:** Air entrapment. When the expiratory flow does not reach zero indicates that the tidal volume was not exhaled completely. This signal suggests air entrapment and the possible presence of auto-PEEP.

When the obstruction is greater, a narrowing in the airway will restrict the gas output in the whole exhalation (not only at the beginning), it does not allow a high expiratory flow, so the gas comes out from the lung in an

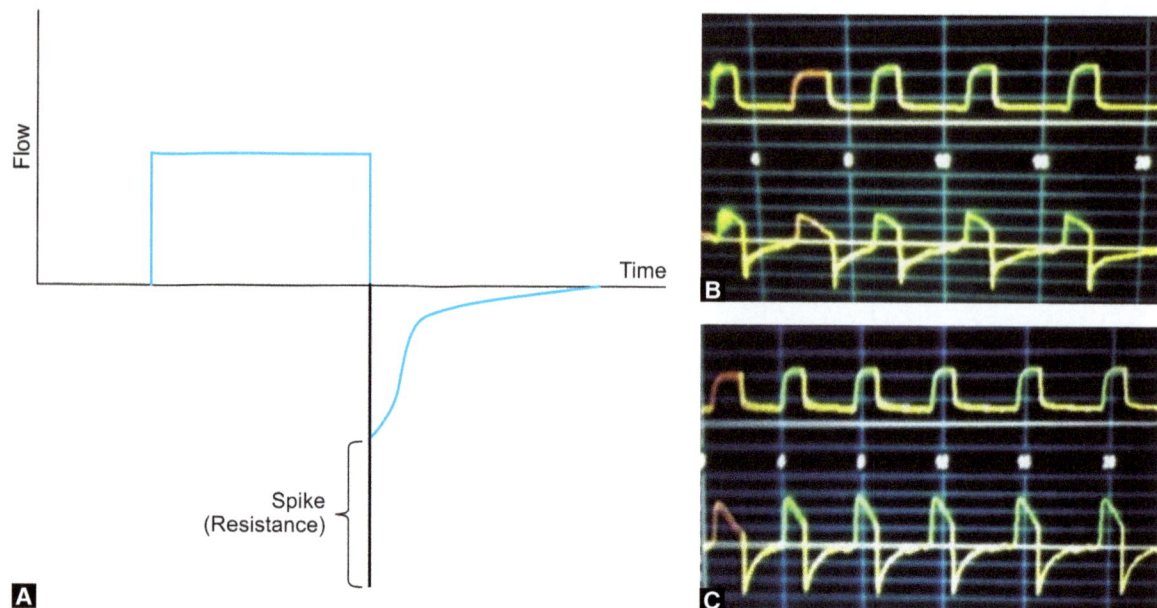

**Figs. 23A to C:** Flow/time (F/t) curve—expiratory resistance. (A) The appearance of a "spike", product of the resistance that suddenly limits the expiratory flow. (B and C) P/t and F/t curve in patients with occluded endotracheal tube: (B) "spikes" in the expiratory flow curves that show resistance to the expiratory flow, which disappear post-endotracheal suction (C).

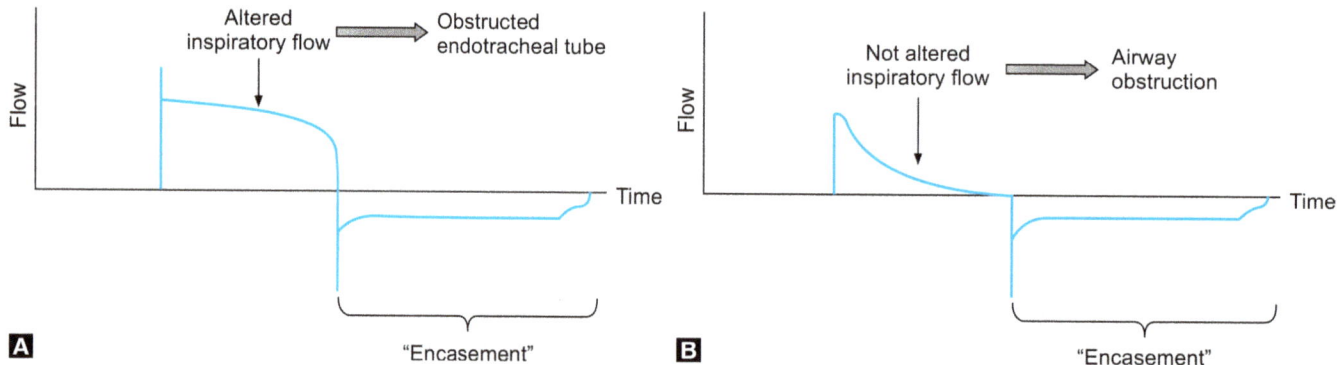

**Figs. 24A and B:** Disturbance of the F/t curve during the airway obstruction. The encasement of the expiratory flow curve and the appearing of the spike show severe obstruction to expiratory air flow. This obstruction can be due to a mucus plug or secretions in the airway, or to bronchospasm. The disturbance in the inspiratory flow curve allows to discriminate where the origin of the disturbance is? If the inspiratory flow curve is also encased and the spike appears, it indicates that there is a resistance as much in the inspiration as in the exhalation, probably caused by endotracheal tube occluded (A). When the inspiratory flow curve is harmless, it would not have disturbances in the inspiratory resistance, so that the increase in the raw is probably caused by a bronchospasm (B).

extended time at a low speed. This gas output at very low flows and in an extended time is named as "encasement" of the expiratory flow curve (Fig. 24A).

The presence of the "encasement" expresses a severe obstruction of the airway or the ETT, which requires an instant attention (Figs. 25A to C). When the encasement and the apparition of the spike also compromise the inspiratory flow curve, it would exist an increased resistance at a global level, both inspiration and exhalation. This phenomenon would show the obstruction in the ETT, usually by mucus plug (other causes include the blockage of the humidifier filter, patients that bite the ETT or too tight ETT fixing systems). When the inspiratory flow curve is not altered, the obstruction can probably be caused by a bronchospasm or some other cause (nor in artificial airway) (Fig. 24B).

Recent studies have proved that the disturbance in the flow curve is more sensitive and early to detect alteration in the resistance to the airway than the increment in the $P_{IP}$.[23]

## LOOPS ANALYSIS

The loops are characterized by establishing two variables in the same ventilatory graphic, with the final purpose

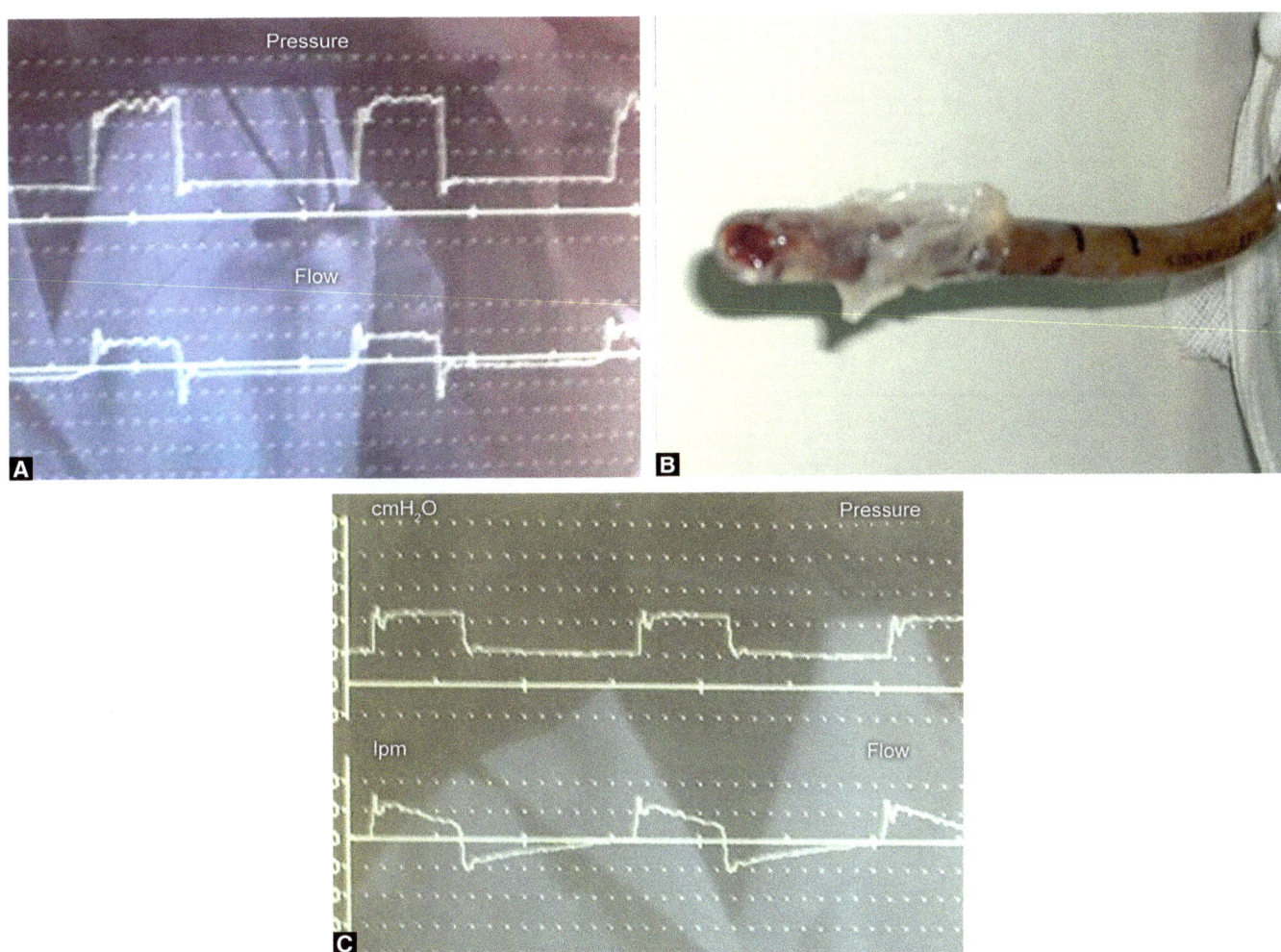

**Figs. 25A to C:** Flow/time (F/t) curve in the endotracheal tube occluded in PC ventilation. (A) F/t curve altered: encasement and spike in the inspiratory and expiratory flow curve. (B) Occluded endotracheal tube. (C) Recovery of the normal F/t curve: inspiratory and expiratory flow decelerating once more. Expiratory curve reaches zero.

of providing information of determined changes in the pulmonary function. Among the loops to be analyzed are:
- Volume/pressure
- Flow/volume.

## Volume/Pressure

In the axis of the ordinate (vertical or Y-axis) the variable volume is located, and in the abscissa axis (horizontal or X-axis) the pressure variable. The curve of this loop is formed in reversed to the movement of the clock hands. Some of the variables that can be observed in the loop are the tidal volume, PEEP and the $P_{IP}$. The V/P loop is related to the compliance of the respiratory system (Fig. 26). It is important to mention that to reach the compliance at the pulmonary level, statics conditions of the system are required, however, the V/P loop is performed in dynamic conditions, so this variable should not be very representative to the Crs.

### Volume Control Ventilation (Constant Flow)

In the inspiratory phase, the lungs fill with air and the pressure increases gradually from the PEEP to hold the constant flow. At this level (Fig. 27), the lower inflection point (LIP) is observed, a zone where the compliance is reduced (little changes in volume with high changes in pressure). The curve in this place presents a tendency to the horizontal plane end, subsequently, it turns to a high compliance zone. These two zones are the ones to be watched in a standard plot.

If during the entry of the volume, the curve appears more horizontal again we could see the higher inflection point (HIP, Fig. 28), a zone with compliance newly reduced,

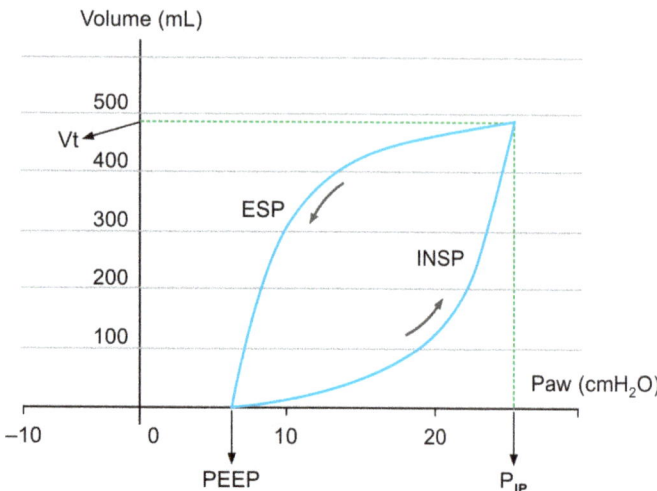

**Fig. 26:** Volume-pressure (V/P) loop in volume control ventilation with constant flow (INSP: inspiration; ESP: expiration phase; PIP: peak inspiratory pressure; PEEP: positive end-expiratory pressure).

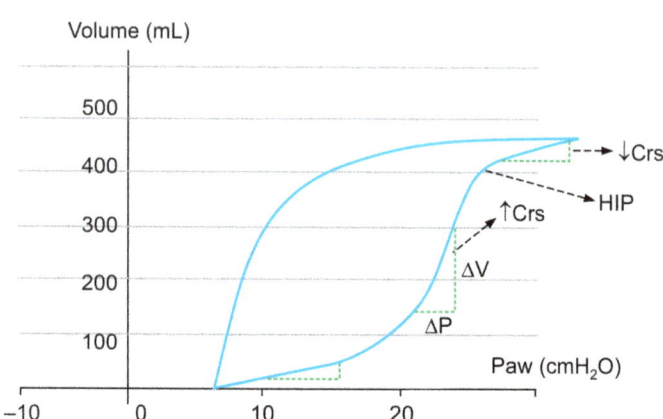

**Fig. 28:** Volume-pressure (V/P) loop: volume control ventilation with constant flow. If the input volume increases, a third zone could appear: higher inflection point (HIP), where the compliance falls once more. This is a sign of pulmonary overstretching.

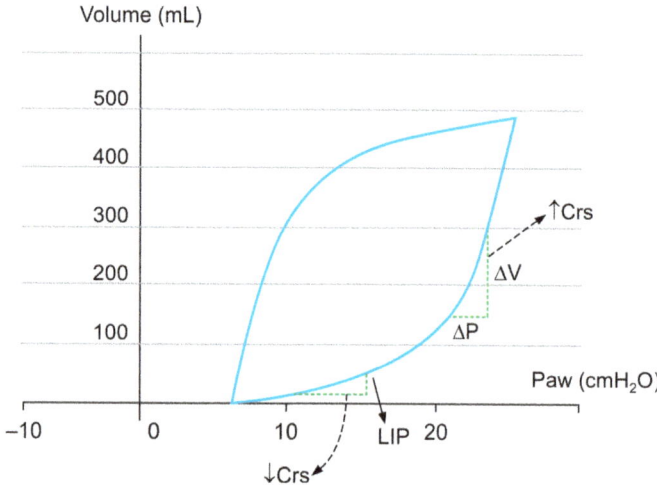

**Fig. 27:** Volume-pressure (V/P) loop in volume control ventilation with constant flow. While the volume begins to enter, the first zone appears, subsequently, it turns to a higher compliance zone (LIP: lower inflection point).

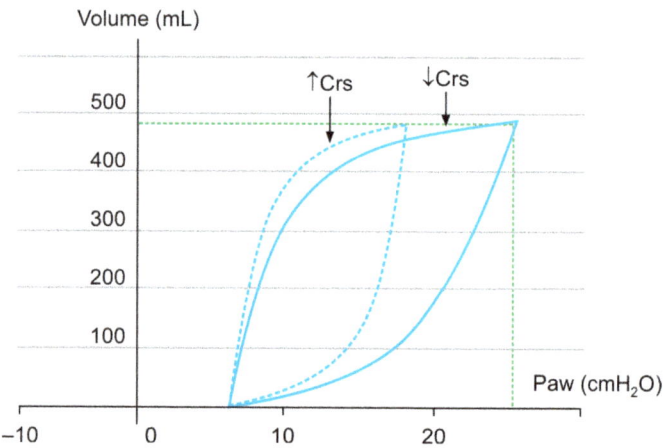

**Fig. 29:** Volume-pressure (V/P) loop: volume control ventilation with constant flow. Two curves can be watched in the same patient with the same ventilatory parameter, but with different compliance: in the discontinuous line, higher compliance.

which could show the overstretching of certain pulmonary regions. It should be noted that to validate this graphic evaluation, it ought to be measured in VC ventilation and constant flow.

### Changes in the compliance

In VC ventilation with constant flow, if a reduction of the compliance is produced (higher pressure to move the same volume), without changing the ventilator parameters, we can see in the P/V loop a displacement to the right (Fig. 29).

It would happen the contrary if there is an increase in the compliance (displacement to the left).

### Volume Control Ventilation (Decelerating Flow)

The ventilator in this mode will usually produce a generally constant pressure, because of the pattern of flow preset. This can be watched in the V/P loop plot, where the airway is rapidly pressurized, and subsequently, the pressure keeps a similar value during the whole inspiration (Fig. 30).

The generated loop presents a similar morphology to a rectangle in vertical position.

### Modality Controlled by Pressure

This loop will show a similar shape to the VC ventilation with decelerating flow (Fig. 30). Since the controlled variable is the pressure, the ventilator pressurizes the airway at a determined speed depending on the rise time applied. Then, when the preset pressure is achieved, it will keep that pressure value and the volume will increase.

### Changes in the compliance

In the PC mode, the changes will be expressed at a dependent variable, which is the volume. In the loop (Fig. 31), two ventilatory curves with different compliance are showed, and one can see differences in the volume obtained at the same pressure.

### Patient's effort in modalities triggered by the patient by pressure

In those modalities triggered by the patient (assisted or spontaneous ventilations), where the respiratory phase trigger can be preset by pressure, the inspiratory effort of the patient can be watched in the pressure/volume loop (Fig. 32). At the beginning the inspiratory effort generates a volume associated to a negative pressure at pulmonary level, once it surpasses the trigger threshold, the ventilator will provide the positive pressure to continue with the inspiratory phase.

## Flow/Volume

In the F/V graphic, the flow is shown in the ordinate axis (vertical) and the volume is shown in the abscissa axis (horizontal). The formation of this loop is in the clock hands direction. In some modern ventilators, it is possible to keep this loop in the memory to subsequently compare them with the possible changes.

### Volume Control Ventilation (Constant Flow)

The curve can be analyzed in a serial way (Fig. 33): in the first circuit (from 0 to 1), an increment in the flow occurs until it reaches the peak inspiratory flow (PIF), from 1 to 2 a constant flow is kept due to the preset ventilator mode, from 2 to 3 the end of the inspiration is produced and at the point 3 the end and beginning of the expiratory phase, then the 3 to 4 the expiratory phase begins reaching the PEF (PEF, 4), later, from 4 to 5 the flow diminishes until reaching zero, as for the x-axis as well as for the y-axis.

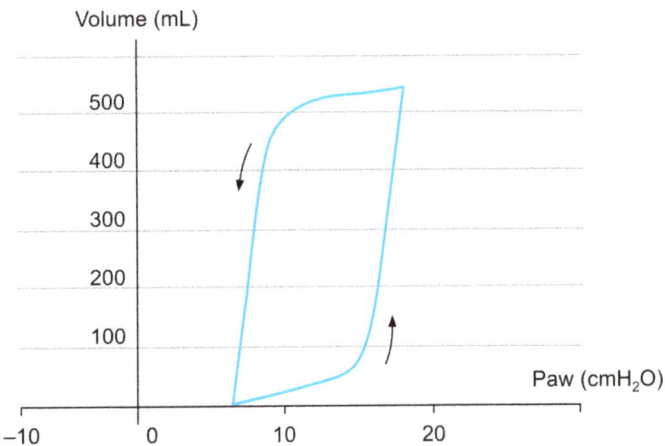

**Fig. 30:** Volume/pressure (V/P) loop: volume control ventilation with decelerating flow or modality controlled by pressure.

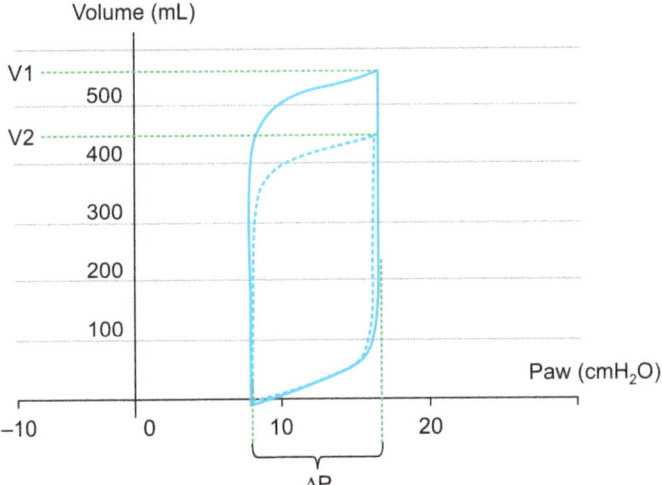

**Fig. 31:** Volume/pressure (V/P) loop: pressure control ventilation. The lower compliance would be watched at the level of the dashed line, since it gets a lower volume (V2) with the same pressure difference (ΔP) when comparing it with a standard curve (V1).

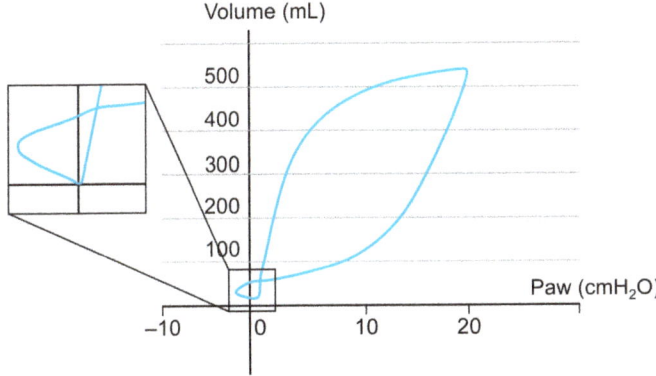

**Fig. 32:** Volume/pressure (V/P) loop: volume control ventilation with constant flow. At the beginning, the pressure is negative because of the patient's inspiratory effort.

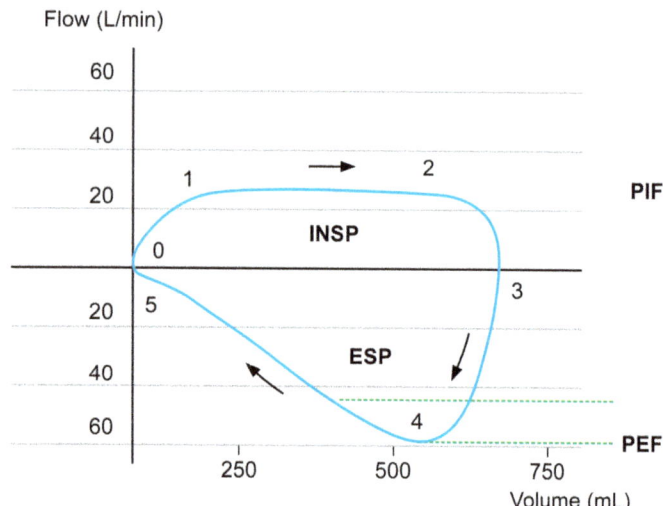

**Fig. 33:** Flow/volume (F/V) loop in volume control ventilation with constant flow (INSP: inspiratory phase; ESP: expiratory phase; PIF: peak inspiratory flow; PEF: peak expiratory flow).

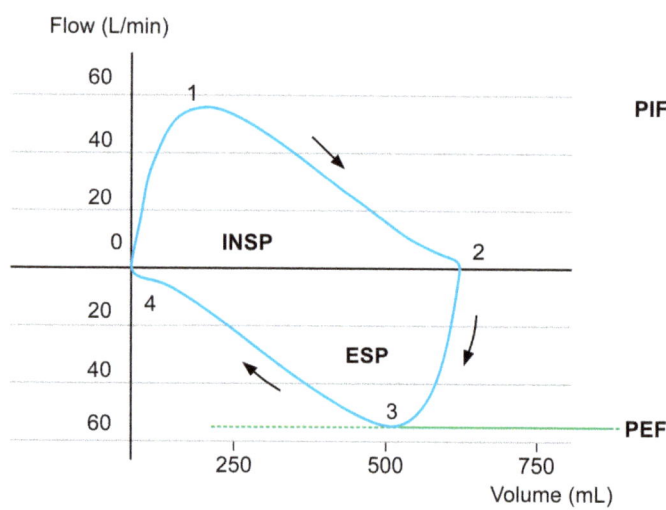

**Fig. 34:** Flow/volume (F/V) loop in pressure control ventilation (INSP: inspiratory phase; ESP: expiratory phase; PIF: peak inspiratory flow; PEF: peak expiratory flow).

### Pressure Control Ventilation

The curve can be analyzed in a serial way (Fig. 34): in the track 0 to 1 an increment in the inspiratory flow is produced until reaching the PIF located in point 1, then, from 1 to 2 a decelerating flow is produced during inspiration, in point 2 the end of the inspiration and the beginning of the exhalation happen, in 2 to 3 the exhalation begins and the PEF appears in point 3; finally, in the track 3 to 4 occurs the decelerating flow during the exhalation to reach zero flow.

### Obstructive Pattern in the Flow/Volume Loop

Using this loop, we can analyze a possible obstruction in the patient, a higher degree of obstruction present in the patient produces lower expiratory flow peak. In the same way that we analyze the obstruction present in the patient, we can evaluate the effect of bronchodilator therapy, since in some ventilator models the F/V loop can be saved and the results after therapy can be compared (Fig. 35).

### Leakage in the Loop System Flow/Volume

One of the ways to detect a possible leakage is to watch the F/V loop in its expiratory phase. We can see in Figure 36 that the volume which enters is higher to the exhale volume, since the expiratory curve does not reach zero.

### Secretions at Airway in Flow/Volume Loop

We can suspect the presence of secretions at airway or liquid in the inlet connections, if in the curve the irregularities are observed, both at the level of the inspiratory and expiratory curves (more frequently in the expiratory curve, Fig. 37).

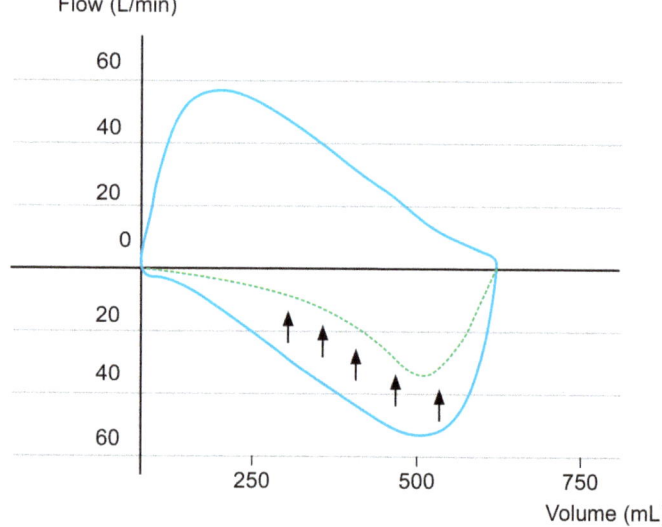

**Fig. 35:** Flow/volume (F/V) loop curve. The displacement of the continuous line curve to the flashing line curve shows a possible obstructive pattern, producing a reduction in the expiratory flows.

## SALIENT POINTS

- The graphic analysis of the mechanical ventilation allows evaluating the respiratory system mechanics and is of vital importance for who works with critical patients.
- The graphics allows the study of mechanical properties of the respiratory system in passive (statics) and active (dynamics) conditions.
- It differentiate the pathological states, especially obstructive and restrictive.

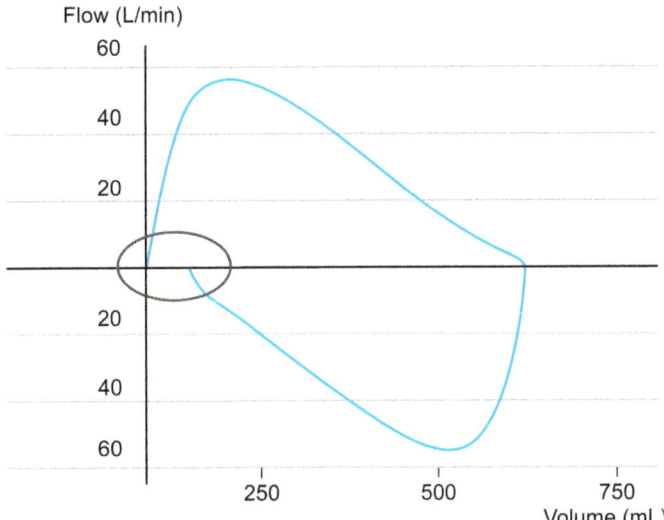

**Fig. 36:** Flow/volume (F/V) loop. We can see that the expiratory curve cuts the abscissa axis (X-axis) in a point higher than zero, this could be detecting the possible presence of leakage in the system.

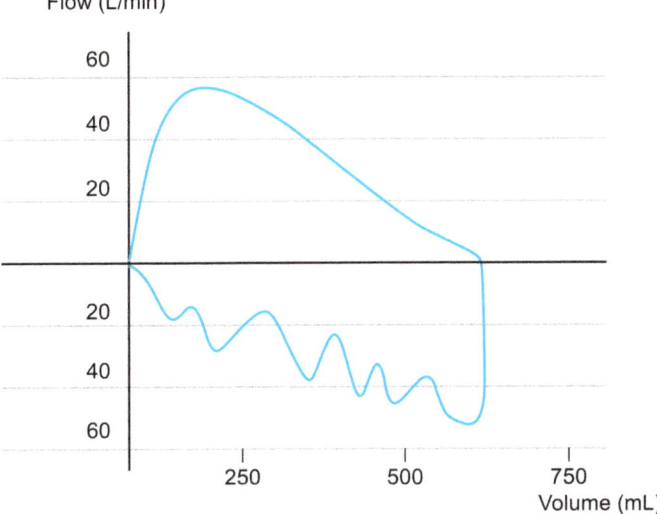

**Fig. 37:** Flow/volume (F/V) loop. In the expiratory curve, you can see irregularities which could make you suspect of possible secretions at airway level or fluids in circuit of ventilator.

- It determine procedures effects in the patient condition (chest physiotherapy, alveolar recruitment maneuvers, bronchodilatation, etc.).
- It optimize the ventilatory assistance.
- Also, avoid complications.
- Finally, we cannot forget that any technology we use will help us to better understand the patient's condition, but the main evaluation tool is our criteria and the clinical reasoning, which must be based upon our expertise and a solid scientific and technical basis.

## REFERENCES

1. Hess DR. Applied respiratory physiology: use of ventilator waveforms and mechanics in the management of critically ill patients. Respir Care. 2005;50(1):26-7.
2. Durbin CG. Applied respiratory physiology: use of ventilator waveforms and mechanics in the management of critically ill patients. Respir Care. 2005;50(2):287-93.
3. Lucangelo U, Bernabe F, Blanch L. Respiratory mechanics derived from signals in the ventilator circuit. Respir Care. 2005;50(1):55-65.
4. MacIntyre NR. Graphical analysis of flow, pressure and volume during mechanical ventilation, 3rd edition. Yorba Linda, CA: Bear Medical Systems. 1991.
5. Harris RS. Pressure-volume curves of the respiratory system. Respir Care. 2005;50(1):78-98.
6. MacIntyre NR, Branson R. Classification of Mechanical Ventilators. In: MacIntyre NR, Branson R (Eds). Mechanical Ventilation, 3th Edition. Philadelphia, Pennsylvania: Saunder Editorial; 2001.
7. Waugh JB, Deshpande VM, Harwood RJ. Rapid Interpretation of Ventilator Waveforms. New Jersey, USA: Prentice Hall; 1999.
8. Hess D, Kacmarek R. Flows, waveforms, I:E ratios. In: Hess D, Kacmarek R (Eds). Essentials of Mechanical Ventilation, 2nd edition. New York: McGraw Hill; 2002.
9. Branson RD, Johannigman JA. What is the evidence base for the newer ventilation modes? Respir Care. 2004;49(7):742-60.
10. Campbell R, Davis B. Pressure-controlled versus volume-controlled ventilation: does it matter? Respir Care. 2002;47(4):416-26.
11. Raoof S. Basics of initial ventilator set-up. In: Raoof S, Khan FA (Eds). Mechanical Ventilation Manual. Philadelphia: American College of Physicians; 1998.
12. Nilsestuen JO, Hargett KD. Using ventilator graphics to identify patient-ventilator asynchrony. Respir Care. 2005;50(2):202-32.
13. MacIntyre NR. Respiratory mechanics in the patient who is weaning from the ventilator. Respir Care. 2005;50(2):275-84.
14. MacIntyre NR. Respiratory system mechanics. In: MacIntyre NR, Branson RD (Eds). Mechanical Ventilation. Philadelphia: Saunders; 2001.
15. Bigatello LM, Davignon KR, Stelfox HT. Respiratory mechanics and ventilator waveforms in the patient with acute lung injury. Respir Care. 2005;50(2):235-44.
16. Chang DW. Compliance: static (Cst). In: Chang DW (Ed). Respiratory Care Calculations, 2nd edition. Albany: Delmar; 1999.
17. Chang DW. Airway resistance: estimated (Raw). In: Chang DW (Ed). Respiratory Care Calculations, 2nd edition. Albany: Delmar; 1999.
18. Main E, Castle R, Newham D, et al. Respiratory physiotherapy vs. suction: the effects on respiratory function in ventilated infants and children. Intensive Care Med. 2004;30:1144-51.

19. MacIntyre NR. Patient-ventilator interactions: optimizing conventional ventilation modes. Respir Care. 2011;56(1):73-84.
20. Pilbeam SP. Basic terms and concepts in mechanical ventilation. In: Pilbeam SP (Ed). Mechanical Ventilation, Physiological and Clinical Applications. Missouri: Mosby; 1998.
21. Blanch L, Bernabe F, Lucangelo U. Measurement of air trapping, intrinsic positive end-expiratory pressure, and dynamic hyperinflation in mechanically ventilated patients. Respir Care. 2005;50(1):110-23.
22. Dhand R. Ventilator graphics and respiratory mechanics in the patient with obstructive lung disease. Respir Care. 2005;50(2):246-59.
23. Kawati R, Lattuada M, Sjöstrand U, et al. Peak airway pressure increase is a late warning sign of partial endotracheal tube obstruction whereas change in expiratory flow is an early warning sign. Anesth Analg. 2005;100(3):889-93.

# CHAPTER 9

# Patient-Ventilator Asynchrony

*Daniel Arellano Sepúlveda, Ivan Ramírez Venegas*

## INTRODUCTION

Patient ventilator interaction is described by Kondili et al.[1] as "an expression of the function of two controllers (the ventilator controlled by the physician and the patient's own respiratory muscle pump) which should be in harmony if the result is to be appropriate for the patient". Therefore, any condition where patient-ventilator interaction is not optimal will be consider patient-ventilator asynchrony (PVA) as defined by Epstein.[2] However, Subira et al. considered that "patient-ventilator exists when the phases of breath delivered by the ventilator do not match those of the patient".[3] This is an example of the current problem associated with understanding PVA. As mentioned by Mireles-Cabodevila and Dugar[4], reviews, trials, and reports use different definitions to describe PVA and the different types of them, which may lead to confusion. That is why the establishment of standard definitions and vocabulary, to describe PVA is needed as mentioned by Ramirez et al. in a multicenter study.[5]

Currently, mechanical ventilators used in the intensive care units (ICUs) show different types of waveforms, such as: pressure/time, flow/time, and volume/time. As mentioned by Kacmarek "the primary reason for these waveforms is to determine if the patient is ventilating in synchrony with the ventilator".[6]

Waveform analysis is a noninvasive and reliable method in identifying PVA, and had been found well correlated with other methods like use of esophageal pressure measurement in identification of PVA.[7]

A significant percentage of patients (approximately 25%) have some type of asynchrony during mechanical ventilation.[7] That is why some authors point out that healthcare professionals that work in the ICU should be competent in identifying PVAs using waveform analysis in order to prevent complications associated with the patient outcome.[5]

However, identifying PVA is not an easy task. In a multicenter study, Ramirez et al.[5] found that 21% out of the 366 health care professionals, which work in ICUs, were able to recognize the three most common types of PVAs (ineffective effort, double triggering, auto-triggering) from video recordings that showed pressure/time and flow/time waveforms. In addition, they found that neither experience nor profession proved to be a relevant factor in identifying asynchrony using waveform analysis. However, they found that specific training in mechanical ventilation was associated with the correct identification of PVA.

## ASYNCHRONY INDEX

Asynchrony index is the percentage of asynchrony breaths per minute.

Asynchrony index = (number of asynchronies/number of total breaths) × 100

Where, number of total breaths includes number of asynchrony events + number of breaths effectively delivered by the mechanical ventilator.[8]

## IMPACT OF ASYNCHRONY ON PATIENT OUTCOME

Several studies have shown the negative impact of PVA on patient outcome. Among the complications associated with PVA are increasing the work of breathing,[9] ineffective effort,[10] dynamic hyperinflation,[11] muscle damage,[11] longer stay in mechanical ventilation and in the ICU,[7,12] sleep disorders,[13] prolonged weaning,[14] patient discomfort, and mortality.[10,15] Negative impact on patient outcome occurs when the asynchrony index is greater than 10%.

## TYPES OF ASYNCHRONY

- Ineffective effort
- Auto-triggering
- Double triggering
- Reverse triggering
- Flow asynchronies
- Premature cycling
- Delayed cycling.

### Ineffective Effort

Ineffective effort is defined as patient efforts that are not sensed by the ventilator or can also be defined as an inspiratory muscle effort not followed by a ventilator breath.[13] This is common in patients with chronic obstructive pulmonary disease (COPD). Ineffective efforts can be identified as a decrease in airway pressure in the pressure/time waveform, caused by the inspiratory effort of the patient, and a simultaneous change in the expiratory flow, which tends to return to zero due to the inspiratory effort of the patient, without the delivery of a breath from the ventilator (Fig. 1). It usually occurs in the expiratory phase (78% of the cases), although can also occur in the inspiratory phase in all modes.[7]

Ineffective effort may occur particularly when patient's COPD receives a large tidal volume, due to an excessive support, on each breath.[7] A large tidal volume will reduce the expiratory time for the patient to exhale causing air trapping and auto-positive end-expiratory pressure (auto-PEEP).[7] In fact, some of the characteristics of the breaths preceding ineffective efforts, due to an excessive support delivered by the ventilator, are: a significant larger tidal volume delivered, higher inspiratory time, shorter expiratory time, shorter respiratory cycle duration, and a higher dynamic PEEPi (intrinsic positive end-expiratory pressure) than the breaths preceding effective breaths.[16] Because of that, overcoming the trigger threshold will be harder for the patient resulting in ineffective triggering. Another cause of ineffective triggering is the inadequate level of trigger sensitivity,[7] muscle weakness,[17] and a decrease respiratory drive.[16] Other factors associated with a high prevalence of ineffective that has been described are: alkaline pH and high values of bicarbonate.[7]

### Auto-triggering

Auto-triggering can be described as breaths delivered to the patient that are neither scheduled nor initiated by the patient inspiratory effort.[13] Auto-triggering can be caused by leaks in the mechanical ventilator circuit,[13] condensation in the circuit (generating transient changes in flow),[13] improper setting of trigger sensitivity (trigger threshold is too sensitive),[13] and cardiac oscillations[18] that can make significant changes in intrathoracic pressure leading to overcome the trigger threshold (Fig. 2). These nonscheduled breaths may cause double triggering, respiratory alkalosis, and hyperinflation.

Auto-triggering can be easily identified in the pressure/time waveform by the lack of patient effort.

### Double Triggering

Double trigger is one of the most common types of patient ventilator asynchronies and can occur in any mode (most common in volume-controlled mode).[7] This type of asynchrony can be described as two consecutive ventilator

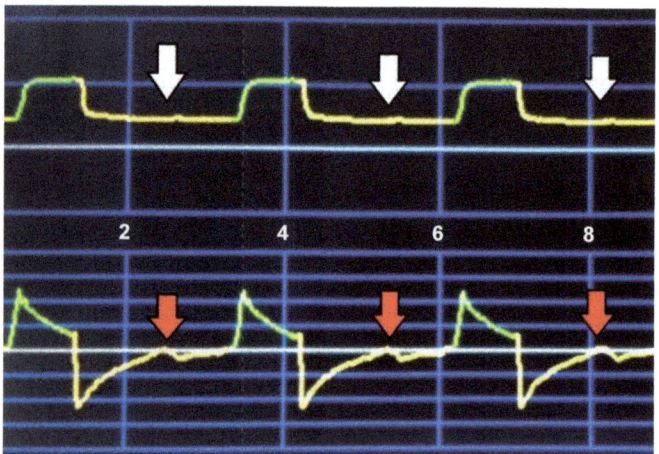

**Fig. 1:** Case of ineffective effort. White arrows indicate a decrease in airway pressure (in the pressure/time waveform). Red arrows indicate the changes in expiratory flow due to the inspiratory effort of the patient in the flow/time waveform.

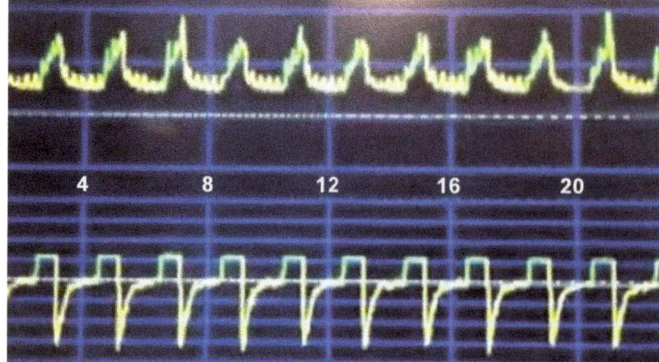

**Fig. 2:** Case of auto-triggering due to circuit condensation. The artifacts, in the pressure/time waveform, are created by the condensation in the mechanical ventilator circuit.

cycles separated by a very short or absent expiratory period (Fig. 3).[7] An absent or a short expiratory time (less than half of the mean inspiratory time) increases the tidal volume delivered by the ventilator because there is not enough expiratory time; this may lead to even double the tidal volume delivered causing overdistension, volume, and barotrauma.[19]

Double triggering can occur when the neural inspiratory time is longer than the inspiratory time program in the ventilator.[7] This means that the patient effort continues after the mechanical ventilator as cycle to expiratory phase. If the patient inspiratory effort can overcome the trigger threshold, in the expiratory phase, the ventilator will deliver a second breath. However, double triggering may also occur when respiratory drive is high and ventilatory support delivered to the patient is insufficient.[7,20]

Double triggering may be, also, caused by auto-triggering and reverse triggering.[21] The last one caused, as described by Akoumianaki et al.,[22] by "the activation of vagally mediated pulmonary reflexes, along with cortical and subcortical influences". This reflex is trigger in response to passive insufflation of the lungs. So, there are three types of double triggering depending on who is triggering the first breath. When the first breath is triggered by the patient, the double triggering occurs due to greater neural inspiratory time in comparison to the programed inspiratory time. This type of double triggering can be solve by increasing the inspiratory time.[22] The second type is when the first breath is auto-triggered and the third type is the double triggering due to reverse triggering.[21] Differentiating the different types of double triggering can be difficult sometimes. That is why a very careful analysis of the first breath is needed, because if the first breath shows a decrease in airway pressure the most likely cause will be a greater neural inspiratory time.

## Reverse Triggering

Reverse triggering is a poorly recognized type of PVA that occurs when the patient's respiratory center is activated in response to a passive insufflation of the lungs.[22] The activation of the respiratory center will generate an inspiratory effort, due to contraction of the diaphragm, during the inspiratory phase.[22] So, as described previously it is a reflex in response to a passive insufflation that creates a pattern in which the inspiratory efforts of the patient occurred over a specific and repetitive phase of the ventilator respiratory cycle. The muscle contraction of the diaphragm may persist, or not, after the inspiratory phase is completed which may lead to double triggering if the inspiratory effort can overcome the sensitivity threshold.[22]

Identifying reverse triggering using waveform analysis is difficult, especially if this type of asynchrony causes double triggering, that is why healthcare professional should evaluate not only the ventilator waveforms but also the patient's breathing pattern simultaneously. So, it is necessary to use other types of waveforms like the esophageal pressure waveform (Fig. 4).

If we analyze the pressure/time, along with the esophageal pressure, waveform the first one will not show a decrease in airway pressure at the beginning of

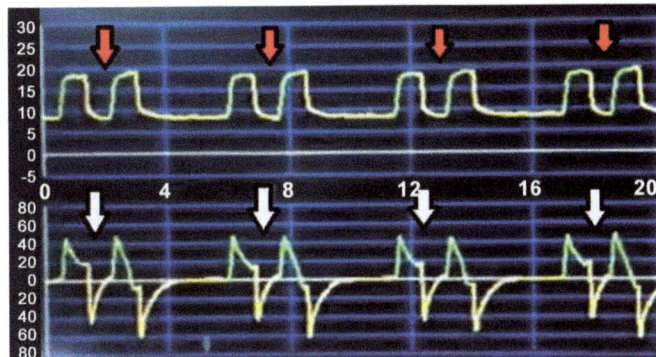

**Fig. 3:** Case of double triggering in a pressure-controlled mode. Red arrows show double triggering in the pressure/time waveform. White arrows show double triggering in the flow/time waveform.

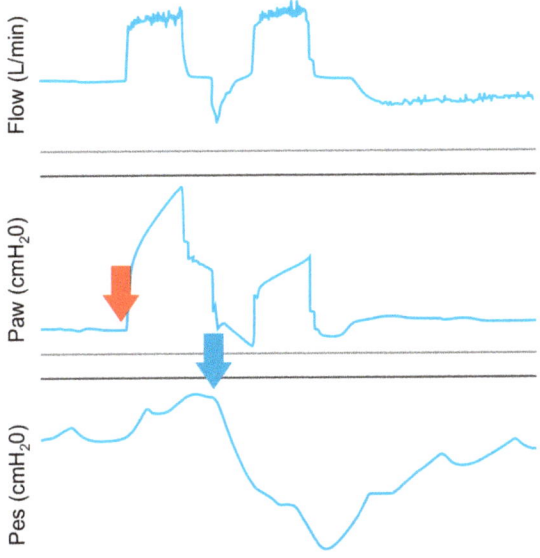

**Fig. 4:** Case of double triggering caused by reverse trigger. Note that the red arrow shows, in the pressure time waveform, the beginning of the inspiratory phase initiated by the mechanical ventilator. The blue arrow shows, in the esophageal pressure waveform, the beginning of the patient inspiratory effort. Note that there is a difference, in time, between the beginning of the patient inspiratory effort and the breath initiated by the mechanical ventilator. This difference is known as phase difference. (Paw: airway pressure; Pes: esophageal pressure)

the inspiratory phase, which means that the breath is not triggered by the patient's effort. However, patient effort will be seen, clearly, in the esophageal pressure waveform once the passive insufflation of the lung activates the reflex that leads to the contraction of the diaphragm.[22] The interval, in time, between the commencement of the mechanical and the neural inspiration is called phase difference.[22] Another important concept to know is the phase angle. A phase angle of 0° means that the inspiratory phase initiated by the ventilator and the patient inspiratory effort begins at the same time. The phase angle can be calculated as phase difference/the total ventilator cycle duration × 360°.[22]

## Flow Asynchronies

Flow asynchrony, also known as "flow starving" or "flow hungry", is a type of asynchrony that occurs when the programed flow in the ventilator does not meet the patient's ventilatory demands especially in patients having high ventilatory demand overall, as well as changes in individual respiratory breath requiring high flow.[23] This inadequate inspiratory flow will increase the work of breathing that can be, easily, identified in the pressure/time waveform as a deformation of this waveform when patients are ventilated in volume-controlled modes. As Branson described, the scalloped-out portion of the pressure/time waveform during a patient-triggered volume breath is a well-recognized sign of flow asynchrony (Fig. 5).[13]

However, flow asynchrony can also occur when the inspiratory flow, delivered by the ventilator, is too high for the patient (a rapid rise time) leading to an abrupt increase in airway pressure at the beginning of the inspiratory phase what is better known as overshooting.[24] Overshooting can cause an early termination of the inspiratory phase and patient discomfort.[24]

This phenomenon can, also, be appeared when a high inspiratory flow is programed in a volume-controlled mode (Fig. 6).[24]

Overshooting can be solved by adjusting the rise time (decreasing the rise time), in pressure-controlled modes and in volume-controlled modes by adjusting the inspiratory flow (decreasing the inspiratory flow) (Figs. 7A and B).[24]

Now, in those cases when the programed flow does not meet patient's demands, flow asynchrony, can be resolved by increasing inspiratory flow, when the patient is on volume-controlled mode, or by changing to a pressure-controlled mode.[25] However, changing to a pressure control mode as shown better results in reducing work of breathing, patient discomfort due to flow asynchrony.[9,25,26]

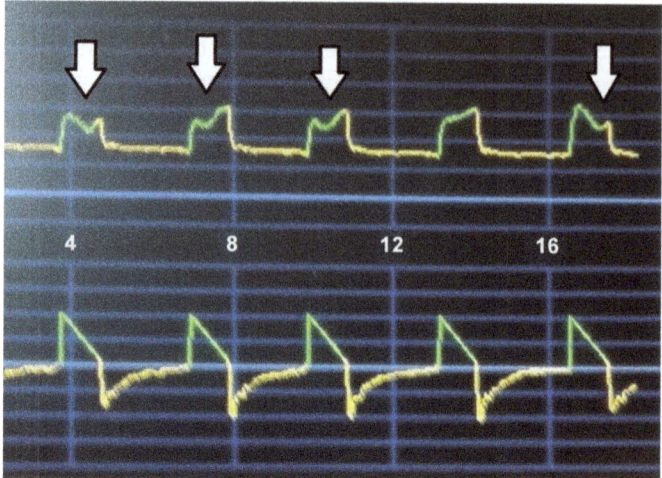

**Fig. 5:** Case of flow asynchrony in a volume-controlled mode. White arrows indicate the phenomenon called "dished out" in the pressure/time waveform. This phenomenon occurs when the flow delivered by the mechanical ventilator does not meet the patient's flow demands.

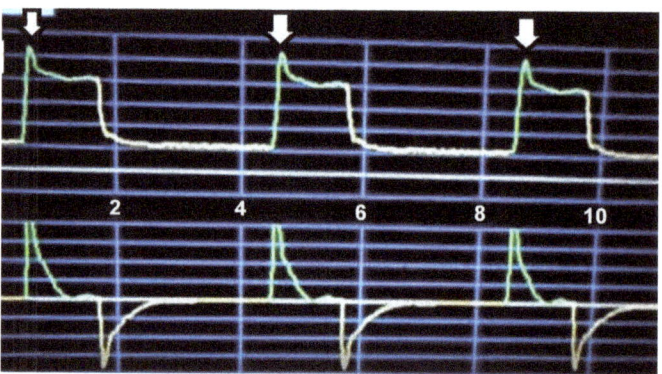

**Fig. 6:** Case of overshooting in a pressure/controlled mode due to rapid rise time. The white arrows indicate an increase in airway pressure at the beginning of the inspiratory phase. This phenomenon can also be present when a high inspiratory flow is programed in a volume-controlled mode.

This is no surprise considering that in volume-controlled modes once the inspiratory flow is programed it does not change in every patient's breath; this is the reason why flow asynchrony occurs in patients ventilated in volume-controlled modes.[27] Unlike volume-controlled mode, in pressure-controlled modes, the flow is variable in each breath.[27]

## Premature Cycling

Premature cycling or premature termination occurs when inspiratory neural time exceeds the ventilatory inspiratory time.[28] As mentioned before, this is one of the causes that

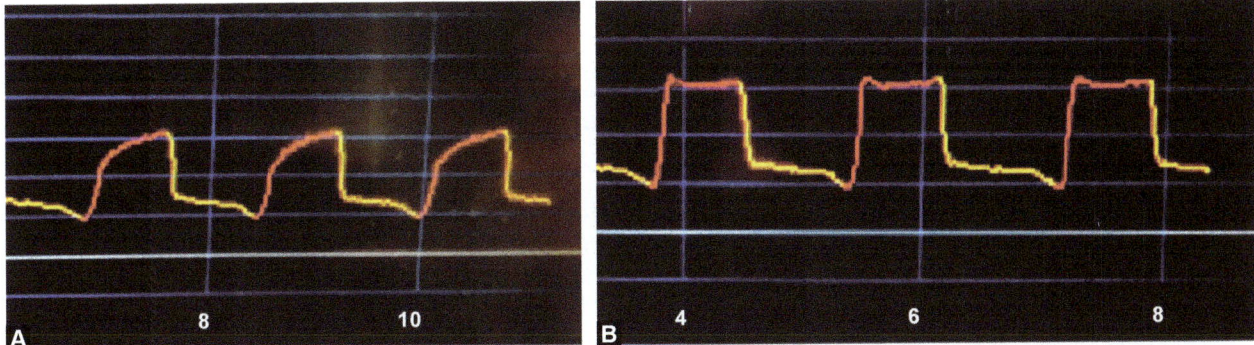

**Figs. 7A and B.** Rise time: It is defined as the time required, by the mechanical ventilator, to achieve the preset pressure during a pressure control mode. (A) A rapid rise time produce a high flow at the start of the breath, resulting in an immediate rise in pressure to the pre-set level, generating a square pressure curve; (B) On the other hand, a slow rise time decrease initial flow delivery, thus delaying the pressure rise to the pre-set. The rise time can be applied to any pressurized mode.

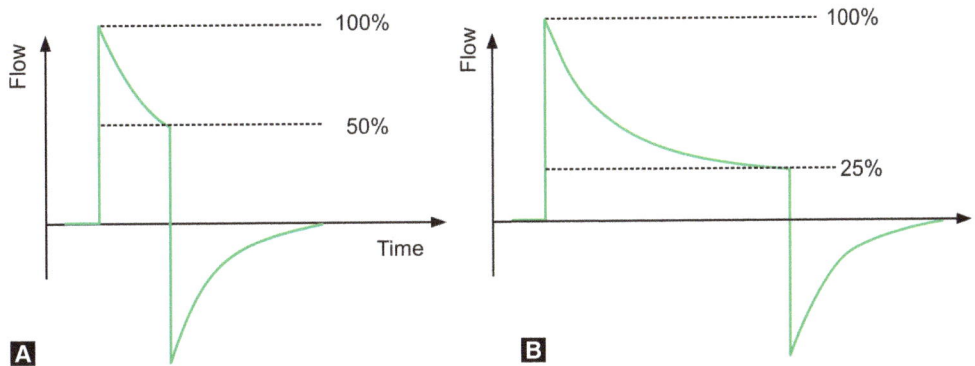

**Figs. 8A and B:** Expiratory sensitivity: It is the form of cycling in the pressure support mode. The cycling occurs when the inspiratory flow decreases to a determined threshold, generally, a percentage of the peak inspiratory flow. (A) If the flow cycling (or expiratory sensibility, $E_{sens}$) is set to 50%, the inspiratory time finish when the inspiratory flow decreases until the 50% of peak inspiratory flow. If the flow cycling is set to 50%, the flow reaches the threshold faster and the inspiratory time is shorter; (B) If the flow cycling is set to 25%, the flow reaches the threshold slowly and the inspiratory time is higher.

also generates double triggering. The difference between premature cycling and double triggering is that, in the first one, the patient's inspiratory effort does not overcome the sensitivity threshold to trigger a second breath like in double triggering.[27]

Several studies have shown the presence of premature cycling in spontaneous modes such as pressure support.[29] In this mode, adjusting a proper cycling criterion is a key factor to consider because, if the percentage of cycling criteria is increased the inspiratory time will decrease which may lead to premature cycling (Figs. 8A and B).[29]

Premature cycling shows a significant decrease in airway pressure in the pressure/time waveform, when the inspiratory phase has ended. Simultaneously, the expiratory flow rapidly returns to zero in the flow/time waveform (Fig. 9).

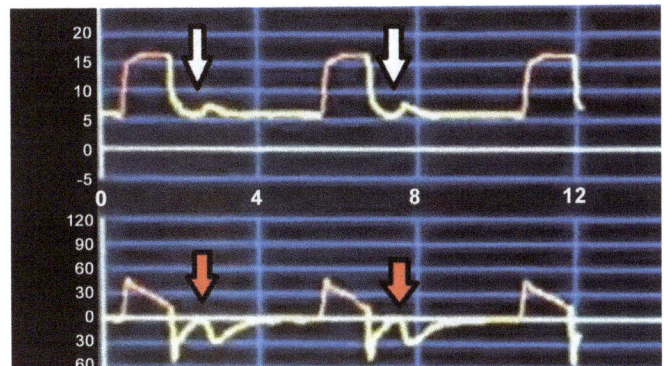

**Fig. 9:** Case of premature cycling in a pressure support mode. White arrows indicate, in the pressure time waveform, a decrease in airway pressure caused by the inspiratory effort of the patient that continues after the mechanical ventilator cycled to expiratory phase. Red arrows indicate a rapid return of the expiratory flow to zero due to the inspiratory effort of the patient in the flow/time waveform.

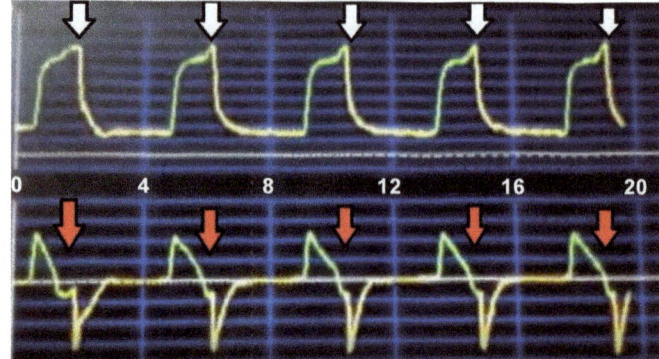

**Fig. 10:** Case of delayed cycling. White arrows indicate an increase in airway pressure at the end of the inspiratory phase due to the activation of the expiratory muscles in the pressure/time waveform. Red arrows indicate an abrupt decrease in the inspiratory flow caused by the muscle contraction in the flow/time waveform.

## Delayed Cycling

Delayed cycling occurs when the ventilator inspiratory time exceeds the patient's inspiratory time.[13] A shorter expiratory time may lead to air trapping and auto-PEEP which may cause ineffective effort.[30,31] Delayed cycling can also cause activation of expiratory muscles in the inspiratory phase.[30] Activation of the expiratory muscles will increase the airway pressure, usually near the end of the inspiratory phase, in the pressure/time waveform and a sudden decrease in inspiratory flow in the flow/time waveform.[27] The correct adjustment in the cycling criteria will make the "spike" in the pressure/time waveform disappear (Fig. 10).

## SALIENT POINTS

- Patient-ventilator asynchrony is a crucial topic for healthcare professionals that work in the ICU.
- Identifying PVA is not an easy task for healthcare professionals.
- The only factor associated with a correct identification of PVA is specific training in the topic.
- Patient-ventilator asynchrony impacts in a deleterious way on patient outcome.
- Currently, there are different definitions and classifications for the different types of asynchronies that may lead to confusion in the healthcare professional team.
- Knowing the cause of PVA is a key factor for proper management.

## REFERENCES

1. Kondili E, Prinianakis G, Georgopoulos D. Patient-ventilator interaction. Br J Anaesth. 2003;91(1):106-19.
2. Epstein SK. How often does patient-ventilator asynchrony occur and what are the consequences? Respir Care. 2011;56(1):25-38.
3. Subirà C, de Haro C, Magrans R, et al. Minimizing asynchronies in mechanical ventilation: Current and future trends. Respir Care. 2018;63(4):464-78.
4. Mireles-Cabodevila E, Dugar S. On the need for standard definitions and education to optimize patient-ventilator interactions. Respir Care. 2017;62(2):248-9.
5. Ramirez II, Arellano DH, Adasme RS. Patient-ventilator asynchrony and standard waveforms: looks can be deceiving-reply. Respir Care. 2017;62(7):1004-5.
6. Kacmarek RM. Mechanical ventilation competencies of the respiratory therapist in 2015 and Beyond. Respir Care. 2013;58(6):1087-96.
7. Thille AW, Rodriguez P, Cabello B, et al. Patient-ventilator asynchrony during assisted mechanical ventilation. Intensive Care Med. 2006;32(10):1515-22.
8. Hess DR. Ventilator waveforms and the physiology of pressure support ventilation. Respir Care. 2005;50(2):166-83.
9. Yang LY, Huang YC, Macintyre NR. Patient–ventilator synchrony during pressure-targeted versus flow-targeted small tidal volume assisted ventilation. J Crit Care. 2007;22(3):252-7.
10. Vaporidi K, Babalis D, Chytas A, et al. Clusters of ineffective efforts during mechanical ventilation: impact on outcome. Intensive Care Med. 2017;43(2):184-91.
11. Nilsestuen JO, Hargett KD. Using ventilator graphics to identify patient-ventilator asynchrony. Respir Care. 2005;50(2):202-34; discussion 232-4.
12. de Wit M, Miller KB, Green DA, et al. Ineffective triggering predicts increased duration of mechanical ventilation. Crit Care Med. 2009;37(10):2740-5.
13. Branson RD, Blakeman TC, Robinson BR. Asynchrony and dyspnea. Respir Care. 2013;58(6):973-89.
14. Chao DC, Scheinhorn DJ, Stearn-Hassenpflug M. Patient-ventilator asynchrony in prolonged mechanical ventilation. Chest. 1997;112(6):1592-9.
15. Blanch L, Villagra A, Sales B, et al. Asynchronies during mechanical ventilation are associated with mortality. Intensive Care Med. 2015;41(4):633-41.
16. Leung P, Jubran A, Tobin MJ. Comparison of assisted ventilator modes on triggering, patient effort, and dyspnea. Am J Respir Crit Care Med. 1997;155(6):1940-8.
17. de Wit M, Pedram S, Best AM, et al. Observational study of patient-ventilator asynchrony and relationship to sedation level. J Crit Care. 2009;24(1):74-80.
18. Imanaka H, Nishimura M, Takeuchi M, et al. Autotriggering caused by cardiogenic oscillation during flow-triggered mechanical ventilation. Crit Care Med. 2000;28(2):402-7.

19. Chanques G, Kress JP, Pohlman A, et al. Impact of ventilator adjustment and sedation-analgesia practices on severe asynchrony in patients ventilated in assist-control mode. Crit Care Med. 2013;41(9):2177-87.
20. Takioka H, Tanaka T, Ishizu T, et al. The effect of breath termination criterion on breathing patterns and the work of breathing during pressure support ventilation. Anesth Analg. 2001;92(1):161-5.
21. Liao KM, Ou CY, Chen CW. Classifying different types of double triggering based on airway pressure and flow deflection in mechanically ventilated patients. Respir Care. 2011;56(4):460-6.
22. Akoumianaki E, Lyazidi A, Rey N, et al. Mechanical ventilation induced reverse-triggered breaths: a frequently unrecognized form of neuromechanical coupling. Chest. 2013;143(4):927-38.
23. Bulleri E, Fusi C, Bambi S, et al. Patient-ventilator asynchronies: types, outcomes and nursing detection skills. Acta Biomed. 2018;89(7-S):6-18.
24. Holanda MA, Vasconcelos RD, Ferreira JC, et al. Patient-ventilator asynchrony. J Bras Pneumol. 2018;44(4):321-33.
25. MacIntyre NR, McConnell R, Cheng KC, et al. Patient-ventilator flow dyssynchrony: flow-limited versus pressure-limited breaths. Crit Care Med. 1997;25(10):1671-7.
26. Kallet RH, Campbell AR, Alonso JA, et al. The effects of pressure control versus volume control assisted ventilation on patient work of breathing in acute lung injury and acute respiratory distress syndrome. Respir Care. 2000;45(9):1085-96.
27. Daniel HA, Ivan IR. Identifying patient-ventilator asynchrony using waveform analysis. Palliat Med Care. 2017;4(4): 1-6.
28. Gilstrap D, MacIntyre NR. Patient-ventilator interactions: Implications for clinical management. Am J Respir Crit Care Med. 2013;188(9):1058-68.
29. Takioka H, Tanaka T, Ishizu T, et al. The effect of breath termination criterion on breathing patterns and the work of breathing during pressure support ventilation. Anesth Analg. 2001;92(1):161-5.
30. Parthasarathy S, Jubran A, Tobin M. Cycling of inspiratory and expiratory muscle groups with the ventilator in airflow limitation. Am J Respir Crit Care Med. 1998;158(5):1471-8.
31. Gentile M. Cycling of the mechanical ventilator breath. Respir Care. 2011;56(1):52-7.

# CHAPTER 10

# Monitoring $O_2$ and $CO_2$ during Mechanical Ventilation

*András Lovas, Zsolt Molnár*

## INTRODUCTION

Commencing mechanical ventilation in the critically ill is one of the most frequently applied organ support modalities in the intensive care unit (ICU). However, on the one hand, it is a lifesaving intervention; but on the other hand, inadequate mechanical ventilation can cause serious harm. To avoid iatrogenic complications, continuous monitoring is mandatory. The two main tasks of mechanical ventilation are the maintenance of adequate oxygenation and the assurance of effective carbon dioxide elimination. Although clinical assessment still has a major role in the observation of ventilated patients, these physical signs can be unspecific and inaccurate. On the contrary, arterial blood gas analysis provides accurate measurement of the partial pressures of these two gases, the reading is sequential. Therefore, in addition to regular blood gas analysis, pulse oximetry and continuous measurement of oxygen and carbon dioxide concentrations, both in the inspired and expired gas, also has a pivotal role in appropriate monitoring during mechanical ventilation.

## OXYGEN MEASUREMENT

### Pulse Oximetry

Pulse oximetry is considered to be the greatest technical advancement on the observation of oxygen level of patients with significant improvement in safety, not just on the ICU and in the operating rooms but also on general wards and during patient transport.[1] This noninvasive technique enables quantification of arterial blood oxygen saturation at the microcapillary level. The main principle of the measurement is the spectrophotometric technique comprehending passing radiation through a sample and determining the quantity of radiation absorbed. On the one hand, its working principle is based on Lambert's law, which states that each layer of equal thickness absorbs an equal fraction of radiation which passes through, and on the other hand, on Beer's law which states that the absorption of radiation by a given thickness of a solution of a given concentration is the same as that of twice the thickness of a solution of half the concentration.

The two main components of a pulse oximeter are the measurement probe and the house. The latter includes the microprocessor for data processing and a display, on which oxygen saturation, pulse rate, and plethysmography waveform are presented. Alarm limits can also be adjusted for low and high readings either for saturation and the pulse rate. An audible signal, with variable pitch proportional to the level of saturation can supplement the monitoring process.

Pulse oximeters assess the ratio of light absorbed at two specific wavelengths—a red light at 660 nm and an infrared light at 940 nm. The lights are emitted from monochromatic light-emitting diodes (LED). The light passes through the tissues toward a photodetector which measures the rate of absorption (Fig. 1). The LEDs are turned on and off at high frequency resulting in sensation

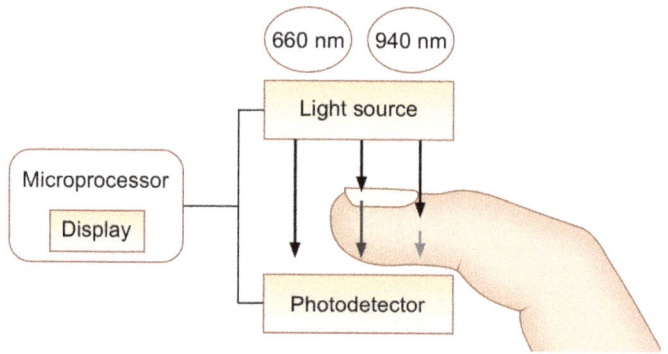

**Fig. 1:** Working principle of the pulse oximeter.

of continuous light emission for the human eyes. The emitted light is absorbed by a nonpulsatile manner by, e.g. venous blood, skin, and soft tissues and a pulsatile manner by arterial blood pulsations. The nonconstant element of the wave is less than 5% of the total signal. The microprocessor is programmed to analyze the changes generated by pulsatile arterial flow evoked by the cardiac cycle. The absorption of the oxygenated and deoxygenated hemoglobin differs on the two wavelengths of 660 nm and 940 nm warranting good sensitivity of the measurements. Where the absorbance of the two hemoglobin forms is identical, is called the isosbestic point. One of these wavelengths is at 805 nm where absorbance depends only on the hemoglobin concentration. The software of the instrument mathematically dissects the components at the two wavelengths both of the constant and nonconstant absorption and only that light which is constantly varying and represents the pulsatile (i.e. arterial) component is used and displayed.

For the reliable assessment of the pulse oximeter measurement several deliberations should be taken into account. Reading is accurate in the 70–100% range as below this level observations are extrapolated. Hypoperfusion, such as in different shock states or grave vasoconstriction at the periphery, can significantly affect the performance and reliability of the device.[2] This is due to the reduced component of the pulsatile absorption what is accountable for just about 1–5% of all reading. Excessive movement of the patient e.g. in agitated states with loss of the measurement probe leads to error as well. The response time of the observation can be as long as 60 seconds with finger probes as readings are averaged in every 10–20 seconds. This means delayed reaction time what can be significant in emergency situations.[3] Carbon monoxide in the arterial blood (due to poisoning or smoking), intravenous administration of certain dyes (indocyanine green, methylene blue), methemoglobinemia, and colored nail varnish can all lead to errors in measurements. Applying multiple wavelengths can eradicate false readings from carboxyhemoglobin and methemoglobinemia (Table 1). The site of application of the measurement probe should be checked and changed in regular intervals as pressure sores can be developed with continuous use.

It is worth to notify that pulse oximetry quantifies the oxygen saturation alone with no direct information of oxygen delivery at the tissue level. However, the measurement of arterial oxygen saturation ($SaO_2$) gives an indication of the oxygen content ($CaO_2$) of the blood taken into account that the hemoglobin concentration (Hb) and its ability to oxygen absorption are known along with partial pressure of $O_2$ ($PaO_2$) in the plasma. Beyond, if cardiac output (CO) is charted, oxygen delivery ($DO_2$) can be precisely estimated by the following equations:

$$DO_2 = CO \times CaO_2$$
$$DO_2 = CO \times (Hb \times 1.39\ mL \times SaO_2 + PaO_2 \times 0.003)$$

where every gram of hemoglobin can bind 1.39 mL of oxygen when hemoglobin is completely saturated. 0.003 is solubility coefficient of oxygen if expressed in mm Hg.

**Table 1:** Sources of error with pulse oximetry.

| | |
|---|---|
| MetHb | False low reading |
| CoHb | False high reading |
| Methylene blue | False low reading |
| Indocyanine green | False low reading |
| Bilirubin | No effect on reading |
| Dark skin | No effect on reading |
| Nail varnish | No or false low reading |

## Clinical Utility of Pulse Oximetry

Worldwide implementation of pulse oximetry as a compulsory tool in intraoperative monitoring during anesthesia had a huge impact on patient safety and reduced anesthesia related morbidity and mortality tremendously. However, there are some important limitations what one should be aware of when interpreting data provided by the device. It is important to note that accuracy is the best in the high ranges (~94%). Below this value, inaccuracy can be as high as compared to the real arterial saturation measured by co-oximetry.[4]

Another important issue is the response time of the sensor. Obtaining the trace and getting the first readings usually takes 5–8 seconds, regardless of the position of the probe, whether it is placed on the finger, earlobe, or the toes. However, during desaturation it has a substantial delay in general—as compared to that of what is ongoing in the blood and this delay also depends on the position of the sensor. The response time delay was found to be 7–20 seconds on the earlobe and 20–35 seconds on the fingers.[4] This should be taken into account when there is rapid desaturation as the real situation in the patient's blood can be much worse than indicated by pulse oximetry readings and aggressive measures to treat and avoid hypoxemia should be implemented immediately.

## Measurement of Oxygen Tension in Blood

Blood gas analyzers can measure the oxygen tension (partial pressure) in any kind of blood sample. This is an invasive measurement as direct puncture is required for sampling or blood can be withdrawn from an indwelling arterial or venous catheter. Specimen should be taken in an anaerobic manner in a heparinized syringe. Analysis should be performed promptly as the oxygen compound of the blood falls steadily due to the metabolism of the cells in the sample.[5]

For oxygen tension measurements, the blood gas analyzer includes an oxygen electrode, the so called Clark electrode. A platinum cathode and a silver anticathode in an electrolyte solution are used for the measurement. The electrodes are polarized with a voltage of 0.6 V. An oxygen-permeable Teflon membrane separates the cell from the sample to prevent contamination of the electrode. Temperature control of the electrode is also important; measurements are implemented at 37.0°C. The number of oxygen molecules that traverse the membrane is proportional to its partial pressure in the sample. At the anticathode, electrons are administered by the reaction of silver with the chloride ions of the potassium chloride electrolyte to donate silver chloride and electrons. At the cathode, $O_2$ mixes with the electrons and $H_2O$, giving an elevation in $OH^-$ concentration:

$$O_2 + 4e + 2H_2O \rightarrow 4OH^-$$

An electric current is produced when the cathode donates electrons to the anticathode. As for every molecule of $O_2$, four electrons are supplied while a current is produced which is directly proportional to the $PO_2$ in the sample. For maintenance, regular calibration of the electrode is required with a standard gas mixture.

When a tiny oxygen electrode is equipped on the spire of a catheter, this enables the nonstop detection of $PO_2$ of blood inside vessels or the heart. As single readings by blood gas analyzers may not be representative, continuous observation and trend assessment aids the evaluation of response for the commenced therapy. This technique has a major role in the ongoing monitoring of central venous or mixed venous saturation assisting the estimation of the balance between the oxygen delivery and consumption of the critically ill. Unfortunately, calibration of these devices still remains a problem because of their subtle design.

### Oxygen Concentration Analyzers

Accurate monitoring of the gas mixture comprehending the concentration of oxygen delivered to the patient via the breathing circuit during mechanical ventilation is fundamental in the prevention of administration of hypoxic gas mixture.

The most widely used detection method is the paramagnetic analyzer with rapid response time. The mechanism of action is based on the fact that oxygen has a paramagnetic property; henceforward can be attracted by a magnetic field. This paramagnetic characteristic arises from the molecular structure as electrons in the outer shell of an oxygen molecule are unpaired. Most other gases, like nitrogen, are weakly diamagnetic and are repelled from a magnetic field. Inside the paramagnetic analyzer two chambers are separated by a sensitive pressure transducer. Measurement gas and reference, room air gas are delivered by sampling tubes to the measuring chamber. A rapidly changing electromagnetic field with a frequency of about 100–110 Hz is created to which the gases are subjected. As the magnetic field attracts and agitates the oxygen molecules, this leads to a change in pressure on both sides of the transducer. The pressure difference across the transducer is proportional to the oxygen partial pressure difference between the reference and sample gas. The pressure force is converted to an electric signal that is displayed as the fraction of inspired and expired oxygen depending on the position of sampling tubes in the breathing circuit. The reading is very accurate and highly sensitive with a continuous function.

The second type of the oxygen concentration analyzers is the galvanic oxygen analyzer which is also called as fuel cell. The analyzer is constructed of a noble metal cathode and a lead anode immerged in a potassium chloride electrolyte solution covered by an oxygen-permeable membrane which separates the sample gas from the fuel cell. As oxygen molecules diffuse through the membrane and the electrolyte solution to the gold cathode, they are generating an electric current proportional to the partial pressure of oxygen in the sampling gas according to the following equations:

$$O_2 + 4e^- + 2H_2O \rightarrow 4OH^-$$
$$Pb + 2OH^- \rightarrow PbO + H_2O + 2e^-$$

The galvanic oxygen analyzer has a slow response time of 20–30 seconds and the accuracy of reading is around ±3%. Continuous exposure to oxygen is avoidable when reading is unnecessary as fuel cell can be exhausted earlier limiting its utilization.

The above detailed Clark electrode can also be used for the measurement of oxygen tension in gas mixtures. In this type of polarographic electrode, the electrolyte is in a form of gel. The main disadvantages of the Clark electrode applied for oxygen tension reading in gas mixtures are the restrained lifetime because of the deterioration of the membrane and the slow response time of 20–30 seconds with limited accuracy of about ±3%.

## Co-oximetry

A co-oximeter is a blood gas analyzer that measures, in addition to the partial pressure of blood gases, the concentration of oxygenated hemoglobin, deoxygenated hemoglobin, carboxyhemoglobin, and methemoglobin as a percentage of the total hemoglobin concentration. Application of co-oximetry can be indicated when a history is consistent with pathologies such as toxin exposure; persistent hypoxemia, which fails to improve for extra oxygen supplementation; when there is a discrepancy between the $PaO_2$ in a blood gas sample and the oxygen saturation on pulse oximetry; or dyshemoglobinemias are presumed. The working principle of the device is based on light absorption technique. Different wavelengths of light are passing through the blood sample and the rate of absorption is measured by the device. The different types of hemoglobin have different absorption properties.[6]

## Near Infrared Spectroscopy

Near infrared spectroscopy (NIRS) provides a noninvasive continuous observation of tissue oxygenation with a limited array at the bedside. The technique is quite similar as described for pulse oximetry. The monitor functions as follows: near infrared light with a spectrum of 700–1,100 nm is generated and emitted by a light source. NIR spectrum has the capability to penetrate into the tissues several centimeters deep. The probe is usually cutaneously attached depending on the interest of region. A sticker of the probe stabilizes the probe and also restricts of surrounding light to enter into the observation field. The depth of the measurement depends on the distance between the light source and the detector, usually in the range of 1 to couple of centimeters with a U-shaped path of the light from the cutaneous light source down to the examined tissue and back to the superficial detector.

The emitted NIRS light is absorbed with different level by pigments like myoglobin and hemoglobin in the tissues. In these situations, the spectrum is changing, depending on the oxygenation status of the pigments. Several detectors are incorporated to the NIRS probe to gather a fraction of light finally returning to the tissue surface. As near infrared spectrum is featured by typical differences in the spectrum of oxygenated and deoxygenated hemoglobin hereby it enables the measurement of the level of tissue oxygenation.

Prevalent application of NIRS is the observation and maintenance of cerebral tissue oxygenation in the operating room during cardiac or carotid vascular surgery or during the management of patients with raised intracranial pressure on the intensive care unit. As near infrared light can penetrate the bones thus the skull, it is possible to assess the regional cortical oxygenation attaching the probe to the forehead of the patient. In certain circumstances, peripheral oxygenation measurements can be performed by NIRS over the region of the thenar eminence or the forearm hereby detecting inadequate tissue oxygenation due to shock state or hypoxemia.

Despite the substantial improvement in the technology of NIRS monitoring over recent years the technique also has several limitations. In contrast to pulse oximetry, even skin pigmentation may play a role in false reading. Hemoglobin and myoglobin share similar optical properties, hence this can also cause misinterpretation of the results. This can be a negligible issue in the measurement of cerebral tissue oxygenation but during thenar and forearm measurements myoglobin may become an eminent source to the complete reading, leading to overestimation of tissue oxygenation as the oxygen affinity is higher to myoglobin than to hemoglobin.[7]

## CARBON DIOXIDE MEASUREMENT

### Measurement of Carbon Dioxide Tension in Blood

Assessment of $PaCO_2$ has a major role in the evaluation of patient's breathing and the guidance of mechanical ventilation. The method of measuring the $PCO_2$ in liquids is based on hydrogen ion measurement as carbon dioxide reacts with water-producing hydrogen ions resulting in a change in pH:

$$CO_2 + H_2O \leftrightarrow H_2CO_3 \leftrightarrow H^+ + HCO_3^-$$

The Severinghaus carbon dioxide electrode consists an electrode, made of glass and sensitive to pH, with a silver/silver chloride reference electrode forming its outer part. The electrodes are immerged in a thin film of sodium bicarbonate. The electrolyte liquid mixture is covered by a carbon dioxide permeable rubber or Teflon membrane which is in direct contact with the blood sample during the measurement. Through the process carbon dioxide diffuses in both directions until equilibrium supervenes across the membrane between the blood sample and the electrolyte solution. The diffused carbon dioxide reacts with the water of the electrolyte solution according to the above detailed equation resulting in alteration of hydrogen ion concentration and hereby pH. The resulting change in pH is detected by the electrode made of glass.

The time lag between the electronic input and output signal of the electrode is pretty slow as diffusion of the carbon dioxide takes around 2–3 minutes across the membrane. If the integrity of the membrane disrupts, it results in inadequate measurement. The electrode should be operated at 37°C. Routine calibration of the electrode should be performed with a standard gas mixture containing known concentration of carbon dioxide. The measured partial pressure of carbon dioxide in blood is just a fine proportion of the total carbon dioxide. The latter also includes carbon dioxide combined as bicarbonate and carbonate buffered by hemoglobin.

### End-tidal Carbon Dioxide Analyzer (Capnography)

Continuously monitoring the concentration of the carbon dioxide in the exhaled gas mixture has paramount importance in tailoring respiratory therapy to the patients' needs. The instrument what serves for this purpose with the help of an infrared analyzer is called the capnograph. The Greek language origin *kapnos*, meaning smoke, composing the term along with the idea that carbon dioxide can be realized as the "smoke" of turnover within the cells.

Gases with molecules containing two or more different type of atoms absorb radiation in the infrared spectrum of light. Each of these gases absorbs radiation at a characteristic wavelength of 4.28 μm specifically for the analysis of carbon dioxide. The components of the capnograph are—a sampling chamber and a photodetector which perceives photons falling on it from an illuminating source radiating the characteristic wavelength after passing through the gas sample. The partial pressure of the carbon dioxide in the sample is proportional to the absorbed amount of infrared light. Finally, the nonabsorbed infrared light falls on a thermopile detector where heat is produced. The change in temperature is measured by a thermometer which is producing the electrical signal of measurement (Fig. 2). Calibration process of the detector can be performed with a gas mixture containing a known concentration of carbon dioxide. Older versions of capnographs provided only the end-tidal carbon dioxide concentration. Newer versions are indicating a continuous capnography trace throughout the respiratory cycle.

There are two main types of capnographs regarding their working principles. The first one is the side stream analyzer that consists a tube for sampling with a rate of 150–200 mL/min conducting the gas mixture to a capnograph. At the end of the patient's breathing system the tube is connected to an adapter. Sampling line should be connected as close to the patient's trachea as possible for the improvement of accurate reading. The response

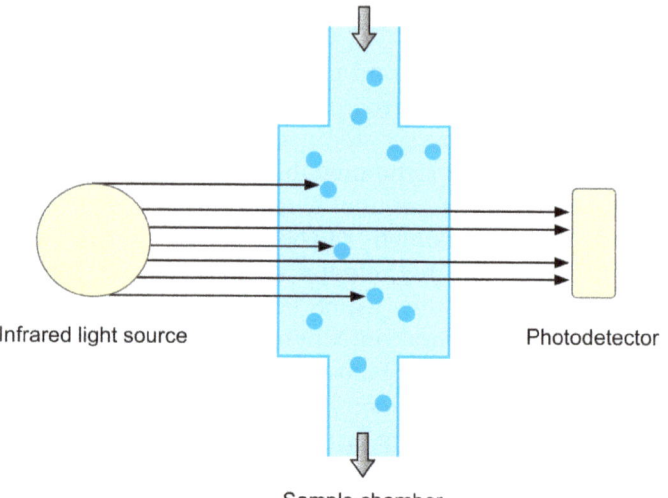

**Fig. 2:** Working principle of the capnograph.

time of the measurement reflects the length of the sampling tube what should be as short as possible for tempering the delay. The other type of the analyzer is called the main stream analyzer. In this case the sampling chamber is connected within the breathing circuit nearby the opening of the expiratory limb of the breathing circuit. Infrared photodetector is directly connected on this sampling chamber so there is no delay because of the transportation of the sample gas. Accordingly, the observed trace is real time.

Reading the whole carbon dioxide concentration trace has several advantages. First of all, respiratory rate can be calculated from the rise and the fall in concentration during the respiratory cycle. Hypo-, normo-, and hyperventilation can be controlled by the measurement as known that the level of end-tidal carbon dioxide is less than the alveolar carbon dioxide concentration which is always extended with alveolar dead space gas from nonperfused alveoli. Alveolar concentration of carbon dioxide is lower than the arterial as blood from nonventilated lung regions mixes with blood from the ventilated parenchyma. This phenomenon gives the ability to estimate changes in alveolar dead-space if both arterial and end-tidal carbon dioxide concentrations are known. Capnograph can aid the diagnosis of undesirable esophageal intubation as no or extremely low level of carbon dioxide is measured. On the contrary, correct position of the endotracheal tube can be confirmed with the detection of continuous carbon dioxide trace. In case of disconnection of the breathing circuit a sudden absence of the end-tidal carbon dioxide is detected what triggers an alarm signal of detachment. A sloping trace of the exhaled carbon dioxide can indicate small airway obstruction (e.g. in COPD, asthma) as the emptying of alveoli is decelerating (Figs. 3A and B). In case when the end-tidal carbon dioxide waveform does not drop back to the baseline rebreathing takes place.[8]

## Volumetric Capnography

Dead space measurement has an essential importance in the proper detection of ventilation-perfusion abnormalities. A relatively new method, the so-called volumetric capnography enables measurement of physiological and alveolar dead space regularly at the bedside. Time-based capnography is detailed in the section above. By contrast, volumetric capnography provides the measurement of expired $CO_2$ what is plotted against the exhaled lung volume during respiration. With the help of this technique assessment of the anatomical source of $CO_2$ is available. A breath-by-breath detection of the volume of lung units is feasible, that are ventilated but nonperfused, along with measurement of alveolar dead space. The latter refers to the lung volume that is ventilated but not perfused.

The rationale for the analysis is similar to that of the nitrogen washout technique developed at the beginning of the 1980s. Newly developed ventilators are equipped by volumetric $CO_2$ detectors that enable computations of mixed expired $CO_2$ pressure and real-time dead space fraction. To perform volumetric capnography data processing software is required to combine the $CO_2$ with the volume signal.[9]

In a clinical setting, alveolar dead space can arise through two main pathophysiological mechanisms. The first one is called over distension of alveoli that can be the result of several causes such as dynamic hyperinflation of the lung, when the expiratory ratio is rather short to entirely empty the ventilated alveoli or when the applied PEEP is higher than the ideal and finally if the delivered tidal volume is too large. All of these processes lead to the reduction in alveolar perfusion due to compression of vessels in the wall of alveoli. During the second scenario pulmonary perfusion is reduced or alterations in the distribution of perfusion are detected caused by either true obstruction of the pulmonary arteries or by decreased cardiac output of the right ventricle.

Volumetric capnography can aid PEEP titration at the bedside. Defining the optimal level of PEEP during mechanical ventilation can avoid further atelectasis of the lung and prevent over distension of the alveoli. Both pathophysiological mechanisms can be monitored by volumetric capnography. Optimal PEEP should render not just the best oxygenation and compliance but at the same time minimal ventilation dead space. By monitoring both sides of the alveolar–capillary boundary, volumetric capnography can be useful in setting the ideal PEEP, along with reduction of ventilator-induced lung injury.[10]

## Gastric Tonometry and Mucosal pH Measurement

For gastric mucosal pH measurement a nasogastric tube is inserted via the esophagus into the stomach. At the tip of the tube a silicon balloon is mounted which is permeable for carbon dioxide. Balloon is filled with air or either saline. A nonpermeable additional channel is connected to this balloon for enabling sample withdrawal. Carbon dioxide pressure inside the balloon levels out with that in the gastric lumen which is representing the pressure within the mucosal cells (Fig. 4). With the help of the Henderson-Hasselbalch equation, intracellular pH can be

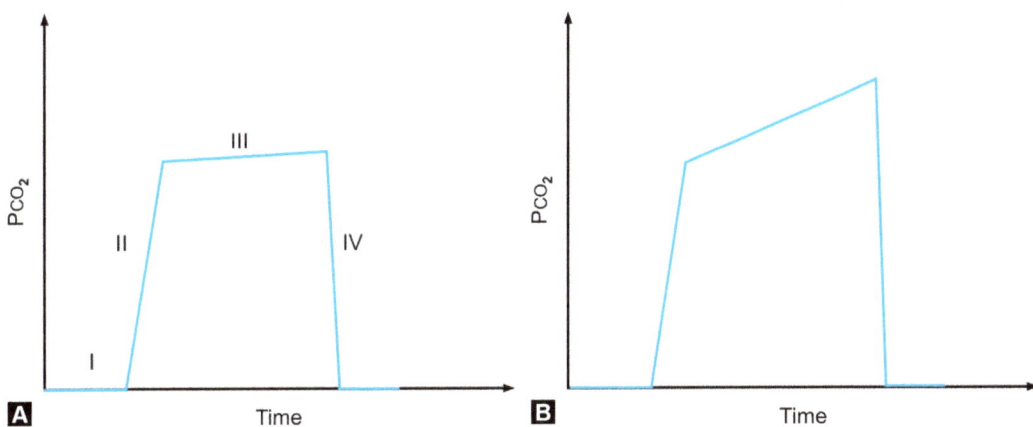

**Figs. 3A and B:** Normal (A) and obstructive (B) capnography traces (I: inspiratory baseline; II: expiratory upstroke; III: alveolar plateau phase; IV: inspiratory down stroke).

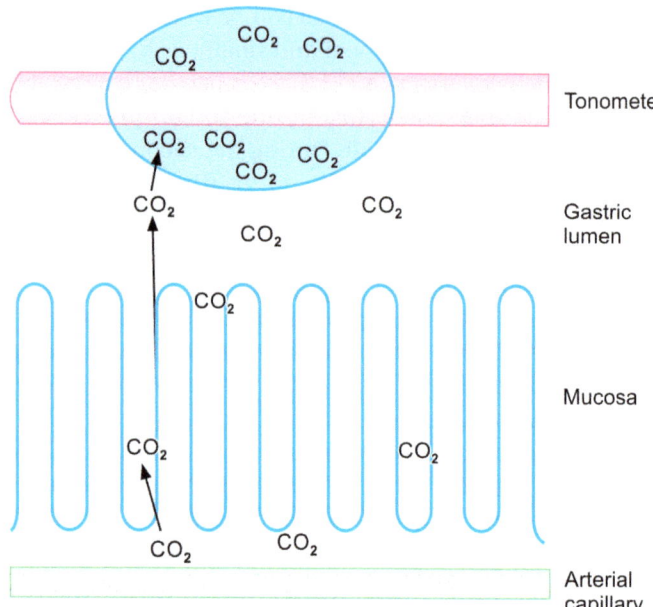

**Fig. 4:** Working principle of the gastric tonometer.

calculated with the help of the carbon dioxide tension in the withdrawn sample if arterial bicarbonate concentration is known. During shock state because of the redistribution of the circulation antedated by splanchnic vasoconstriction hypoperfusion of the gastrointestinal system may occur. Therefore, the rate of splanchnic blood flow and the level of shock can be estimated via gastric mucosal pH measurement.

In automatic tonometry systems a pump is transferring the sample from the balloon in certain time intervals. Automatically taken samples are analyzed with the help of the above detailed infrared principle. Air is recycled back into the balloon to avoid carbon dioxide depletion hence improving equilibration time. The measurement provides the reading of the carbon dioxide partial pressure in the lumen of the stomach which can be the predictor of gut hypoperfusion.[11] If a double-lumen catheter is used, continuous measurement can be performed in case of the ongoing recirculation of the sample. In this case, response time is relatively slow around 5 minutes.

## SALIENT POINTS

- The simple and noninvasive technique of pulse oximetry has significantly improved patient safety.
- Blood gas analyzers enable accurate measurement of the partial pressure of oxygen and carbon dioxide in a blood sample.
- Co-oximetry provides the measurement of the concentration of oxygenated and deoxygenated hemoglobin, carboxyhemoglobin along with methemoglobin as a percentage of the total hemoglobin.
- Near infrared spectroscopy provides a noninvasive continuous monitoring of tissue oxygenation.
- Oxygen content analyzers can prevent the administration of hypoxic gas mixtures hence improving patient safety.
- Time and volume based capnography have a pivotal importance in tailoring respiratory therapy.
- Gastric tonometry can be the predictor of gut hypoperfusion.

## REFERENCES

1. Lam T, Nagappa M, Wong J, et al. Continuous pulse oximetry and capnography monitoring for postoperative respiratory depression and adverse events: A systematic review and meta-analysis. Anesth Analg. 2017;125(6):2019-29.
2. Shafique M, Kyriacou PA, Pal SK. Investigation of pulse oximeter failure rates during artificial hypoperfusion utilising a custom made multimode pulse oximetry sensor. Conf Proc IEEE Eng Med Biol Soc. 2011;2011:4352-5.
3. Baquero H, Alviz R, Castillo A, et al. Avoiding hyperoxia during neonatal resuscitation: time to response of different $SpO_2$ monitors. Acta Paediatr. 2011;100(4):515-8.
4. Webb RK, Ralston AC, Runciman WB. Potential errors in pulse oximetry. II. Effects of changes in saturation and signal quality. Anaesthesia. 1991;46(3):207-12.
5. Toffaletti JG, Rackley CR. Monitoring oxygen status. Adv Clin Chem. 2016;77:103-24.
6. Brunelle JA, Degtiarov AM, Moran RF, et al. Simultaneous measurement of total hemoglobin and its derivatives in blood using co-oximeters: analytical principles; their application in selecting analytical wavelengths and reference methods; a comparison of the results of the choices made. Scand J Clin Lab Invest Suppl. 1996;224:47-69.
7. Scheeren TWL, Schober P, Schwarte LA. Monitoring tissue oxygenation by near infrared spectroscopy (NIRS): background and current applications. J Clin Monit Comput. 2012;26(4):279-87.
8. Nagler J, Krauss B. Capnography: a valuable tool for airway management. Emerg Med Clin North Am. 2008;26(4):881-97.
9. Verscheure S, Massion PB, Verschuren F, et al. Volumetric capnography: lessons from the past and current clinical applications. Crit Care. 2016;20(1):184.
10. Tusman G, Groisman I, Fiolo FE, et al. Noninvasive monitoring of lung recruitment maneuvers in morbidly obese patients: the role of pulse oximetry and volumetric capnography. Anesth Analg. 2014;118(1):137-44.
11. Ackland GL, Grocott MP, Mythen MG. Understanding gastrointestinal perfusion in critical care: so near, and yet so far. Crit Care. 2000;4(5):269-81.

**CHAPTER 11**

# Lung Recruitment Maneuvers

*Abdul Wahab, Shalini Donthi, Salim Surani, Rahul Kashyap*

## INTRODUCTION

Acute respiratory distress syndrome (ARDS) alters the mechanics and gas exchange due to underlying inflammatory process. Hypoxemia and inflammatory process lead to multiple organ failure that is associated with significant morbidity and mortality.[1] ARDS patients require mechanical ventilation to survive. Mechanical ventilation can cause lung injury due to alveolar overdistension as the functional lung size is small in ARDS patients. As a result, lung protective ventilation strategy with low tidal volume (6 mL/kg of predicted body weight) and lowest possible plateau pressure (≤30 cmH$_2$O) is mainstay of treatment for ARDS.[2] Lung recruitment maneuvers (LRM) are used to improve oxygenation and compliance of lungs and to prevent ventilator-induced lung injury (VILI). Studies have shown survival benefits from volume and pressure limitation. Clinical benefits of LRM are still uncertain. A variety of recruitment maneuvers have been described, each with its pros and cons. Here we present a brief review of current literature available related to different LRM.

## DEFINITION OF RECRUITMENT MANEUVERS

An LRM is transient increase in the airway pressure intended to open collapsed alveoli and keep them opened. Critically ill patients with ARDS have decreased functional lung size due to interstitial and alveolar edema, collapse, and consolidation. Decreased functional lung size increases the risk of VILI. LRMs are aimed to increase end expiratory lung volume which can increase oxygenation and protect against VILI.[3-5]

## METHODS OF RECRUITMENT MANEUVERS

Lung recruitment is a physiologic and dynamic process to reopen the collapsed part of the lung. It can be achieved by a variety of methods. It is still uncertain which method is the best for lung recruitment. Different lung recruitment methods are described in Box 1.

### Sustained Inflation

It is the most commonly used recruitment maneuver. In this method ventilator is set to continuous positive airway pressure (CPAP) and pressure is increased to 30–40 cm H$_2$O for 30–40 seconds.[5-7] In the meanwhile it is essential to monitor patient for adverse effects. Sustained inflation can improve oxygenation and respiratory compliance, and prevent derecruitment. But association with better outcomes in ARDS patients has not been found.[8-10]

### Stepwise or Staircase

In this method lung recruitment is accomplished through incremental positive end-expiratory pressure (PEEP) titration keeping a balance between recruitment and overdistension. PEEP is increased by 2–5 cmH$_2$O in stepwise manner. Each step is 3–5 minutes unless an adverse effect is noted. Volume control ventilation is used with a fixed tidal volume of 6 mL/kg of ideal body weight. PEEP is

---

**Box 1:** Various lung recruitment methods.

- Lung recruitment maneuvers
- Sustained inflation
- Stepwise or staircase recruitment
- Sigh
- Prone positioning
- Ventilator modes as recruitment maneuvers
  – Airway pressure release ventilation (APRV)
  – High frequency oscillatory ventilation (HFOV)

(APRV: airway pressure release ventilation; HFOV: high frequency oscillatory ventilation)

increased if there is evidence of lung recruitment. In case of positive response there will be decreased driving pressure, plateau pressure less than 30 cmH$_2$O, and increased oxygen saturation by pulse oximetry. PEEP is decreased to the previous step if there is overdistension—increased driving pressure, plateau pressure more than 30 cmH$_2$O, decreased oxygen saturation, and hypotension. This method is considered better than sustained inflation as recruitment can be achieved by it with low risk of hyperinflation and hemodynamic compromise.[5-7,10-13]

## Sigh

Sigh function is available in different ventilators and can be used for lung recruitment, particularly in patients on pressure support ventilation. Sigh can be provided via certain modes on ventilators such as PCV+ called biphasic positive airway pressure or BiLevel mode. This method can be achieved in different ways. One way to add sigh to pressure support ventilation is using biphasic positive airway pressure at 35 cmH$_2$O for 3-4 seconds at rates of 2 sighs/min, 1 sigh/min, and 1 sigh/2 min.[5-7] Alternative way is the extended sigh method which consists of inflation phase, pause, and deflation phase. During the inflation phase, tidal volume ($V_T$) is decreased from 8 to 2 mL/kg and PEEP is increased from 10 to 25 cmH$_2$O in stepwise manner; each step is of approximately 30 seconds. As PEEP of 25 cmH$_2$O and $V_T$ of 2 mL/kg are reached, a pause is taken and continuous positive airway pressure of 30 cmH$_2$O is applied for 30 seconds. During deflation phase, reverse sequence is applied back to baseline settings.[14] Sigh recruits alveoli in both dependent and nondependent areas that improve oxygenation and also recruited lung volume.[3,12,14,15]

## Prone Positioning

Prone positioning has been in use for many years to improve oxygenation as it reduces intrapulmonary shunt and promotes ventilation and perfusion matching by change in their redistribution.[16,17]

Human and animal studies have shown that both ventilation and perfusion are unevenly distributed within the lungs and are affected by postural changes.[18-20] In supine position there is progressive decrease in the alveolar size along the vertical axis and resultant collapse of dorsal regions at the end of expiration creates ventilation gradient. Gravity, distribution of lung tissue in the chest cavity, regional distension and compression of lung parenchyma, and pressure by abdominal contents play role in ventilation heterogeneity.[21,22] Prone positioning decreases ventilation heterogeneity by redistribution of lung tissue. Large portion of lung tissue is contained in the dorsal chest.[23] Even though prone position redistributes some lung mass to ventral chest, lung parenchyma compressed by tissue above it and by the heart is relatively less in prone position than in supine. Also intra-abdominal pressure has less influence on the intrathoracic pressure in prone than supine position.[22,23] As a consequence prone position increases ventilation in dorsal regions with some decrease in the ventral regions and decreases the ventilation gradient.[21,24] As compared to normal individuals, patients with ARDS have much greater ventilation heterogeneity and gradient in the supine position due to increased lung weight. Prone positioning significantly decreases ventilation heterogeneity and makes it more homogeneous and this has been shown by imaging studies.[25]

Blood flow in different regions of the lungs is influenced by factors such as alveolar and vascular pressures, hydrostatic pressure, vascular resistance, endothelial nitric oxide production, and vascular geometry.[26,27] Significant perfusion heterogeneity exists in lungs similar to ventilation heterogeneity. Studies have shown that dorsal lung region have favorable blood flow as compared to other areas and this perfusion bias persists irrespective of the posture and is unaffected by gravity.[28,29] Increased endothelial nitric oxide production, more available pulmonary vasculature to accommodate cardiac output and difference in conductance due to vascular geometry are the possible mechanisms for increased blood flow in the dorsal lung region. It has been reported that despite persistent dorsal perfusion bias pulmonary perfusion becomes more homogenous in prone position as compared to supine position.[30]

So in prone position ventilation and perfusion become more homogeneous and ventilation/perfusion matching is much stronger that results in improved oxygenation in patients with ARDS and survival benefits.[7,16,17,31-34]

Other than better ventilation perfusion matching, prone positioning decreases the risk of VILI by reducing lung strain and atelectasis, enhances clearance of edema and upper airway secretions, and improves right ventricular function by decreasing pulmonary vascular resistance.[21,24]

## Ventilator Modes as Recruitment Maneuvers

Certain ventilator modes can be used for lung recruitment. Two of those are described below:

### Airway Pressure release Ventilation (APRV)

APRV is a type of partial ventilatory mode which allows spontaneous breathing at any phase of ventilation cycle and provides high airway pressure with an intermittent pressure release.[35] High pressure in APRV can recruit alveoli and spontaneous breathing can improve recruitment in the dorsal caudal lung regions. APRV might improve oxygenation but mortality benefit has not been shown. This method does have the potential to cause lung injury due to probable high transalveolar distending pressure during spontaneous breathing.[35-38]

### High Frequency Oscillatory Ventilation (HFOV)

HFOV delivers small tidal volume and high airway pressure and has been used to promote lung recruitment. It is sometimes used as an alternative in patients with acute respiratory distress syndrome but not as first line. Studies have not shown survival benefit of HFOV as compared to conventional ventilation.[5,39,40]

## ADVANTAGES AND DISADVANTAGES OF RECRUITMENT MANEUVERS

Advantages and disadvantages of recruitment maneuvers are described in Table 1.

## RECRUITMENT MANEUVERS AND PEEP TITRATION

Acute respiratory distress syndrome decreases functional lung size. Aim of LRMs and PEEP titration is to recruit alveoli, improve oxygenation, and decrease the risk of

**Table 1:** Advantages and disadvantages of lung recruitment maneuvers (LRM).

| LRM | Advantage | Disadvantage | Recommended (ATS/ESICM/SCCM) |
|---|---|---|---|
| Sustained inflation | • Improves oxygenation<br>• Decreases atelectasis<br>• Decreases decruitment[5,6,8,10,28] | Can—<br>• Cause hypotension<br>• Reduce clearance of alveolar fluid<br>• Increase risk of barotrauma<br>• Increase intracranial pressure[4,7,29,30] | Recommended in ARDS patients (conditional recommendation)[31] |
| Stepwise or staircase | • Improves oxygenation and lung compliance<br>• Less risk of hemodynamic instability and over-distension as compared to sustained inflation[3-6] | • Risk of hyperinflation<br>• Risk of hemodynamic instability[8,9,32] | Recommended in ARDS patients (conditional recommendation)[31] |
| Prone positioning | • Improves oxygenation<br>• Improves lung recruitment: Increases end-expiratory lung volume, increases ventilation perfusion matching, decreases ventilator induced lung injury<br>• Decreases mortality in patients with severe ARDS[16-20] | • Risk of endotracheal tube obstruction<br>• Increased rate of pressure sore[7,31] | Recommended for >12 hours/day in patients with severe ARDS (strong recommendation)[31] |
| Sigh | • Improves oxygenation<br>• Recruits alveoli in both dependent and nondependent areas of lungs<br>• Reduces regional ventilation heterogeneity<br>• Considered as more physiologic as compared to other LRMs[6,14,15,33] | • Can cause excessive strain[14] | Recommended in ARDS patients (conditional recommendation)[31] |
| Airway pressure release ventilation | • Allows spontaneous breathing<br>• Improves alveolar recruitment[22,24,25] | • Increases risk of lung injury[5,23] | Not recommended for use in ARDS patients[7] |
| High frequency oscillatory ventilation | • Can recruit collapsed alveoli and decrease tidal stress and strain[34,35] | • Requires heavy sedation<br>• Increases mortality[26,27,34,35] | Not to be used routinely in patients with moderate or severe ARDS (Strong recommendation)[31] |

(ARDS: acute respiratory distress syndrome; ATS: American Thoracic Society; ESICM: European Society of Intensive Care Medicine; LRM: lung recruitment maneuvers; SCCM: Society of Critical Care Medicine)

VILI. Randomized controlled trials have shown that higher PEEP strategy can lead to improved oxygenation in ARDS patients without complications but controversy about survival benefits of high PEEP in certain patient population still remains.[2,41] A PEEP less than 5 cmH₂O can be harmful in ARDS patients.[42] In ARDS patients not only the pressure and volume can induce VILI, frequent opening and closing of the alveoli (atelectrauma) also pose a major risk.[43] Rationale behind using high PEEP is to keep alveoli open at the end of expiration and reduce atelectrauma and the risk of VILI.[44] Current guidelines recommend low tidal volume and high PEEP or at least avoidance of low PEEP in patients with ARDS as a lung protective ventilation strategy. Conclusive evidence supports the survival benefits of using low tidal volume ventilation in ARDS patients but there is lack of such evidence about using high PEEP in ARDS.[2] It has been reported that in patients with mild form of acute lung injury or ARDS, high PEEP can be associated with longer duration of mechanical ventilation.[41] High PEEP levels can improve gas exchange significantly in certain patients with ARDS but may not bring any improvement in others and even can cause hemodynamic disturbance. It is fine balance between improving gas exchange and avoiding barotrauma to set optimal PEEP. Thus random application of high or low PEEP in any patients with lung injury may not be beneficial. Optimal PEEP in appropriate patient population can be set by targeted oxygenation and compliance, using pressure volume curves, stress index, lung volumes, imaging (computerized tomography and ultrasound), and esophageal manometry.[5]

## DERECRUITMENT

Derecruitment is defined as the amount of poorly and normally aerated tissue that becomes nonaerated at the end of expiration. End-expiratory collapse is considered to be depended on the tidal volume, preceding inspiratory pressure, and pressure at the end of expiration.[45] At low tidal volume lung parenchyma may stay collapsed during deflation because it does not get sufficient airway pressure during inspiration to open. As reported by Pelosi et al.[45] and Crotti et al.[46] at high tidal volume end-expiratory collapse was more at PEEP of 5 cmH₂O as compare to a PEEP of 15 cmH₂O.

## RECRUITMENT MANEUVERS AND VENTILATOR-INDUCED LUNG INJURY

Acute respiratory distress syndrome patients exhibit small functional lung volume due to alveolar collapse, edema, and consolidation. LRMs reduce atelectasis and increase end-expiratory lung volume which leads to decrease strain on the alveoli and thus reduce VILI.[3,6,47] Analysis of computed tomography (CT) scan images of ARDS patients showed that dependent areas are affected more, some areas are nonaerated others are poorly aerated and some have normal aeration. LRMs along with appropriate PEEP can reduce regional heterogeneity and decrease risk of VILI. LRMs not only reduce atelectasis but also increase alveolar fluid clearance. As shown by Jabaudon, et al.[48] LRMs lead to a drop in the plasma soluble form of the receptor for advanced glycation end-product (sRAGE) in ARDS patients. It is a marker of alveolar type I cell injury and correlates with the severity and outcome in ARDS patients, and has been found to have inverse relation to alveolar fluid clearance rate. Possible mechanisms by which LRMs can increase alveolar fluid clearance are by increasing the surface area for fluid reabsorption and by increasing alveolar pressure which can affect hydrostatic pressure and decrease fluid penetration to the alveolar space.[6] LRMs can also increase the risk of VILI by overdistension and excessive strain.[14]

## FUTURE TRIALS AND FUTURE DIRECTIONS

There are several clinical trials (Table 2) underway measuring various ways to do lung recruitment and measuring its effect in wide variety of patient population.

## CONCLUSION

Lung recruitment maneuvers have been proposed as a part of lung protective ventilation strategy for many years. Studies have shown that LRMs are associated with physiologic benefits but clinical benefits are still uncertain. Physiologic benefits achieved with LRMs are short-term unless followed by higher PEEP.[3,5,6,49] Combination of LRMs and higher PEEP can lead to significant lung recruitment and prevent VILI. So, if a recruitment maneuver is effective and is followed by higher PEEP it can be beneficial in patients with ARDS. Hemodynamic effects due to recruitment maneuvers are transient and barotrauma is found to be rare. Future studies are needed to separate effects of LRMs from co-interventions such as PEEP.[5,50] Research is also needed to identify preferred recruitment maneuver with regards to pressure, PEEP titration and duration, and also to severity of ARDS.

## SALIENT POINTS

- Controversy remains regarding the beneficial use of lung recruitment maneuvers due to insufficient evidence.

**Table 2:** Future lung recruitment maneuvers trials (as of July 30th, 2018).

| Sl N. | Trial name: US National Clinical Trial (NCT) Number | Primary Aim |
|---|---|---|
| 1 | Lung protective one-lung ventilation with fix and variable tidal volume: NCT03364465 | To compare constant tidal volume with recruitment maneuver vs. variable tidal volume with recruitment maneuvers in patients undergoing thoracic surgery to see if there is protection against postoperative pulmonary complications and improved oxygenation |
| 2 | Lung recruitment improves right ventricle performance: NCT02795208 | To see whether LRM improves the performance of the right ventricle by comparing two groups one received standard protective ventilation and other group received same ventilator pattern following lung recruitment |
| 3 | Open-lung protective ventilation in cardiac surgery (PROVECS): NCT02866578 | To assess the postoperative outcome during first seven days following cardiac surgery with open lung approach (RM, PEEP) and conventional approach without RM |
| 4 | Effect low pressure pneumoperitoneum and pulmonary recruitment on postoperative pain: NCT03069586 | To see if there is additional decrease on the postoperative pain in two groups with or without addition of RM to a low pressure pneumoperitoneum |
| 5 | Alveolar recruitment maneuver during pneumoperitoneum: NCT03331471 | To compare the incidence of pulmonary complications with and without applying LRM during pneumoperitoneum in elderly patients undergoing laparoscopic surgery |
| 6 | Protective ventilation with high vs. low PEEP during one-lung ventilation for thoracic surgery: NCT02963025 | To see whether LRM with high PEEP vs. low PEEP prevent any postoperative pulmonary complications in patients undergoing thoracic surgery under standardized one lung ventilation |
| 7 | Open-lung strategy in critically ill morbid obese patients: NCT02503241 | After performance of the RM, describing the lung mechanics and heart lung interaction at titrated PEEP levels with the help of TTE and electric impedance tomography imaging in morbidly intubated and mechanically ventilated patients |
| 8 | Individualized perioperative open-lung ventilatory strategy with high vs. conventional inspiratory oxygen fraction (iPROVE-$O^2$): NCT02776046 | To see whether high $FiO_2$ is better than conventional $FiO_2$ within perioperative individualized ventilation strategy to reduce the incidence of surgical site infection |
| 9 | Effect of pulmonary recruitment maneuver (PRM) on pain and nausea after laparoscopic cholecystectomy: NCT03026543 | To see the effect on postoperative pain and nausea after the application of pulmonary recruitment maneuver following laparoscopic cholecystectomy |
| 10 | High vs. low positive end expiratory pressure with alveolar recruitment maneuver in laparoscopic bariatric surgeries: NCT03505632 | To see whether low PEEP with frequent RM is better than conventional mechanical ventilation with high PEEP in terms of lung compliance, improvement of intraoperative oxygenation, lower dead space in patients undergoing laparoscopic bariatric surgeries |
| 11 | Open-lung strategy, gas distribution and right heart function in ARDS patients: NCT03202641 | To compare two PEEP titration techniques (one is PEEP selected based on low PEEP/high $FiO_2$ table, other is LRM plus PEEP titration), in intubated and mechanically ventilated ARDS patients, and measuring the outcomes (primary is the driving pressure, other outcomes are chest wall and lung elastance, dead space, ventilation/perfusion matching, etc.) |
| 12 | Hemodynamic changes induced by alveolar recruitment maneuver with respect to volemic state in colon surgery: NCT03468764 | To see whether after performance of LRM, the hemodynamic changes (heart rate, BP, saturation) differs between hypovolemic and normovolemic patients |

(LRM: lung recruitment maneuvers; NCT: national clinical trial; PEEP: positive end expiratory pressure; PROVECS: protective ventilation in cardiac surgery; PRM: pulmonary recruitment maneuver; RM: recruitment maneuvers; TTE: transthoracic echocardiogram)

- Recruitment maneuvers can be considered in appropriate patients.
- Hemodynamic changes associated with recruitment maneuvers are usually short term.
- Recruitment maneuvers with appropriate PEEP can improve oxygenation and decrease the risk of VILI.
- Appropriate PEEP is usually necessary to maintain recruitment achieved by a recruitment maneuver.

- Positive end expiratory pressure should be titrated appropriately in ARDS patients as a balance between recruitment and barotrauma.
- Studies have shown improvement in oxygenation with high PEEP in patients with moderate and severe ARDS but evidence for survival benefit is still lacking.

## REFERENCES

1. Gattinoni L, Caironi P, Cressoni M, et al. Lung recruitment in patients with the acute respiratory distress syndrome. N Engl J Med. 2006;354(17):1775-86.
2. Brower RG, Matthay MA, Morris A, et al. Acute Respiratory Distress Syndrome Network. Ventilation with lower tidal volumes as compared with traditional tidal volumes for acute lung injury and the acute respiratory distress syndrome. N Engl J Med. 2000;342(18):1301-8.
3. Goligher EC, Hodgson CL, Adhikari NK, et al. Lung recruitment maneuvers for adult patients with acute respiratory distress syndrome. A systematic review and meta-analysis. Ann Am Thorac Soc. 2017;14(Suppl 4):S304-11.
4. Marini JJ. Recruitment by sustained inflation: Time for a change. Intensive Care Med. 2011;37(10):1572-4.
5. Hess DR. Recruitment maneuvers and PEEP titration. Respir Care. 2015;60(11):1688-704.
6. Constantin JM, Godet T, Jabaudon M, et al. Recruitment maneuvers in acute respiratory distress syndrome. Ann Transl Med. 2017;5(14):290.
7. Nguyen A. Use of recruitment maneuvers in patients with acute respiratory distress syndrome. Dimens Crit Care Nurs. 2018;37(3):135-43.
8. Brower RG, Morris A, MacIntire N, et al. Blood Institute, National Institutes of Health. Effects of recruitment maneuvers in patients with acute lung injury and acute respiratory distress syndrome ventilated with high positive end-expiratory pressure. Crit Care Med. 2003;31(11):2592-7.
9. Constantin JM, Jaber S, Futier E, et al. Respiratory effects of different recruitment maneuvers in acute respiratory distress syndrome. Crit Care. 2008;12(2):R50.
10. Hess DR, Bigatello LM. Lung recruitment: The role of recruitment maneuvers. Respir Care. 2002;47(3):308-18.
11. Borges JB, Okamoto VN, Matos GF, et al. Reversibility of lung collapse and hypoxemia in early acute respiratory distress syndrome. Am J Respir Crit Care Med. 2006;174(3):268-78.
12. Lim SC, Adams AB, Simonson DA, et al. Transient hemodynamic effects of recruitment maneuvers in three experimental models of acute lung injury. Crit Care Med. 2004;32(12):2378-84.
13. Meade MO, Cook DJ, Guyatt GH, et al. Lung Open Ventilation Study Investigators. Ventilation strategy using low tidal volumes, recruitment maneuvers, and high positive end-expiratory pressure for acute lung injury and acute respiratory distress syndrome: A randomized controlled trial. JAMA. 2008;299(6):637-45.
14. Lim CM, Koh Y, Park W, et al. Mechanistic scheme and effect of "extended sigh" as a recruitment maneuver in patients with acute respiratory distress syndrome: A preliminary study. Crit Care Med. 2001;29(6):1255-60.
15. Patroniti N, Foti G, Cortinovis B, et al. Sigh improves gas exchange and lung volume in patients with acute respiratory distress syndrome undergoing pressure support ventilation. Anesthesiology. 2002;96(4):788-94.
16. Gattinoni L, Taccone P, Carlesso E, et al. Prone position in acute respiratory distress syndrome. Rationale, indications, and limits. Am J Respir Crit Care Med. 2013;188(11):1286-93.
17. Guérin C, Reignier J, Richard JC, et al. PROSEVA Study Group. Prone positioning in severe acute respiratory distress syndrome. N Engl J Med. 2013;368(23):2159-68.
18. Glazier JB, Hughes JM, Maloney JE, et al. Vertical gradient of alveolar size in dog lungs frozen in situ. J Physiol. 1966;186(2):114p-5p.
19. Kaneko K, Milic-Emili J, Dolovich MB, et al. Regional distribution of ventilation and perfusion as a function of body position. J Appl Physiol. 1966;21(3):767-77.
20. Henderson AC, Sá RC, Theilmann RJ, et al. The gravitational distribution of ventilation-perfusion ratio is more uniform in prone than supine posture in the normal human lung. J Appl Physiol (1985). 2013;115(3):313-24.
21. Johnson NJ, Luks AM, Glenny RW. Gas exchange in the prone posture. Respir Care. 2017;62(8):1097-110.
22. Pelosi P, Tubiolo D, Mascheroni D, et al. Effects of the prone position on respiratory mechanics and gas exchange during acute lung injury. Am J Respir Crit Care Med. 1998;157(2):387-93.
23. Gattinoni L, Pelosi P, Vitale G, et al. Body position changes redistribute lung computed-tomographic density in patients with acute respiratory failure. Anesthesiology. 1991;74(1):15-23.
24. Kallet RH. A comprehensive review of prone position in ARDS. Respir Care. 2015;60(11):1660-87.
25. Gattinoni L, Pelosi P, Valenza F, et al. Patient positioning in acute respiratory failure. In: Tobin M (Ed). Principles and Practice of Mechanical Ventilation. New York: McGraw-Hill; 1994. pp. 1067-76.
26. Hlastala MP, Glenny RW. Vascular structure determines pulmonary blood flow distribution. News Physiol Sci. 1999;14(5):182-6.
27. Rimeika D, Nyrén S, Wiklund NP, et al. Regulation of regional lung perfusion by nitric oxide. Am J Respir Crit Care Med. 2004;170(4):450-5.
28. Burrowes KS, Tawhai MH. Computational predictions of pulmonary blood flow gradients: Gravity versus structure. Respir Physiol Neurobiol. 2006;154(3):515-23.
29. Nyrén S, Radell P, Lindahl SG, et al. Lung ventilation and perfusion in prone and supine postures with reference to anesthetized and mechanically ventilated healthy volunteers. Anesthesiology. 2010;112(3):682-7.
30. Wiener CM, Kirk W, Albert RK. Prone position reverses gravitational distribution of perfusion in dog lungs with oleic acid-induced injury. J Appl Physiol (1985). 1990;68(4):1386-92.
31. Guerin C, Baboi L, Richard JC. Mechanisms of the effects of prone positioning in acute respiratory distress syndrome. Intensive Care Med. 2014;40(11):1634-42.

32. Lee JM, Bae W, Lee YJ, et al. The efficacy and safety of prone positional ventilation in acute respiratory distress syndrome: Updated study-level meta-analysis of 11 randomized controlled trials. Crit Care Med. 2014;42(5):1252-62.
33. Mentzelopoulos SD, Roussos C, Zakynthinos SG. Prone position reduces lung stress and strain in severe acute respiratory distress syndrome. Eur Respir J. 2005;25(3):534-44.
34. Sud S, Friedrich JO, Taccone P, et al. Prone ventilation reduces mortality in patients with acute respiratory failure and severe hypoxemia: Systematic review and meta-analysis. Intensive Care Med. 2010;36(4):585-99.
35. Varpula T, Valta P, Niemi R, et al. Airway pressure release ventilation as a primary ventilatory mode in acute respiratory distress syndrome. Acta Anaesthesiol Scand. 2004;48(6):722-31.
36. Maung AA, Schuster KM, Kaplan LJ, et al. Compared to conventional ventilation, airway pressure release ventilation may increase ventilator days in trauma patients. J Trauma Acute Care Surg. 2012;73(2):507-10.
37. Maxwell RA, Green JM, Waldrop J, et al. A randomized prospective trial of airway pressure release ventilation and low tidal volume ventilation in adult trauma patients with acute respiratory failure. J Trauma. 2010;69(3):501-11.
38. Mireles-Cabodevila E, Kacmarek RM. Should airway pressure release ventilation be the primary mode in ARDS? Respir Care. 2016;61(6):761-73.
39. Young D, Lamb SE, Shah S, et al. High-frequency oscillation for acute respiratory distress syndrome. N Engl J Med. 2013;368(9):806-13.
40. Sud S, Sud M, Friedrich JO, et al. High-frequency oscillatory ventilation versus conventional ventilation for acute respiratory distress syndrome. Cochrane Database Syst Rev. 2016;4:CD004085.
41. Briel M, Meade M, Mercat A, et al. Higher vs lower positive end-expiratory pressure in patients with acute lung injury and acute respiratory distress syndrome: Systematic review and meta-analysis. JAMA. 2010;303(9):865-73.
42. Ferguson ND, Frutos-Vivar F, Esteban A, et al. Airway pressures, tidal volumes, and mortality in patients with acute respiratory distress syndrome. Crit Care Med. 2005;33(1):21-30.
43. Bates JH, Smith BJ. Ventilator-induced lung injury and lung mechanics. Ann Transl Med. 2018;6(19):378.
44. Falke KJ, Pontoppidan H, Kumar A, et al. Ventilation with end-expiratory pressure in acute lung disease. J Clin Invest. 1972;51(9):2315-23.
45. Pelosi P, Goldner M, McKibben A, et al. Recruitment and derecruitment during acute respiratory failure: An experimental study. Am J Respir Crit Care Med. 2001;164(1):122-30.
46. Crotti S, Mascheroni D, Caironi P, et al. Recruitment and derecruitment during acute respiratory failure: A clinical study. Am J Respir Crit Care Med. 2001;164(1):131-40.
47. Cavalcanti AB, Suzumura ÉA, Laranjeira LN, et al. Writing group for the alveolar recruitment for acute respiratory distress syndrome trial (ART) Investigators. Effect of lung recruitment and titrated positive end-expiratory pressure (PEEP) vs Low PEEP on mortality in patients with acute respiratory distress syndrome: A randomized clinical trial. JAMA. 2017;318(14):1335-45.
48. Jabaudon M, Hamroun N, Roszyk L, et al. Effects of a recruitment maneuver on plasma levels of soluble RAGE in patients with diffuse acute respiratory distress syndrome: A prospective randomized crossover study. Intensive Care Med. 2015;41(5):846-55.
49. Arnal JM, Paquet J, Wysocki M, et al. Optimal duration of a sustained inflation recruitment maneuver in ARDS patients. Intensive Care Med. 2011;37(10):1588-94.
50. Fan E, Del Sorbo L, Goligher EC, et al. American Thoracic Society, European Society of Intensive Care Medicine, and Society of Critical Care Medicine. An Official American Thoracic Society/European Society of Intensive Care Medicine/Society of Critical Care Medicine Clinical Practice Guideline: Mechanical Ventilation in Adult Patients with Acute Respiratory Distress Syndrome. Am J Respir Crit Care Med. 2017;195(9):1253-63.

# CHAPTER 12

# Heart Lung Interactions during Mechanical Ventilation

*JV Divatia, Jacob George Pulinilkunnathil*

## CASE

A 56-year-old gentleman with a history of ischemic heart disease was being managed in wards as a case of bilateral pneumonia for 3 days. He remained febrile and tachypneic and over the past 3 hours, was not maintaining saturation even on nonrebreathing mask at 15 L of oxygen. He was shifted to the ICU and chest X-ray was suggestive of acute respiratory distress syndrome (ARDS). In view of worsening respiratory status, he was intubated and initiated on lung protective ventilation (6 mL/kg Tidal volume, PEEP 15, $FiO_2$ 100%). He remained hypotensive despite an initial fluid resuscitation with 1 liter of lactated Ringers' solution. An arterial line and central line were secured. The CVP measured was 16 mm Hg. The pulse pressure variation (PPV) as derived from arterial line was 16%. Bed side echocardiography showed a left ventricular ejection fraction of 45% with normal right ventricular function and no pericardial effusion.

- His CVP at end of expiration is 16—does it mean that he does not need fluids?
- The PPV is 16%—does it mean he is hypovolemic or fluid responsive?
- Under what circumstances is the PPV not reliable as an indicator of fluid responsiveness?

## DETERMINANTS OF HEART-LUNG INTERACTION

The cardiac chambers and lungs are enclosed together in a closed thoracic cavity and are under the constant influence of the surrounding intrathoracic pressure and its variations. Changes in the pressure or volume of the thoracic cavity will affect the pulmonary parenchyma and also the cardiac function. Phasic variations of intrathoracic pressure and volume that occur during positive pressure ventilation make these interactions more prominent.

A proper understanding of these interactions not only helps in anticipating the complications of ventilation, but also assists in predicting treatment effects such as that of fluid administration and helps in day to day practice to make appropriate decisions in managing critically ill patients in ICU. The physiological changes and the clinical applications of heart lung interactions are described in the chapter. Table 1 explains the common terminologies used throughout the chapter.

**Table 1:** Understanding the terms that are to be used in the article.

| | |
|---|---|
| Heart lung interactions | Changes in cardiovascular physiology brought around by changes in lungs volume as a result of changes in intrathoracic pressure during respiration. |
| Transmural Pressure | The difference between the internal expanding forces and the external collapsing forces. So, for a cardiac chamber, the transmural pressure is the pressure inside the chamber minus the intrathoracic pressure. (intraluminal pressure—pleural pressure) |
| Transpulmonary pressure | The transmural pressure of the alveoli is called transpulmonary pressure. It is the airway pressure minus the intrapleural pressure. |
| Mean systemic filling pressure (MSFP) | The mean pressure in the central circulation after cessation of cardiac function and complete redistribution of blood. It is related to the effective blood volume, compliance of blood vessels and the pressure the blood volume exerts on the vasculature. The MSFP—CVP gradient determines the venous return to the heart.[1] |
| Ventricular interdependence | The mechanism by which volume or pressure overloading of either ventricle affects the function of the other ventricle is called ventricular interdependence. |

MSFP: mean systemic filling pressure; CVP: central venous pressure

# Chapter 12
## Heart Lung Interactions during Mechanical Ventilation

The major determinants of heart-lung interactions are:
- Changes in intrathoracic pressure (ITP) that affects the right ventricular preload and the left ventricular afterload.
- Changes in lung volume that modulates humoral responses, autonomic tone, pulmonary vascular resistance (PVR), and effects a compression of the heart in the cardiac fossa.
- *Ventricular interdependence*: A series effect occurs because the left ventricular (LV) preload depends on the right ventricular (RV) output; a parallel effect occurs because both ventricles are enclosed in the pericardium which limits their expansion resulting in bowing of the interventricular septum towards the side of lesser pressure.
- Changes in intra-abdominal pressure due to the movements of the diaphragm.

## HEMODYNAMIC EFFECTS DUE TO CHANGES IN INTRATHORACIC PRESSURE

### Effect of Intrathoracic Pressure on Venous Return

When the intrathoracic pressure increases, it is transmitted to the right atrium, and the gradient between mean systemic filling pressure (MSFP) and right atrial pressure reduces. This results in a significant reduction in the venous return and hence a reduced right ventricular output.[1] This effect is more significant in hypovolemic patients and is one of the causes of immediate hypotension after initiation of ventilation. The human body maintains the venous return by an increased sympathetic tone (secondary to lung inflation) that causes venoconstriction which maintains the MSFP—right atrial pressure gradient. The descent of diaphragm during inspiration increases the intra-abdominal pressure, compresses the splanchnic circulation, and also aids in maintaining the venous return to thorax.[2]

In severely hypovolemic patients, with a low transmural pressure gradient to begin with, any positive intrathoracic pressure that gets transmitted into the abdomen may collapse the veins at the entry point into thorax, reducing the venous return, and causing a severe reduction in cardiac output.[2] For this reason, it is necessary to preload hypovolemic patients prior to intubation and initiation of ventilation. Preloading with crystalloids increases the intravascular volume, maintains the transmural pressure and MSFP thereby maintaining the venous return to the right side of heart.

When the intrathoracic pressure reduces, the reduction in intrathoracic pressure is transmitted to the right atria. The MSFP-right atrial pressure gradient increases, resulting in increased venous return and an increase in RV preload (Fig. 1). At one point, the venous return is limited and does not increase with further decrease of ITP. This check on the venous return at sub atmospheric values of ITP happens due to the collapse of the great vessels just prior to their entry into the thorax. This check is physiologically important as tachypneic patients with large negative swings of ITP will otherwise have an increased intrathoracic volume in resulting severe pulmonary edema.

### Effect of Intrathoracic Pressure on Ventricular Function

The ventricular output depends upon the ventricular contractility, myocardial stretch produced by the end-diastolic volume (EDV), and the transmural pressure of the left ventricle. With positive-pressure ventilation, the venous return to the rght side of the heart reduces and the afterload to the RV increases. Thus, the right ventricular output is reduced. The reduction in venous return and RV output eventually reduces the preload to the left heart resulting in low left LV end-diastolic volume (LVEDV). However, the positive intrapleural pressure decreases the transmural pressure and left ventricular afterload and thus improving ejection of the left ventricle.[3]

These physiological changes induced by positive-pressure ventilation simulates the effects of vasodilator therapy and can be used to manage heart failure. The effects of positive-pressure ventilation on biventricular function are summarized in Flowchart 1.

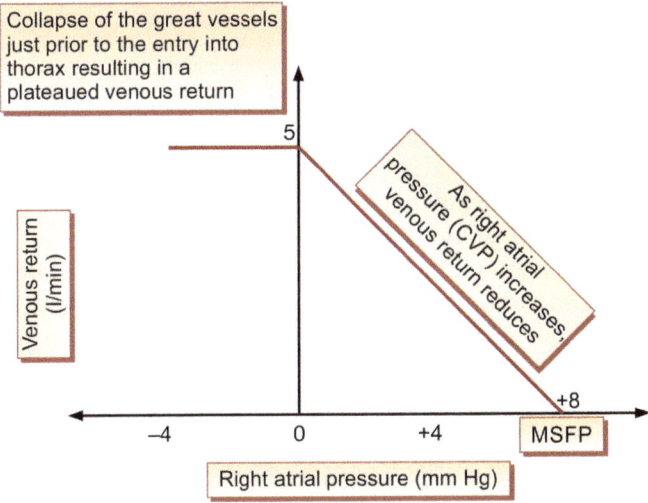

**Fig. 1:** The relationship between right atrial pressure, mean systemic filling pressure (MSFP) and venous return.

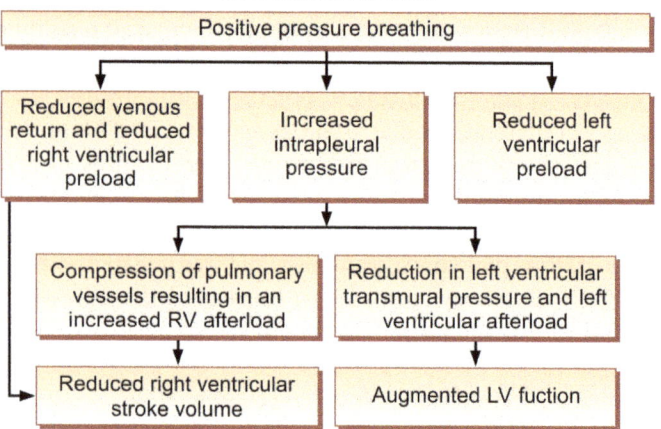

**Flowchart 1:** Effects of positive pressure ventilation (PPV) on biventricular function.

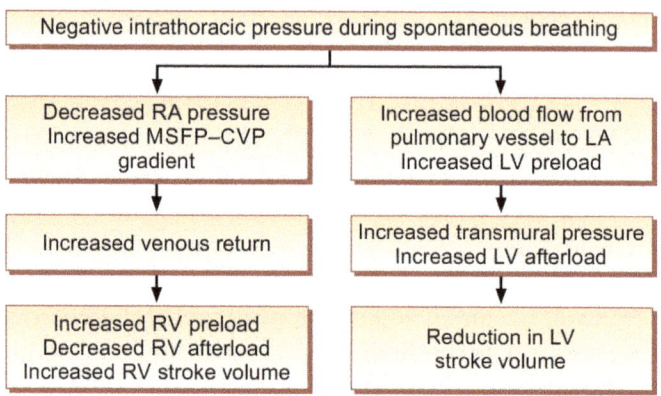

**Flowchart 2:** Effects of intrathoracic pressure (ITP) during spontaneous breathing on biventricular function.

As the intrathoracic pressure becomes negative (as in extreme tachypnea or removal of positive pressure support), the LV transmural pressure increases resulting in an increased afterload and increased impedance to LV output. Similarly, the transmural pressure across the intrathoracic aorta is increased, also increasing LV afterload. On the other hand, a reduction in intrathoracic pressure favors venous return, and increased intrathoracic blood volume.[3] Hence, during weaning from mechanical ventilation, as the positive pressure ventilation is being reduced, the venous return and the RV preload increases while the LV output is impeded by an increase in LV transmural pressure. This may result in increased accumulation of intrathoracic blood volume, pulmonary edema, and failure to wean. The effects of intra thoracic pressure swings on biventricular function during spontaneous ventilation are summarized in Flowchart 2.

## HEMODYNAMIC EFFECTS DUE TO CHANGES IN LUNG VOLUME

### Changes due to a Change in Autonomic Tone

Lung inflation with normal tidal volumes exert a vagolytic effect resulting in tachycardia (sinus arrythmias). However, if the lungs are inflated with a volume more than 10 mL/kg, it can result in bradycardia with vasodilation. Positive pressure ventilation causes an increased prostaglandin synthesis along with a reduced ANP synthesis resulting in weight gain from salt and water retention.[4]

### Effects of Changes in Lung Volume on Cardiovascular System

During positive-pressure ventilation, as the lungs expand, the pulmonary vessels are squeezed, resulting in a transiently increased blood volume entering the left atrium. This effect on preload is short lived and is over-shadowed by the effects of positive intra thoracic pressure on venous return—resulting in a net reduced preload to both atria. Similarly, during spontaneous breathing, the dilation of pulmonary vessels results in pooling of blood in the pulmonary circulation and reduced left atrial preload. But eventually, due to an increased venous return and increased right ventricular stroke volume, the left atrial preload also increases with time. Another feature of clinical significance with increased lung volume is a reduced diastolic compliance of the heart. With positive-pressure ventilation, the inflated lungs compress the heart in the cardiac fossa and reduces the cardiac volume resulting in a reduction in diastolic compliance. This effect is more significant during ventilation with high peep and recruitment maneuvers or any ventilation with an increased mean airway pressure.[5]

### Effects of Changes in Lung Volume on Pulmonary Vascular Resistance

At lung volume below the functional residual capacity (FRC), the tortuosity of extra-alveolar vessels increases causing kinking of these vessels resulting in an increased pulmonary vascular resistance (PVR). The regional hypoxia induced by atelectasis also acts as a stimulus for pulmonary vasoconstriction and increased PVR. As the lung is inflated from residual volume towards FRC, the extra-alveolar vessel resistance reduces, but alveolar capillary PVR increases due to compression of the intra alveolar vessels by the distended alveoli. At high lung volumes, PVR is increased as overdistended alveoli compress the alveolar capillaries. The net PVR is least at FRC and increases above and below the FRC.[6] RV afterload is determined mainly by the PVR. Increases in PVR can occur during mechanical ventilation with high PEEP or tidal volume because of hyperinflation which can precipitate RV failure acutely.[6]

## HEMODYNAMIC EFFECTS DUE TO VENTRICULAR INTERDEPENDENCE

Both ventricles are enclosed together in the pericardium, separated by the interventricular septum. They are connected by the pulmonary circulation in series in such a way that the output of one ventricle directly influences the preload of the other. The pericardium limits dilatation of cardiac chambers and in case of pressure or volume overload of either chamber, compromise is attained by the interventricular septum bowing towards the side of less strain. This mechanism by which volume or pressure overloading of either ventricle affect the function of the other ventricle is called ventricular interdependence.

### Series Effect

During positive-pressure ventilation, the phasic changes in lung volume and intrathoracic pressure results in changes in the right atrial pressure, venous return, and intrathoracic blood volume. With PPV, during inspiration the RV preload and RV stroke volume reduces which is reflected as a reduced LV preload after about three heart beats. If the left ventricle is preload-responsive, then the LV output is also reduced transiently in accordance to the reduced preload.[7] These phasic variations in LV stroke volume (stroke volume variation, SVV) or its surrogate arterial pulse pressure (systolic pressure variation (SPV) and pulse pressure variation (PPV), respectively) during ventilation can easily identify patients who will be volume responsive (Fig. 2).

### Parallel Effect

Normally the LV pressure exceeds the RV pressure and the interventricular septum is usually central. In cases of rise in RV volume or pressure, the RV accommodates the changes by dilation. In deep inspiration in spontaneously breathing person, the negative intrathoracic pressure acts as a pump that pumps in blood from the peripheral venous system, thereby increasing RV preload and RVEDV.[8] There is a shift of the septum into the LV cavity, with reduction in pulmonary venous return (Fig. 3). Similarly, if there is a pericardial effusion that prevents expansion of the volume of the cardiac chambers, the LV diastolic compliance, LV filling, LVEDV, and LV output decrease, especially during inspiration, when the venous return and RV filling increase. This is manifested at bedside as an exaggerated drop in systolic pressure during inspiration in a spontaneously breathing patient, called pulsus paradoxus.

## CLINICAL APPLICATIONS OF HEART-LUNG INTERACTION

### Pulsus Paradoxus

Pulsus paradoxus is a physiological phenomenon best explained based on ventricular interdependence. As ITP becomes negative during inspiration, the venous return increases and volume overload of the right ventricle results in a shift of the interventricular septum towards the left ventricle. This reduces the diastolic compliance of left ventricle, reduces LVEDV and a fall in left ventricle stroke volume that manifests as a fall in systolic pressure. This systolic reduction in blood pressure during normal inspiration is further accentuated in patients with active breathing efforts with great negative swings of intrathoracic pressure and can be a marker of disease severity, e.g. status asthmaticus and pericardial diseases.[9]

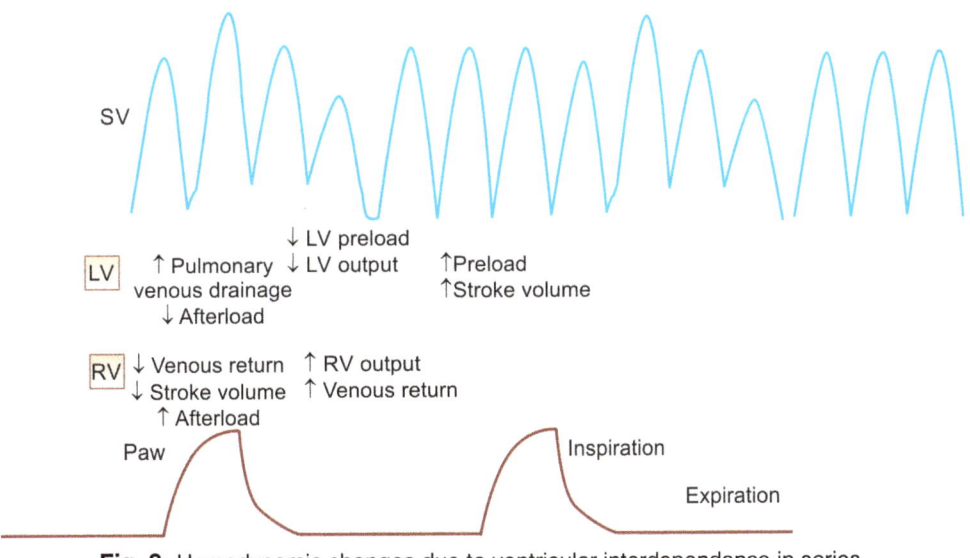

**Fig. 2:** Hemodynamic changes due to ventricular interdependence in series.

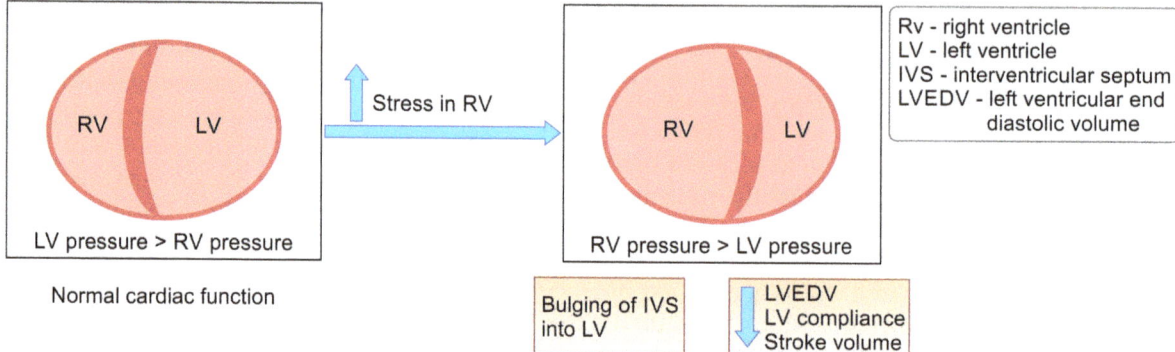

**Fig. 3:** Ventricular interdependence in parallel.
(RV: right ventricle; LV: left ventricle; IVS: interventricular septum; LVEDV: left ventricular end diastolic volume)

### Reverse Pulsus Paradoxus

A paradoxical increase in systolic pressure during inspiration followed by a decrease in systolic pressure during expiration is called reversed pulsus paradoxus. This is due to an augmentation in left ventricular function due to a significant reduction in left ventricular afterload in patients with relative hypervolemia such as LV systolic failure.

### Kussmaul's Sign

During spontaneous breathing, inspiration results in reduced intrathoracic and right atrial pressure, increased MSFP—right atria pressure gradient and increased venous return. The right atrial pressure and CVP will remain low only if the right ventricle is compliant and the right ventricular outflow matches the venous inflow. In conditions of poor RV compliance (RV failure/RV infarction) or in conditions of increased RV afterload (pulmonary embolism) an increased venous return during inspiration will increase the right atrial pressure and CVP. This paradoxical rise of CVP during inspiration is called Kussmaul's sign.[10]

### Negative Pressure Pulmonary Edema

In cases where there is a markedly negative intrathoracic pressure—such as breathing against an obstructed glottis—there is a marked increase in the venous return. The left ventricular transmural pressure will increase significantly, and the left ventricular outflow is impeded. This combination of increased venous return associated with a reduced left ventricular outflow results in increased intrathoracic blood volume, increased venous hydrostatic pressure causing increased transudation at the capillary end with lymphatic outflow. As the lymphatic drainage is outpaced by the increased venous return, fluid leaks into the pulmonary interstitium resulting in negative pressure pulmonary edema.[11]

### Hemodynamic Response to Prone Positioning

In patients with severe ARDS, hypoxia and high PEEP may impair the RV function. Prone positioning may help to offset these adverse effects. During prone positioning, although the chest wall compliance reduces, the lung compliance improves, and the net thoracic compliance also increases. Diaphragmatic descent will increase the intra-abdominal pressure and MSFP, maintaining the MSFP-CVP gradient and venous return. Prone positioning opens the collapsed dorsal alveoli and improves oxygenation by reducing pulmonary shunt. As atelectasis and oxygenation improves, the PVR reduces and the RV afterload reduces. By ventricular interdependence, a reduction in RV afterload translates into better LV function.[12]

### Effect on Positive Pressure on CVP

Increased intrathoracic pressure also increases the measured central venous pressure (CVP) and pulmonary artery occlusion pressure (PAOP). The increased intrathoracic pressure during ventilation and PEEP application will be partially transmitted to the right atria also. Therefore, the CVP measured in a patient on positive-pressure ventilation and PEEP may be spuriously higher. It is difficult to quantify the proportion of intrathoracic pressure that is transmitted to the CVP although transmission indices based on pulmonary compliance has been proposed by Teboul, et al.[13] As the beneficial effect of PEEP on lung recruitment is rapidly lost when PEEP is removed and difficult to regain, removing the set PEEP for the sole purpose of measuring CVP is not advocated. A pragmatic approach will be to keep in mind that although PEEP increases CVP, tracking the changes in CVP values than individual measurements of CVP would be more rewarding. Very high PEEP or tidal volume can cause hyperinflation which worsens the hypoxia induced PVR and can precipitate RV failure acutely which will also result in high values of CVP.

## Predicting Fluid Responsiveness

During respiration there is a cyclic change in the intrathoracic pressure causing cyclic changes in right ventricular and left ventricular function. Any decrease in RV stroke volume will decrease left ventricular (LV) preload after 2–3 breaths as they are connected to each other in series. This cyclical change in preload acts as an auto fluid challenge to the left ventricle and demonstrates the current cardiac function and fluid responsiveness. These are identified at the bedside as systolic pressure variation (SPV), stroke volume variation (SVV), and pulse pressure variation (PPV), and are increasingly used to determine fluid responsiveness.[7] Both pulse pressure variation (PPV) and stroke volume variation (SVV) can be calculated at bedside by commercially available minimally invasive monitors using inbuilt mathematical algorithms (Fig. 4).

### Understanding How SVV or PPV Act as a Marker of Preload Responsiveness

The SPV/PPV/SVV are made up by an increase from baseline (delta up) and a decrease in tracing from the baseline (delta down). Delta-up is due to an increase in left ventricular output assisted by positive pressure inspiration and delta-down is the decrease in left ventricular output due to an exaggerated hypovolemia induced by positive pleural pressure.[14] In euvolemic patients, both components will be equally contributing towards PPV and SVV (Fig. 5).

In patients with a high SPV/PPV/SVV predominantly due to a delta up, relative hypervolemia or an afterload dependent LV must be suspected, whereas in patients with a PPV/SVV predominantly due to delta down, hypovolemia and preload responsiveness should be suspected. So, while diuretics might be indicated in the initial case, fluid administration remains the treatment in the latter.

PPV and SVV are relatively easy, minimally invasive accurate markers of cardiac function and preload responsiveness if the caveats are recognized (Tables 2 and 3). However, neither PPV nor SVV should be taken as a universal marker of hypovolemia, and patients with high PPV or SVV should be given fluids only if there are signs of hypoperfusion, and no obvious contraindications for fluid therapy. A persistently high PPV or SVV or a PPV or SVV

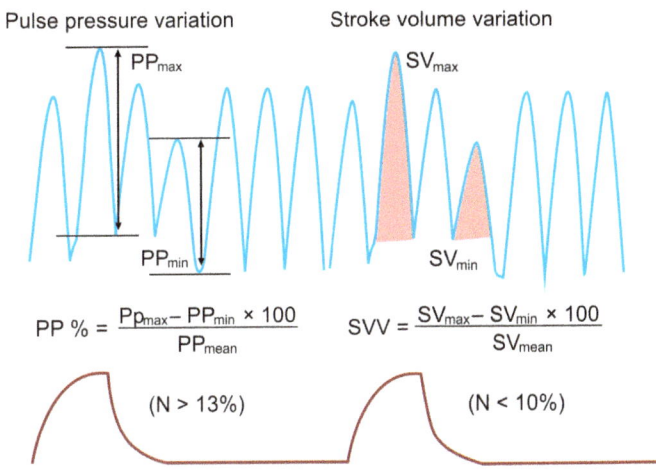

**Fig. 4:** Calculation of pulse pressure variation (PPV) and stroke volume variation (SVV) (N: normal).

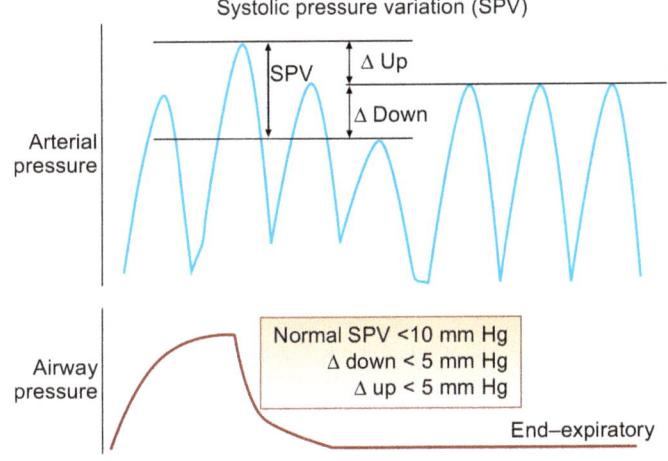

**Fig. 5:** Delta up and delta down in normal subjects.

value that fails to reduce with fluid therapy should alert the physician towards the possibility of underlying cardiac dysfunction or relative hypervolemia.

### Tidal Volume Challenge Test

Both PPV and SVV lose their ability to predict preload responsiveness during lung protective low tidal volume ventilation. In the current era of lung protective ventilation, this limits the applicability of these indices in the ICU significantly. The tests proposed to overcome the limitations of PPV and SVV (passive leg raising test and end expiratory occlusion test or mini fluid challenge) require continuous cardiac output monitoring, are not applicable in a certain group of patients such as intra-abdominal hypertension, or patients with raised intracranial pressure and may still carry hazards of fluid overload. A modification of PPV—the tidal volume challenge test (ΔPPV) helps overcome this

**Table 2:** Factors affecting pulse pressure variation (PPV)—apart from preload.[15]

| | |
|---|---|
| Tidal volume | Increased tidal volume increases the phasic change in intrathoracic pressure and increase PPV and SVV<br>Low tidal volumes lack the ability to induce adequate swings in intrathoracic pressure and PPV and SVV may remain falsely negative even in preload responders |
| PEEP | A high PEEP reduces cardiac output but does not affect PPV and SVV |
| Lung compliance | Increased lung compliance will transmit airway pressure to the intrathoracic pressure and result in increased PPV and SVV, while reduced lung compliance will not produce swings in intrapleural pressures. Hence PPV and SVV will remain falsely low |
| Heart rate | Bradycardia or a low pulse rate to respiratory rate ratio less than 3.6 in patients with ARDS (Acute respiratory distress syndrome) falsely reduces the changes in preload, thereby causing a false negative PPV/SVV |
| Heart Rhythm | Not validated in varying LV output states of arrhythmia |
| Ventricular function | RV failure—increased PPV and SVV while the heart is not responsive to fluid administration<br>isolated left ventricular failure—increased PPV and SVV<br>SVV and PPV are reliable only in case of biventricular fluid responsiveness |
| Arterial elastance | With varying degree of arterial compliance, discordant values of PPV and SVV might be obtained. Not clearly understood[16] |

PPV: pulse pressure variation; SVV: stroke volume variation

**Table 3:** Clinical use of pulse pressure variation (PPV) and stroke volume variation (SVV).

| Clinical use of PPV and SVV[17] | Caveats of PPV or SVV[17] |
|---|---|
| In patients with normal biventricular function, a SVV >10% and a PPV> 13–15% predicts preload responsiveness | All breaths must be completely controlled, with no spontaneous breathing activity, having a tidal volume of at least 8 ml/kg and no cardiac arrythmia. |
| An increasing PPV/SVV during attempts of deresuscitation will be an early predictor of relative/absolute hypovolemia and further fluid removal might be deleterious in these patients. | PPV and SVV are not validated in patients with ARDS or having a compliance lower than 30 ml/cm of $H_2O$ |
| PPV and SVV might identify patients with significant dynamic hyperinflation due to bronchospasm. | Confounding factors such as open chest, intra-abdominal hypertension etc. should be absent while measuring these dynamic variables. |

PPV: pulse pressure variation; SVV: stroke volume variation; ARDS: Acute respiratory distress syndrome

limitation of low tidal volume in using PPV.[12] During the tidal volume challenge (ventilating to 6 mL/kg tidal volume followed by a transient increase to 8 mL/kg tidal volume for a minute and then ventilating back at 6 mL/kg) an absolute change in PPV by 3.5%, or SVV by 2.5%, accurately identified preload responders. In patients who had a high PPV, and receiving fluids, a reduction of the PPV after fluid bolus ($\Delta PPV_{fluid\ bolus}$) of 1.5% reliably discriminated preload responders from nonresponders (PPV due to delta down than delta up). Tidal volume challenge test is exciting and promising in the sense that it is minimally invasive, cheap, does not require patient mobilization, and produces no major swings in intrathoracic pressure. It has to be clearly remembered that apart from low tidal volume, all the other caveats of PPV stand true for tidal volume challenge test also.

### Dynamic Changes in CVP to Identify Preload Responders in Spontaneously Breathing Patients

Spontaneously breathing patients who are preload responsive can be identified by an inspiratory decrease of CVP by 2 mm of Hg during spontaneous breathing. In clinical practice, the converse of this statement is important. Patients with no significant inspiratory reduction in the CVP (<2 cm $H_2O$) are unlikely to be fluid responders. However, before concluding on test results of dynamic CVP, the adequacy of inspiratory efforts should be considered. Correct identification of a positive test depends on identifying a fall in the whole CVP wave form as assessed at the base of the "a" wave and taking care not to misinterpret the release of an active expiration as a fall in CVP. This has been validated only in spontaneously breathing patients and not in patients on mechanical ventilation.[18]

### Other Tests that Depend on Heart Lung Interactions to Predict Fluid Responsiveness

- *Vena caval variation:* The variation in vena caval diameter in accordance with respiration can be easily measured by bedside echocardiography, either at superior vena cava (SVC) or inferior vena cava (IVC) distal to the entry of portal vein. A diameter variation of 36% in SVC as measured by transesophageal echocardiography and an IVC distensibility of 12% as measured on transthoracic echocardiography accurately predict preload responsiveness. The clinical utility of vena caval variations is that they may be used in patients with atrial fibrillation, a shortcoming for PPV and SVV. Low tidal volume and poor lung compliance seems to be limiting factor as like for PPV and SVV.[17]

- *End expiratory occlusion test:* In preload responsive patients, a prolonged expiratory hold (>15 secs) transiently increases the venous return and cardiac preload by abolishing the dip in venous return due to positive pressure. This is a relatively easy maneuver and has been validated in patients with low lung compliance, cardiac arrhythmias, and also in spontaneously breathing patients who are able to do an expiratory hold for 15 seconds. An increase in cardiac output as manifested by an increase in aortic flow rate-time index (VTI) more than 5% can be assumed as a biventricular preload responsiveness.[17]

## Management of Cardiogenic Pulmonary Edema

The pathophysiology of cardiogenic pulmonary edema can be best described as 1) reduced left ventricle function due to a relative hypervolemia or impaired contractility or an increased afterload, 2) low cardiac state resulting in hypoxemia that in turn increases myocardial stress and ischemia, and 3) wide intrathoracic swings associated with tachypnea increasing venous return to the thorax. Positive pressure effectively acts on each step as explained in Flowchart 3.
- An increased intrathoracic positive pressure decreases the venous return and the preload of the heart.
- An increased intrathoracic positive pressure reduces the transmural pressure, thereby reducing afterload, and augmenting the left ventricular ejection and cardiac output.
- As hypoxia and respiratory muscles are also supported, the work of breathing reduces resulting in a reduction in the wide fluctuations of intrathoracic pressure. The positive pressure opens up areas of peripheral collapse, augmenting oxygenation and reduces the hypoxia induced vasoconstriction and PVR. In short, the effects of positive-pressure ventilation are similar to that of a vasodilatory drug in reducing the preload and afterload of a failing heart and in addition, it also supports the respiratory muscles and mitigates respiratory fatigue.
- *Pulmonary edema of weaning:* When patients with borderline cardiac reserve are planned for weaning, as spontaneous breathing is resumed, the left ventricular afterload increases, and the work of left ventricle increases. The reduction in intrathoracic pressure increases the venous return to the heart and the patient is at risk of pulmonary edema (Flowchart 2). The net effect is an increased intrathoracic blood volume and decreased left ventricular function both resulting in increased pulmonary hydrostatic pressure and pulmonary edema in patients with poor cardiac function. Development of pulmonary edema is associated with a drop in the lung volume and lung compliance, requiring greater respiratory effort for inspiration. These efforts in virtue of deep inspiratory efforts, reduce the ITP and decrease the transmural pressure, thereby increasing the afterload. The increased afterload causes more pulmonary edema and the vicious cycle continues. In such patients, weaning or attempts to weaning causes an increased myocardial oxygen demand, increased respiratory muscle load and increased oxygen demand due to pulmonary edema. Such patients if identified early will benefit from reduction in preload and afterload or will require positive pressure support even after extubation, such as with noninvasive ventilation.

## Case Revisit

The screening ECHO revealed normal biventricular function (even though there is history of ischemic heart disease). There is evidence of circulatory failure, as

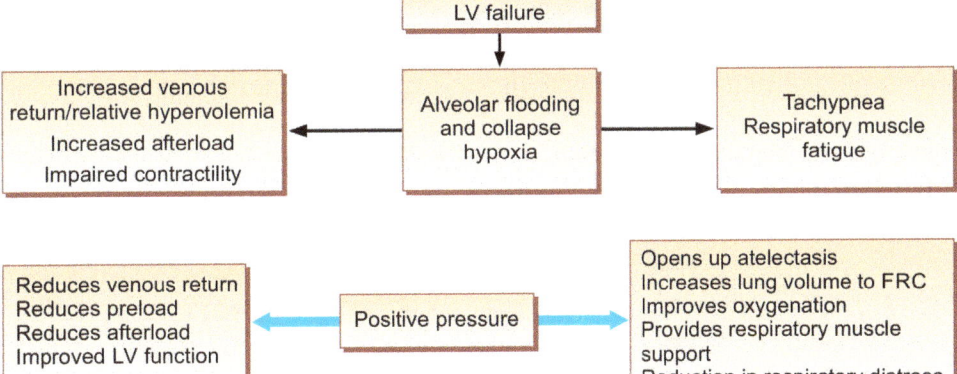

**Flowchart 3:** Effects of positive pressure ventilation in pulmonary edema.

evidenced by hypotension, for which no cardiac cause could be elucidated. The high PEEP and positive-pressure ventilation may have caused an accentuated reduction in the venous return, further worsening the hypotension. In these situations of high PEEP and ventilation, a single value of CVP, irrespective of its magnitude cannot predict volume status or preload responsiveness. A high PPV suggests preload dependency. Fluids may be administered in this patient, monitoring the gas exchange, and oxygenation. In the situation of worsening oxygenation with fluids, other measures to optimize cardiac output and blood pressure need to be undertaken. In case the oxygenation is not worsened significantly, further fluid boluses maybe administered under careful monitoring, if the patient has signs of persisting circulatory insufficiency, and still remains preload responsive.

## CONCLUSION

The heart lung interactions occurring due to positive-pressure ventilation can be beneficial or detrimental. In the presence of preexisting pulmonary disease, hypovolemia or RV dysfunction, the detrimental effects are pronounced. However, the same interactions can be successfully used for benefit in select cases such as cardiac failure. Early identification of patient disease states and prediction of the possible heart lung interactions is important for further hemodynamic monitoring and to optimize ventilatory management in critically ill patients.

## SALIENT POINTS

- Understanding heart lung interactions helps to identify hypovolemia and preload responders in patients on PPV.
- In patients undergoing positive-pressure ventilation, it is difficult to predict the exact effect of positive pressure on CVP. This limits the use of CVP as a predictor of fluid status and fluid responsiveness. The trends of CVP and effects of fluid bolus on CVP can still be useful at the bedside.
- PPV and SVV have high sensitivity and specificity for identifying fluid responders – provided the prerequisites for their measurement are met.
- A failing right ventricle or fluid overloaded left ventricle can result in falsely positive PPV and SVV.
- In patients ventilated with lung protective strategy, tidal volume challenge test may be used to circumvent the disadvantage of low tidal volumes.

## REFERENCES

1. Henderson WR, Griesdale DE, Walley KR, et al. Clinical review: Guyton—the role of mean circulatory filling pressure and right atrial pressure in controlling cardiac output. Crit Care. 2010;14(6):243.
2. Takata M, Wise RA, Robotham JL. Effects of abdominal pressure on venous return: Abdominal vascular zone conditions. J Appl Physiol (1985). 1990;69(6):1961-72.
3. Grübler MR, Wigger O, Berger D, et al. Basic concepts of heart-lung interactions during mechanical ventilation. Swiss Med Wkly. 2017;147:w14491.
4. Pinsky MR. Heart-lung interactions. Curr Opin Crit Care. 2007;13:528-31.
5. Gomez H, Pinsky MR. Effect of mechanical ventilation on heart-lung interactions. In: Tobin MJ (Ed). Principles and Practice of Mechanical Ventilation, 3rd edition. Columbus: McGraw-Hill Education; 2012.
6. Cherpanath TG, Lagrand WK, Schultz MJ, et al. Cardiopulmonary interactions during mechanical ventilation in critically ill patients. Neth Heart J. 2013;21(4):166-72.
7. Michard F, Teboul JL. Using heart-lung interactions to assess fluid responsiveness during mechanical ventilation. Crit Care. 2000;4(5):282-9.
8. Jardin F, Vieillard-Baron A. Monitoring of right-sided heart function. Curr Opin Crit Care. 2005;11(3):271-9.
9. Hamzaoui O, Monnet X, Teboul JL. Pulsus paradoxus. Eur Respir J. 2013;42(6):1696-705.
10. Mansoor AM, Karlapudi SP. Images in clinical medicine. Kussmaul's sign. N Engl J Med. 2015;372(2):e3.
11. Bhattacharya M, Kallet RH, Ware LB, et al. Negative-pressure pulmonary edema. Chest. 2016;150(4):927-33.
12. Kenny JS. Predicting the haemodynamic response to prone positioning: A novel and simultaneous analysis of the guyton and rahn diagrams. Crit Care Horizons. 2017:1-7.
13. Teboul JL, Pinsky MR, Mercat A, et al. Estimating cardiac filling pressure in mechanically ventilated patients with hyperinflation. Crit Care Med. 2000;28(11):3631-6.
14. Cannesson M, Aboy M, Hofer CK, et al. Pulse pressure variation: Where are we today? J Clin Monit Comput. 2011;25(1):45-56.
15. Kubitz JC, Reuter DA. Using heart-lung interactions for functional hemodynamic monitoring: Important factors beyond preload. Intensive Care Med. 2007;d:511-9.
16. Pinsky MR. Functional haemodynamic monitoring. Curr Opin Crit Care. 2014;20(3):288-93.
17. Monnet X, Teboul JL. Assessment of fluid responsiveness: recent advances. Curr Opin Crit Care. 2018;24(3):190-5
18. Magder S. Hemodynamic monitoring in the mechanically ventilated patient. Curr Opin Crit Care. 2011;17(1):36-42.

# CHAPTER 13

# Monitoring Pressures during Mechanical Ventilation

*Nadia Corcione, Marco Albanese, Elena Spinelli, Tommaso Mauri*

## INTRODUCTION

Respiratory monitoring is a fundamental tool to evaluate lung mechanic and its pathological changes in critically ill patients, functioning as guide to personalize both invasive and noninvasive mechanical ventilation. In this chapter, we will focus on the main pressures that may be measured in a ventilated patient, including a synthetic explanation about the physiological principle and the clinical meaning of each parameter.

## AIRWAY PRESSURE

Airway pressure (Paw), measured at airways opening, depends on the forces applied to the respiratory system by mechanical ventilation. Paw reflects the interaction between lung and ventilator, as expressed by respiratory system equation of motion:

$$Paw = (Vt/Crs) + (Flow \times Rrs) + (Pmus) + (PEEP)$$

where:
- Vt = Tidal volume (mL)
- Crs = Respiratory system compliance (mL/cmH$_2$O)
- Rrs = Respiratory system resistance (cmH$_2$O × L/sec)
- Pmus = Muscle pressure (cmH$_2$O)
- PEEP = Positive end-expiratory pressure (cmH$_2$O)

Thus, at each moment of a respiratory cycle, Paw corresponds to the sum of resistive load (Flow × Rrs) + elastic load (Vt/Crs) + pressure generated by respiratory muscles (if spontaneous efforts are present) + PEEP (both externally applied PEEP and intrinsic PEEP, if present). The dynamic inspiratory Paw values (i.e. in presence of inspiratory flow) may reach very high values (50–60 cmH$_2$O), especially if Rrs is increased, without causing excessive lung injury; on the other hand, the static inspiratory Paw value (i.e. no-flow condition) considered as maximum limit to reach during mechanical ventilation is ≤30 cmH$_2$O.

## PEAK AND PLATEAU PRESSURE

End-inspiratory airway occlusion consists in the simultaneous closure of inspiratory and expiratory valves of the ventilator circuit, at the end of inspiration; the maneuver is performed by pushing for 3–5 seconds the inspiratory hold ventilator button during controlled ventilation. When the occlusion is achieved during square flow volume controlled ventilation, a rapid flow-drop is observed, Paw falling from the highest airway-pressure level, named Ppeak, to a lower level named P1; the latter is measured when the flow reaches zero. The flow-drop is proportional to the resistive load imposed on inspiration. Starting from the P1 level, a further slow drop of airway pressure occurs; it is caused by pendelluft[1] (air redistribution between lung compartments with different filling-time constants) and by tissue-relaxation phenomena. The new, constant, and end-inspiratory level reached is the plateau pressure (Pplat), corresponds to end-inspiratory elastic load of the respiratory system (Fig. 1). Pplat is the estimate closest to the higher transalveolar pressure value, during the respiratory cycle. The limit of Pplat for the prevention of volutrauma is ≤30 cmH$_2$O. The current paradigm attributes ventilator-induced lung injury (VILI), amongst other factors, to the alveolar overstretching caused by very high-volume ventilation (volutrauma).[2,3] Furthermore, the measurement of Pplat allows calculation of Crs, corresponding to the ratio between the changes in lung volume for unitary change in airway pressure (ΔV/ΔPaw); respiratory system elastance is defined as Crs reciprocal (1/Crs). Physiologically, Ppeak is only slightly higher than Pplat and, for each level of Ppeak–Pplat difference, Ppeak and Pplat rise together in a proportional manner, if Vt is increased or if Crs is decreased. Conversely, if Ppeak rises with no changes in Pplat, increased Raw or elevated inspiratory flow values should be suspected.

## MEAN AIRWAY PRESSURE

Mean airway pressure ($Paw_{mean}$) is the average pressure exerted on airway and lungs during the ventilatory cycle; $Paw_{mean}$ is affected by many variables in mechanical ventilation:
- Inspiratory pressure
- PEEP and auto-PEEP
- Inspiration to expiration ratio
- Inspiratory pressure waveform

$Paw_{mean}$ closely reflects mean alveolar pressure (Palv), in absence of significant airway obstruction.[4] The closer it approximates Palv, the more relevant it becomes, being mean alveolar pressure a major determinant of both respiratory and hemodynamic effects of ventilation. Typical $Paw_{mean}$ values for passively ventilated patients ranges from 5 to 10 $cmH_2O$ in normal subjects, from 20 to 30 $cmH_2O$ if Crs is markedly reduced and from 10 to 20 $cmH_2O$ in presence of airflow obstruction.

## POSITIVE END-EXPIRATORY PRESSURE

An end-expiratory airway occlusion maneuver consists in the simultaneous closure of inspiratory and expiratory ventilator's valves at the end of expiration, during controlled ventilation. The maneuver is obtained by holding for 3–5 seconds the end-expiratory occlusion button. During this period, airway pressure re-equilibrates in all lung compartments, so that Paw will correspond to average PEEP level. In the presence of gas trapping, Paw will rise from set PEEP to total PEEP and this rise is named auto-PEEP (Fig. 1).

For mild to severe forms of acute hypoxemic respiratory failure, PEEP ≥5 $cmH_2O$ is needed in order to improve oxygenation, but debates still happen about the so-called "optimal" PEEP[5] and its determinants.[6,7] PEEP should maximize gas exchanges by minimizing the end-expiratory atelectasis while limiting the end-inspiratory overdistension. Different methods of setting PEEP in hypoxemic respiratory failure have been proposed; in some cases, the primary goal is the improvement of oxygenation, whereas in others lung-protective ventilation strategies are privileged, even at the price of sub-optimal oxygenation. Each method has both advantages and shortcomings. Below, we report a brief description of the methods mainly used in clinical practice.

### Strategies to Select PEEP

#### ARDSnet Protocol

This strategy is based on increasing the PEEP levels when high $FiO_2$ values are needed to obtain a viable $SpO_2$, as reported in Table 1. The clinical trial performed by the acute respiratory distress syndrome (ARDS) Network in 2004,[8] on patients affected by ARDS, aimed to compare the mortality between patients ventilated according to the Table 1 settings (lower $FiO_2$, higher PEEP) and patients ventilated with higher $FiO_2$ and lower PEEP levels. No significant difference in mortality was found.

A possible explanation is that this over-simplistic approach cannot always guarantee success—the lack of correlation between PEEP levels and respiratory mechanic could result in a suboptimal lung recruitment (atelectasis) or in alveolar overdistension (increased lung stress).[9,10] Moreover, the elevated PEEP values recommended in the higher $FiO_2$ range may worsen ventilation to perfusion ratio (increase in dead space fraction), with a detrimental effect on right ventricular function (increase in afterload and pulmonary hypertension) possibly until acute Cor Pulmonale.[11] However, testing high PEEP levels in patients

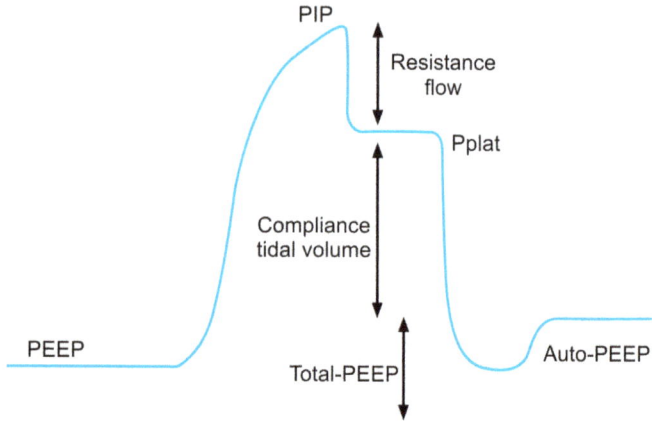

**Fig. 1:** Airway pressure trace of a volume-targeted breath, after performing an end-inspiratory airway occlusion maneuver. Flow is interrupted at the end of inspiration, allowing the measurement of the quasi-static pressures of respiratory system. PEEP: positive end-expiratory pressure; PIP: peak inspiratory pressure; Pplat: end-inspiratory plateau pressure; auto-PEEP: pressure exerted by the incompletely exhaled air, in presence of small-airways obstruction (difference between total PEEP and PEEP applied).

**Table 1:** ARDSnet ventilation-guide panel to select higher PEEP/lower $FiO_2$ values.[8]

| $FiO_2$ | 0.3 | 0.3 | 0.3 | 0.3 | 0.3 | 0.4 | 0.4 | 0.5 | 0.5 | 0.5–0.8 | 0.8 | 0.9 | 1.0 | 1.0 |
|---|---|---|---|---|---|---|---|---|---|---|---|---|---|---|
| PEEP | 5 | 8 | 10 | 12 | 14 | 14 | 16 | 16 | 18 | 20 | 22 | 22 | 22 | 24 |

(PEEP: positive end-expiratory pressure).

requiring higher $FiO_2$ may be considered as a reasonable option, especially in the emergency setting.

### Highest Compliance

Assuming Crs as an index of lung response to mechanical recruitment, PEEP is set to the value corresponding to maximal Crs. Both increasing and decreasing PEEP value beyond this point will worsen Crs by overdistension or derecruitment, respectively.

The clinical protocol, in brief, might be as follows:
- A recruitment maneuver is performed.
- Static compliance (that is Vt/Pplat-PEEPtot, at the end of a 4 seconds end-inspiratory hold) should be measured after each 2–3 $cmH_2O$ PEEP decrease of 2–3 $cmH_2O$ from a level usually corresponding to 20–25 $cmH_2O$.
- The PEEP level to which corresponds the highest static Crs will be set in the ventilator.

This approach has been recently questioned from both a physiological point of view (mismatch between the highest static compliance and the best gas exchanges) and from a clinical perspective (increased mortality in ARDS patients group treated with this approach vs. standard lower PEEP levels).[12]

### Transpulmonary Pressure

Transpulmonary pressure ($P_L$) results from the difference applied across the lungs at any time-point during the respiratory cycle (Fig. 2). $P_L$ is calculated as the difference between airway pressure (Paw, in dynamic conditions) or pressure inside the alveoli (approximated to Pplat plus total PEEP, in static conditions) and pleural pressure (which cannot be directly measured, being the esophageal pressure a reasonable surrogate). Thus, esophageal pressure catheter placement and esophageal pressure traces monitoring are needed in order to measure $P_L$.

Negative end-expiratory $P_L$ ($P_L$ <0 $cmH_2O$) increases the risk of alveolar derecruitment and atelectasis, whereas high end-inspiratory $P_L$ (>25 $cmH_2O$) leads to alveolar overdistension, with additional VILI. Based on these observations, a bedside method to select optimal PEEP has been implemented:[13]
- PEEP is set to keep end-expiratory $P_L$ around 0–10 $cmH_2O$;
- Or the highest PEEP yielding end-inspiratory $P_L \leq 25$ $cmH_2O$, which will also be associated with the least negative end-expiratory $P_L$.

Another approach to set PEEP, ever based on $P_L$, distinguishes the measure of respiratory system elastance from the measure of lung elastance (Ers and $E_L$, respectively), in order to calculate the percentage of airway pressure applied to lung parenchyma at the end of inspiration.[14] In details:
- End-inspiratory $P_L$ is calculated as
$$P_L = Pplat \times E_L/Ers$$
- PEEP is set to obtain an end-inspiratory $P_L \leq 25$ $cmH_2O$.

The method of titrating PEEP according to the $P_L$ values has a strong physiological rationale: $P_L$ measures de facto the mechanical stress applied to the lung under mechanical ventilation, allowing personalized rather than average PEEP selection. However, technical limitations of esophageal pressure monitoring and assumptions about pleural pressure value at zero airway pressure might limit their validity.[15]

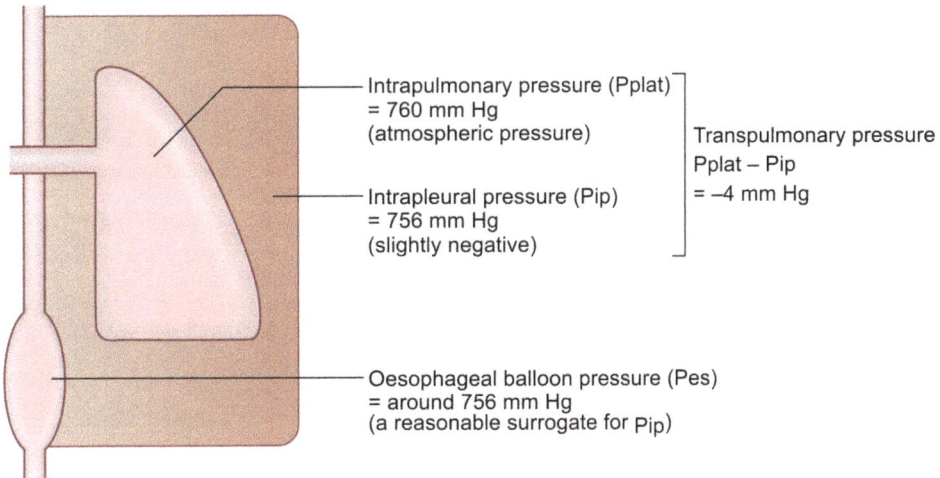

**Fig. 2:** Physiological pressures of respiratory system.

## Evaluation of Lung Recruitment by CT Scan

It is possible to determine the optimal PEEP through the evaluation of thoracic CT scans performed in ARDS patient, at different pressure levels. For example, a significant reduction of nonaerated lung area after a recruitment maneuvers at 45 cmH$_2$O, could indicate that high PEEP level is preferable[16] (Fig. 3). However, CT remains an undesirable option because of excessive exposure to radiations, as well as the logistics and the necessity of dynamic PEEP titration along the ventilation time-course.[17] Conversely, CT is useful to set PEEP in patients needing repeated scans for clinically unsolved issues.

## Electrical Impedance Tomography as Measure of Improved Regional Respiratory Mechanics

Electrical impedance tomography (EIT) is a new, noninvasive imaging method, based on changes in electrical properties of a section of chest tissues, induced by the respiratory cycle. The data are inferred from a series of superficial skin electrodes (belt) measurements and are used to create dynamic tomographic image of the examined lung portion (around half of the whole lungs in an adult) (Fig. 4). Assessing the dynamic changes in electrical impedance of different thoracic regions allows regional measure of ventilation. Indeed, EIT is useful primarily in the evaluation of air distribution across the lung (i.e. detection of ventilation dyshomogeneities), as well as changes in dependent and nondependent regional lung compliance. PEEP level associated with the more homogenous air distribution (reduced regional stress) + improvement of lung compliance in dependent regions (recruitment) + no changes of lung compliance in nondependent region (no overdistension), could be chosen as the optimal PEEP.[18] At last, through EIT use, it is possible to obtain radiation-free dynamic lung images during mechanical ventilation, allowing quicker real time adjustments in ventilation parameters.[19]

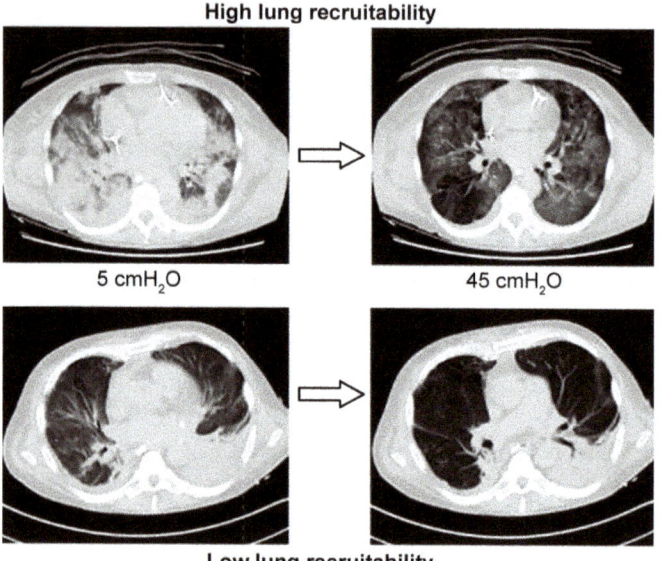

**Fig. 3:** Example of lung CT scan of patients with high or low potential of lung recruitment. Arrows depict the morphologic change from a condition of low airway pressure (i.e. 5 cmH$_2$O), to one of high airway pressure (i.e. 45 cmH$_2$O). Higher PEEP should be considered in the case of high recruitability. (modified with permission from: Umbrello M. et al. Int J Mol Sci 2017).

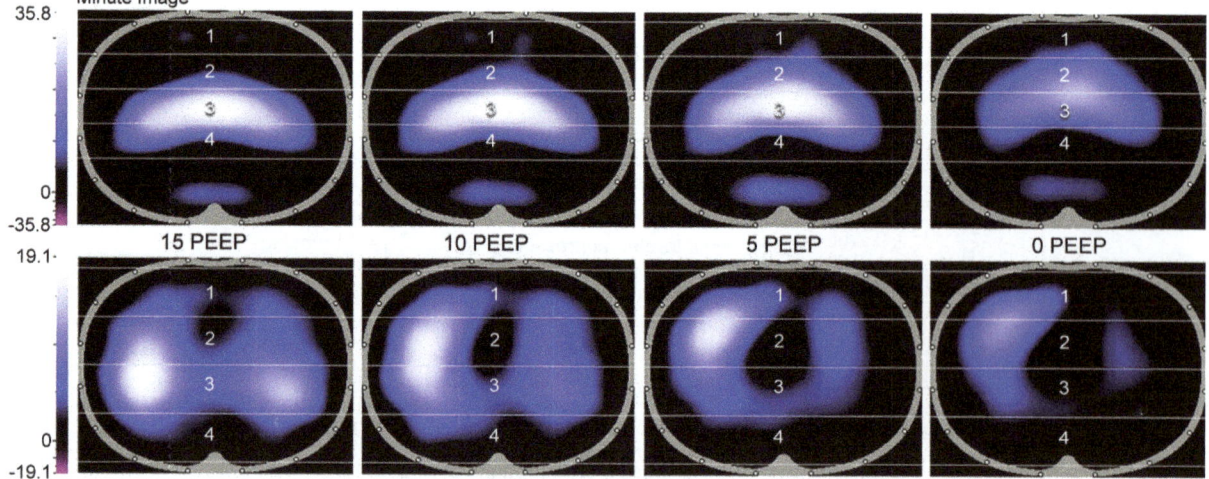

**Fig. 4:** Electrical impedance tomography images, showing the distribution of ventilation at different PEEP levels. Different PEEP are tested to detect the one associated with the lowest heterogeneity in air distribution across the lung.
*Source:* Bikker IG, et al. Crit Care 2011;15(4):R193.

## DRIVING PRESSURE

Mechanical ventilation is a well-recognized cause of lung damage; it is better known as VILI.[20,21] The first mechanism of VILI is the alveolar wall rupture because of excessive distension during ventilation (volutrauma). Volutrauma depends on the interaction between the size of tidal volume and the size of residual ventilated lung.[21] Pneumothorax, subcutaneous emphysema, pneumomediastinum, and gas embolism are further complications. Given that Crs is strongly correlated to the end-expiratory aerated volume during acute lung injury, airway driving pressure expresses Vt normalized to functional lung, representing a simple bedside assessment of lung strain. Driving pressure ($\Delta P$) may be routinely calculated during controlled ventilation (no-inspiratory efforts) as follows: Pplat minus total PEEP. Then, $\Delta P$ reflects the sum of cyclic deformations of lung parenchyma imposed on ventilated, preserved alveolar units. Cyclic strain predicts pulmonary injury better than Vt per kilogram of ideal body weight, likely because the size of functional lung during a disease state, is better expressed by Crs than by ideal body weight. Cyclic strain, VILI, and survival index should all be correlated with $\Delta P$ rather than with Vt.[22] Driving pressure <15 cmH$_2$O minimizes lung strain and, in ARDS patients, this threshold is strongly associated with improved long-term survival.[23]

## ESOPHAGEAL AND TRANSPULMONARY PRESSURE

Esophageal pressure (Pes) is a surrogate of pleural pressure (Ppl) and is measured using a dedicated catheter equipped at the tip with an esophageal balloon. Paw minus Pes is an accurate estimation of transpulmonary pressure ($P_L$) in surrounding balloon catheter region. Respiratory mechanic, lung volume, lung and chest elastance, abdominal pressure, posture, esophageal smooth muscle wall contractions, and intrinsic balloon properties can influence Pes absolute values. Moreover, pleural pressure, and thus esophageal pressure, changes within the pleural space due to both gravitational gradients and lung regional inhomogeneity. However, data from literature suggest that Pes remains an effective, acceptable surrogate of mean Ppl. To this end, the correct placement and the adequate inflation of the esophageal balloon cover a primary role. The esophageal balloon must be placed in the lower third of esophagus. To be sure about the correct catheter positioning, two tests may be performed—(1) Positive pressure occlusion test by compressing the thorax of a passively-ventilated patients, during an end-expiratory pause and (2) Baydur test is performed in pressure support ventilation through airway occlusion during an inspiratory effort. Specifically, in the first case, sedated and paralyzed patients are subjected to an external manual pressure on the rib cage and esophageal and airway pressure changes are recorded during the expiratory pause (positive pressure occlusion test). In the second case, during spontaneous breathing, an inspiratory pause is performed and the subsequent esophageal pressure swings are recorded. In both cases, a ratio between the changes in esophageal and airway pressure ($\Delta Pes/\Delta Paw$) close to unity, validates the correct catheter positioning.

The difference between Paw and Ppl defines the transpulmonary pressure ($P_L$). $P_L$ allows to separate the pressure delivered to the lungs from the one acting on chest wall and abdomen.[24,13] $P_L$ is the measure of the stress applied by mechanical ventilation onto parenchymal lung structures, thus representing one of the main determinants of VILI. Measuring $P_L$ at patient's bedside is a useful guide in ventilation settings, ranging from the choice of the optimal PEEP (see above) to the reduction of Pplat and the selection of a personalized driving transpulmonary pressure, with a potential impact on ARDS survival.[25]

## LUNG STRESS AND STRAIN

Lung stress and strain are the main determinants of VILI, resulting both from an excessive transpulmonary pressure (stress) and from a dearranged ratio between lung volume variations and functional residual capacity (strain). In physic, stress reflects the internal distribution of the counterforces per unit area, as reaction and balance to an external load; translated to the lung, stress corresponds to the lung distending pressure. Strain is defined as the system deformation divided by the initial condition and reflects the relationship between tidal volume and the mechanical characteristics of lung ventilated-area. Stress and strain are reciprocally linked, as showed by the formula:

$$\text{Stress} = k \times \text{strain}$$

This equation, referred to the respiratory system, becomes:

$$\text{Transpulmonary pressure } (P_L) = k \times VT/FRC$$

Then, higher transpulmonary pressures correspond to larger deformation of the lung. The best clinical surrogates of stress and strain are: (1) $P_L$ calculated as Paw – Pes and (2) $\Delta P$ calculated as Pplat – PEEPtot. Again, transpulmonary and driving pressure might be key to decrease the risk of VILI in patients suffering from acute hypoxemic respiratory failure.

## INSPIRATORY PRESSURE DURING SPONTANEOUS BREATHING

In spontaneously breathing patients, lung stress and strain largely depends from patient's inspiratory efforts rather than from mechanical ventilation settings.[26] Thus, the measurement of pressures closely reflecting the patient's effort, is fundamental to set protective assisted mechanical ventilation.

### Airway Occlusion Pressure (P0.1)

The airway occlusion pressure (P0.1) is the pressure developed in an occluded airway within 100 msec after the beginning of inspiration.[27] P0.1 is a good measure of respiratory center output, (i.e. patient's respiratory drive), even in the presence of respiratory muscles fatigue. High P0.1 values (>5 cmH$_2$O) indicate insufficient levels of support and the risk of acute exhaustion, while lower values (<2 cmH$_2$O) reflect an excessive respiratory assistance by the ventilator, both during assist-controlled and spontaneous modes of ventilation.[28]

### Inspiratory Muscle Pressure Index (PMI)

During assisted mechanical ventilation, the difference between airway pressure right before the beginning of an inspiratory occlusion (Ppeak) and the end-inspiratory elastic recoil plateau pressure (Pplat) reflects the end-inspiratory muscle pressure (Pmus), which is correlated with the intensity of inspiratory effort. This difference is named Pmus index (PMI).[29] A PMI threshold of 6 cmH$_2$O is the level of inspiratory effort currently considered as reasonable clinical target.

### Esophageal Pressure Swing (ΔPes)

ΔPes is the difference between Pes measured at the end of expiration and Pes measured at the end of inspiration. ΔPes defines the dynamic pressure change across the lungs, applied by the active patient's inspiratory activity. Measuring ΔPes allows accurate estimation of dynamic driving transpulmonary pressure (by adding the dynamic airway driving pressure) (Fig. 5) and of the inspiratory patient's effort, with 15–20 cmH$_2$O and 5–8 cmH$_2$O as acceptable thresholds, respectively.[30]

### SALIENT POINTS

- Measuring bedside ventilation pressures of a patient in mechanical ventilation gives to clinician an array of

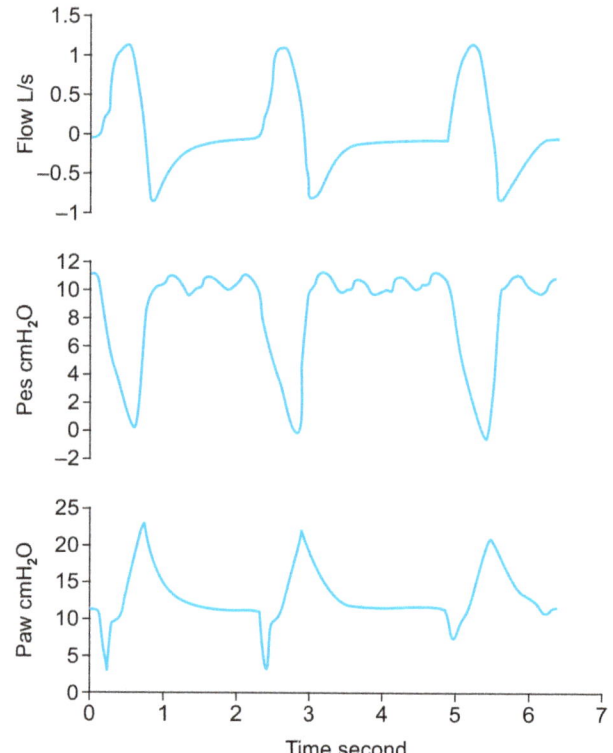

**Fig. 5:** Example of Flow, Paw and Pes swings during pressure support ventilation.

powerful tools to understand the severity of the disease and select the most appropriate settings to decrease the risk of additional injury and ventilation failure.

- In ARDS patients, a PEEP level balancing alveolar recruitment and overdistention should be sought. Recruitment maneuvers and higher PEEP levels are useful in order to obtain a lung protection and not just to improve oxygenation.

- Driving pressure represents the Vt corrected for the Crs. In ARDS, using driving pressure may be a more accurate way to select Vt and minimize lung strain during mechanical ventilation.

- Transpulmonary pressure is computed as the difference between airway pressure and pleural pressure and allows to differentiate the pressure loads onto the lung and chestwall. High transpulmonary pressure indicate high lung stress and increased risk of VILI.

- In patients on spontaneous breathing, effort is the main determinant of transpulmonary pressure and long-term endurance, thus close monitoring should be applied to fully exploit the benefits associated with active inspiration.

## REFERENCES

1. Greenblatt EE, Butler JP, Venegas JG, et al. Pendelluft in the bronchial tree. J Appl Physiol (1985). 2014;117(9):979-88.
2. Hubmayr RD, Kallet RH. Understanding pulmonary stress-strain relationships in severe ARDS and its implications for designing a safer approach to setting the ventilator. Respir Care. 2018;63(2):219-26.
3. Dornhorst AC, Leathart GL. A method of assessing the mechanical properties of lungs and air-passages. Lancet. 1952;2(6725):109-11.
4. Valta P, Corbeil C, Chassé M, et al. Mean airway pressure as an index of mean alveolar pressure. Am J Respir Crit Care Med. 1996;153(6 Pt 1):1825-30.
5. Ranieri VM, Rubenfeld GD, Thompson BT, et al. ARDS Definition Task Force. Acute respiratory distress syndrome: the Berlin Definition. JAMA. 2012;307(23):2526-33.
6. Gattinoni L, Carlesso E, Cressoni M. Selecting the 'right' positive end-expiratory pressure level. Curr Opin Crit Care. 2015;21(1):50-7
7. Briel M, Meade M, Mercat A, et al. Higher vs lower positive end-expiratory pressure in patients with acute lung injury and acute respiratory distress syndrome: systematic review and meta-analysis. JAMA. 2010;303(9):865-73.
8. Brower RG, Lanken PN, MacIntyre N, et al. National Heart, Lung, and Blood Institute ARDS Clinical Trials Network. Higher vs. lower positive end-expiratory pressures in patients with the acute respiratory distress syndrome. N Engl J Med. 2004;351(4):327-36.
9. Brower RG, Matthay MA, Morris A, et al. Acute Respiratory Distress Syndrome Network. Ventilation with lower tidal volumes as compared with traditional tidal volumes for acute lung injury and the acute respiratory distress syndrome. N Engl J Med. 2000;342(18):1301-8.
10. Grasso S, Stripoli T, De Michele M, et al. ARDSnet ventilatory protocol and alveolar hyperinflation: role of positive end-expiratory pressure. Am J Respir Crit Care Med. 2007;176(8):761-7.
11. Repessé X, Vieillard-Baron A. Right heart function during acute respiratory distress syndrome. Ann Transl Med. 2017;5(14):295.
12. Cavalcanti AB, Suzumura ÉA, Laranjeira LN, et al. Writing Group for the Alveolar Recruitment for Acute Respiratory Distress Syndrome Trial (ART) Investigators. Effect of lung recruitment and titrated Positive End-Expiratory Pressure (PEEP) vs. Low PEEP on mortality in patients with acute respiratory distress syndrome: A randomized clinical trial. JAMA. 2017;318(14):1335-45.
13. Talmor D, Sarge T, Malhotra A, et al. Mechanical ventilation guided by esophageal pressure in acute lung injury. N Engl J Med. 2008;359(20):2095-104.
14. Grasso S, Terragni P, Birocco A, et al. ECMO criteria for influenza A (H1N1)-associated ARDS: role of transpulmonary pressure. Intensive Care Med. 2012;38(3):395-403.
15. Cherniack RM, Farhi LE, Armstrong BW, Proctor DF. A comparison of esophageal and intrapleural pressure in man. J Appl Physiol. 1955;8(2):203-11.
16. Crotti S, Mascheroni D, Caironi P, et al. Recruitment and derecruitment during acute respiratory failure: a clinical study. Am J Respir Crit Care Med. 2001;164(1):131-40.
17. Cressoni M, Gallazzi E, Chiurazzi C, et al. Limits of normality of quantitative thoracic CT analysis. Crit Care. 2013;17(3):R93.
18. Mauri T, Eronia N, Turrini C, et al. Bedside assessment of the effects of positive end-expiratory pressure on lung inflation and recruitment by the helium dilution technique and electrical impedance tomography. Intensive Care Med. 2016;42(10):1576-87.
19. Lowhagen K, Lundin S, Stenqvist O. Regional intratidal gas distribution in acute lung injury and acute respiratory distress syndrome assessed by electric impedance tomography. Minerva Anestesiol. 2010;76(12):1024-35.
20. Gattinoni L, Tonetti T, Quintel M. Regional physiology of ARDS. Crit Care. 2017;21(Suppl 3):312.
21. Sahetya SK, Mancebo J, Brower RG. Fifty years of research in ARDS. Vt selection in acute respiratory distress syndrome. Am J Respir Crit Care Med. 2017;196(12):1519-25.
22. Amato MB, Meade MO, Slutsky AS, et al. Driving pressure and survival in the acute respiratory distress syndrome. N Engl J Med. 2015;372(8):747-55.
23. Costa EL, Slutsky AS, Amato MB. Driving pressure as a key ventilation variable. N Engl J Med. 2015;372(21):2072.
24. Jubran A, Grant BJ, Laghi F, et al. Weaning prediction: esophageal pressure monitoring complements readiness testing. Am J Respir Crit Care Med. 2005;171(11):1252-9.
25. Baedorf Kassis E, Loring SH, Talmor D. Mortality and pulmonary mechanics in relation to respiratory system and transpulmonary driving pressures in ARDS. Intensive Care Med. 2016;42(8):1206-13.
26. Mauri T, Cambiaghi B, Spinelli E, et al. Spontaneous breathing: a double-edged sword to handle with care. Ann Transl Med. 2017;5(14):292.
27. Alberti A, Gallo F, Fongaro A, et al. P0.1 is a useful parameter in setting the level of pressure support ventilation. Intensive Care Med. 1995;21(7):547-53.
28. Telias I, Damiani F, Brochard L. The airway occlusion pressure ($P_{0.1}$) to monitor respiratory drive during mechanical ventilation: increasing awareness of a not-so-new problem. Intensive Care Med. 2018;44(9):1532-5.
29. Foti G, Cereda M, Banfi G, et al. End-inspiratory airway occlusion: a method to assess the pressure developed by inspiratory muscles in patients with acute lung injury undergoing pressure support. Am J Respir Crit Care Med. 1997;156(4 Pt 1):1210-6.
30. Mauri T, Yoshida T, Bellani G, et al. PLeUral pressure working Group (PLUG—Acute Respiratory Failure section of the European Society of Intensive Care Medicine). Esophageal and transpulmonary pressure in the clinical setting: meaning, usefulness and perspectives. Intensive Care Med. 2016;42(9):1360-73.

# CHAPTER 14

# Inspiratory Effort Assessment in Ventilated Patient

*Sai Saran PV*

## INTRODUCTION

Weaning failure in critically ill mechanically ventilated patients increases the intensive care unit (ICU) length of stay, consuming ICU resources, thereby increasing morbidity and mortality.[1] Around 30-40% of the patients can fail initial weaning attempt and can still remain dependent on ventilator support by 7 days, classified as "difficult weaning" and around 6-15% of patients enter a phase after more than three failed spontaneous breathing trials (SBTs) or take more than 7 days after the first SBT, still on ventilator support, classified as "prolonged weaning".[2-4] Few of these patients end up requiring prolonged ventilatory support (≥6 hours/day for >3 weeks).[5] Time spent in weaning phase accounts for 50% of total duration of respiratory support.[6] Interestingly many patients will be kept on ventilator support unnecessarily, because of improper assessment of patients in the "ready to wean phase".[7]

Liberation from mechanical ventilation is usually done after an successful SBT standardized for a period of 30-120 minutes, but even then up to 21% of patients who pass an SBT may still fail requiring reintubation and initiation of mechanical ventilation.[8] This is because SBT passage for 120 minutes cannot ensure the respiratory system's efficiency to spontaneously breathe later on for prolonged periods. This method of weaning is not having strong evidence especially in patients with prolonged weaning.[9]

Inspiration, an active respiratory process, respiratory muscle endurance (skeletal muscle performance over a period of time), along with good expiratory effort forms the key to successful liberation from mechanical ventilator, apart from correction of underlying pathophysiology of the patient.[10] Although weaning failure is multifactorial, assessment of inspiratory effort and respiratory muscle strength bedside in mechanically ventilated is a challenge to intensive care physician. Factors like poor peak expiratory flow (cough strength), increased airway resistance, reduced compliance, impairment in gas exchange, cardiac dysfunction, electrolyte disturbances, infection and other neurological issues like excess sedation or delirium which can lead to difficulty in liberation, can be diagnosed and treated accordingly, but the assessment of inspiratory effort is not standardized.[11-13]

## ASSESSMENT OF INSPIRATORY EFFORTS IN VENTILATED PATIENTS

Assessment of inspiratory effort assessment in mechanically ventilated patients is under evolution from simple estimate of peak inspiratory flow (PIF) rate by disconnecting ventilator and attaching spirometer to the endotracheal tube, the least square fitting method[14,15] to the advanced microprocessor driven controls like $P_{01}$ (inspiratory depression of airways pressure achieved after first 100 ms of occlusion) and techniques like measuring electrical activity at diaphragm through specially designed catheters inserted through esophagus. This step is key to titrate the ventilator assistance required and prevent complications like muscle atrophy or patient ventilator asynchrony.[16] We classify them as noninvasive and invasive methods (Table 1).

### Noninvasive Methods

#### Maximum Inspiratory Pressure

Maximum inspiratory pressure (PImax or MIP) is the negative pressure generated by skeletal muscles of inspiration (60-70% contribution from diaphragm), an usual pulmonary function test done in cooperative patients with reproducibility.[17] It was first assessed by

**Table 1:** Summary of various techniques to assess inspiratory effort in mechanically ventilated.

| Technique | Description/Method | Interpretation (adequate) | Advantages | Limitations | References |
|---|---|---|---|---|---|
| **1. Noninvasive:** | | | | | |
| a. PImax or MIP | Patient's maximum inspiratory effort against a closed shutter (usually obtained by inspiratory hold for at least 20 s) | More than $-75$ cm in men and $-50$ cmH$_2$O in women | Noninvasive | Requires patient complete cooperation Interindividual variation | 17-19 |
| b. P$_{01}$ | Inspiratory pressure generation after first 100 ms of effort against a closed circuit, quasi-occlusion (closed inspiratory valve) measured through pressure transducer with a high speed recorder | More than $-4$ cm to $-6$ cmH$_2$O | Noninvasive Easily available on ventilator screen with continuous display Assess central respiratory drive Can be assessed in poorly cooperative | Requires pressure trigger with an opening time and demand valve (Not available in all ventilators) Cannot be correlated with P$_{oes}$ as there will be time-delay | 23-25 |
| c. Increasing flow trigger (FT) | FT increased from 1 L/min to 8 L/min (15 min at each level) with similar pressure support and flow cycling to abort autotriggering P$_{01}$, Pes and PTP was estimated | Increasing FT increased PTP | Available on all ventilators | Trivial effect on inspiratory effort | 28 |
| d. Increasing pressure trigger (PT) | Pressure trigger from $-1$ to $-10$ cmH$_2$O and assessing how many breaths are triggered | If in 1 min 1–2 breaths are lost at $-9$ cmH$_2$O: considered adequate instantaneous effort | Available on all ventilators Provide inspiratory muscle training | No clinical trials | 15, 29 |
| e. Diaphragm USG | Assessment of diaphragm thickening and motion assessed through a low frequency probe (3–5 MHz) held against the highest point of diaphragm with M-mode application | Motion at least 1.1 cm and thickness at least 4.7 cm | Noninvasive Nonvolitional | Operator dependent Poor window (obese patients, recent surgery with dressings) Abdominal distention | 30-33 |
| **2. Invasive:** | | | | | |
| a. Electrical/magnetic phrenic nerve stimulation | A magnetic coil placed in posterior cervical area at 7th cervical vertebra stimulates phrenic nerve and movement of one hemidiaphragm | Pdi after B/L magnetic stimulation has a lower limit of 20 cmH$_2$O | Nonvolitional, hence can be used in patients who are not able to understand and obey commands | Not available easily Mostly used for research purpose Pain, seizures (electrical stimulation) Two coils bilaterally to record both hemidiaphragm movements | 34-37 |
| b. Pdi (Pga – Pes) | Transdiaphragmatic pressure (Pdi) is estimated through air-filled latex balloon catheters or fluid-filled catheters or microtransducer catheters, with balloon in esophagus (Pes) and stomach (Pga), respectively | Pes is an approximate surrogate of pleural pressure Pdi indicates inspiratory muscle strength as diaphragm account for 70% of inspiratory muscle strength | Estimate of pleural pressure Nonvolitional | Invasiveness Esophageal and gastric balloons Confirmation of correct position Not available easily | 14, 38, 39 |

*Contd...*

| Technique | Description/Method | Interpretation (adequate) | Advantages | Limitations | References |
|---|---|---|---|---|---|
| c. EAdi | Electromyographic activity in diaphragm (EAdi) assessed through placement of specially designed catheter in esophagus | Normal values still not established | Visual estimation of trends in EAdi and setting of optimal NAVA level Nearest invasive approach to diaphragm with minimal side effects Nonvolitional | Invasive Costly | 40-43 |

(PImax or MIP: maximum inspiratory pressure; $P_{01}$: inspiratory pressure generation after first 100 ms of effort against a closed circuit; $P_{oes}$: esophageal pressure; PTP: pressure-time product; Pga: gastric pressure; NAVA: neurally adjusted ventilator assist).

Marini JJ et al. in 1986, in 20 critically ill patients by two techniques, one involving total airway occlusion and other involving occlusion of inspiratory valve. This landmark study concluded that the technique, duration of occlusion and patient cooperation form the key to this method of inspiratory effort assessment. Higher MIP was generated with occlusion of inspiratory valve for a period of 20-25 seconds with approximately 10 efforts.[18] Later, Caruso P et al. done crossover designed trial comparing the above two methods in 54 consecutive patients achieved similar results and concluding that the best MIP measurement is with unidirectional valve occlusion called "PImax$_{(UV)}$".[19] Later many integrative indices came up with increasing diagnostic accuracy like "timed inspiratory effort" (TIE), which assesses the ability of generating PImax over a certain time period of 60 seconds with increased diagnostic predictability in weaning especially in patients with neurologic and neuromuscular disorders.[20,21]

Although this technique enables testing of respiratory reflexes (chemical drive due to changes in $PaCO_2$) and endogenous drive, it subjects the patients to asphyxia, especially in awake patients.[19] This technique cannot be done in patients at risk of barotrauma, intracranial pressure changes or predisposition to arrhythmia and with untrained staff. Even it cannot assess the endurance of inspiratory muscles which is crucial for successful liberation from the ventilator.[22]

### Negative Pressure during First 100 Milliseconds of Occlusion ($P_{01}$)

This parameter which has continuous display on ventilator screen is an noninvasive tool to assess the inspiratory drive of the patient, helping in titration of sedation-analgesia in mechanically ventilated and weaning.[23] Historically known since 1975 by Whitelaw and Taylor studies, continuous modifications in the demand valve with quick response, quasi-purpose occlusion and no interruption to natural breathing rhythm, made this parameter be incorporated in majority of the modern day ventilators.[24,25] Study by Truwit JD et al. highlighted the importance of such parameter even in noncooperative patients, for determining MIP in which addition of dead space [1/3rd of tidal volume (Vt)] in patients with $P_{01}$ less than 2 cm $H_2O$ (inadequate drive) helped to determine MIP, while patients who had $P_{01}$ greater than 2 cm $H_2O$ were able to generate adequate MIP.[26] Its combination with MIP ($P_{01}$/PImax) increased the reliability further.[27] This parameter can be assessed "online", no need to disconnect the ventilator.

### Flow Trigger

Assessing inspiratory activity through alteration of flow trigger (FT) is another way. But the evidence is not supportive as the study by Ou CY et al. in nine patients using increasing FT from 1 L/min to 8 L/min and assessing pressure-time product (PTP), inspiratory effort and inspiratory work of breathing failed to reflect increase in inspiratory effort or inspiratory work of breathing. But there was reduction of autotrigger with alteration of FT.[28] It will be difficult to comment on the role of FT activity in assessment of inspiratory effort with this small number of patients.

### Pressure Trigger

Increasing negative pressure trigger (PT) is another method of assessing inspiratory effort although with scarce literature. This can be a better option to reflect increase in inspiratory effort when compared to FT as it is a known fact that PT requires more inspiratory effort.[15] Through this activity, the maximum trigger activity of the patient along with the endurance of respiratory muscles can be assessed. This forms the type of inspiratory muscle training which is of help in difficult and prolonged weaning.[29]

## Diaphragm Ultrasound

Diaphragm plays a crucial role in inspiratory effort and its atrophy leads to prolonged mechanical ventilation. An emerging noninvasive tool available at bedside the inspiratory effort of patients both volitional and nonvolitional through low frequency (3–5 MHz) probe placed at highest point of diaphragm. M-mode measures the excursion of diaphragm (EXdi) in cm (Figs. 1A and B) and zone of apposition of diaphragm to rib cage, the diaphragm thickness or thickening fraction (TFdi).[30] There is good intra- and interobserver reproducibility in assessing diaphragmatic excursion was around 88–99% in ICU patients,[31] even thickness assessment showed good correlation in spontaneously breathing patients off ventilator support.[32] Of-course limitations like lack of proper acoustic window, perpendicular placement to the EXdi line, correlation with the changing ventilatory supports to identify which part of excursion is due to ventilator unless we have esophageal pressure (Pes) measurements. In the recent study by Dubé BP et al. where the diaphragmatic parameters measured through ultrasound were compared with phrenic nerve stimulation guided tracheal pressure (Ptr) measurements. EXdi and TFdi did not correlative with Ptr in assist control ventilation (ACV), but in pressure support ventilation (PSV) they were strongly correlative and act as predictors for the length of mechanical ventilation.[33] With quick learning curve and with its other advantages like lack of specialized expertise with complex interpretation (esophageal catheters, magnetic resonance stimulation), this tool acts promising in patients on partial ventilator support (spontaneously breathing).

## Invasive Methods

### Electromagnetic Stimulation

Stimulation of cervical phrenic nerves with electrical current or magnetic resonance and assessing the transdiaphragmatic twitch pressure (Pdi tw), needs a mention though less used in ICU. It has an advantage of not requiring cooperation from the patient (nonvolitional). While both techniques (electrical and magnetic) have similar specificity; electrical stimulation is rarely employed due to its known adverse effects like pain, induction of seizures.[34,35] From the landmark article by Levine S et al., we know that mechanical ventilation for even few hours can lead to significant atrophy of diaphragm muscle fibers called as ventilator-induced diaphragmatic dysfunction (VIDD).[13] Magnetic phrenic nerve stimulation is done by creating magnetic field by placing coils in the posterior cervical region at 7th cervical vertebra and recording Pdi tw requiring placement of esophageal and gastric catheters with transducer-filled balloons. Methods to lessen the robustness and invasiveness of this technique by Watson AC et al. followed by Cattapan SE et al. studies to assess the correlation of twitch airway pressure (Paw tw) and Pdi tw failed.[34,36] The study by Laghi F et al. giving the impression that after magnetic stimulation of phrenic nerves the Pdi

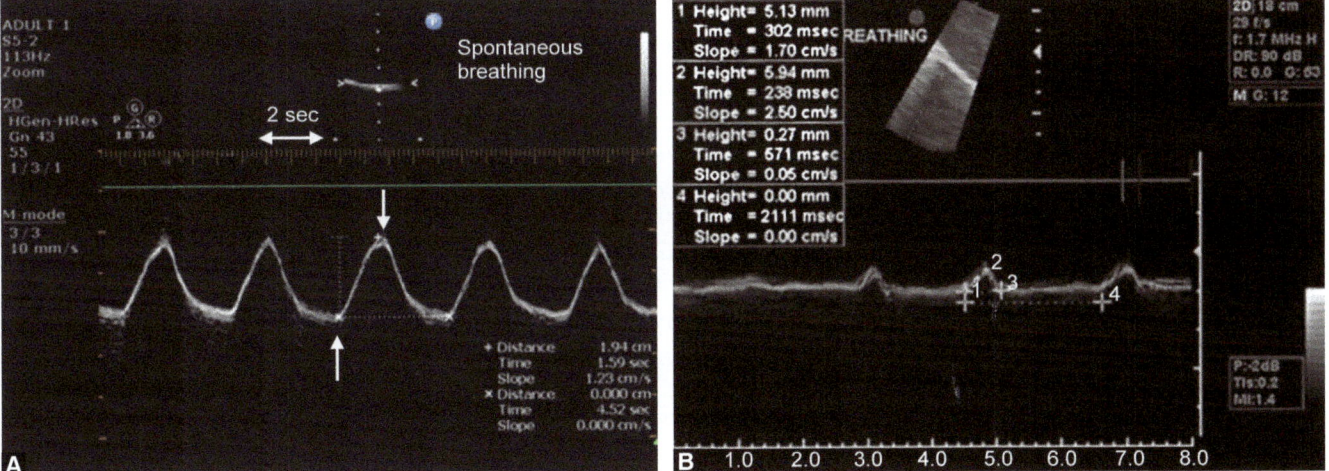

**Figs. 1A and B:** (A) Application of M-mode sonography by using 3.5–5 MHz probe to visualize diaphragmatic excursion (the distance between the two arrows (1.9 cm). (B) The figure revealing decreased excursion (0.5 cm) in a patient with critical illness neuromyopathy.
*Source*: Adapted with permission from Springer Nature. Matamis D, Soilemezi E, Tsagourias M, et al. Sonographic evaluation of the diaphragm in critically ill patients. Technique and clinical applications. Intensive Care Med. 2013;39:801-10.

generated was only about 35% when compared to healthy adults highlights the amount of muscle atrophy that can be there in mechanically ventilated patients. Later study by Jaber S et al. measuring twitch Ptr reduces progressively as the period of mechanical ventilation exists provides strong evidence for VIDD.[37] These techniques help us to diagnose the so-called "hidden difficulties of weaning failure".[12] Predominantly used as research tool, as it has to overcome the noise, costs and other technical difficulties in ICU environment,[36] magnetic resonance techniques still are being used in assessing how much diaphragmatic parameters assessed through ultrasound correlate with phrenic nerve stimulation.[33]

### Esophageal and Gastric Catheter Guided Pleural Pressure Measurement

Esophageal estimate of pleural pressure is renowned technique since 1949 with air-filled latex catheters, fluid-filled catheters or microtransducer catheters.[38] Transdiaphragmatic pressure (Tdi) which is the difference between gastric pressure (Pga) and Pes. Proper positioning of these catheters inserted in esophagus is confirmed by visual estimation of the waveforms (negative deflection of Pes and mirror image of Pga during inspiration) or with "dynamic occlusion test" (Fig. 2).[38] Pes gives an estimate of fraction of airway pressure (Paw) required to overcome lung and chest wall elastance, yielding the assessment of hidden level of patient's muscular activity contribution to ventilator scalars. Relative contribution of diaphragm to inspiration can be assessed through indices like ΔPga/ΔPdi proposed by Gilbert R et al., the higher the value the greater the contribution of diaphragm. The advantage being its nearest accurate to intrapleural pressure through which transpulmonary pressure ($P_L$) can be estimated, PTP of the esophageal pressure (PTPes) estimation and the limitations being its invasiveness, interruptions due to esophagus peristalsis and the availability of catheters are implacable.[39] Despite the presence of abundant evidence with regards to its usefulness in acute respiratory distress syndrome (titration of positive end-expiratory pressure (PEEP), patient-ventilator synchrony and weaning failure (to assess muscle activity), its use in ICU is still less.[38] In fact, the ventilation strategy of the physicians can change if they were to know the Pes and $P_L$ values.[40]

### Neurally adjusted Ventilatory Assist Guided EAdi Measurement

It employs interpretation of electrical activity of the diaphragm (EAdi), through placement of Edi catheter into esophagus, assessing "the neural respiratory drive". For measurement of inspiratory effort, this technique can be promising but requires the placement of a specially designed catheter.[41] The diaphragm electromyography assessed through this catheter measures $EAdi_{peak}$ which gives information regarding the respiratory drive and $EAdi_{AUC}$—the area under the inspiratory portion of the

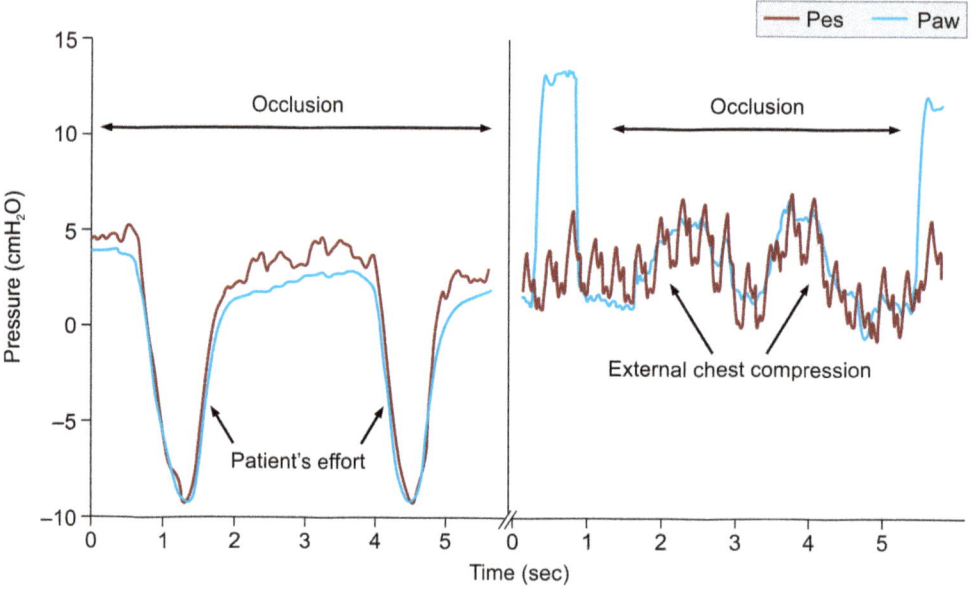

**Fig. 2:** Occlusion test in a spontaneously breathing patient—by occluding the airway during patient effort (left) and in a paralyzed patient—airway occluded while applying external chest compression (right). Airway pressure (red) axis has been shifted to achieve overlap with esophageal pressure (blue).
*Source:* Adapted with permission from American Thoracic Society (Copyright 2017). Akoumianaki E, Maggiore SM, Valenza F, et al. The application of esophageal pressure measurement in patients with respiratory failure. Am J Respir Crit Care Med. 2014;189:520-31.

curve (respiratory muscle endurance). In the study by Muttini S et al., ratio between these two parameters (P/I index) increased in patients with weaning failure.[41] Paw/EAdi ratio gives an estimate of neural inspiratory effort [neuromuscular efficiency (NME)]. Neuroventilatory efficiency is obtained from ratio between Vt and EAdi. These indices have been used to predict extubation success.[42] Although majority of the literature on neurally adjusted ventilatory assist (NAVA) are on synchrony and titration of optimal NAVA level during SBT trials,[43] estimation of diaphragmatic activity as its measurement is an added benefit of NAVA. Disadvantages including proper positioning, interpretation, availability, and costs of course apply here too.

## CONCLUSION

Weaning patients from ventilator require multipronged approach among which assessment of inspiratory effort is one of the important and challenging tasks in mechanically ventilated patients. Among the methods available at bedside measurement of PIF, $P_{01}$ and diaphragm ultrasonography appear promising. Among the invasive methods Pes monitoring and magnetic stimulation appear and can be used to compare and correlate the above methods. NAVA mode paves the way for future to assist in weaning through its continuous assessment of neuromechanical efficiency and neuroventilatory efficiency.

## SALIENT POINTS

- Weaning failure in critically ill mechanically ventilated patients increases the ICU length of stay, consuming ICU resources, thereby increasing morbidity and mortality.
- Inspiration, an active respiratory process, respiratory muscle endurance (skeletal muscle performance over a period of time), along with good expiratory effort forms the key to successful liberation from mechanical ventilator, apart from correction of underlying pathophysiology of the patient.
- Weaning patients from ventilator require multipronged approach among which assessment of inspiratory effort is one of the important and challenging tasks in mechanically ventilated patients.
- Assessment of inspiratory effort in mechanically ventilated patients is key to titrate the ventilator assistance required and prevent complications like muscle atrophy or patient ventilator asynchrony.
- Inspiratory effort can be assessed through noninvasive methods like measurement of PImax or MIP, negative pressure during first 100 ms of occlusion ($P_{01}$), FT, PT and ultrasonography of the diaphragm measuring excursion and zone of apposition.
- Inspiratory effort can be assessed through invasive methods like electromagnetic stimulation, esophageal and gastric catheter guided pleural pressure measurement and NAVA guided EAdi measurement.
- Neurally adjusted ventilatory assist mode paves the way for future to assist in weaning through its continuous assessment of neuromechanical efficiency and neuroventilatory efficiency.

## REFERENCES

1. Epstein SK. Weaning from ventilatory support. Curr Opin Crit Care 2009;15(1):36-43.
2. Boles J, Bion J, Connors A, et al. Weaning from mechanical ventilation. Eur Respir J. 2007;29:1033-56.
3. Esteban A, Frutos F, Tobin MJ, et al. A comparison of four methods of weaning patients from mechanical ventilation. Spanish Lung Failure Collaborative Group. N Engl J Med. 1995;332:345-50.
4. Brochard L, Rauss A, Benito S, et al. Comparison of three methods of gradual withdrawal from ventilatory during weaning from mechanical ventilation. Am J Respir Crit Care Med. 1994;150:896-903.
5. MacIntyre NR, Epstein SK, Carson S, et al. Management of patients requiring prolonged mechanical ventilation: report of a NAMDRC consensus conference. Chest. 2005;128:3937-54.
6. Esteban A, Anzueto A, Frutos F, et al. Characteristics and outcomes in adult patients receiving mechanical ventilation: a 28-day international study. JAMA. 2002;287:345-55.
7. Epstein SK, Nevins ML, Chung J. Effect of unplanned extubation on outcome of mechanical ventilation. Am J Respir Crit Care Med. 2000;161:1912-6.
8. Rothaar RC, Epstein SK. Extubation failure: magnitude of the problem, impact on outcomes, and prevention. Curr Opin Crit Care. 2003;9:59-66.
9. Scheinhorn DJ, Chao DC, Stearn-Hassenpflug M, et al. Outcomes in post-ICU mechanical ventilation: a therapist-implemented weaning protocol. Chest. 2001;119:236-42.
10. Caruso P, Albuquerque AL, Santana PV, et al. Diagnostic methods to assess inspiratory and expiratory muscle strength. J Bras Pneumol. 2015;41:110-23.
11. Jiang C, Esquinas A, Mina B. Evaluation of cough peak expiratory flow as a predictor of successful mechanical ventilation discontinuation: a narrative review of the literature. J Intensive Care. 2017;5:33.
12. Perren A, Brochard L. Managing the apparent and hidden difficulties of weaning from mechanical ventilation. Intensive Care Med. 2013;39:1885-95.

13. Levine S, Nguyen T, Taylor N, et al. Rapid disuse atrophy of diaphragm fibers in mechanically ventilated humans. N Engl J Med. 2008;358:1327-35.
14. Iotti GA, Braschi A, Brunner JX, et al. Respiratory mechanics by least squares fitting in mechanically ventilated patients: applications during paralysis and during pressure support ventilation. Intensive Care Med. 1995;21:406-13.
15. Konyukov YA, Kuwayama N, Fukuoka T, et al. Effects of different triggering systems and external PEEP on trigger capability of the ventilator. Intensive Care Med. 1996;22:363-8.
16. Laghi F. Assessment of respiratory output in mechanically ventilated patients. Respir Care Clin N Am. 2005;11:173-99.
17. Foti G, Cereda M, Banfi G, et al. End-inspiratory airway occlusion: a method to assess the pressure developed by inspiratory muscles in patients with acute lung injury undergoing pressure support. Am J Respir Crit Care. 1997;156(41):1210-6.
18. Marini JJ, Smith TC, Lamb V. Estimation of inspiratory muscle strength in mechanically ventilated patients: the measurement of maximal inspiratory pressure. J Crit Care. 1986;1:32-8.
19. Caruso P, Friedrich C, Denari SD, et al. The unidirectional valve is the best method to determine maximal inspiratory pressure during weaning. Chest. 1999;115:1096-101.
20. de Souza LC, Guimaraes FS, Lugon JR. The timed inspiratory effort: a promising index of mechanical ventilation weaning for patients with neurologic or neuromuscular diseases. Respir Care. 2015;60:231-8.
21. de Souza LC, Lugon JR, Guimaraes FS. Evaluation of a new index of mechanical ventilation weaning: the timed inspiratory effort. J Intensive Care Med. 2015;30:37-43.
22. Loring SH, Malhotra A. Inspiratory efforts during mechanical ventilation. Chest. 2007;131:646-8.
23. Conti G, Antonelli M, Arzano S, et al. Equipment review: measurement of occlusion pressures in critically ill patients. Crit Care. 1997;1(3):89-93.
24. Whitelaw WA, Derenne JP, Milic-Emili J. Occlusion pressure as a measure of respiratory center output in conscious man. Respir Physiol. 1975;23:181-99.
25. Taylor R, Marini JJ, Smith T, et al. Bedside estimation of respiratory drive during machine-assisted ventilation. Am Rev Respir Dis. 1987;135:A51.
26. Truwit JD, Marini JJ. Validation of a technique to assess maximal inspiratory pressure in poorly cooperative patients. Chest. 1992;102:1216-9.
27. Fernández R, Cabrera J, Calaf N, et al. P 0.1/PIMax: an index for assessing respiratory capacity in acute respiratory failure. Intensive Care Med. 1990;16:175-9.
28. Ou CY, Yang SC, Chen CW. Influence of different flow-triggering levels on the breathing effort of mechanically ventilated patients. Minerva Anestesiol. 2012;78:996-1004.
29. Moodie L, Reeve J, Elkins M. Inspiratory muscle training increases inspiratory muscle strength in patients weaning from mechanical ventilation: a systematic review. J Physiother. 2011;57:213-20.
30. Matamis D, Soilemezi E, Tsagourias M, et al. Sonographic evaluation of the diaphragm in critically ill patients. Technique and clinical applications. Intensive Care Med. 2013;39:801-10.
31. Kim WY, Suh HJ, Hong SB, et al. Diaphragm dysfunction assessed by ultrasonography: influence on weaning from mechanical ventilation. Crit Care Med. 2011;39:2627-30.
32. Vivier E, Mekontso Dessap A, Dimassi S, et al. Diaphragm ultrasonography to estimate the work of breathing during non-invasive ventilation. Intensive Care Med. 2012;38:796-803.
33. Dubé BP, Dres M, Mayaux J, et al. Ultrasound evaluation of diaphragm function in mechanically ventilated patients: comparison to phrenic stimulation and prognostic implications. Thorax. 2017;72(9):811-8.
34. Cattapan SE, Laghi F, Tobin MJ. Can diaphragmatic contractility be assessed by airway twitch pressure in mechanically ventilated patients? Thorax. 2003;58:58-62.
35. Wragg S, Aquilina R, Moran J, et al. Comparison of cervical magnetic stimulation and bilateral percutaneous electrical stimulation of the phrenic nerves in normal subjects. Eur Respir J. 1994;7:1788-92.
36. Watson AC, Hughes PD, Louise Harris M, et al. Measurement of twitch transdiaphragmatic, esophageal, and endotracheal tube pressure with bilateral anterolateral magnetic phrenic nerve stimulation in patients in the intensive care unit. Crit Care Med. 2001;29:1325-31.
37. Jaber S, Petrof BJ, Jung B, et al. Rapidly progressive diaphragmatic weakness and injury during mechanical ventilation in humans. Am J Respir Crit Care Med. 2011;183:364-71.
38. Akoumianaki E, Maggiore SM, Valenza F, et al. The application of esophageal pressure measurement in patients with respiratory failure. Am J Respir Crit Care Med. 2014;189:520-31.
39. Laporta D, Grassino A. Assessment of transdiaphragmatic pressure in humans. J Appl Physiol. 1985;58:1469-76.
40. Oppersma E, Hatam N, Doorduin J, et al. Functional assessment of the diaphragm by speckle tracking ultrasound during inspiratory loading. J Appl Physiol. 2017;123(5):1063-70.
41. Muttini S, Villani PG, Trimarco R, et al. Relation between peak and integral of the diaphragm electromyographic activity at different levels of support during weaning from mechanical ventilation: a physiologic study. J Crit Care. 2015;30:7-12.
42. Liu HG, Liu L, Tang R, et al. A pilot study of diaphragmatic function evaluated as predictors of weaning in chronic obstructive pulmonary disease patients. Zhonghua Nei Ke Za Zhi. 2011;50:459-64.
43. Rozé H, Lafrikh A, Perrier V, et al. Daily titration of neurally adjusted ventilatory assist using the diaphragm electrical activity. Intensive Care Med. 2011;37:1087-94.

# CHAPTER 15

# Ventilator-induced Lung Injury

*Renata de Souza Mendes, Pedro Leme Silva, Paolo Pelosi, Patricia RM Rocco*

## INTRODUCTION

The main objectives of mechanical ventilation are to reduce the workload of the respiratory muscles and maintain satisfactory blood gas exchange while lung function or level of consciousness are restored after acute organ dysfunction or surgery.[1] Despite the benefits of mechanical ventilation in many clinical situations, it can cause pulmonary structural damage[1] and hemodynamic instability.[2] It is not unusual for death to occur after the initiation of mechanical ventilation despite satisfactory blood gas exchange. This is in line with a series of deleterious effects of mechanical ventilation, including increases in inflammatory infiltration and vascular permeability, hyaline membrane formation, and pulmonary edema. This constellation of features is called ventilator-induced lung injury (VILI).[3]

During positive mechanical ventilation, the interaction of several mechanical forces acting on the pulmonary structures leads to cell sensitization, prompting biochemical and biomolecular alterations which ultimately lead to VILI.[4] If the mechanical stimulus exceeds what the lung tissues can support, injury to pulmonary structures occurs. These nonphysiological lung tissue stretches can lead to biological events that foster release of inflammatory mediators, alterations in gene expression, and upregulation or downregulation of synthesis of several extracellular matrix molecules.[5,6]

So-called protective ventilation strategies have been shown to minimize VILI and modify mortality rates in some clinical settings, such as the acute respiratory distress syndrome (ARDS).[7] Therefore, understanding the physiological and biological consequences of mechanical ventilation and being familiar with clinical strategies in order to prevent and minimize lung damage is an important issue in critically ill patients.

## SPONTANEOUS BREATHING: HOW DOES IT WORK?

Spontaneous breathing (i.e. under normal conditions and in the upright position) consists of air exchange between the atmosphere and alveoli through the action of the respiratory muscles. This transfer occurs en bloc from a high-pressure into a low-pressure region, as shown in Figure 1. During spontaneous breathing, air moves into and out of the respiratory system with fluctuations in transrespiratory pressure ($P_{TR}$). The alveolar pressure ($P_{alv}$) is alternately less than or greater than atmospheric pressure ($P_{atm}$). Periodically, since $P_{alv}$ is lower than $P_{atm}$, the airflow direction is inward (inspiration), whereas when $P_{alv}$ is higher than $P_{atm}$, outward airflow (expiration) occurs.

$$P_{TR} = P_{alv} - P_{atm} \qquad (Eq.\ 1)$$

For educational purposes, the respiratory system can be divided into two compartments—the lungs and the chest wall. The latter represents the thoracic and abdominal structures that move as a result of respiratory muscle contractions. Therefore, the transthoracic pressure ($P_{CW}$) in this compartment is directly related to pleural pressure ($P_{pl}$) and $P_{atm}$. Under passive conditions, since $P_{pl}$ is negative, the $P_{CW}$ (which represents the expanding force) is also negative. During inspiration, as $P_{pl}$ becomes even more negative, the expanding force increases, leading to thoracic cavity expansion and an increase in lung volume. During expiration, the chest wall relaxes and moves toward its elastic equilibrium:

$$P_{CW} = P_{pl} - P_{atm} \qquad (Eq.\ 2)$$

$P_{alv}$ is ultimately altered by the contraction or relaxation of the thoracic respiratory muscles, which increases or decreases lung volume, respectively. The lungs behave as elastic structures, and the volume depends both on transpulmonary pressure ($P_L$) and on inherent lung

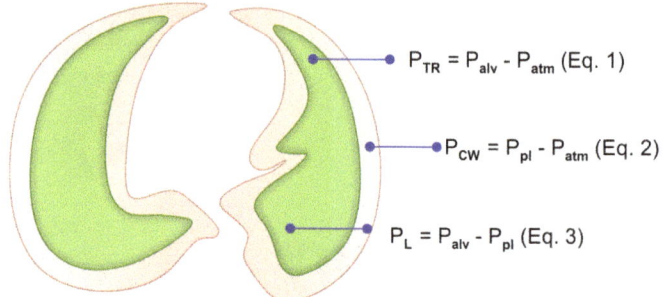

**Fig. 1:** Schematic drawing showing the transrespiratory ($P_{TR}$), transthoracic ($P_{CW}$), and transpulmonary ($P_L$) pressures during spontaneous breathing. According to fluctuations in $P_L$, alveolar pressure ($P_{alv}$) is alternately less (inspiratory) and greater (expiration) than atmospheric pressure ($P_{atm}$). Under passive conditions, since pleural pressure ($P_{pl}$) is negative, the $P_{CW}$ is also negative, which represents the expanding force. During inspiration, as $P_{pl}$ becomes even more negative, the expanding force is greater, which results in chest-wall expansion and increased lung volume. As the chest wall expands due to respiratory muscle contraction, $P_{pl}$ decreases, while $P_L$ becomes more positive. During normal expiration, the respiratory muscles relax, and the elastic recoil of the lungs drives passive expiration.

compliance. During inspiration, the respiratory muscles contract, and as the chest wall expands, $P_{pl}$ decreases, while $P_L$ becomes more positive.

$$P_L = P_{alv} - P_{pl} \qquad (Eq.\ 3)$$

During normal expiration, there is a gradual relaxation of the respiratory muscles, and, through the elastic property of the lungs, expiration occurs toward functional residual capacity (FRC). At FRC, the respiratory system is in elastic equilibrium. When airflow becomes zero, the main force that maintains lung inflation is $P_{TP}$. Therefore, it is clear that the lung volume and transpulmonary pressure are interrelated.

## PATHOPHYSIOLOGY OF VILI: STRESS, STRAIN, AND STRESS RAISERS

Three main mechanisms compete toward lung injury in mechanical ventilation. They are—(1) overdistension due to high tidal volume ($V_T$) or airway pressure ($P_{aw}$), causing volutrauma and barotrauma, respectively; (2) recruitment and derecruitment of alveolar units within every breath, leading to dynamic strain; and (3) concentration of stress between adjacent walls shared by open and closed alveoli due to collapse or edema.[8,9] These mechanical injuries may lead to a secondary inflammation cascade called biotrauma, which is characterized by decompartmentalization of inflammatory markers formerly located in the alveolar space, which can then translocate into the adjacent bloodstream, ultimately resulting in distal organ injury.[6]

Nowadays, the role of alveolar overdistension as a primary mechanism of VILI is questioned because many studies, from cell cultures understretch[10] to large-animal models,[11] have shown that not only alveolar overdistension *per se* but also dynamic alveolar amplitude facilitate VILI development. A landmark paper showed that $V_T$ or $P_{aw}$ high enough to cause overdistension did not lead to lung damage if positive end-expiratory pressure (PEEP) was applied.[12] Interestingly, this experimental design was replicated focusing on right ventricle function and demonstrated dysfunction after injurious ventilation.[13]

Strain and stress describe local deformations and the tension generated by a given force acting on a body, and they can be used to discriminate between the forces acting on the lungs during mechanical ventilation.[4] Strain defines the displacement (or tidal volume) divided by the basal distortion (or end-expiratory lung volume).[11] On the other hand, stress, in respiratory physiology, is directly inferred as the change in transpulmonary pressure. In this line, meta-analyses of clinical studies have shown that high levels of airway driving pressure, which represent the normalization of $V_T$ by the respiratory system compliance, are associated with mortality in ARDS.[14]

Adjustment of mechanical ventilation to stabilize the pulmonary parenchyma during expiration is crucial to reduce alveolar recruitment/derecruitment and thereby reduce lung injury. Many studies have shown that preventing dynamic strain by restricting thoracic movement does not cause VILI in small animals.[12,15]

Harmful thresholds of nonphysiological strain and stress have been studied in healthy pigs. VILI was found to occur when the strain was greater than 1.5–2.[11] Protti et al. compared ventilatory strategies with the same overall strain of 2.5, but varying the dynamic components of the strategies. They found that the presence of pulmonary edema depended not only on overall strain, but also on its dynamic components.[16] A combination of low levels of dynamic strain and high levels of static strain was associated with lower mortality, better pulmonary mechanics, better oxygenation, less histological damage, and less inflammation.[16] Thus, the authors suggested that the dynamic stress caused by recruitment/derecruitment rather than alveolar overdistension itself would be the primary trigger of VILI. This is in contrast to observations made by our group, in which volutrauma was found to increase inflammatory mediators compared to atelectrauma at comparably low $V_T$ and lower driving pressure. This suggests that static stress and strain represent the most important components leading to VILI.[17]

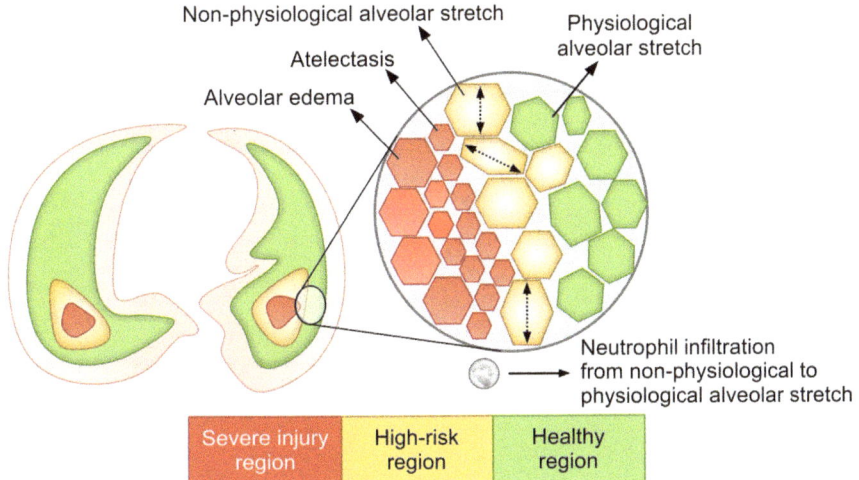

**Fig. 2:** Mechanism of stress raisers. Local atelectatic or edema-filled alveolar units (severe injury region, red) can act as a stress concentrator, generating structural alveolar injury, and inflammation in surrounding tissues at risk of injury (yellow). The lung area at risk may spread toward the healthy region (green). Atelectatic or edema-filled alveolar units acting as a stress concentrator may also induce neutrophil migration from nonphysiological to physiological alveolar stretch.

One mediator that has been recently associated with VILI is the formation of stress raisers.[18] These are formed by the expansion of heterogeneous pulmonary parenchyma, as open alveoli share the same wall of surrounding collapsed areas due to lung interdependence. This, in turn, can amplify alveolar wall distension, which is proportional to alveolar heterogeneities or inhomogeneities.[8] Interestingly, areas of heterogeneity or inhomogeneity correlate positively with severity and, thus, mortality in patients with ARDS.[8] A specific region of atelectasis accumulates stress, which, in turn, can lead to alveolar damage and inflammation (neutrophilic infiltration in the peri-atelectatic and edematous areas) in the surrounding lung tissue (Fig. 2).[8,9]

Mechanical ventilation can amplify stress raisers in the lung, which is consistent with a loss of surfactant function and increase in surface tension.[19] Over time, the monotonous regularity of $V_T$ may favor this pathologic mechanism by limiting surfactant release by type II alveolar epithelial cells.[20] This is observed during low $V_T$ with inadequate PEEP levels, which can cause overall lung volume reduction, and may lead to heterogeneous alveolar ventilation, stress raisers, and excessive local strain.[21]

## PRINCIPLES OF MECHANICAL VENTILATION AND POTENTIAL MECHANISMS OF INJURY

Positive-pressure mechanical ventilation has no similarity with the spontaneous breathing process observed in humans. During quiet spontaneous breathing, it is expected that healthy humans will vary their own breathing pattern by increasing the amplitude and time expended at inspiration or expiration,[22] and that respiratory rate (RR) will fluctuate as necessary. On the other hand, positive-pressure mechanical ventilation adjustments rely on $V_T$, PEEP, RR, fraction of inspired oxygen ($FiO_2$), and inspiratory airway flow (V'). Depending on how these variables are adjusted, they may trigger or facilitate damage to lung tissue. Clinically, it is difficult to establish the onset or degree of injury induced or aggravated by the ventilatory strategy.

In healthy lung tissue, the $P_L$ increment generated by the contraction of the respiratory muscles is transmitted throughout the alveolar surface, admitting the lung as a pure elastic system.[23] In diseased lung tissue, it has been observed that the driving pressure generated by diaphragm contraction increases lung volume in dependent areas and reduces it in the nondependent areas. Since no gain in $V_T$ was observed during this time frame, this phenomenon reflects the *pendelluft*.[24] In the injured lung, *pendelluft* occurs more often with a more negative $P_{pl}$ and it is proportional to the degree of spontaneous effort during positive-pressure mechanical ventilation. Modest inspiratory efforts can recruit the areas of collapse,[24] but excess efforts can lead to local overstretch (due to higher transpulmonary pressure) and *pendelluft*.[24,25]

The mechanisms associated with VILI may be exacerbated if mechanical breath variables are improperly adjusted (Fig. 3). In order to prevent VILI, the shortest possible duration of mechanical ventilation should be

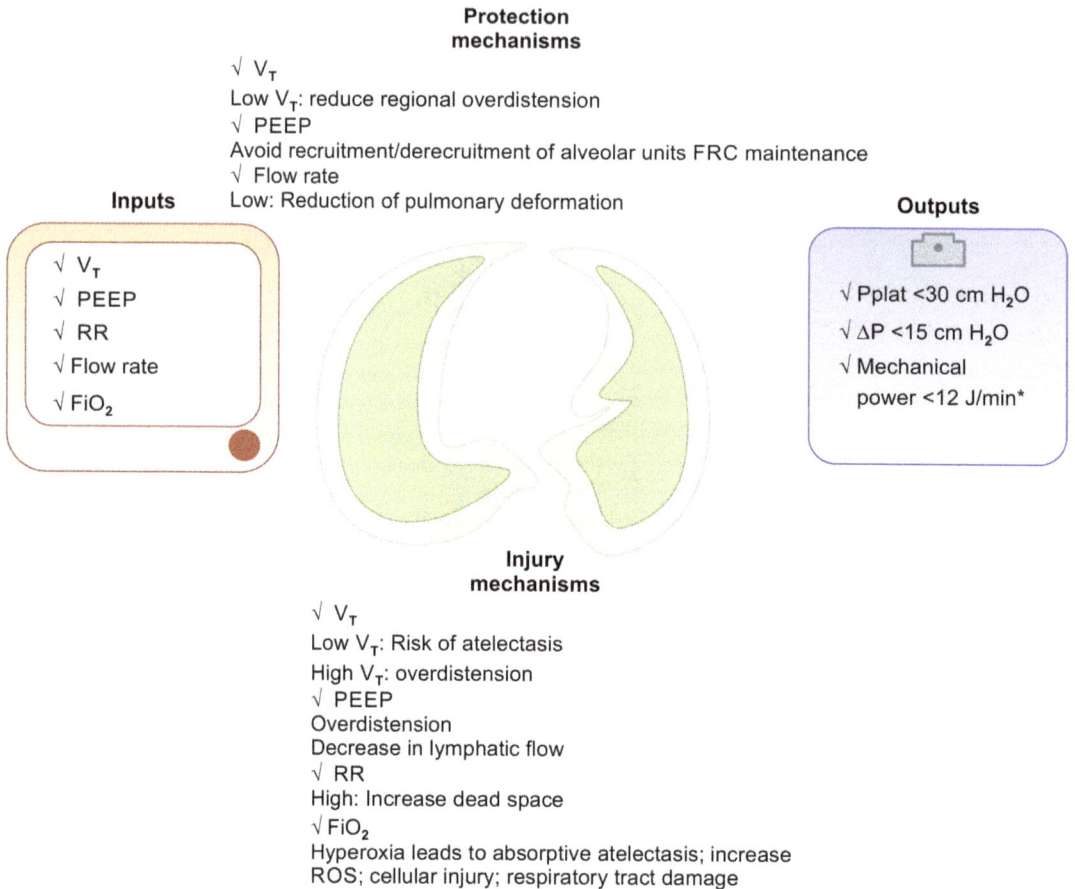

**Fig. 3:** Mechanical ventilator settings (inputs) and readouts (outputs) that can be gathered and monitored. Proposed protective mechanisms are shown for each input. $V_T$: tidal volume; PEEP: positive end-expiratory pressure; $FiO_2$: fraction of inspired oxygen; FRC: functional residual capacity; RR: respiratory rate; Pplat: plateau pressure; ΔP: driving pressure; ROS: reactive oxygen species. *Power threshold associated with lung damage in experimental models.

advocated.[1,26] Thus, constant global monitoring should be in place to determine whether mechanical ventilation is still actually required.

## Inputs

### *Tidal Volume ($V_T$)*

Tidal volume is adjusted during positive-pressure ventilation and most studies adjust it according to predicted body weight in an attempt to standardize $V_T$ to the expected anatomical size of the lungs. However, in disease states such as ARDS, the area of the lung able to ventilate is reduced, which is consistent with the reduction in respiratory system compliance.

In surgical patients, the use of a small $V_T$ with 5 cm $H_2O$ of PEEP or higher and a plateau pressure lower than 30 cm $H_2O$ was associated with better outcomes (lower mortality, shorter period of mechanical ventilation, reduced hospital stay, and less lung damage) when compared to high volumes (>10 mL/kg).[27,28] As previously noted, regional lung overdistension is an important driver of VILI development. Unfortunately, these local asymmetric overdistensions are difficult to recognize at the bedside. Nevertheless, once recognized, $V_T$ limits should be clearly instituted in order to prevent overdistension,[1] despite the negative consequences of this strategy, which include hypercapnia.[29] However, even after setting a low $V_T$, there is a risk of promoting recruitment and derecruitment of alveolar units, especially if the end-expiratory pressure is inadequately low. Therefore, lung damage is a composite of features known as atelectrauma, which consists of alveolar collapse, edema, and hyaline membrane formation.[19] Atelectrauma is more exuberant in asymmetric lung areas, as demonstrated by the force required to open alveolar units at the edges of atelectatic regions, which can be four to five times greater than in healthy lung areas.[30]

Protective ventilation set at low $V_T$ ($V_T$ range lower than 7 mL/kg predicted body weight) was also beneficial in the intensive care unit (ICU) population without lung injury. Patients ventilated with a low $V_T$ strategy have shown fewer pulmonary complications and, consequently, shorter ICU and hospital stay, as well as lower hospital mortality.[31] Therefore, gentle ventilation of aerated lungs while keeping them moderately collapsed may produce less lung damage.[32]

### Positive End-expiratory Pressure

During general anesthesia, the lung volume reduces, which may predispose to alveolar collapse. In this scenario, PEEP application may prevent alveolar collapse at end-expiration, since the presence of the orotracheal tube means that airway sealing by the glottis and the cough mechanism are nonfunctional during mechanical ventilation.[33] Furthermore, PEEP can prevent opening and closing of alveolar units, which can cause atelectrauma.[34]

Many mechanisms involved in the prevention of VILI have been attributed to PEEP—(1) prevention of atelectrauma;[35] (2) counterbalancing the increased lung mass resulting from edema, inflammation, and maintenance of normal FRC;[35] (3) increased lymphatic flow, which drains lung edema toward thoracic lymph ducts;[36] and (4) alveolar stabilization, preventing generation of stress raisers.[19]

In the landmark PROVHILO trial, patients undergoing abdominal surgery were divided into two groups, which received a similar $V_T$ level (8 mL/kg) but either low PEEP (2 cm $H_2O$) without recruitment maneuvers or high PEEP (12 cm $H_2O$) with recruitment maneuvers. The authors found no difference between groups regarding the primary outcome (postoperative pulmonary complications). They also showed that those patients exposed to high PEEP with recruitment maneuvers experienced more episodes of hypotension and required higher doses of vasopressors.[37]

Animal studies of ARDS demonstrated the need for a higher PEEP to ensure protective ventilation and minimize VILI. These studies raised the concept of "opening the lung" through recruitment maneuvers and "keeping it open" and avoiding atelectasis by maintaining alveolar recruitment.[12,38] It has been shown that, in the most severe cases of ARDS, high PEEP levels are associated with better clinical outcomes, such as lower mortality, shorter mechanical ventilation time, and shorter ICU stay.[39] However, considering all patients with ARDS, over the entire spectrum of severity, evidence from randomized trials and meta-analyses suggest absence of any mortality benefit associated with high PEEP levels (>15 cm $H_2O$) compared with low PEEP levels (5–15 cm $H_2O$).[40,41] A clinical study that compared lung recruitment and PEEP titration versus low PEEP strategy in patients with moderate-to-severe ARDS showed increased 28-day all-cause mortality in the recruitment group.[42]

Sahetya and Brower argue that the incongruity between experimental and clinical results in relation to recruitment maneuvers in ARDS patients can occur because their application may be beneficial for the lung, but not necessarily for the patient as a whole. This may be due to its hemodynamic repercussions (increased intracardiac pressures, reduced venous return, and cardiac output) or to the aggressive recruitment maneuver strategies used, which may influence clinical outcomes negatively.[32] Sahetya and Brower also suggest that a strategy of permissive atelectasis with lung resting may be best for the patient.[32]

Currently, the bedside use of thoracic electrical impedance tomography can help guide breath-by-breath adjustment of regional ventilation, including the decision to implement alveolar recruitment maneuvers, as well as monitor for alveolar collapse and hyperinflation in ICU patients[43-45] or support permissive atelectasis. However, additional studies are warranted in order to evaluate the impact of this technology on clinical outcomes.

### Respiratory Rate

Respiratory rate is also set at the mechanical ventilator to keep an adequate minute volume proportional to the patient's metabolic demands. On the one hand, in order to maintain $CO_2$ levels within safe range, RR should be set to a higher level;[7] on the other hand, this can alter the ratio of inspiration to expiration, which can raise the concern of intrinsic PEEP due to short expiratory time.

Acute respiratory distress syndrome patients usually have high levels of dead space, and the most common and easy approach to reverse this is to increase RR. This practice of increasing RR to decrease $CO_2$ levels has been tested in mechanically ventilated ARDS patients. Vieillard-Baron, et al. compared two levels of RR (15 bpm versus 30 bpm) under low plateau pressures (<25 cm $H_2O$) between them. $PaCO_2$ was similar between groups. Interestingly, dead space increased in the 30 bpm group, but not in the 15 bpm group, which is consistent with auto-PEEP due to a reduction in expiratory period, leading to worse right ventricular function.[46]

Increased RR can cause lung injury similar to the atelectrauma mechanism.[47] This can be explained by the number of stress and strain cycles generated into the lung to induce VILI.[48] Thus, RR reduction may prevent VILI.[48]

## Inspiratory Flow Rate

Inspiratory flow can also be adjusted during artificial ventilation, which is an additional potential cause of lung damage.[49,50] High inspiratory flow rates can lead to VILI due to local stress accumulation.[51] The mechanism whereby inspiratory flow contributes to VILI may be influenced by viscoelastic tissue properties. High inspiratory flow can cause lung damage due to viscoelastic accommodation, as there will be no time to dissipate forces when inflation occurs very rapidly. This usually occurs in diseases in which the lungs are affected asymmetrically. It has been shown that different inspiratory flows at comparable $V_T$ levels can modify alveolar surface tension.[52] High inspiratory flow can lead to substantial deformation of the pulmonary parenchyma and of the bronchial epithelial cells,[52] and may predispose to release interleukin 8 (IL-8) and activate mitogen-activated protein kinase, even at mild lung deformation. Additionally, even in healthy animals, high inspiratory flow rates have been shown to alter the respiratory system mechanics and increase the expression of procollagen type III (PCIII).[52] Therefore, controlling inspiratory flow might provide additional lung protection.[53]

## Fraction of Inspired Oxygen

Oxygen supplementation is necessary for all mechanically ventilated patients. However, it is important to remember that hyperoxia leads to histological changes in the lung similar to those induced by ARDS.[54]

Hyperoxia appears to damage lung cells by increasing production of reactive oxygen species (ROS) such as the superoxide anion, hydroxyl radical, and hydrogen peroxide.[55,56] Along with an increase in ROS production and depletion of host antioxidant defenses, intracellular molecules can mount a response that ultimately leads to cell death.[56] Furthermore, ROS can trigger the inflammatory cascade, leading to secondary cellular injury and apoptosis.[57,58]

Hyperoxia also influences the respiratory tract by increasing susceptibility to mucus plugging, atelectasis, and secondary infection, as it impairs mucociliary motion capacity and blunts the bactericidal capacity of immune defense cells.[59,60]

High $FiO_2$ leads to a replacement of nitrogen by oxygen, which can result in alveolar closure (atelectasis) once oxygen is absorbed.[61] Thus, it is important to titrate $FiO_2$ according to arterial oxygen saturation more than 90% or a $PaO_2$ of 60–65 mm Hg, in order to avoid this damage.[62]

## Outputs: Monitoring of Mechanical Ventilation Parameters to Minimize VILI

Respiratory system plateau pressure (Pplat), driving pressure (ΔP), and, more recently, mechanical energy and power have been associated with VILI (Fig. 3). These mechanical ventilation parameters are implicated in both volutrauma and atelectrauma, two mechanisms of mechanical lung injury that can lead to biotrauma. Therefore, Pplat, ΔP, energy, and power should be monitored to prevent VILI progression in critically ill patients.

### Plateau Pressure (Pplat)

Pplat is measured during the inspiratory pause (3–5 seconds) on the ventilator, while the respiratory muscles are relaxed. It denotes the elastic recoil of the respiratory system, and once it is achieved, the $P_{alv}$ is equilibrated throughout the respiratory system. Accordingly, low Pplat values are associated with less alveolar distension.[63] Optimal Pplat values have not been determined clearly in patients without ARDS. Nevertheless, in patients with ARDS, although there is no absolute threshold, previous studies have shown that a Pplat less than 30 cm $H_2O$ is associated with lower mortality.[7] Interestingly, it has been shown that Pplat less than 28 cm $H_2O$ may be more beneficial in those ARDS patients with a large nonaerated portion of the lungs.[64] However, some patients may develop dynamic hyperinflation even with low $V_T$ (6 mL/kg) and Pplat (<30 cm $H_2O$).[64] Therefore, Pplat may not reflect a reliable safe threshold in regards to the development of VILI, but rather a continuous variable that should be kept as low as possible.

### Driving Pressure (ΔP)

The protective ventilation strategy composed of low $V_T$ and adequate PEEP levels has been associated with positive clinical outcomes in critically ill patients. However, many patients ventilated with these parameters are exposed to supraphysiological forces that may induce or compound lung damage.[64,65]

Amato et al. pointed out that respiratory system compliance measurement is linked to the surface area that remains functional (i.e. able to be ventilated) during lung disease. Normalizing the $V_T$ to respiratory system compliance instead of predicted body weight gives the driving pressure. The authors found that ΔP best stratified risk of mortality in ARDS patients.[14]

The ARDSnet study found that ΔP more than 15 cm $H_2O$ was associated with poor outcomes in ARDS patients,[14] while other variables commonly associated with mortality, such as $V_T$, Pplat, and PEEP, did not correlate with increased mortality. Increasing PEEP will lead to different effects on ΔP, depending on how the lung is injured. ΔP reduces if high PEEP levels lead to lung recruitment. However, if no recruitment happens after increasing PEEP, lung tissues will become overinflated and the ΔP will not change, or may even increase. ΔP represents an important parameter to adequately adjust mechanical ventilation in both uninjured[66] and injured[67] lungs. Similar inferences can be made in intraoperative settings.[68] Furthermore, high ΔP levels have been associated with postoperative pulmonary complications when lung-protective mechanical ventilation strategies were not applied.[68,69]

### Transpulmonary Pressure ($P_L$)

As previously discussed, transpulmonary pressure ($P_L$) is the difference between the airway and pleural pressures. The importance of $P_L$ is to divide the pressure acting on the lungs from that acting on the chest wall or abdomen. In clinical practice, the variation in pleural pressure corresponds to variation in esophageal pressure ($P_{eso}$), as measured by esophageal balloon manometry. The measurement of $P_L$ has been proposed because—(1) it expresses the contribution of the chest wall to the airway pressure; (2) it can determine the pressure threshold to maintain the lung open;[70] (3) it can assess patient effort and, as consequently, the $P_L$ generated during partial ventilatory support.[71] Many clinical conditions can change the chest wall mechanics, which, in turn, increases pleural pressure.[72] The transpulmonary driving pressure ($ΔP_L$) is defined as the difference between $P_L$ at end-inspiration ($P_{Lend-insp}$) and $P_L$ at end-expiration ($P_{Lend-exp}$). $ΔP_L$ measurements have some advantages: (1) $ΔP_L$ removes the stress caused by PEEP, which does not necessarily contribute to lung injury and sometimes can mitigate it;[16] (2) $ΔP_L$ eliminates the distending pressure used to move the chest wall observed in respiratory-system ΔP. Hence, it seems that $ΔP_L$ could be a better indicative of VILI risk and may even be a better predictor of clinical outcomes than $ΔP$.[73] $ΔP_L$ is calculated as:

$$ΔP_L = (P_{Plat} - P_{ESO, end-insp}) - (PEEP_{TOT} - P_{ESO, end-exp}) \quad (Eq.\ 4)$$

### The Concept of Energy

As discussed above, $V_T$ and Pplat are associated with the development of VILI. $V_T$ can influence pulmonary tissue strain, while Pplat influences respiratory-system stress.[74] In addition to strain and stress, factors such as respiratory rate and inspiratory flow may contribute to VILI, and have been underappreciated within the actual mechanical ventilation scenario compared to $V_T$, ΔP or Pplat.[75-77] To minimize VILI, high $V_T$ and/or Pplat should be avoided; however, the role of "mechanical energy" (i.e. mechanical transfer from the ventilator to the lung structures) is uncertain.[48] Taken together, all of these factors generate the mechanical energy applied to the respiratory system during a single breath cycle. The energy per tidal cycle (airways + lung) is defined as the total area between the inspiratory limb of $ΔP_L$ (x) versus the volume axis (y), measured in Joules (J). In order to compute the actual energy transfer toward the lungs, some components should be subtracted, such as—(1) the chest wall; (2) the endotracheal tube and tracheobronchial tree; and (3) the energy recovered at the mouth.

### Mechanical Power and Intensity

The frequency with which mechanical energy is applied to the lungs is called mechanical power. In a recent study,[48] several mechanical power data ranges were applied to the respiratory system. This was done by decreasing and/or increasing the RR and maintaining the $V_T$ and $P_L$ constant, which made it possible to identify a power threshold for VILI. The study showed that widespread edema developed only when the mechanical power exceeded 12 J/min in healthy pigs. In a lung injury scenario, lung collapse results in a reduction of the lung surface area able to be ventilated, this requires more airway pressure and airflow. In this scenario, mechanical power will increase without significant changes in $V_T$. This problematic cycle might explain the increase in lung damage as the mechanical power is amplified. A better understanding of mechanical power and related factors, such as temperature, flow, and RR, will further advance our understanding of VILI.

The so-called intensity (i.e. mechanical power normalized to the lung tissue able to be ventilated) should also be measured. Intensity may be similar between volutrauma and opening/closing of alveolar units depending on the mechanical power.[78] If power increases with no important changes in lung surface area, the intensity will be higher. On the other hand, if both power and lung surface area increase (e.g. due to lung recruitment), the intensity may decrease or even remain unchanged.

## CONCLUSION

The best strategy to avoid VILI is to minimize the duration of mechanical ventilation. Thus, patients should be routinely reassessed to determine whether mechanical ventilation is still necessary. While positive pressure is required, ventilator variables ($V_T$, PEEP, RR, flow rate, and $FiO_2$) should be individualized and constantly monitored. Ventilator readouts are also essential to monitor the effect of the predefined parameters—Pplat, ΔP, and mechanical power—in order to reduce VILI.

## SALIENT POINTS

- Mechanical ventilation is applied in order to reduce the workload of the respiratory muscles and maintain satisfactory blood gas exchange.
- However, mechanical ventilation may cause pulmonary structural damage, known as VILI.
- The mechanisms associated with VILI may be exacerbated if mechanical breath variables, such as $V_T$, PEEP, RR, inspiratory flow rate, and $FiO_2$ are inadequate adjusted.
- In order to minimize VILI, the following parameters need to be tightly monitored—respiratory system plateau pressure, driving pressure, and transpulmonary pressure.
- More recently, new ventilator parameters are under investigation, such as mechanical energy, power, and intensity.

## REFERENCES

1. Slutsky AS, Ranieri VM. Ventilator-induced lung injury. N Engl J Med. 2013;369(22):2126-36.
2. Shekerdemian L, Bohn D. Cardiovascular effects of mechanical ventilation. Arch Dis Child. 1999;80(5):475-80.
3. Avignon PD, Hedenstrom G, Hedman C. Pulmonary complications in respirator patients. Acta Med Scand Suppl. 1956;316:86-90.
4. Gattinoni L, Carlesso E, Cadringher P, et al. Physical and biological triggers of ventilator-induced lung injury and its prevention. Eur Respir J Suppl. 2003;47:15s-25s.
5. Garcia CS, Prota LF, Morales MM, et al. Understanding the mechanisms of lung mechanical stress. Braz J Med Biol Res. 2006;39(6):697-706.
6. Santos CC, Zhang H, Liu M, et al. Bench-to-bedside review: Biotrauma and modulation of the innate immune response. Crit Care. 2005;9(3):280-6.
7. Brower RG, Matthay MA, Morris A, et al. Acute Respiratory Distress Syndrome Network. Ventilation with lower tidal volumes as compared with traditional tidal volumes for acute lung injury and the acute respiratory distress syndrome. N Engl J Med. 2000;342(18):1301-8.
8. Cressoni M, Cadringher P, Chiurazzi C, et al. Lung inhomogeneity in patients with acute respiratory distress syndrome. Am J Respir Crit Care Med. 2014;189(2):149-58.
9. Retamal J, Bergamini BC, Carvalho AR, et al. Non-lobar atelectasis generates inflammation and structural alveolar injury in the surrounding healthy tissue during mechanical ventilation. Crit Care. 2014;18(5):505.
10. Tschumperlin DJ, Oswari J, Margulies AS. Deformation-induced injury of alveolar epithelial cells. Effect of frequency, duration, and amplitude. Am J Respir Crit Care Med. 2000;162(2 Pt 1):357-62.
11. Protti A, Cressoni M, Santini A, et al. Lung stress and strain during mechanical ventilation: any safe threshold? Am J Respir Crit Care Med. 2011;183(10):1354-62.
12. Dreyfuss D, Soler P, Basset G, et al. High inflation pressure pulmonary edema. Respective effects of high airway pressure, high tidal volume, and positive end-expiratory pressure. Am Rev Respir Dis. 1988;137(5):1159-64.
13. Schmitt JM, Vieillard-Baron A, Augarde R, et al. Positive end-expiratory pressure titration in acute respiratory distress syndrome patients: impact on right ventricular outflow impedance evaluated by pulmonary artery doppler flow velocity measurements. Crit Care Med. 2001;29(6):1154-8.
14. Amato MB, Meade MO, Slutsky AS, et al. Driving pressure and survival in the acute respiratory distress syndrome. N Engl J Med. 2015;372(8):747-55.
15. Seah AS, Grant KA, Aliyeva M, et al. Quantifying the roles of tidal volume and PEEP in the pathogenesis of ventilator-induced lung injury. Ann Biomed Eng. 2011;39(5):1505-16.
16. Protti A, Andreis DT, Monti M, et al. Lung stress and strain during mechanical ventilation: any difference between statics and dynamics? Crit Care Med. 2013;41(4):1046-55.
17. Güldner A, Braune A, Ball L, et al. Comparative effects of volutrauma and atelectrauma on lung inflammation in experimental acute respiratory distress syndrome. Crit Care Med. 2016;44(9):e854-65.
18. Gattinoni L, Carlesso E, Caironi P. Stress and strain within the lung. Curr Opin Crit Care. 2012;18(1):42-7.
19. Albert RK. The role of ventilation-induced surfactant dysfunction and atelectasis in causing acute respiratory distress syndrome. Am J Respir Crit Care Med. 2012;185(7):702-8.
20. Fanelli V, Mascia L, Puntorieri V, et al. Pulmonary atelectasis during low stretch ventilation: "open lung" versus "lung rest" strategy. Crit Care Med. 2009;37(3):1046-53.
21. Wolthuis EK, Vlaar AP, Choi G, et al. Mechanical ventilation using non-injurious ventilation settings causes lung injury in the absence of pre-existing lung injury in healthy mice. Crit Care. 2009;13(1):R1.
22. Tobin MJ, Mador MJ, Guenther SM, et al. Variability of resting respiratory drive and timing in healthy subjects. J Appl Physiol (1985). 1988;65(1):309-17.
23. D'Angelo E, Agostoni E. Continuous recording of pleural surface pressure at various sites. Respir Physiol. 1973;19(3):356-68.
24. Yoshida T, Torsani V, Gomes S, et al. Spontaneous effort causes occult pendelluft during mechanical ventilation. Am J Respir Crit Care Med. 2013;188(12):1420-7.
25. Hraiech S, Yoshida T, Papazian L. Balancing neuromuscular blockade versus preserved muscle activity. Curr Opin Crit Care. 2015;21(1):26-33.
26. Bellani G, Laffey JG, Pham T, et al. LUNG SAFE Investigators; ESICM Trials Group. Epidemiology, patterns of care, and

mortality for patients with acute respiratory distress syndrome in intensive care units in 50 countries. JAMA. 2016;315(8): 788-800.
27. Guay J, Ochroch EA. Intraoperative use of low volume ventilation to decrease postoperative mortality, mechanical ventilation, lengths of stay and lung injury in patients without acute lung injury. Cochrane Database Syst Rev. 2015;(12):CD011151.
28. Ladha K, Vidal Melo MF, McLean DJ, et al. Intraoperative protective mechanical ventilation and risk of postoperative respiratory complications: hospital based registry study. BMJ. 2015;351:h3646.
29. Nin N, Muriel A, Peñuelas O, et al. VENTILA Group. Severe hypercapnia and outcome of mechanically ventilated patients with moderate or severe acute respiratory distress syndrome. Intensive Care Med. 2017;43(2):200-8.
30. Mead J, Takishima T, Leith D. Stress distribution in lungs: a model of pulmonary elasticity. J Appl Physiol. 1970;28(5): 596-608.
31. Neto AS, Simonis FD, Barbas CS, et al. PROtective Ventilation Network Investigators. Lung-protective ventilation with low tidal volumes and the occurrence of pulmonary complications in patients without acute respiratory distress syndrome: a systematic review and individual patient data analysis. Crit Care Med. 2015;43(10):2155-63.
32. Sahetya SK, Brower RG. Lung recruitment and titrated PEEP in moderate to severe ARDS. Is the door closing on the open lung? JAMA. 2017;318(14):1327-9.
33. Manzano F, Fernández-Mondéjar E, Colmenero M, et al. Positive end-expiratory pressure reduces incidence of ventilator-associated pneumonia in nonhypoxemic patients. Crit Care Med. 2008;36(8):2225-31.
34. Slutsky AS, Villar J, Pesenti A. Happy 50th birthday ARDS! Intensive Care Med. 2016;42(5):637-9.
35. Dreyfuss D, Saumon G. Ventilator-induced lung injury: lessons from experimental studies. Am J Respir Crit Care Med. 1998;157(1):294-323.
36. Fernández Mondéjar E, Vazquez Mata G, Cárdenas A, et al. Ventilation with positive end-expiratory pressure reduces extravascular lung water and increases lymphatic flow in hydrostatic pulmonary edema. Crit Care Med. 1996;24(9):1562-7.
37. Hemmes SN, Gama de Abreu M, Pelosi P, et al. PROVE Network Investigators for the Clinical Trial Network of the European Society of Anaesthesiology. High versus low positive end-expiratory pressure during general anaesthesia for open abdominal surgery (PROVHILO trial): a multicentre randomised controlled trial. Lancet. 2014;384(9942):495-503.
38. Muscedere JG, Mullen JB, Gan K, et al. Tidal ventilation at low airway pressures can augment lung injury. Am J Respir Crit Care Med. 1994;149(5):1327-34.
39. Briel M, Meade M, Mercat A, et al. Higher vs lower positive end-expiratory pressure in patients with acute lung injury and acute respiratory distress syndrome: systematic review and meta-analysis. JAMA. 2010;303(9):865-73.
40. Brower RG, Lanken PN, MacIntyre N, et al. Higher versus lower positive end-expiratory pressures in patients with the acute respiratory distress syndrome. N Engl J Med. 2004;351(4):327-36.
41. Meade MO, Cook DJ, Guyatt GH, et al. Lung Open Ventilation Study Investigators. Ventilation strategy using low tidal volumes, recruitment maneuvers, and high positive end-expiratory pressure for acute lung injury and acute respiratory distress syndrome: a randomized controlled trial. JAMA. 2008;299(6):637-45.
42. Cavalcanti AB, Suzumura ÉA, Laranjeira LN, et al. Writing Group for the Alveolar Recruitment for Acute Respiratory Distress Syndrome Trial (ART) Investigators. Effect of lung recruitment and titrated positive end-expiratory pressure (PEEP) vs low PEEP on mortality in patients with acute respiratory distress syndrome: A randomized clinical trial. JAMA. 2017;318(14):1335-45.
43. Rosa RG, Rutzen W, Madeira L, et al. Use of thoracic electrical impedance tomography as an auxiliary tool for alveolar recruitment maneuvers in acute respiratory distress syndrome: case report and brief literature review. Rev Bras Ter Intensiva. 2015;27(4):406-11.
44. Bikker IG, Preis C, Egal M, et al. Electrical impedance tomography measured at two thoracic levels can visualize the ventilation distribution changes at the bedside during a decremental positive end-expiratory lung pressure trial. Crit Care. 2011;15(4):R193.
45. Costa EL, Borges JB, Melo A, et al. Bedside estimation of recruitable alveolar collapse and hyperdistension by electrical impedance tomography. Intensive Care Med. 2009;35(6):1132-7.
46. Vieillard-Baron A, Prin S, Augarde R, et al. Increasing respiratory rate to improve CO2 clearance during mechanical ventilation is not a panacea in acute respiratory failure. Crit Care Med. 2002;30(7):1407-12.
47. Carrasco Loza R, Villamizar Rodríguez G, Medel Fernández N. Ventilator-induced lung injury (VILI) in acute respiratory distress syndrome (ARDS): Volutrauma and molecular effects. Open Respir Med J. 2015;9:112-9.
48. Cressoni M, Gotti M, Chiurazzi C, et al. Mechanical power and development of ventilator-induced lung injury. Anesthesiology. 2016;124(5):1100-8.
49. Rich PB, Reickert CA, Sawada S, et al. Effect of rate and inspiratory flow on ventilator-induced lung injury. J Trauma. 2000;49(5):903-11.
50. Maeda Y, Fujino Y, Uchiyama A, et al. Effects of peak inspiratory flow on development of ventilator-induced lung injury in rabbits. Anesthesiology. 2004;101(3):722-8.
51. Protti A, Maraffi T, Milesi M, et al. Role of strain rate in the pathogenesis of ventilator-induced lung edema. Crit Care Med. 2016;44(9):e838-45.
52. Garcia CS, Abreu SC, Soares RM, et al. Pulmonary morphofunctional effects of mechanical ventilation with high inspiratory air flow. Crit Care Med. 2008;36(1):232-9.
53. Kotani M, Kotani T, Li Z, et al. Reduced inspiratory flow attenuates IL-8 release and MAPK activation of lung overstretch. Eur Respir J. 2004;24(2):238-46.
54. Quinn DA, Moufarrej RK, Volokhov A, et al. Interactions of lung stretch, hyperoxia, and MIP-2 production in ventilator-induced lung injury. J Appl Physiol. (1985). 2002;93(2):517-25.
55. Freeman BA, Crapo JD. Hyperoxia increases oxygen radical production in rat lungs and lung mitochondria. J Biol Chem. 1981;256(21):10986-92.

56. Winslow RM. Oxygen: the poison is in the dose. Transfusion. 2013;53(2):424-37.
57. Barazzone C, Horowitz S, Donati YR, et al. Oxygen toxicity in mouse lung: pathways to cell death. Am J Respir Cell Mol Biol. 1998;19(4):573-81.
58. Mantell LL, Lee PJ. Signal transduction pathways in hyperoxia-induced lung cell death. Mol Genet Metab. 2000;71(1-2):359-70.
59. Sackner MA, Hirsch JA, Epstein S, et al. Effect of oxygen in graded concentrations upon tracheal mucous velocity. A study in anesthetized dogs. Chest. 1976;69(2):164-7.
60. Griffith DE, Garcia JG, James HL, et al. Hyperoxic exposure in humans. Effects of 50 percent oxygen on alveolar macrophage leukotriene B4 synthesis. Chest. 1992;101(2):392-7.
61. Carvalho CR, de Paula Pinto Schettino G, Maranhão B, et al. Hyperoxia and lung disease. Curr Opin Pulm Med. 1998;4(5):300-4.
62. Santos C, Ferrer M, Roca J, et al. Pulmonary gas exchange response to oxygen breathing in acute lung injury. Am J Respir Crit Care Med. 2000;161(1):26-31.
63. Oba Y, Salzman GA. Ventilation with lower tidal volumes as compared with traditional tidal volumes for acute lung injury. N Engl J Med. 2000;343(11):813-14.
64. Terragni PP, Rosboch G, Tealdi A, et al. Tidal hyperinflation during low tidal volume ventilation in acute respiratory distress syndrome. Am J Respir Crit Care Med. 2007;175(2):160-6.
65. Bellani G, Guerra L, Musch G, et al. Lung regional metabolic activity and gas volume changes induced by tidal ventilation in patients with acute lung injury. Am J Respir Crit Care Med. 2011;183(9):1193-9.
66. Guldner A, Kiss T, Serpa Neto A, et al. Intraoperative protective mechanical ventilation for prevention of postoperative pulmonary complications: a comprehensive review of the role of tidal volume, positive end-expiratory pressure, and lung recruitment maneuvers. Anesthesiology. 2015;123(3): 692-713.
67. Samary CS, Santos RS, Santos CL, et al. Biological impact of transpulmonary driving pressure in experimental acute respiratory distress syndrome. Anesthesiology. 2015;123(2): 423-33.
68. Neto AS, Hemmes SN, Barbas CS, et al. PROVE Network Investigators. Association between driving pressure and development of postoperative pulmonary complications in patients undergoing mechanical ventilation for general anaesthesia: a meta-analysis of individual patient data. Lancet Respir Med. 2016;4(4):272-80.
69. Neto AS, Hemmes SN, Barbas CS, et al. PROVE Network Investigators. Incidence of mortality and morbidity related to postoperative lung injury in patients who have undergone abdominal or thoracic surgery: a systematic review and meta-analysis. Lancet Respir Med. 2014;2(12):1007-15.
70. Talmor D, Sarge T, Malhotra A, et al. Mechanical ventilation guided by esophageal pressure in acute lung injury. N Engl J Med. 2008;359(20):2095-104.
71. Grieco DL, Chen L, Brochard L. Transpulmonary pressure: importance and limits. Ann Transl Med. 2017;5(14):285.
72. Ranieri VM, Brienza N, Santostasi S, et al. Impairment of lung and chest wall mechanics in patients with acute respiratory distress syndrome: role of abdominal distension. Am J Respir Crit Care Med. 1997;156(4 Pt 1):1082-91.
73. Baedorf Kassis E, Loring SH, Talmor D. Mortality and pulmonary mechanics in relation to respiratory system and transpulmonary driving pressures in ARDS. Intensive Care Med. 2016;42(8):1206-13.
74. Liu Q, Li W, Zeng QS, et al. Lung stress and strain during mechanical ventilation in animals with and without pulmonary acute respiratory distress syndrome. J Surg Res. 2013;181(2):300-7.
75. Suzuki S, Hotchkiss JR, Takahashi T, et al. Effect of core body temperature on ventilator-induced lung injury. Crit Care Med. 2004;32(1):144-9.
76. Rich PB, Douillet CD, Hurd H, et al. Effect of ventilatory rate on airway cytokine levels and lung injury. J Surg Res. 2003;113(1):139-45.
77. Simonson DA, Adams AB, Wright LA, et al. Effects of ventilatory pattern on experimental lung injury caused by high airway pressure. Crit Care Med. 2004;32(3):781-6.
78. Samary CS, Silva PL, Gama de Abreu M, et al. Ventilator-induced lung injury: Power to the mechanical power. Anesthesiology. 2016;125(5):1070-1.

# CHAPTER 16

# Ventilator-induced Diaphragm Dysfunction

*Tom Schepens, Ewan C Goligher*

## INTRODUCTION

Muscle weakness is common in patients admitted to the intensive care unit (ICU), affecting both limb muscles and respiratory muscles.[1] This loss of muscle capacity impacts the length of ventilation and the probability of survival.[2,3]

Multiple factors contribute to muscle weakness, including critical illness-related factors and treatment-related factors. Recent evidence suggests that mechanical ventilation (MV) itself may be responsible for a substantial proportion of the diaphragm dysfunction observed in critically ill patients. This entity is called ventilator-induced diaphragm dysfunction (VIDD).

## DIAPHRAGM ANATOMY AND FUNCTION

The diaphragm is the most important muscle of inspiration. It is a thin, dome-shaped muscle that inserts into the lower ribs, xiphoid process, and lumbar vertebrae, separating the thoracic and abdominal cavities. The muscle is composed of three separate segments—a central noncontractile tendon, the costal diaphragm, and the crural diaphragm. The costal diaphragm inserts into the ribs and xiphoid process; it runs parallel to the ribcage before curving along the lungs.[4] The crural diaphragm inserts into the first three lumbar vertebrae. At the center of the diaphragm we find a noncontractile tendon (Fig. 1).

The diaphragm is composed of both slow (Type I) and fast twitch (Type IIa and IIx) fiber types in approximately equal proportions.[5] Innervation of the diaphragm derives from the phrenic nerves, which originate within cervical nerve roots 3–5. Blood supply to the diaphragm arises from anastomoses between the phrenic artery and internal mammary arteries and between branches of the phrenic artery and the intercostal arteries.[6] The venous anatomy parallels the arterial circulation.

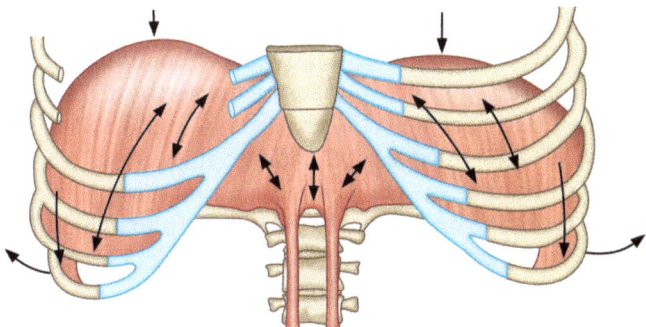

**Fig. 1:** Diaphragm anatomy showing the functional arrangement of the costal and crural diaphragm with respect to their various interactions with the different components of the chest wall. Arrows show the direction of muscle action. Because the costal diaphragm inserts onto the rib cage, its action can elevate the lower ribs, while the action of the crural diaphragm, which inserts onto the lumbar spine, acts only to lower the dome of the diaphragm.

As a consequence of its anatomical arrangement, shortening of diaphragm muscle fibers results in a piston-like action, drawing the lungs downward, and pushing the abdominal content downward and forward during inspiration.[7,8] The abdominal contents resist this downward displacement, generating an increase in intraabdominal pressure. This pressure propels the ribs upward and outward,[9] resulting in an increase in the transverse diameter of the thorax (Fig. 1).

The pressure gradient generated across the diaphragm (i.e. between the thoracic and abdominal cavities) during its contraction is referred to as the transdiaphragmatic pressure (Pdi). It can be calculated by measuring the pressure in the stomach (gastric pressure, Pga) and the esophageal pressure (Pes), where by convention Pdi = Pga − Pes.[10]

During normal tidal breathing, the diaphragm moves downward about a centimeter. This distance can easily increase to over 10 cm, allowing a great level of adaptation to physiologic needs. Expiration is normally a passive motion, although active expiration is possible by contracting the abdominal muscles and pushing the diaphragm upward.

Other inspiratory muscles, referred to as accessory muscles because they are marginally activated during tidal breathing, include the scalene, sternocleidomastoid, and external intercostal muscles. The external intercostal muscles pull the ribs upward and forward, increasing the lateral and anteroposterior diameters of the thorax. The scalene muscles elevate the first two ribs and the sternocleidomastoids raise the sternum.

## DIAPHRAGM DYSFUNCTION IN THE ICU

Patients who are admitted to an ICU frequently exhibit weakness of respiratory muscles including the diaphragm at the beginning of their ICU stay. Demoule and colleagues found that 64% of ventilated patients already had significant respiratory muscle weakness on admission.[11] This loss of respiratory muscular capacity results in an inability to tolerate relatively small increases in work of breathing, impairing a patient's capability to separate from the ventilator.[12]

### Impact on Outcomes

Several studies have examined the maximal force generating capacity of the diaphragm in patients admitted to the ICU and found a clear association between diaphragm dysfunction and an increased risk of mortality or prolonged MV.[2,3] Kim and colleagues demonstrated diaphragm dysfunction in 29% of patients in the ICU, and it was associated with a significantly higher risk of difficult weaning and longer ICU and hospital stay.[13] Similar results were reported by Dres and colleagues, who demonstrated that at the moment when patients were assessed for extubation readiness, 63% had diaphragm dysfunction, 34% had limb muscle weakness, and 21% had a combination of both. In that study, worse diaphragm function was independently associated with weaning failure and mortality, while presence of limb muscle weakness was associated with longer duration of MV and hospital stay.[14] Furthermore, diaphragm weakness at the time of extubation was associated with an increased risk of mortality one year after extubation in a study by Medrinal.[15] In order to explain this high incidence of diaphragm dysfunction in the ICU, we need to consider factors related to both critical illness and ICU interventions.

### Systemic Causes

Sepsis is one of the most prominent important mechanisms, and is associated with marked reductions in diaphragm strength.[3] A number of pathways link sepsis to muscle weakness, including proinflammatory cytokines,[16] oxidative stress,[17] and activation of proteolytic pathways.[18] One study demonstrated that sepsis has a more profound impact on the diaphragm than on other muscles.[19]

Many medications that are routinely used in an ICU may have a negative effect on diaphragm muscle strength. These include neuromuscular blocking agents, corticosteroids, and aminoglycosides.[20,21] Other factors that could be associated with diaphragm dysfunction include metabolic derangements such as acidosis and hypokalemia.[22] Preexisting systemic conditions like malnutrition or endocrinopathies may also contribute to diaphragm dysfunction in the critically ill.[21]

### Neuromuscular Causes

Mechanical ventilation alters the geometry of the chest wall and diaphragm, generally shortening the resting diaphragm length by inflating the thorax. This by itself can impair diaphragm muscle function, especially in combination with dynamic hyperinflation due to frequent increases in airway resistance in acute respiratory failure.

The above-mentioned systemic factors, together with immobility and microvascular injury, have a combined effect on the muscles (myopathy) and nerves (neuropathy) of an ICU patient. Those effects are known as critical illness polymyoneuropathy (CIPMN) or ICU-acquired weakness (ICU-AW)[23,24] (Flowchart 1) and may contribute to diaphragm weakness. In patients receiving ventilation for 7 or more days, diaphragm strength was correlated with peripheral muscle function measured by the Medical Research Council score, suggesting that CIPMN can affect the phrenic nerves and diaphragm as well as the limb muscles.[1]

### Mechanical Ventilation: The Concept of Ventilator-induced Diaphragm Dysfunction

Although CIPMN may affect the diaphragm, several observations suggest that it is not the main cause of diaphragm weakness in ventilated patients. Certain histological features typical of CIPMN (selective loss of thick filaments, patchy necrosis, and regeneration) have not been demonstrated in the diaphragm of ventilated patients to this point. Moreover, diaphragm injury occurs very early (hours

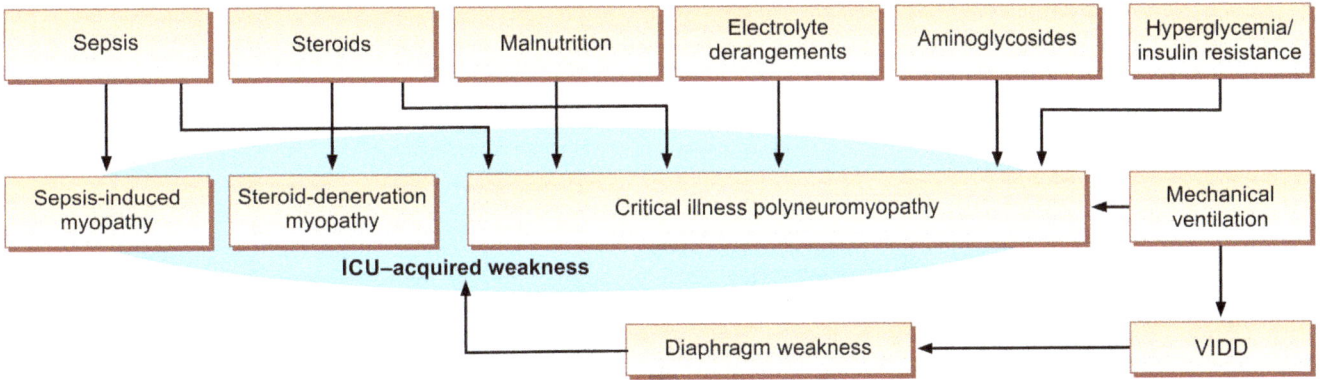

**Flowchart 1:** Risk factors contributing to the development of diaphragm dysfunction. Different pathophysiological mechanisms define separate entities. In ICU patients, several factors intertwine and are frequently simultaneously present.

to days) after initiating MV, whereas the effect of CIPNM on skeletal muscles that are equally inactive during MV usually takes weeks to develop.[25] A growing body of evidence suggests that MV itself may be responsible for the structural injury, atrophy, and dysfunction observed in the diaphragm in critically ill patients, giving rise to the concept of ventilator-induced diaphragm dysfunction (VIDD).[26] VIDD constitutes a vicious cycle of ventilator-dependence: acute respiratory failure renders the patient ventilator-dependent, and injurious MV weakens the respiratory muscles thus perpetuating ventilator-dependence. VIDD therefore increases the risk of persistent ventilator dependence and associated morbidity and mortality.[27] The evidence linking MV to diaphragm injury is two-fold—MV is strongly associated with structural and functional abnormalities of the diaphragm, and there are several putative mechanisms with strong experimental support by which MV could cause diaphragm injury.

Multiple studies have demonstrated atrophy specifically affecting the diaphragm (but not other axial skeletal muscles) in histological samples of patients that were ventilated for an extended period of time.[5,28] In these studies, the magnitude of injury was correlated with the duration of MV.[28-31] Taken together, these studies provide strong evidence that MV can cause clinically important diaphragm injury and dysfunction.

## PATHOPHYSIOLOGY OF VENTILATOR-INDUCED DIAPHRAGM DYSFUNCTION

### Oxidative Stress

Considerable progress has been made in delineating the molecular pathways linking diaphragm inactivity and MV to diaphragm injury and dysfunction (Flowchart 2). In animal models, an essential element in the development of VIDD is oxidative stress in the diaphragm, caused by an excess amount of mitochondrial reactive oxygen species (ROS).[32-35] Mechanisms involved include upregulation of transcription factors of the forkhead box O (FOXO) and signal transducer and activator of transcription (STAT) families.[32,36,37] Other signaling molecules are involved as well, and include nuclear factor kappa-light-chain-enhancer of activated B cells (NF-κB)[38] and different altered proteolysis pathways like the calpains-caspases and ubiquitin-proteasome pathways, both of which are activated by oxidative stress.[39,40] The role of oxidative stress is supported by the observation that treatment with various antioxidant agents attenuate VIDD in experimental models.[41-44]

It is more difficult to identify specific mechanisms that link MV to oxidative stress.[45] Some elements that are known to play a role include the disruption of the normal mitochondrial fission/fusion balance and the potential toxic effects of fatty acids on mitochondria, both of which are present in inactive skeletal muscles.[46,47] This hypothesis was supported by studies that demonstrated mitochondrial DNA damage and increased intramyocellular lipid accumulation in diaphragms with VIDD.[33] A decrease in blood flow to the diaphragm and resulting decrease in $pO_2$ could potentially worsen this mitochondrial damage. Titin, a key structural protein in muscle, might also act as a force transducer to sense mechanical loading or unloading and modulate cellular protein synthetic controls.[48]

It is unclear what the exact role of autophagy is in VIDD. Autophagy is a proteolytic process and it is known to be upregulated in humans during MV.[37] Increased autophagy seems to be beneficial in an early stage of VIDD,[49] but whether it is harmful or beneficial in the later stages of VIDD remains unknown.

The precise molecular mechanisms responsible for the activation of proteolytic systems in the clinical setting

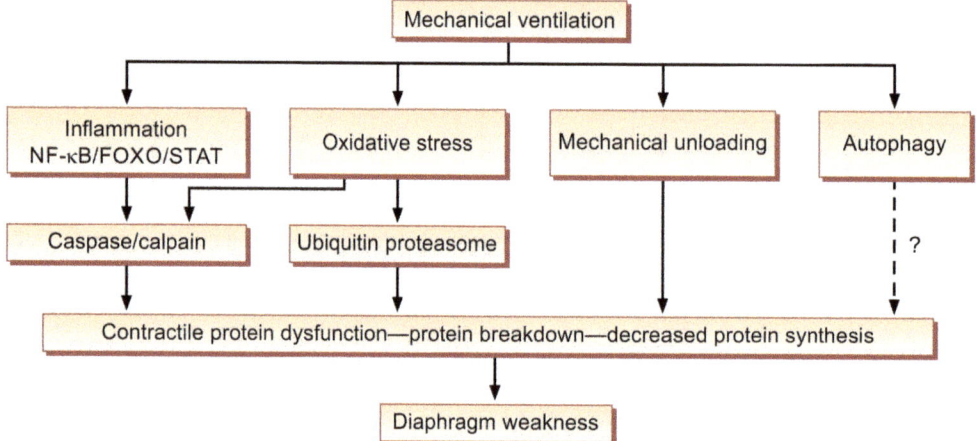

**Flowchart 2:** Pathways linking mechanical ventilation to diaphragm weakness. (NF-κB: nuclear factor kappa-light-chain-enhancer of activated B cells; FOXO: forkhead box O; STAT: signal transducer and activator of transcription).

remain uncertain. In fact, recent work suggests that patients with diaphragm injury and atrophy do not manifest signs of oxidative stress on histology.[50] Much remains to be learned about the basic biology of VIDD.

### Diaphragm Inactivity

While the complex biology underlying VIDD remains uncertain, the physiological mechanisms are reasonably well understood. Both *in vitro* and *in vivo* experiments in animal models demonstrated that controlled mechanical ventilation (CMV) results in diaphragm disuse leading to a rapid loss of muscle mass and muscle fiber contractility beginning within mere hours of starting the ventilation.[51-54] The detrimental effect of diaphragm inactivity is further supported by experimental observations that diaphragm atrophy and dysfunction can be attenuated by maintaining some level of diaphragm activity during ventilation. VIDD was less severe, and proteolysis was unaltered, in animals receiving assisted MV compared to CMV.[55,56] Adaptive support ventilation prevented diaphragm atrophy and weakness in piglets.[57] Nevertheless, mode is a secondary concern—the primary determinant of the development of atrophy is the level of inspiratory effort—ventilator mode matters insofar as it modifies the patient's effort.[30] Clinicians should not assume that the patient's inspiratory effort level is adequate merely because the patient is ventilated in a partially assisted mode such as pressure support ventilation (PSV).

### Concentric Diaphragm Loading

Two types of diaphragm activity can result in injury. These include an excessive amount of muscle activity (concentric loading) as well as muscle activity during muscle lengthening (eccentric loading).

There is strong evidence that excess respiratory muscle loads can cause diaphragm inflammation, injury, and ultimately, dysfunction and failure.[58-60] Diaphragm injury due to both chronic and acute inspiratory loading has been documented histologically in humans, e.g. both in healthy subjects and in patients with chronic obstructive pulmonary disease (COPD).[61] The initiation of MV significantly reduces circulating cytokines in COPD patients during acute exacerbations, possibly as a consequence of reducing diaphragm load.[62] However, it remains unclear whether load-induced injury occurs frequently during MV in the clinical setting. The load required for injury is surprisingly low in some studies[63] and the inflamed respiratory muscles of patients with sepsis and acute respiratory failure are likely highly susceptible to load-induced injury.[64]

### Eccentric Diaphragm Loading

Low levels of eccentric contractile activity are common during resting tidal ventilation, as both inspiratory and expiratory muscle groups are simultaneously activated to control air flow to a fine degree.[65] However, eccentric contractile activity can cause significant muscle injury and are generally much more injurious than concentric loads.[66] Animal models have demonstrated the injurious effects of eccentric contractions.[67,68] But this has not yet been documented in humans. In mechanically ventilated patients, the diaphragm may be exposed to eccentric contractile injury during episodes of certain forms of patient-ventilator dyssynchrony (e.g. ineffective efforts).[69]

Because lung volume is falling as the diaphragm contracts, such contractions may occasionally be eccentric and diaphragm injury may result. Similarly, reverse triggering dyssynchrony leads to diaphragm contractile activation while the ventilator is already switching from inspiration to expiration.[70] Eccentric diaphragm contractions may also occur in the context of expiratory braking, where the diaphragm is activated to prevent excessive loss of lung volume and development of atelectasis.[71,72] Whether this theoretical form of injurious muscle loading has any important clinical impact remains uncertain.

## CLINICAL PRESENTATION AND DIAGNOSIS OF VENTILATOR-INDUCED DIAPHRAGM DYSFUNCTION

Diagnosing VIDD is a challenging task, and its presence may remain unnoticed if the patient can be separated from the ventilator (weaned) uneventfully. Diaphragm weakness should be considered in the setting of prolonged weaning, or repeated episode of respiratory failure. In mechanically ventilated patients, certain physical and radiological findings may indicate the presence of VIDD.[73] Abdominal paradox, an inward movement of the abdomen during inspiration, is associated with diaphragm or bilateral phrenic nerve injury.[21] An elevated (hemi) diaphragm on chest radiograph may signify diaphragm weakness. Unilateral elevation may point to a phrenic nerve injury, whereas bilateral elevation may be pointing to severe diaphragm weakness. Finally, hypercapnic respiratory failure in a patient without apparent parenchymal lung disease should lead clinicians to investigate the possibility of significant diaphragm weakness.

### Diagnostic Approach and Monitoring Tools

Because of technical complexity, monitoring diaphragm function is not widely employed as part of routine clinical practice. Some commonly used methods to evaluate global respiratory muscle dysfunction do not necessarily reflect diaphragm function. Confounding from a lack of volitional effort is a key challenge in mechanically ventilated patients. For example, the maximum inspiratory pressure (Pi, max) is easy to obtain, but a low value may be a result of submaximal effort by the patient.

#### Pressure Measurements

The Gilbert index is a test that was developed to test for diaphragm paresis or paralysis after cardiac surgery. It measures the ratio of $\Delta Pga$ (the inspiratory swing in gastric pressure) to $\Delta Pdi$ (the inspiratory swing in transdiaphragmatic pressure) during resting (unsupported) breathing.[74] $\Delta Pga/\Delta Pdi$ is closely related to the magnitude of abdominal displacement during inspiration relative to total chest wall displacement. When the diaphragm moves upward (instead of downward) during inspiration, this index will take a negative value. Negative values of the Gilbert index measured during resting tidal breathing are diagnostic of severe diaphragm weakness.[75,76] Clinicians should bear in mind that vigorous accessory muscle effort may lower the Gilbert index, and measurements should be obtained during resting tidal breathing.[77]

The best accepted method for measuring diaphragm strength in anesthetized patients is magnetic twitch stimulation of the phrenic nerve while measuring the transdiaphragmatic pressure. This can be recorded with double-balloon catheters with one balloon in the stomach and one in the esophagus. This technique is labor-intensive and technically challenging, with a number of important technical pitfalls.[63]

#### Neuromuscular Coupling

Alternatively, we can assess the neuromuscular coupling (NMC) as a parameter for diaphragm function. NMC is the ratio of diaphragm pressure generation (Pdi) to the neural stimulus activating the diaphragm (i.e. diaphragm electric activity, Edi).[78] NMC is a novel and potentially feasible and reliable method of monitoring respiratory muscle function. Because it takes the neural stimulus to the diaphragm into account, NMC may be independent of volitional inspiratory effort, potentially overcoming a key limitation of standard methods of assessing diaphragm function as discussed above. In a number of early studies, the relationship between Pdi and Edi was found to be curvilinear or quasilinear,[79] but studies in ventilated patients have obtained varying results.[80,81]

#### Biopsies

Given the anatomical location of the diaphragm, it is evidently not feasible to obtain serial biopsies to describe changes over time in diaphragm function. Nevertheless, this technique has provided us with essential information on diaphragm function and structure in an animal model of VIDD.

#### Ultrasound

One novel and potentially more useful monitoring technique for diaphragm function is ultrasound.[82] Two techniques have been described—thickness and thickening fraction using B-mode measurements, or excursion using M-mode measurements.[83,84]

Normal values of diaphragm excursion measured by ultrasound for various inspiratory maneuvers have been published[85] and the reproducibility of this technique is excellent.[85] Diminished diaphragm excursion has been shown to be diagnostic of diaphragm dysfunction.[76]

The second ultrasonographic approach for diagnosing diaphragm dysfunction is to measure diaphragm thickness and thickening during inspiration using a high frequency linear array transducer positioned in the 8th or 9th intercostal space between the mid- and anterior axillary lines, the so-called zone of apposition.[86] The percentage increase in thickness during inspiration—the diaphragm thickening fraction, TFdi, is related to shortening of the diaphragm during inspiration.[87] TFdi, therefore, provides a surrogate estimate of diaphragm shortening during inspiratory effort, and TFdi during a maximal inspiratory effort is correlated with diaphragm function.[88-90] This technique has good reproducibility in ventilated patients[91] but its relation to maximal pressure generation requires further research. Serial measurements of thickness may demonstrate atrophy as an element of diaphragm dysfunction, but will not provide information on structural changes responsible for these sonographic changes.

## PREVENTION OF VENTILATOR-INDUCED DIAPHRAGM DYSFUNCTION

### Diaphragm-protective Ventilation Concepts

As discussed above, diaphragm injury may result from either excessive or insufficient (or mistimed) diaphragm contractile activity (reflecting patient inspiratory effort) during ventilation. The patient's inspiratory effort can be modified in a number of ways, e.g. by increasing driving pressures, changing the ventilation mode, or altering the type and dose of sedation.[30] The optimal level of inspiratory effort to prevent the development of VIDD has been uncertain, particularly because preserving inspiratory effort may result in patient self-inflicted lung injury[92] or excess respiratory muscle oxygen consumption.[93,94] Recent clinical observations suggest that an inspiratory effort level similar to that of healthy subjects breathing at rest is associated with relatively stable diaphragm thickness. Importantly, patients with this level of inspiratory effort during the early course of ventilation were shown to have the shortest duration of ventilation and ICU admission.[27] This suggests that this range of inspiratory effort might be the optimal target for diaphragm-protective ventilation. Future trials are required to confirm this hypothesis.

An alternate approach is to use external stimulation of the phrenic nerve to activate the diaphragm during MV. An interesting study in sheep showed reduced atrophy and muscle fiber injury in the stimulated hemidiaphragm after 72 hours of MV,[95] and a study in pigs showed some protective effect of transvenous phrenic nerve pacing on diaphragm strength.[96] In patients who underwent cardiothoracic surgery and short intervals of unilateral phrenic nerve stimulation during this procedure, researchers found increased mitochondrial respiration rates in the stimulated hemidiaphragm.[97]

### How to Monitor Diaphragm Activity?

We can either monitor the activity of a muscle by looking at the movement with ultrasound, measuring the electric activity generated by the muscle with electromyography (EMG) or by measuring the pressures generated by muscle contraction.

- *Pressure measurements*: The pressure generated by all the respiratory muscles can be measured. Different parameters, like the transdiaphragmatic pressure (Pdi), airway occlusion pressure (P0.1), and pressure-time product (PTP) have been developed. Measuring them often requires a balloon catheter to be inserted in the patient's esophagus.
- *Electromyography*: Either esophageal, intramuscular, or transcutaneous electromyographic measurements can be used, and show a good correlation to the patient's inspiratory effort.[80] Esophageal electrodes have recently gained more attention by its use as the control signal for Neurally Adjusted Ventilatory Assist (NAVA).[98]
- *Ultrasound*: Ultrasound evaluation of thickening during inspiration is a novel and promising method to assess diaphragm activity (Figs. 2A to C). Diaphragm thickening correlates with inspiratory pressure development,[88,99] inspiratory volume[86], and work of breathing.[100,101]

### Pharmacological Interventions

As our insight into the pathways by which MV results in diaphragm dysfunction increases, pharmacological strategies are starting to appear in small studies using animal models. One of the options includes the use of mitochondria-targeted antioxidants.[35] Other strategies have been developed as well, using Janus kinase-signal transducer and activator of transcription (JAK-STAT3) inhibitors,[102,103] and drugs which target this pathway are already in clinical development. Modulating proteolysis pathways, including autophagy,[49] is another option. Finally, the possible beneficial use of a troponin-activator drug acting at the muscle fiber level is being investigated as well.[104] It is well known that long-term use of corticosteroids

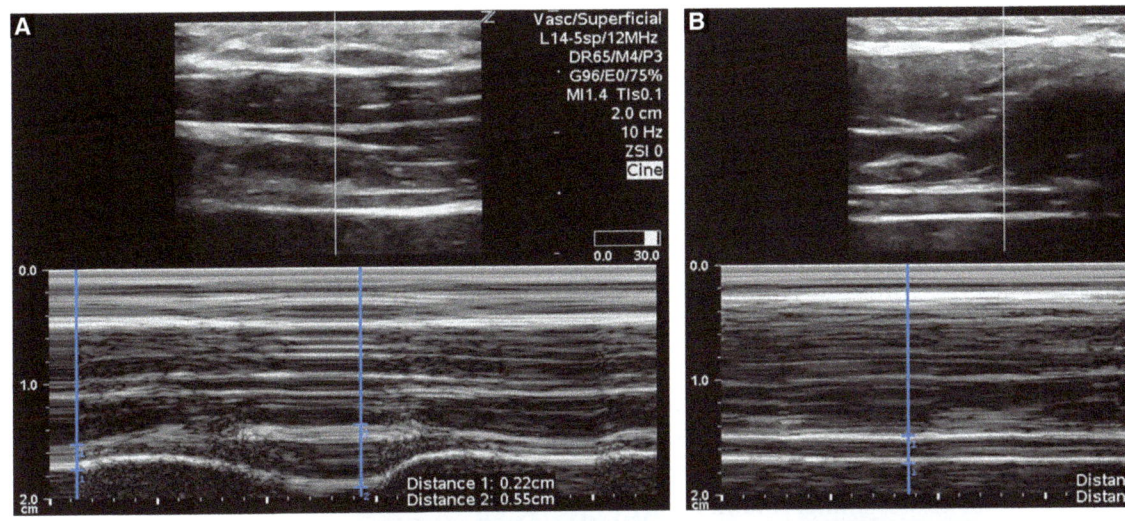
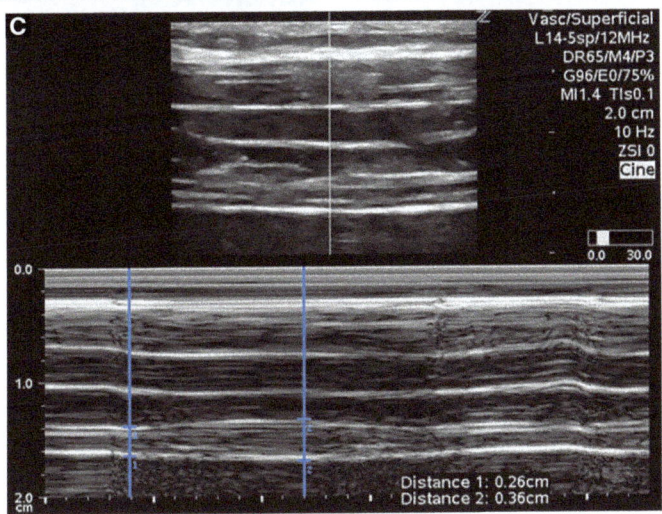

**Figs. 2A to C:** M-mode ultrasound images of the diaphragm during assisted mechanical ventilation, and measurements of the thickness (blue vertical lines) during expiration (Distance 1) and inspiration (Distance 2). (A) Under-support with a thickening fraction of 150%; (B) Over-support with a thickening fraction of 4%; and (C) Adequate support with a thickening fraction of 38%.

is associated with (diaphragm) muscle atrophy,[105] but some studies suggest that short-term use of corticosteroids may have a beneficial effect on the occurence of VIDD.[106,107]

## Other Protective Factors

The possibility to strengthen the diaphragm before exposing it to the risk of VIDD was tested in a rat model.[108] In this trial, a 1-hour endurance exercise for 10 days prior to MV increased the antioxidant capacity and upregulated heat shock proteins in the diaphragm, which would serve to protect against VIDD.

Hypercapnia seems to protect against VIDD. Piglets with hypercapnic acidosis during MV showed preserved diaphragmatic function after 3 days of MV.[109] Its specific mechanism is thus far incompletely understood.

Nevertheless, respiratory acidosis may worsen diaphragm function[110,111] and the appropiate use of hypercapnia is uncertain.

Finally, some drugs are known to have a positive effect on diaphragm strength, like levosimendan and theophylline,[112,113] but these do not protect the diaphragm from VIDD as such.

## RECOVERY FROM VENTILATOR-INDUCED DIAPHRAGM DYSFUNCTION

There is little information about the recovery of diaphragm function after discontinuation of MV, or about the recovery during assisted MV. A study in a rodent model subjected animals to 12 hours of CMV, after which they restarted spontaneous breathing. They still had impaired diaphragm muscle function 12 hours after extubation, but regained full strength 24 hours after extubation.[114] In one study in ventilated critically ill humans, the diaphragm thickness stayed stable in most of the patients during the first few days after separation from the ventilator.[30] In other patients from the same cohort, the diaphragm thickness returned toward baseline following extubation.

### Role of Inspiratory Muscle Training

Diaphragm weakness might be reversed by inspiratory muscle training (IMT). The effectiveness of IMT on weaning outcomes was demonstrated in a trial in patients who failed previous weaning attempts.[115] In this study, the IMT group improved maximal inspiratory pressure by approximately 35% after 2 weeks of training. Another trial found that IMT resulted in larger tidal volumes and a slower respiratory rate during weaning, shortening weaning times.[116] Although promising, those were studies in small cohorts and larger trials are warranted to confirm those results.

## CONCLUSION

Respiratory muscle weakness, especially weakness of the diaphragm, is a major cause of prolonged ventilator dependence and excess morbidity and mortality in critically ill patients. Mechanical ventilation is a major cause of diaphragm weakness in acute respiratory failure, leading to the concept of ventilator-induced dysfunction. Some 15 years of research has shed important insights on the molecular mechanisms linking MV with diaphragm dysfunction. New options have emerged to assess both diaphragm function and activity in critically ill patients, most notably ultrasound. Therapeutic options mainly focus on maintaining appropriate levels of diaphragm activity during ventilation, but in future may also include pharmacological strategies or inspiratory muscle training. We are slowly beginning to understand the concept of muscle-protective ventilation, paving the way to accelerate successful liberation from ventilator, in critically ill patients.

## SALIENT POINTS

- Respiratory muscle weakness is common in mechanically ventilated patients. This weakness is associated with significantly worse short-term and long-term outcomes.
- Among other factors, MV per se is an important cause of diaphragm weakness, a phenomenon referred to as VIDD.
- Various pathophysiological processes link MV to the development of diaphragm weakness, including inflammation, oxidative stress, and excessive or insufficient unloading of the diaphragm.
- Several monitoring techniques, including ultrasound, facilitate the assessment of diaphragm function and activity in critically ill patients.
- Several potential therapies are the subject of active investigation, including ventilation strategies, rehabilitation strategies, and pharmacological agents.
- Diaphragm-protective ventilation is an important new concept in the field. Future trials are required to confirm the feasibility and effectiveness of this approach to preventing diaphragm weakness during critical illness.

## REFERENCES

1. De Jonghe B, Bastuji-Garin S, Durand MC, et al. Groupe de Réflexion et d'Etude des Neuromyopathies en Réanimation. Respiratory weakness is associated with limb weakness and delayed weaning in critical illness. Crit Care Med. 2007;35(9):2007-15.
2. Hermans G, Agten A, Testelmans D, et al. Increased duration of mechanical ventilation is associated with decreased diaphragmatic force: a prospective observational study. Crit Care. 2010;14(4):R127.
3. Supinski GS, Callahan LA. Diaphragm weakness in mechanically ventilated critically ill patients. Crit Care. 2013;17(3):R120.
4. Mead J. Functional significance of the area of apposition of diaphragm to rib cage [proceedings]. Am Rev Respir Dis. 1979;119(2 Pt 2):31-2.
5. Levine S, Nguyen T, Taylor N, et al. Rapid disuse atrophy of diaphragm fibers in mechanically ventilated humans. N Engl J Med. 2008;358(13):1327-35.
6. Comtois A, Gorczyca W, Grassino A. Anatomy of diaphragmatic circulation. J Appl Physiol (1985). 1987;62(1):238-44.
7. Troyer A, Loring SH. Action of the Respiratory Muscles. Hoboken, NJ, USA: John Wiley & Sons, Inc; 2011.
8. Gauthier AP, Verbanck S, Estenne M, et al. Three-dimensional reconstruction of the in vivo human diaphragm shape at different lung volumes. J Appl Physiol (1985). 1994;76(2):495-506.
9. Goldman MD, Mead J. Mechanical interaction between the diaphragm and rib cage. J Appl Physiol. 1973;35(2):197-204.
10. Agostoni E, Rahn H. Abdominal and thoracic pressures at different lung volumes. J Appl Physiol. 1960;15:1087-92.
11. Demoule A, Jung B, Prodanovic H, et al. Diaphragm dysfunction on admission to the intensive care unit: prevalence, risk factors, and prognostic impact-a prospective study. Am J Respir Crit Care Med. 2013;188(2):213-9.
12. Watson AC, Hughes PD, Louise Harris M, et al. Measurement of twitch transdiaphragmatic, esophageal, and endotracheal tube pressure with bilateral anterolateral magnetic phrenic nerve stimulation in patients in the intensive care unit. Crit Care Med. 2001;29(7):1325-31.

13. Kim WY, Suh HJ, Hong SB, et al. Diaphragm dysfunction assessed by ultrasonography: Influence on weaning from mechanical ventilation. Crit Care Med. 2011;39(12):2627-30.
14. Dres M, Dubé BP, Mayaux J, et al. Coexistence and impact of limb muscle and diaphragm weakness at time of liberation from mechanical ventilation in medical intensive care unit patients. Am J Respir Crit Care Med. 2017;195(1):57-66.
15. Medrinal C, Prieur G, Frenoy É, et al. Respiratory weakness after mechanical ventilation is associated with one-year mortality—a prospective study. Crit Care. 2016;20(1):1-7.
16. Maes K, Stamiris A, Thomas D, et al. Effects of controlled mechanical ventilation on sepsis-induced diaphragm dysfunction in rats. Crit Care Med. 2014;42(12):e772-82.
17. Callahan LA, Nethery D, Stofan D, et al. Free radical-induced contractile protein dysfunction in endotoxin-induced sepsis. Am J Respir Cell Mol Biol. 2001;24(2):210-7.
18. Supinski GS, Wang W, Callahan LA. Caspase and calpain activation both contribute to sepsis-induced diaphragmatic weakness. J Appl Physiol (1985). 2009;107(5):1389-96.
19. Jung B, Nougaret S, Conseil M, et al. Sepsis is associated with a preferential diaphragmatic atrophy: a critically ill patient study using tridimensional computed tomography. Anesthesiology. 2014;120(5):1182-91.
20. Testelmans D, Maes K, Wouters P, et al. Rocuronium exacerbates mechanical ventilation-induced diaphragm dysfunction in rats. Crit Care Med. 2006;34(12):3018-23.
21. Laghi F, Tobin MJ. Disorders of the respiratory muscles. Am J Respir Crit Care Med. 2003;168(1):10-48.
22. Tobin MJ, Laghi F, Jubran A. Narrative review: ventilator-induced respiratory muscle weakness. Ann Intern Med. 2010;153(4):240-5.
23. Latronico N, Bolton CF. Critical illness polyneuropathy and myopathy: a major cause of muscle weakness and paralysis. Lancet Neurol. 2011;10(10):931-41.
24. Fan E, Cheek F, Chlan L, et al. ATS Committee on ICU-acquired Weakness in Adults; American Thoracic Society. An Official American Thoracic Society Clinical Practice Guideline: the diagnosis of intensive care unit-acquired weakness in adults. Am J Respir Crit Care Med. 2014;190(12):1437-46.
25. Visser LH. Critical illness polyneuropathy and myopathy: clinical features, risk factors and prognosis. Eur J Neurol. 2006;13(11):1203-12.
26. Vassilakopoulos T, Petrof BJ. Ventilator-induced diaphragmatic dysfunction. Am J Respir Crit Care Med. 2004;169(3):336-41.
27. Goligher EC, Dres M, Fan E, et al. Mechanical ventilation-induced diaphragm atrophy strongly impacts clinical outcomes. Am J Respir Crit Care Med. 2018;197(2):204-13.
28. Jaber S, Petrof BJ, Jung B, et al. Rapidly progressive diaphragmatic weakness and injury during mechanical ventilation in humans. Am J Respir Crit Care Med. 2011;183(3):364-71.
29. Grosu HB, Lee YI, Lee J, et al. Diaphragm muscle thinning in patients who are mechanically ventilated patients. Chest. 2012;142(6):1455-60.
30. Goligher EC, Fan E, Herridge MS, et al. Evolution of diaphragm thickness during mechanical ventilation: impact of inspiratory effort. Am J Respir Crit Care Med. 2015;192(9):1080-8.
31. Schepens T, Verbrugghe W, Dams K, et al. The course of diaphragm atrophy in ventilated patients assessed with ultrasound: a longitudinal cohort study. Crit Care. 2015;19:422.
32. Tang H, Lee M, Budak MT, et al. Intrinsic apoptosis in mechanically ventilated human diaphragm: linkage to a novel Fos/FoxO1/Stat3-Bim axis. FASEB J. 2011;25(9):2921-36.
33. Picard M, Jung B, Liang F, et al. Mitochondrial dysfunction and lipid accumulation in the human diaphragm during mechanical ventilation. Am J Respir Crit Care Med. 2013;186(11):1140-9.
34. Kavazis AN, Talbert EE, Smuder AJ, et al. Mechanical ventilation induces diaphragmatic mitochondrial dysfunction and increased oxidant production. Free Radic Biol Med. 2009;46(6):842-50.
35. Powers SK, Hudson MB, Nelson WB, et al. Mitochondria-targeted antioxidants protect against mechanical ventilation-induced diaphragm weakness. Crit Care Med. 2011;39(7):1749-59.
36. Levine S, Biswas C, Dierov J, et al. Increased proteolysis, myosin depletion, and atrophic AKT-FOXO signaling in human diaphragm disuse. Am J Respir Crit Care Med. 2011;183(4):483-90.
37. Hussain SN, Mofarrahi M, Sigala I, et al. Mechanical ventilation-induced diaphragm disuse in humans triggers autophagy. Am J Respir Crit Care Med. 2010;182(11):1377-86.
38. Smuder AJ, Hudson MB, Nelson WB, et al. Nuclear factor-κB signaling contributes to mechanical ventilation-induced diaphragm weakness. Crit Care Med. 2012;40(3):927-34.
39. Smuder AJ, Sollanek KJ, Min K, et al. Inhibition of forkhead box O-specific transcription prevents mechanical ventilation-induced diaphragm dysfunction. Crit Care Med. 2015;43(5):e133-42.
40. Agten A, Maes K, Thomas D, et al. Bortezomib partially protects the rat diaphragm from ventilator-induced diaphragm dysfunction. Crit Care Med. 2012;40(8):2449-55.
41. Betters JL, Criswell DS, Shanely RA, et al. Trolox attenuates mechanical ventilation-induced diaphragmatic dysfunction and proteolysis. Am J Respir Crit Care Med. 2004;170(11):1179-84.
42. McClung JM, Kavazis AN, Whidden MA, et al. Antioxidant administration attenuates mechanical ventilation-induced rat diaphragm muscle atrophy independent of protein kinase B (PKB-Akt) signalling. J Physiol. 2007;585(Pt 1):203-15.
43. Whidden MA, Smuder AJ, Wu M, et al. Oxidative stress is required for mechanical ventilation-induced protease activation in the diaphragm. J Appl Physiol (1685). 2010;108(5):1376-82.
44. Agten A, Maes K, Smuder A, et al. N-Acetylcysteine protects the rat diaphragm from the decreased contractility associated with controlled mechanical ventilation. Crit Care Med. 2011;39(4):777-82.
45. Powers SK, Wiggs MP, Duarte JA, et al. Mitochondrial signaling contributes to disuse muscle atrophy. Am J Physiol Endocrinol Metab. 2012;303(1):E31-9.
46. Schönfeld P, Wojtczak L. Fatty acids as modulators of the cellular production of reactive oxygen species. Free Radic Biol Med. 2008;45(3):231-41.

47. Romanello V, Sandri M. Mitochondrial biogenesis and fragmentation as regulators of protein degradation in striated muscles. J Mol Cell Cardiol. 2013;55:64-72.
48. van Hees HW, Schellekens WJ, Andrade Acuña GL, et al. Titin and diaphragm dysfunction in mechanically ventilated rats. Intensive Care Med. 2012;38(4):702-9.
49. Azuelos I, Jung B, Picard M, et al. Relationship between autophagy and ventilator-induced diaphragmatic dysfunction. Anesthesiology. 2015;122(6):1349-61.
50. van den Berg M, Hooijman PE, Beishuizen A, et al. Diaphragm atrophy and weakness in the absence of mitochondrial dysfunction in the critically ill. Am J Respir Crit Care Med. 2017;196(12):1544-58.
51. Anzueto A, Peters JI, Tobin MJ, et al. Effects of prolonged controlled mechanical ventilation on diaphragmatic function in healthy adult baboons. Crit Care Med. 1997;25(7):1187-90.
52. Powers SK, Shanely RA, Coombes JS, et al. Mechanical ventilation results in progressive contractile dysfunction in the diaphragm. J Appl Physiol (1985). 2002;92(5):1851-8.
53. Sassoon CSH, Caiozzo VJ, Manka A, et al. Altered diaphragm contractile properties with controlled mechanical ventilation. J Appl Physiol (1985). 2002;92(6):2585-95.
54. Yang L, Luo J, Bourdon J, et al. Controlled mechanical ventilation leads to remodeling of the rat diaphragm. Am J Respir Crit Care Med. 2002;166(8):1135-40.
55. Sassoon CS, Zhu E, Caiozzo VJ. Assist-control mechanical ventilation attenuates ventilator-induced diaphragmatic dysfunction. Am J Respir Crit Care Med. 2004;170(6):626-32.
56. Futier E, Constantin JM, Combaret L, et al. Pressure support ventilation attenuates ventilator-induced protein modifications in the diaphragm. Crit Care. 2008;12(5):R116.
57. Jung B, Constantin JM, Rossel N, et al. Adaptive support ventilation prevents ventilator-induced diaphragmatic dysfunction in piglet: an in vivo and in vitro study. Anesthesiology. 2010;112(6):1435-43.
58. Reid WD, Huang J, Bryson S, et al. Diaphragm injury and myofibrillar structure induced by resistive loading. J Appl Physiol (1985). 1994;76(1):176-84.
59. Jiang TX, Reid WD, Belcastro A, et al. Load dependence of secondary diaphragm inflammation and injury after acute inspiratory loading. Am J Respir Crit Care Med. 2012;157(1):230-6.
60. Jiang TX, Reid WD, Road JD. Delayed diaphragm injury and diaphragm force production. Am J Respir Crit Care Med. 2012;157 (3 Pt 1):736-42.
61. Orozco-Levi M, Lloreta J, Minguella J, et al. Injury of the human diaphragm associated with exertion and chronic obstructive pulmonary disease. Am J Respir Crit Care Med. 2001;164(9):1734-9.
62. Hillas G, Perlikos F, Toumpanakis D, et al. Controlled mechanical ventilation attenuates the systemic inflammation of severe chronic obstructive pulmonary disease exacerbations. Am J Respir Crit Care Med. 2016;193(6):696-8.
63. Laghi F, Cattapan SE, Jubran A, et al. Is weaning failure caused by low-frequency fatigue of the diaphragm? Am J Respir Crit Care Med. 2003;167(2):120-7.
64. Ebihara S, Hussain SNA, Danialou G, et al. Mechanical ventilation protects against diaphragm injury in sepsis: interaction of oxidative and mechanical stresses. Am J Respir Crit Care Med. 2012;165(2):221-8.
65. Sieck GC, Ferreira LF, Reid MB, et al. Mechanical properties of respiratory muscles. Compr Physiol. 2013;3(4):1553-67.
66. Proske U, Morgan DL. Muscle damage from eccentric exercise: mechanism, mechanical signs, adaptation and clinical applications. J Physiol. 2001;537(Pt 2):333-45.
67. Watchko JF, Johnson BD, Gosselin LE, et al. Age-related differences in diaphragm muscle injury after lengthening activations. J Appl Physiol (1985). 1994;77(5):2125-33.
68. Gea J, Zhu E, Gáldiz JB, et al. Functional consequences of eccentric contractions of the diaphragm. Arch Bronconeumol. 2009;45(2):68-74.
69. Thille AW, Rodriguez P, Cabello B, et al. Patient-ventilator asynchrony during assisted mechanical ventilation. Intensive Care Med. 2006;32(10):1515-22.
70. Akoumianaki E, Lyazidi A, Rey N, et al. Mechanical ventilation-induced reverse-triggered breaths: a frequently unrecognized form of neuromechanical coupling. Chest. 2013;143(4):927-38.
71. Pellegrini M, Hedenstierna G, Roneus A, et al. The diaphragm acts as a brake during expiration to prevent lung collapse. Am J Respir Crit Care Med. 2017;195(12):1608-16.
72. Baydur A. Decay of inspiratory muscle pressure during expiration in anesthetized kyphoscoliosis patients. J Appl Physiol (1985). 1992;72(2):712-20.
73. Supinski GS, Morris PE, Dhar S, et al. Diaphragm dysfunction in critical illness. Chest. 2018;153(4):1040-51.
74. Gilbert R, Auchincloss JH Jr, Peppi D. Relationship of rib cage and abdomen motion to diaphragm function during quiet breathing. Chest. 1981;80(5):607-12.
75. Diehl JL, Lofaso F, Deleuze P, et al. Clinically relevant diaphragmatic dysfunction after cardiac operations. J Thorac Cardiovasc Surg. 1994;107(2-):487-98.
76. Lerolle N, Guérot E, Dimassi S, et al. Ultrasonographic diagnostic criterion for severe diaphragmatic dysfunction after cardiac surgery. Chest. 2009;135(2):401-7.
77. Tobin MJ, Guenther SM, Perez W, et al. Konno-Mead analysis of ribcage-abdominal motion during successful and unsuccessful trials of weaning from mechanical ventilation1. Am Rev Respir Dis. 1987;135(6):1320-8.
78. American Thoracic Society/European Respiratory Society. ATS/ERS Statement on respiratory muscle testing. Am J Respir Crit Care Med. 2002;166(4):518-624.
79. Goldman MD, Grassino A, Mead J, et al. Mechanics of the human diaphragm during voluntary contraction: dynamics. J Appl Physiol Respir Environ Exerc Physiol. 1978;44(6):840-8.
80. Bellani G, Mauri T, Coppadoro A, et al. Estimation of patient's inspiratory effort from the electrical activity of the diaphragm. Crit Care Med. 2013;41(6):1483-91.
81. Akoumianaki E, Prinianakis G, Kondili E, et al. Physiologic comparison of neurally adjusted ventilator assist, proportional assist and pressure support ventilation in critically ill patients. Respir Physiol Neurobiol. 2014;203:82-9.
82. Jorens PG, Schepens T. Ultrasound: a novel translational tool to study diaphragmatic dysfunction in critical illness. Ann Transl Med. 2016;4(24):515.

83. Sarwal A, Walker FO, Cartwright MS. Neuromuscular ultrasound for evaluation of the diaphragm. Muscle Nerve. 2013;47(3):319-29.
84. Matamis D, Soilemezi E, Tsagourias M, et al. Sonographic evaluation of the diaphragm in critically ill patients. Technique and clinical applications. Intensive Care Med. 2013;39(5):801-10.
85. Boussuges A, Gole Y, Blanc P. Diaphragmatic motion studied by m-mode ultrasonography: methods, reproducibility, and normal values. Chest. 2009;135(2):391-400.
86. Cohn D, Benditt JO, Eveloff S, et al. Diaphragm thickening during inspiration. J Appl Physiol (1985). 1997;83(1):291-6.
87. Wait JL, Johnson RL. Patterns of shortening and thickening of the human diaphragm. J Appl Physiol (1985). 1997;83(4):1123-32.
88. Ueki J, De Bruin PF, Pride NB. In vivo assessment of diaphragm contraction by ultrasound in normal subjects. Thorax. 1995;50(11):1157-61.
89. de Bruin PF, Ueki J, Watson A, et al. Size and strength of the respiratory and quadriceps muscles in patients with chronic asthma. Eur Respir J. 1997;10:59-64.
90. Ferrari G, De Filippi G, Elia F. Diaphragm ultrasound as a new index of discontinuation from mechanical ventilation. Crit Ultrasound J. 2014;6(1):8.
91. Goligher EC, Laghi F, Detsky ME, et al. Measuring diaphragm thickness with ultrasound in mechanically ventilated patients: feasibility, reproducibility and validity. Intensive Care Med. 2015;41(4):642-9.
92. Brochard L, Slutsky A, Pesenti A. Mechanical ventilation to minimize progression of lung injury in acute respiratory failure. Am J Respir Crit Care Med. 2017;195(4):438-42.
93. Field S, Kelly SM, Macklem PT. The oxygen cost of breathing in patients with cardiorespiratory disease. Am Rev Respir Dis. 1982;126(1):9-13.
94. Aubier M, Viires N, Syllie G, et al. Respiratory muscle contribution to lactic acidosis in low cardiac output. Am Rev Respir Dis. 1982;126(4):648-52.
95. Masmoudi H, Coirault C, Demoule A, et al. Can phrenic stimulation protect the diaphragm from mechanical ventilation-induced damage? Eur Respir J. 2013;42(1):280-3.
96. Reynolds SC, Meyyappan R, Thakkar V, et al. Mitigation of ventilator-induced diaphragm atrophy by transvenous phrenic nerve stimulation. Am J Respir Crit Care Med. 2017;195(3):339-48.
97. Martin AD, Joseph AM, Beaver TM, et al. Effect of intermittent phrenic nerve stimulation during cardiothoracic surgery on mitochondrial respiration in the human diaphragm. Crit Care Med. 2014;42(2):e152-6.
98. Sinderby C, Navalesi P, Beck J, et al. Neural control of mechanical ventilation in respiratory failure. Nat Med. 1999;5(12):1433-6.
99. Dubé BP, Dres M, Mayaux J, et al. Ultrasound evaluation of diaphragm function in mechanically ventilated patients: comparison to phrenic stimulation and prognostic implications. Thorax. 2017;72:811-8.
100. Vivier E, Mekontso Dessap A, Dimassi S, et al. Diaphragm ultrasonography to estimate the work of breathing during non-invasive ventilation. Intensive Care Med. 2012;38(5):796-803.
101. Umbrello M, Formenti P, Longhi D, et al. Diaphragm ultrasound as indicator of respiratory effort in critically ill patients undergoing assisted mechanical ventilation: a pilot clinical study. Crit Care. 2015;19:161.
102. Smith IJ, Godinez GL, Singh BK, et al. Inhibition of Janus Kinase signaling during controlled mechanical ventilation prevents ventilation-induced diaphragm dysfunction. FASEB J. 2014;28(7):2790-803.
103. Tang H, Smith IJ, Hussain SN, et al. The JAK-STAT pathway is critical in ventilator-induced diaphragm dysfunction. Mol Med. 2015;20:579-89.
104. Hooijman PE, Beishuizen A, de Waard MC, et al. Diaphragm fiber strength is reduced in critically ill patients and restored by a troponin activator. Am J Respir Crit Care Med. 2014;189(7):863-5.
105. Dekhuijzen PN, Gayan-Ramirez G, de Bock V, et al. Triamcinolone and prednisolone affect contractile properties and histopathology of rat diaphragm differently. J Clin Invest. 1993;92(3):1534-42.
106. Maes K, Agten A, Smuder A, et al. Corticosteroid effects on ventilator-induced diaphragm dysfunction in anesthetized rats depend on the dose administered. Respir Res. 2010;11:178.
107. Sassoon CS, Zhu E, Fang L, et al. Interactive effects of corticosteroid and mechanical ventilation on diaphragm muscle function. Muscle Nerve. 2011;43(1):103-11.
108. Smuder AJ, Min K, Hudson MB, et al. Endurance exercise attenuates ventilator-induced diaphragm dysfunction. J Appl Physiol (1985). 2012;112(3):501-10.
109. Jung B, Sebbane M, Le Goff C, et al. Moderate and prolonged hypercapnic acidosis may protect against ventilator-induced diaphragmatic dysfunction in healthy piglet: an in vivo study. Crit Care. 2013;17(1):R15.
110. Juan G, Calverley P, Talamo C, et al. Effect of carbon dioxide on diaphragmatic function in human beings. N Engl J Med. 1984;310(14):874-9.
111. Michelet P, Carreira S, Demoule A, et al. Effects of acute respiratory and metabolic acidosis on diaphragm muscle obtained from rats. Anesthesiology. 2015;122(4):876-83.
112. Kim WY, Park SH, Kim WY, et al. Effect of theophylline on ventilator-induced diaphragmatic dysfunction. J Crit Care. 2016;33:145-50.
113. Doorduin J, Sinderby CA, Beck J, et al. The calcium sensitizer levosimendan improves human diaphragm function. Am J Respir Crit Care Med. 2012;185(1):90-5.
114. Bruells CS, Bergs I, Rossaint R, et al. Recovery of diaphragm function following mechanical ventilation in a rodent model. PLoS One. 2014;9(1):e87460.
115. Martin AD, Smith BK, Davenport PD, et al. Inspiratory muscle strength training improves weaning outcome in failure to wean patients: a randomized trial. Crit Care. 2011;15(2):R84.
116. Cader SA, Vale RG, Castro JC, et al. Inspiratory muscle training improves maximal inspiratory pressure and may assist weaning in older intubated patients: a randomised trial. J Physiother. 2010;56(3):171-7.

# CHAPTER 17

# Weaning from Mechanical Ventilation

*Abhay Vakil, Bryan Anderson, Kirtivardhan Vashistha, Rahul Kashyap*

## INTRODUCTION

Critically ill patients often require ventilatory support while underlying disease processes are addressed. Invasive or mechanical ventilation is one means of providing that support. Once the patient has been deemed ready for consideration of weaning from this support, proper steps must be taken to ensure safety with extubation. Delay in weaning is likely to cause more harm to the patient and may result in a variety of adverse outcomes including ventilator-associated pneumonia, ventilator-induced lung injury, respiratory muscle fatigue and atrophy, fewer ventilator free days, lengthier intensive care unit (ICU) stays, and even increase mortality. There is some variation in approach from clinician to clinician; however there have been landmark studies that support some methods of weaning from the ventilation over others. These methods are supported in clinical guideline recommendations published by the American Thoracic Society (ATS) as well as the European Respiratory Society (ERS) and will be discussed further.[1,2]

## DEFINITIONS

Weaning from mechanical ventilation is defined as a sudden or a step by step process of disengaging the patient from the ventilator.[2] It could be classified further:
- *Simple*: Comprises of patients who are weaned off in the first attempt and do not face any difficulties during or after extubation.
- *Difficult*: Comprises of patients who are unable to wean off in the first attempt and for successful weaning, require up to three spontaneous breathing trials (SBTs) or 7 days from first SBT.
- *Prolonged*: Includes patients who take more than 7 days after the first weaning attempt to wean off successfully. In defining weaning success or failure, time duration is one of the important factors.
- *Weaning success*: It is defined as successful extubation without any need of ventilatory support 48 hours after discontinuation.[2]
- *Weaning failure*: It is defined as when the patient is unable to pass a SBT or when reintubation and/or mechanical ventilation is indicated within 48 hours after extubation.[2]

## GENERAL APPROACH

A 2007 task force published guidelines on weaning from mechanical ventilation.[2] They outlined several stages through which the process of mechanical ventilation should typically proceed, from intubation through liberation from mechanical ventilation and potential reintubation. These six stages provide a helpful framework to understand the process. This chapter generally follows the same order as these stages, which are as follows:
- *Stage 1:* Treatment of acute respiratory failure
- *Stage 2:* Suspicion that weaning may be possible—this begins when the physician believes there is a reasonable probability of weaning success
- *Stage 3:* Assessment of readiness to wean—confirms the suspicion that weaning is possible through clinical and objective tests
- *Stage 4:* Spontaneous breathing trial
- *Stage 5:* Liberation from mechanical ventilation (also known as extubation)
- *Stage 6:* Reintubation, if needed.

## Stage 1

This is not addressed in this chapter as it regards the decision to place patients on mechanical ventilation.

## Stage 2

This is the first step of initiation of the weaning process. The biggest delay in extubation is usually at stage 2, when a physician fails to recognize the potential for weaning success. It has been demonstrated that relying on a physician's clinical judgment or "intuition" poorly identifies those capable of being weaned. One study showed that relying on clinical judgment for determining success of weaning had only 50% positive predictive value and 67% negative predictive value, indicating a bias toward ventilator dependency.[3] The physician subsequently fails to assess readiness to wean and mechanical ventilation is prolonged. Delay in weaning results in increased cost of care and higher risks of complications.[4] Thus, it is encouraged to move aggressively through stage 2 and into stage 3, as soon as the reason for respiratory failure or condition requiring mechanical ventilation has begun to improve.

## Stage 3: Assessing Readiness for Weaning

Assessing readiness for weaning (stage 3 above) occurs before performing a SBT. It is a process of determining who is ready to be weaned from the ventilator. As soon as there is suspicion that a patient is potentially weanable, readiness for weaning should be assessed daily. This is based on both clinical assessment and objective data.[2]

First and foremost the cause of the patient's respiratory failure should have been addressed and treated. Once the underlying cause has been addressed, there are a variety of reasons patients may remain dependent on MV. MacIntyre et al. suggest the following system-based categorization as basic etiologies of respiratory failure and ventilator dependency: neurologic, respiratory, cardiovascular, and psychological.[5] These four categories are reflected in the following recommendations:

- There should be evidence of reversal of the underlying cause of respiratory failure.
- The patient should have adequate oxygenation. No exact value for oxygenation has been rigorously established. It is reasonable however to target the following approximate values: $PaO_2/FiO_2$ >150 mm Hg, $SpO_2$ >90% while receiving $FiO_2$ of 40% or less and positive end-expiratory pressure (PEEP) of 5–8 $cmH_2O$.
- pH should be greater or equal to 7.25.
- The patient demonstrates hemodynamic stability without evidence of active myocardial ischemia or clinically significant hypotension. Rationale for this recommendation is based on the fact that the process of extubation will produce hemodynamic changes and increase cardiovascular demand. A reasonable goal for blood pressure would be to keep systolic blood pressure >90 mm Hg and <180 mm Hg. The use of vasoactive medications (i.e. vasopressors) is not a contraindication to weaning from mechanical ventilation as long as the dose is low. Higher reliance of vasoactive medications to achieve goal blood pressures is likely to result in increased respiratory and cardiovascular demand once the patient has been liberated from mechanical ventilation.
- The patients demonstrate capacity to initiate their own breath. This may be impaired for a variety of reasons including excessive sedation, acute or chronic neurologic diseases, critical care myopathy, severe electrolyte disturbances, potential airway obstructions, etc.
- The patient has an adequate cough and does not have excessive secretions. Cough strength is usually assessed by inserting the suctioning tubing through the endotracheal tube and into the trachea. This should result in a cough response by the patient. Absence of cough may result in reintubation due to aspiration and respiratory failure.

Other factors one might consider in assessing readiness for weaning are also related to the potential for increased metabolic demand as well as potential for extubation failure. These include adequate hemoglobin (>7 g/dL), absence of fever, and adequate mental status. Occasionally there are other factors that prohibit extubation, e.g. planned procedures and repeated surgeries. In these circumstances one should weigh the risks and benefits of prolonged mechanical ventilation against the potential for extubation with its attendant risks.

### *Weaning Predictors*

Weaning predictors are objective data gathered to determine readiness for weaning. These are tests conducted to predict likelihood of successful weaning. No single weaning predictor can guarantee success or failure of liberation from mechanical ventilation. Additionally, none should be used in isolation without the use of the clinical factors mentioned above. There have been many proposed tools for weaning prediction. The use of each varies depending on the clinician and institution. Rapid shallow breathing index (RSBI) is the most commonly used and has been used in published guidelines, in part because of its ease of use. Here we will review a few of the most commonly used weaning predictors:

- *Rapid shallow breathing index*
  First introduced in 1991 by Yang et al. RSBI is presently the most popular of weaning predictors. It is the ratio of respiratory frequency to tidal volume (in liters), expressed as f/Vt. As originally described, it is ideally calculated while a patient is breathing room air spontaneously for 1 minute in duration. As such, outcomes will vary from the original publication if it is being calculated while the patient is receiving pressure support ventilation (PSV), continuous positive airway pressure (CPAP), or other weaning modes of ventilation. Nevertheless, it remains a useful tool. Other studies have examined this as well.[3] At an RSBI greater than 105, there is a 95% negative predictive value of failing extubation. Below this level, there is a 78% positive predictive value for successfully weaning from mechanical ventilation. Thus it is best used to determine who is likely to fail weaning.
- *Minute ventilation (Ve)*
  Similar to RSBI, minute ventilation is calculated using respiratory rate and tidal volume: f × Vt. Normal values typically lie around 5-6 L/min. It is expected that very high minute ventilation would indicate increased metabolic demand or work of breathing, and thus predict weaning failure. A 2001 review[6] of weaning predictors determined that minute ventilation poorly predicts weaning outcome. However, high minute ventilation may portend failure of weaning.
- *Respiratory rate*
  Monitoring of respiratory rate is often intuitive. Indeed, it may be considered as part of clinical assessment. Nevertheless, several studies have demonstrated that rates >38 are more likely to predict failure of weaning, especially when used in concert with other weaning predictors.[4]
- *Maximal inspiratory pressure (MIP)*
  This is a measure of the patient's force of maximal inhalation. It is performed by manometry testing on the endotracheal tube. The patient is asked to inhale maximally and the negative pressure is measured in cm of $H_2O$. The more negative values demonstrate a greater maximal inspiratory capability by the patient and roughly reflect patient strength of respiration. Values less than equal to −20 $cmH_2O$ indicate higher likelihood of weaning failure. Very negative values have not definitively shown to be strong predictors of weaning success.[4] Patient cooperation may make this test difficult.

As mentioned previously, there are many other weaning predictors not described here. These include, but are not limited to occlusion pressure, work of breathing, compliance, oxygenation, gastric mucosal acidosis, inspiratory effort quotient, CROP index (compliance, respiratory rate, oxygenation, and pressure), pressure time product, weaning index, etc. Some of these tools attempt to integrate multiple physiologic scores and are more complicated to calculate. None has been singled out as a superior stand-alone test. Each has advantages and disadvantages.

## Stage 4: Spontaneous Breathing Trial

After readiness assessment has been performed and the patient is deemed a suitable candidate for weaning, a SBT should be conducted (Flowchart 1). This is also referred to as "weaning", and corresponds to stage 4 above. It is the process whereby a patient assumes more responsibility for respirations as the support from the ventilator is reduced. This can be done by decreasing the pressure support received, or decreasing the number of supported breaths.

Because intubated patients commonly require sedation, the SBT is usually performed concurrently with cessation of sedation. This allows for more adequate patient effort and assessment of neurologic status. Conducting sedation holiday and SBT together has been shown in randomized controlled trials (RCTs) to reduce both total ventilator days as well as mortality.[7]

### Methods of Conducting SBT

In general, most patients deemed appropriate for weaning can undergo a SBT once daily, for 30-120 minutes, on PSV with a pressure of 5-8 $cmH_2O$. Successful SBT is followed by extubation.

There are several ways of manipulating the ventilator to conduct the SBT. One can gradually decrease the number of supported breaths while intermittent mandatory ventilation (IMV) is used. Alternatively, providing less pressure in a pressure support mode may be used. Another choice is to disconnect the ventilator altogether and allow the patient to breathe through a T-piece. Although some trends and methods of SBT are preferred over others and are supported in published guidelines, no one method has been definitively deemed superior to others.

In the 1990s the question of whether to conduct a timed SBT versus a more gradual weaning of the vent was addressed in RCTs.[8,9] Esteban et al. found, in an RCT

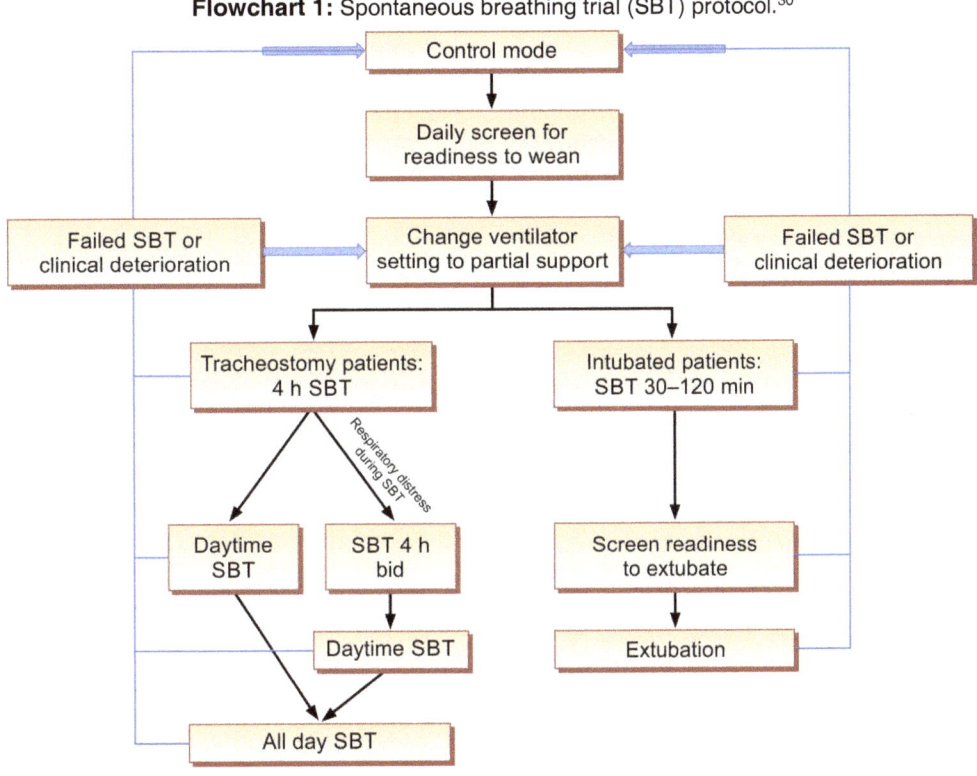

**Flowchart 1:** Spontaneous breathing trial (SBT) protocol.[30]

*Source:* Reproduced with permission from 'The Chinese Medical Association'; Copyright holder of Reference 30.

comparing four different weaning methods, that once-daily SBT leads to extubation more quickly than other methods. This was opposed to the idea that a continuous and gradual weaning of the vent may be better tolerated. Brochard et al. showed less weaning failure occurred when trial of PSV was used over IMV or T-piece.[8] From these and other studies, once a daily spontaneous trial of pressure support or T-piece has become the more accepted and popularized method of weaning. Indeed, in many ICUs the once-daily SBT has become a protocolized part of care of the intubated patient. In such circumstances, all patients that have been deemed appropriate candidates for weaning are scheduled to have sedation holiday and SBT concurrently in the morning on a daily basis until extubation is achieved.

A 2017 clinical practice guideline published by the American College of Chest Physician/American Thoracic Society (ACCP/ATS) conducted a review of the literature relative to SBTs.[1] They identified four prospective RCTs testing whether use of T-piece or modest PSV was superior. The breathing trials were conducted over a period of 30 minutes to 2 hours. Pressure support was "modest", set at 5–8 cmH$_2$O. Successful weaning was defined as no reintubation or noninvasive ventilation at 48 hours. The summary of these studies was that SBT was more successful with pressure support rather than T-piece. Such SBTs had higher rates of extubation success and there was a trend toward lower ICU mortality. This data culminated in the recommendation that SBT be conducted with pressure augmentation of 5 to 8 cmH$_2$O.

There are legitimate arguments to be made for alternative methods of conducting SBTs. For example, it logically follows that use of T-piece, which provides no extra pressure support, may require more effort by the patient. For this reason, a subset of patients who can pass a SBT with PSV may fail with T-piece trial. This may identify some patients who are not fully ready for extubation. It is imperative, as always, that appropriate clinical judgment be used.

The duration of SBT is usually between 30 minutes and 120 minutes. This is simply because several studies have used these durations. There is no definitively established best duration. In general, 30 minutes is probably sufficient. Those who have failed a SBT of 30 minutes duration may benefit from longer subsequent SBTs.

It is important to be able to determine weaning success versus failure. This determination is usually made on the basis of change in vital signs, ventilator parameters, and/or mental status. The development of significant tachycardia, tachypnea, fever, hemodynamic changes, change in oxygenation, poor tidal volumes, or mental status change should alert the physician that the patient is failing the SBT (Table 1). In such circumstances, the SBT should be terminated. There are not strict guidelines regarding these values. In previous weaning trials, however, some of these values included heart rate greater than 140 or a change of at least 20%, respiratory rate greater than 35, oxygen saturation less than 90%, systolic blood pressure greater than 180 or less than 90, agitation, diaphoresis, or anxiety.[8,9]

In cause evaluation for weaning failure, there must be a systematic approach to identify underlying problem (Table 2). Although it has been addressed in the readiness assessment noted previously, there should be proper evaluation of the patient's cough and quantity of secretions as well as alertness prior to extubation. Cough is usually assessed qualitatively rather than quantitatively by stimulus to the trachea. Although peak flow rate during cough may be measured, this is not required. It has been shown in several observational studies that there is a direct correlation between the strength of the cough and success of weaning.[10,11] Similarly correlated is the patient's ability to cough on command and follow other commands. Additionally the presence of excessive secretions (oral and endotracheal) is reason for concern as this has been correlated with extubation failure.[12] These patients are at elevated risk of aspiration and recurrent respiration failure with resultant reintubation.

Some patients are known to fail weaning due to laryngeal edema. These patients may require reintubation in order to maintain a secure and patent airway. A cuff leak test is an easy way to assess laryngeal edema. There are variations of this test. The basic test is conducted by deflating the cuff on the endotracheal tube and assessing for the passage of air around the tube when the patient initiates a breath. This can be done by listening with a stethoscope to the larynx, or may be detectable by listening for air passage by the patient's mouth. If one wishes to quantify the degree of air leak, one can observe the difference between inspired and expired tidal volume on the ventilator. Lack of air leak suggests the possibility of laryngeal edema, although the sensitivity and specificity of this determination is questionable.

Recent guidelines recommended performing a cuff leak in mechanically ventilated adults who meet extubation criteria and are deemed high risk for post-extubation stridor. This was a conditional recommendation with low certainty in the evidence.[1] Patients who were considered to be high risk for post-extubation stridor include patients who experienced a traumatic intubation, were intubated more than 6 days, have a large endotracheal tube, are female, or were reintubated after an unplanned extubation. Pooled analysis of data showed that sensitivity of the cuff leak test was only 52% and specificity was 92%.[13] Because not all patients who lack a cuff leak actually have laryngeal edema, there is a danger that performing the test will delay extubation unnecessarily. Nevertheless, it is probably good practice to perform a cuff leak test on high-risk patients, as noted above. The benefit being avoidance of both; reintubation and stridor, due to decreased laryngeal edema.

If there is no cuff leak, possible laryngeal edema may be treated with glucocorticoids. Glucocorticoids should be given at least 4 hours prior to extubation.[1] This has been shown to decrease both post-extubation stridor as well

**Table 1:** Signs and symptoms of spontaneous breathing trial failure.

| | Variable |
|---|---|
| Clinical assessment and subjective indices | • Agitation and anxiety<br>• Depressed mental status<br>• Diaphoresis<br>• Cyanosis<br>• Evidence of increasing effort:<br>  – Increased accessory muscle activity<br>  – Facial signs of distress<br>  – Dyspnea |
| Objective measurements | • $PaO_2 \leq 50–60$ mm Hg on $FiO_2 \geq 0.5$ or $SaO_2 <90\%$<br>• $PaCO_2 >50$ mm Hg or an increase in $PaCO_2 >8$ mm Hg<br>• pH <7.32 or a decrease in pH $\geq 0.07$ pH units<br>• $f_R/V_T >105$ breaths minutes$^{-1}$ L$^{-1}$<br>• $f_R >35$ breaths min$^{-1}$ or increased by $\geq 50\%$<br>• $f_C >140$ beats min$^{-1}$ or increased by $\geq 20\%$<br>• Systolic BP >180 mm Hg or increased by $\geq 20\%$<br>• Systolic BP $\leq 90$ mm Hg<br>• Cardiac arrhythmias |

($PaO_2$: arterial oxygen tension; $FiO_2$: inspiratory oxygen fraction; $SaO_2$: arterial oxygen saturation; $PaCO_2$: arterial carbon dioxide tension; $f_R$: respiratory frequency; $V_T$: tidal volume; $f_C$: cardiac frequency; BP: blood pressure; 1 mm Hg = 0.133 kPa)

*Source:* Reproduced with permission from "European Respiratory Society", copyright holder of Reference 2.

**Table 2:** A systematic approach to cause evaluation for weaning failure.

| | System | Look out for |
|---|---|---|
| Central and peripheral nervous system | Neurophysiological | • Delirium, anxiety, depression |
| | Decreased respiratory drive | • Sedative/hypnotic medications<br>• Primary CNS disease<br>• Metabolic alkalosis |
| | Peripheral dysfunction | • Electrolytes: Potassium, phosphate level<br>• Critical illness neuromyopathy<br>• Ventilator-induced diaphragm dysfunction<br>• Primary causes of neuromuscular weakness |
| Cardiovascular system | Pre-existing cardiac dysfunction | • Review history |
| | Acute myocardial dysfunction | • Septic cardiomyopathy<br>• Stress cardiomyopathy<br>• Increased metabolic demand<br>• Dynamic hyperinflation |
| Respiratory system | Decreased compliance | • Respiratory: Due to ventilator acquired pneumonia, cardiogenic or non-cardiogenic edema, pulmonary fibrosis, pulmonary hemorrhages, diffuse pulmonary infiltrates<br>• Extrapulmonary: Abdominal compartment syndrome |
| | Increased resistive load | • Bronchospasm<br>• Glottic edema<br>• Increased airway secretions<br>• Small endotracheal tube size |
| Metabolic system | | • Electrolytes: Potassium, magnesium level<br>• Metabolic disturbances: Role of corticosteroids, thyroid function, hyperglycemia |
| Nutrition | | • Overweight, malnutrition<br>• Electrolytes: Potassium, phosphate level<br>• Ventilator-induced diaphragm dysfunction |
| Hematological system | | • Hemoglobin |

(CNS: central nervous system; SBT: spontaneous breathing trial).

as reintubation rates.[14-16] 40 mg of methylprednisolone given 4 hours prior to extubation may be sufficient. If a higher dose is desired, another possible regimen is 20 mg methylprednisolone given every 4 hours starting 12 hours before extubation.[14,17]

## Stage 5: Extubation

In recent years there has been more research into methods of respiratory support after liberation from mechanical ventilation. Historically patients were placed on oxygen mask or nasal cannula. More recently, patients are increasingly being placed on noninvasive ventilation (NIV) or high flow humidified oxygen.

Noninvasive ventilation is likely to benefit patients at high risk for weaning failure. It may also benefit those with hypercapnia, chronic obstructive pulmonary disease (COPD), or chronic heart failure (CHF). A meta-analysis showed that the use of NIV post-extubation was associated with shorter hospital and ICU stay, and may also be related to improved mortality. Importantly, its use was *not* associated with increased risk of weaning failure or reintubation.[18] The benefits of NIV are best seen when applied immediately after extubation rather than waiting until the patient appears to be failing extubation. If delayed, some data indicates NIV could be potentially harmful.[19] Recently published joint European Respiratory Society/American Thoracic Society (ERS/ATS) clinical practice guidelines on the use of NIV give specific recommendations for its use in the post-extubation setting. They recommend the use of NIV to *prevent* post-extubation respiratory failure, but not as a rescue therapy in those who develop respiratory failure after extubation.[20] This reinforces the practice of using NIV immediately post extubation if it is to be used at all, and not delaying its use. Using NIV in a delayed manner may unnecessarily delay reintubation.

Respiratory support with high flow nasal cannula (HFNC) following extubation is less well established. A RCT showed that in low-risk patients, use of HFNC cannula reduced rates of reintubation at 72 hours compared with standard oxygen therapy.[21] This is only one trial and did not include high-risk patients. There was also no comparison with NIV. A second randomised clinical trial (RCT) used HFNC in relatively hypoxic patients, post-extubation, and compared this with venture mask use. This also showed improved reintubation rates with HFNC, although no mortality difference was seen. These two studies indicate that there may be a role for HFNC post extubation; however it should not be used as a substitute for NIV.

## WEANING AFTER PROLONG MECHANICAL VENTILATION

In critically ill patients on mechanical ventilation, weaning process in itself is a big challenge with weaning failure rates around 31%, ranging from 26% to 42%.[4,8,9] All patients with difficult or prolonged weaning process should be assessed for reversible causes and the physician should choose an appropriate mode of ventilation to:
- Maintain a good equilibrium between respiratory system capacity and load
- To reduce the chances of diaphragm muscle atrophy
- Help in the process of weaning.

Pressure assisted ventilation or assist-control ventilation should be used in patients with difficult and/or prolonged weaning process.[9] NIV is likely to benefit patients at high risk for weaning failure too. It may also benefit those with hypercapnia, COPD, or CHF to decrease the duration of intubation.[19] CPAP has shown some promise in patients with hypoxic respiratory failure after major surgery.[19]

One study showed that approximately 10% of patients in the ICU experience prolonged weaning failure and consume a large chunk of financial resources (~50%).[22] Other studies showed having 20% of the patients in the medical ICU on mechanical ventilation after 21 days.[22]

After having assessed for all the reversible causes which might be coming in the way of a successful weaning process, clinical outcomes in these patients are dependent on the nature of the comorbidities and the underlying primary pathology. Patient groups with neuromuscular and chest wall disorders when compared with the ones having COPD had less favorable outcomes but the COPD group had the highest mortality rate.[23]

These patients need individualization of weaning process, and these options might be considered during their management.

### Tracheostomy

These patients should be tracheotomized for prolonged mechanical ventilation for an easier airway management, patient comfort and communication, decreased sedative use, improved weaning outcomes and respiratory mechanics, reduced trauma to oropharyngeal pathway, and reduction in rates of pneumonia (ventilator-related).[2,24]

### Specialized Weaning Units

These groups of patients can benefit from specialized weaning units who can properly care for the ones on prolonged mechanical ventilation with the required focus, expertise, and organizational resources. They can act like a "bridge to home" and decrease the ICU-related clinical, social morbidity, and utilization of financial resources.[2] They can function in two types:[2]
1. Step-down units or noninvasive respiratory care units
2. Regional weaning centers.

### Home Ventilation

A subgroup of patients can benefit from home ventilation which can be provided in the form of NIV. A study done in 2002 showed that almost 32% of the population with COPD required home NIV.[25]

### Rehabilitation

Critically ill patients, especially the ones on prolonged mechanical ventilation, may experience physical deconditioning,[26] e.g. neuromyopathies, muscle atrophy, weakness, fatigue, etc. and active rehabilitation efforts with a focus on improving the quality of life and restoring the previous baseline health can improve clinical outcomes for these patients.[27]

### Terminal Care for the Ventilator-dependent Patients

Several studies have showed that a routine palliative care/ethics consult improves the quality of decision-making regarding the withdrawing mechanical ventilation in this patient group.[28,29] This type of an aid especially in a scenario where the patients lack decision-making capacity can help reach a goal-concordant care and a desired outcome.

## CONCLUSION

Weaning from mechanical ventilation is an essential aspect of critically ill patients. It begins with recognition that weaning is a possibility. As soon as the possibility is realized, readiness for weaning should be assessed based on clinical factors as well as weaning predictors. When ready, weaning should be undertaken. SBTs with pressure support should be used in the majority of patients unless there is reason to use an alternative approach. If the SBT is successful, the patient should be undertaken. Consideration of extubation to NIV can be given to high-risk patients or those with hypercapnia, COPD, or CHF. Once extubated, patients should be closely monitored for signs of respiratory failure and potential need for reintubation.

## SALIENT POINTS

- Weaning from mechanical ventilation is defined as a sudden or a step by step process of disengaging the patient from the ventilator. On the basis of the time and efforts required, weaning process can be grouped into being simple, difficult or prolonged.
- Weaning failure is defined as when the patient is unable to pass a SBT or when reintubation and/or mechanical ventilation is indicated within 48 hours after extubation.
- Process of weaning involves treatment of acute respiratory failure → suspicion that weaning may be possible → assessment of readiness to wean → spontaneous breathing trial → extubation → reintubation, if needed.
- Weaning predictors include RSBI, minute ventilation, respiratory rate, and maximal inspiratory pressure (MIP).
- Signs and symptoms of SBT failure include agitation and anxiety, depressed mental status, diaphoresis, cyanosis, and evidence of increased respiratory effort.
- Causes of weaning failure include increased respiratory load, increased cardiac load, neuromuscular causes, neurophysiological causes, metabolic causes, nutritional causes-anemia, etc.
- Pressure-assisted ventilation or assist-control ventilation should be used in patients with difficult and/or prolonged weaning process. NIV should be used in COPD patients and CPAP in hypoxic respiratory failure after major surgery.

## REFERENCES

1. Girard TD, Alhazzani W, Kress JP, et al. An Official American Thoracic Society/American College of Chest Physicians Clinical Practice Guideline: Liberation from Mechanical Ventilation in Critically Ill Adults. Rehabilitation Protocols, Ventilator Liberation Protocols, and Cuff Leak Tests. Am J Respir Crit Care Med. 2017;195(1):120-33.
2. Boles JM, Bion J, Connors A, et al. Weaning from mechanical ventilation. Eur Respir J. 2007;29(5):1033-56.
3. Stroetz RW, Hubmayr RD. Tidal volume maintenance during weaning with pressure support. Am J Respir Crit Care Med. 1995;152(3):1034-40.
4. Ely EW, Baker AM, Dunagan DP, et al. Effect on the duration of mechanical ventilation of identifying patients capable of breathing spontaneously. N Engl J Med. 1996;335(25):1864-9.
5. MacIntyre NR, Cook DJ, Ely EW Jr, et al. Evidence-based guidelines for weaning and discontinuing ventilatory support: a collective task force facilitated by the American College of Chest Physicians; the American Association for Respiratory Care; and the American College of Critical Care Medicine. Chest. 2001;120(6 Suppl):375S-95S.
6. Meade M, Guyatt G, Cook D, et al. Predicting success in weaning from mechanical ventilation. Chest. 2001;120 (6 Suppl):400S-24S.
7. Girard TD, Kress JP, Fuchs BD. Efficacy and safety of a paired sedation and ventilator weaning protocol for mechanically ventilated patients in intensive care (Awakening and Breathing Controlled trial): a randomised controlled trial. Lancet. 2008;371(9607):126-34.
8. Brochard L, Rauss A, Benito S, et al. Comparison of three methods of gradual withdrawal from ventilatory support during weaning from mechanical ventilation. Am J Respir Crit Care Med. 1994;150(4):896-903.
9. Esteban A, Frutos F, Tobin MJ, et al. A comparison of four methods of weaning patients from mechanical ventilation. Spanish Lung Failure Collaborative Group. N Engl J Med. 1995;332(6):345-50.
10. Salam A, Tilluckdharry L, Amoateng-Adjepong Y, et al. Neurologic status, cough, secretions and extubation outcomes. Intensive Care Med. 2004;30(7):1334-9.
11. Beuret P, Roux C, Auclair A, et al. Interest of an objective evaluation of cough during weaning from mechanical ventilation. Intensive Care Med. 2009;35(6):1090-3.
12. Thille AW, Boissier F, Ben Ghezala H, et al. Risk factors for and prediction by caregivers of extubation failure in ICU patients: a prospective study. Crit Care Med. 2015;43(3):613-20.
13. Ochoa ME, Marín Mdel C, Frutos-Vivar F, et al. Cuff-leak test for the diagnosis of upper airway obstruction in adults: a systematic review and meta-analysis. Intensive Care Med. 2009;35(7):1171-9.
14. François B, Bellissant E, Gissot V, et al. 12-h pretreatment with methylprednisolone versus placebo for prevention of postextubation laryngeal oedema: a randomised double-blind trial. Lancet. 2007;369(9567):1083-9.
15. Cheng KC, Hou CC, Huang HC, et al. Intravenous injection of methylprednisolone reduces the incidence of postextubation stridor in intensive care unit patients. Crit Care Med. 2006;34(5):1345-50.
16. Cheng KC, Chen CM, Tan CK, et al. Methylprednisolone reduces the rates of postextubation stridor and reintubation associated with attenuated cytokine responses in critically ill patients. Minerva Anestesiol. 2011;77(5):503-9.
17. Ladeira MT, Vital FM, Andriolo RB, et al. Pressure support versus T-tube for weaning from mechanical ventilation in adults. Cochrane Database Syst Rev. 2014;(5):CD006056.
18. Burns KE, Adhikari NK, Keenan SP, et al. Noninvasive positive pressure ventilation as a weaning strategy for intubated adults with respiratory failure. Cochrane Database Syst Rev. 2010;(8):CD004127.

19. Esteban A, Frutos-Vivar F, Ferguson ND, et al. Noninvasive positive-pressure ventilation for respiratory failure after extubation. N Engl J Med. 2004;350(24):2452-60.
20. Rochwerg B, Brochard L, Elliott MW, et al. Official ERS/ATS clinical practice guidelines: noninvasive ventilation for acute respiratory failure. Eur Respir J. 2017;50(2).
21. Maggiore SM, Idone FA, Vaschetto R, et al. Nasal high-flow versus Venturi mask oxygen therapy after extubation. Effects on oxygenation, comfort, and clinical outcome. Am J Respir Crit Care Med. 2014;190(3):282-8.
22. Cohen IL, Booth FV. Cost containment and mechanical ventilation in the United States. New Horiz. 1994;2(3):283-90.
23. Pilcher DV, Bailey MJ, Treacher DF, et al. Outcomes, cost and long term survival of patients referred to a regional weaning centre. Thorax. 2005;60(3):187-92.
24. Kurek CJ, Cohen IL, Lambrinos J, et al. Clinical and economic outcome of patients undergoing tracheostomy for prolonged mechanical ventilation in New York State during 1993: analysis of 6,353 cases under diagnosis-related group 483. Crit Care Med. 1997;25(6):983-8.
25. Schönhofer B, Euteneuer S, Nava S, et al. Survival of mechanically ventilated patients admitted to a specialised weaning centre. Intensive Care Med. 2002;28(7):908-16.
26. Herridge MS, Cheung AM, Tansey CM, et al. One-year outcomes in survivors of the acute respiratory distress syndrome. N Engl J Med. 2003;348(8):683-93.
27. Jones C, Skirrow P, Griffiths RD, et al. Rehabilitation after critical illness: a randomized, controlled trial. Crit Care Med. 2003;31(10):2456-61.
28. Dowdy MD, Robertson C, Bander JA. A study of proactive ethics consultation for critically and terminally ill patients with extended lengths of stay. Crit Care Med. 1998;26(2):252-9.
29. Schneiderman LJ, Gilmer T, Teetzel HD, et al. Effect of ethics consultations on nonbeneficial life-sustaining treatments in the intensive care setting: a randomized controlled trial. JAMA. 2003;290(9):1166-72.
30. Lee YC, Wang HC, Hsu CL, et al. The importance of tracheostomy to the weaning success in patients with conscious disturbance in the respiratory care center. J Chin Med Assoc. 2016;79(2):72-6.

# CHAPTER 18

# Aerosol Drug Delivery in Ventilated Patient

*O Kalchiem-Dekel, MG Allison, A Sachdeva*

## INTRODUCTION

Delivery of aerosolized drugs to mechanically ventilated patients differs significantly from the delivery of similar medications to spontaneously breathing patients. Several important factors result in significant difference in aerosol delivery and lung deposition between spontaneously breathing and mechanically ventilated patients. These include the ventilator-generated driving force, the ventilator circuit, the need for adaptive devices, and the varied nature of the underlying disease processes resulting in the need for mechanical ventilation. Other factors that affect the efficacy of drug delivery and deposition in the lungs in mechanically ventilated patients include the properties of the delivery device, molecular composition and properties of the drug, as well as the mode of mechanical ventilation, type of artificial airway, location of the delivery device along the ventilator circuit, and temperature and humidity of the cycled air. Understanding these differences is essential in order to provide adequate dosing and delivery of aerosolized medications to ventilated patients.

Although standardized protocols are often implemented in many centers, surveys have previously demonstrated that the practice of aerosolized drug administration can in fact vary both between intensive care units (ICUs) and between providers within the same ICU.[1] Many factors affect this therapeutic intervention. As such, maintaining standardized and evidence-based techniques for delivery of aerosols to mechanically ventilated patients is likely to maximize therapeutic efficacy by optimizing drug deposition at target receptors within the airways and the lungs and providing consistent and reproducible dosing, while maintaining patient safety.

Indeed, for many years, delivery of inhaled medications to mechanically ventilated patients was hampered by low lung deposition with rates of 10–15% of the total prescribed, or nominal, dose. More recently, experimental models have clarified some aspects of the mechanisms involved in drug delivery and deposition.[2] This has led to the development of new devices and more advanced techniques that allow more efficient delivery of up to 70% of the nominal medication dose into the lower respiratory tract, even surpassing the deposition fraction frequently achieved in spontaneously breathing patients.

This chapter focuses on practical aspects of aerosol delivery in mechanically ventilated patients, emphasizing commonly used drugs and delivery systems that are commercially available for routine application in the ICU setting.

## FACTORS AFFECTING ADEQUATE AEROSOL DELIVERY IN MECHANICAL VENTILATED PATIENTS

The factors affecting the efficiency of aerosol deposition within the respiratory system can be classified into patient related (e.g. airway anatomy, respiratory physiology, differential aeration of lung regions, and underlying pulmonary pathology) and nonpatient related (e.g. chemo-physical characteristics of the aerosolized drug, dosing, delivery system, position of the delivery device along the mechanical ventilator circuit, ventilation mode and settings, and degree of air humidification). Moreover, pulmonary diseases differ in the target site for drug delivery. To illustrate, in obstructive airway diseases, including chronic obstructive pulmonary disease (COPD) and asthma, target bronchodilator receptors can be mainly found in the proximal bronchial tree (up to the 10-generation branching), whereas in other conditions such as bacterial pneumonia or pulmonary hypertension, the relevant drug targets may be more distal and situated mainly in the alveolar ducts, alveoli, and even the pulmonary microcirculation. In addition, the physical characteristics of particle deposition vary significantly along the tracheo-broncho-bronchiolo-alveolar tree. Whereas inertial impaction dominates along the first 10 airway generations, gravitational sedimentation dominates along airway generations 11-16, and Brownian diffusion motion dominates particle deposition in the respiratory bronchioles, alveolar ducts, and alveoli. The depth of penetration into the respiratory tree and thus the mechanism of deposition are dependent mainly on particle size.[3] Hence, establishing a firm clinical-pharmacological correlation is critical in the treatment decision-making process.

## Patient-related Factors

### Pulmonary Anatomy

Even among healthy volunteers, drug deposition has been shown to favor the right lung[4] and this pattern is accentuated in the mechanically ventilated critically ill patient, regardless of underlying lung involvement.[5] Moreover, when critical illness combines with pulmonary disease, proximal aerosol deposition should be expected.[6] To illustrate, in patients with obstructive lung disease due to bronchoconstriction or endoluminal bronchial secretions, the decrease in airway cross-sectional area results in higher flow velocities and hence increased turbulence, leading to increased proximal drug deposition.[7] Additionally, obesity or obstructive lung conditions result in air flow diversion into less-obstructed airways. This nonuniform distribution of drug delivery may also result in diversion of the aerosol from the areas of disease and into the more healthy respiratory zones.[8] In a similar vein, the abnormal airway architecture of bronchiectasis can result in modified airflow dynamics and alter the patterns of drug deposition and distribution within the respiratory system.[9]

### Airway Clearance Mechanisms

Altered mucus composition, impairment of the mucociliary clearance apparatus, mucus impaction, and resultant airway narrowing and turbulent airflows are inherent to bronchiectatic lung diseases, such as cystic fibrosis (CF), but are also described in obstructive lung diseases, such as asthma and COPD. These factors can impair aerosolized drug deposition by entrapping drug molecules within the thick mucus layer, promoting more proximal aerosol deposition and thus reducing the effective drug dose at target sites.[3]

### Lung Aeration

Differential lung aeration exists both in the upright and the recumbent positions. While particle deposition tends to favor the apical zones of the lung in the upright position, the anterior lung portions have been shown to be favored in the supine position.[10] Moreover, different pulmonary disease states may involve the lung in a heterogeneous manner, promoting differential airflow patterns and thus heterogeneous aerosol deposition. For example, acute respiratory distress syndrome (ARDS) is associated with relative surfactant deficiency and regional atelectasis. Naturally, aerosol deposition in the atelectatic lung units is reduced.[11] In patients who are unable to remain seated during aerosol administration, these data form the rationale for the recommendation to perform aerosolized drug delivery while the patient's head is elevated at 30° to the semirecumbent position if possible.[12]

## Nonpatient-related Factors

### Physical Drug Properties

Particle size as defined by mass median aerodynamic diameter (MMAD) is a major determinant of both nominal delivered dose and area of distribution and deposition. In general, aerosols with MMAD in the range of 5-10 μm deposit mainly in the large conducting airways, particles in the range of 1-5 μm deposit in the smaller airways, and more than 50% of 3 μm or smaller-sized particles deposit in the alveoli.[6] For beta-agonists, the particle size of less than or equal to 5 but more than 1.5 μm has been associated with a favorable therapeutic effect; particles less than or equal to 1.5 μm have been shown to result in less favorable response, perhaps as a result of overtly distal deposition.[13,14] For the inhaled muscarinic antagonist, ipratropium bromide, favorable therapeutic effect has been observed with particle MMAD of up to 7.7 μm, likely due to a more proximal position of target receptors within the bronchial tree.[15] Importantly, while smaller particles may penetrate deeper, they also contain smaller amount of active drug. Hence, the complex relation between particle MMAD and nominal dose has a major potential impact on overall therapeutic drug efficacy.

Adding further to the complexity of aerosol delivery is the concept of airway humidity. For hygroscopic particles, natural or artificial humidification of inhaled air results in an increase in particle size, thus resulting in altered deposition kinetics. The degree of particle growth depends on initial particle size, e.g. the relative increase in size is most significant in the particles with the smallest initial size. Temperature also affects the magnitude of change in particle size with greater size increase at relatively higher temperatures.[16] Therefore, for certain hygroscopic medications such as albuterol sulfate, heating and humidification of the ventilator circuit are likely to have a detrimental effect on drug delivery,[17] which needs to be taken into consideration. This impact of heat and humidity may potentially be overcome by increasing the nominal dose.[12]

## Drug Dose

Even with meticulous methodology in delivery system assembly and drug administration, one should anticipate some nominal dose loss along the ventilator circuit, artificial airway, and large conducting airways, i.e. the trachea and mainstem bronchi. Dose adjustments may be required to compensate for this loss. The degree of adjustment depends on factors such as the type of medication, delivery device, and underlying disease pathophysiology. While not a fundamental characteristic of pressurized metered-dose inhaler (pMDI), drug retainment in the range of 3–50% of the nominal dose is common to all forms of nebulizers (discussed in later section). Of the dose that leaves the nebulizer chamber, between 10% and 40% of the medication is likely to get trapped within the ventilator circuit, never reaching the artificial airway.[18] Deposition within the artificial and large conducting airways accounts for additional 1–27% of nominal dose loss.[18] Furthermore, between 7% and 20% of the nominal dose is eliminated during expiration.[18] Dose increase may seem like a simple solution to this problem, however it presents a dilemma of increased risk for drug adverse reactions and requirement for longer nebulization time, which may not be tolerated by all critically ill patients. Therefore, drug dosing should probably be determined based on clinical-pharmacological correlation and on a case-to-case basis, depending on delivery system, drug formulation, and underlying patient condition. Consultation with a clinical pharmacologist with expertise in care of critically ill patients may be indispensable in these cases.

## Ventilator Settings

Given the multitude of ventilation modes available, there is no one agreed upon setting for optimal delivery of aerosols. Currently, no guidelines are available to support the decision as to the best ventilation mode that will assure adequate aerosol delivery. As a general rule, the more turbulent the flow, the more drug is likely to be deposited along the ventilator circuit, the artificial airway, and the large conductive airways, resulting in less effective medication dose deposited along the distal airways and in the alveoli. At the same time, some ventilator settings, thought to be optimal for aerosol delivery, may not be tolerated by severely hypoxemic patients. Therefore, any adjustment in ventilator settings made for the purpose of aerosol delivery must be weighed against patient requirements and clinical status. Table 1 provides current evidence regarding preferred ventilator settings for efficient aerosol delivery. For delivery of medications via a mesh nebulizer, volume-controlled ventilation has been shown to be superior to pressure support mode in one study;[19] however, in a separate study, aerosol administration via a pMDI was not shown to vary significantly when comparing volume-controlled, pressure support, and continuous positive airway pressure modes.[20] Similarly, for nebulized but not pMDI-delivered drugs, higher bias flow of 5.0 L/min (LPM) compared with lower bias flow of 2.0 LPM has been associated with reduced efficacy of delivery.[17] This phenomenon is accounted by increased aerosol washout into the expiratory limb with higher bias flow rates. A decelerating flow pattern was shown to be inferior to constant flow pattern for nebulized aerosol delivery.[21] Settings that are demonstrated to have a favorable result

**Table 1:** Ventilator settings shown to be associated with improved distal aerosol delivery.

| Setting | pMDI | Jet nebulizer | Vibrating mesh nebulizer |
| --- | --- | --- | --- |
| Tidal volume | ≥ 500 mL[19] | ≥ 500 mL[21] | ≥ 500 mL[20,21] |
| Duty cycle ($T_{inspiration}:T_{total}$ Ratio) | 0.3–0.5[2,19] | 0.3–0.5[22,23] | 0.3[28] |
| Inspiratory flow rate | 15–40 L/min[2,24] | 15–40 L/min[25,31] | 30 L/min[19,20] |
| Constant versus decelerating flow pattern | No difference[19,26] | Constant[26] | Constant[17] |
| Bias flow | Not affected[17] | ≤ 10 L/min[21] 2 L/min[17] | ≤ 10 L/min[20,21] 2 L/min[17] |
| Additional settings | Holding chamber[2,24] Synchronization with inspiration[19,27] | Spacer chamber[23] Synchronization with inspiration[21] | Synchronization with inspiration[21] |

(pMDI: pressurized metered-dose inhaler)

on aerosol deposition when delivered via pMDI include inspiratory flow rate of less than 60 LPM and preferably between 15 LPM and 40 LPM, likely secondary to reduction in turbulent flow;[22,23] longer inspiratory to total cycle time ratio (duty cycle) of 0.3 to 0.5 when compared with lower ratios; and tidal volume more than or equal to 500 mL.[20] In one animal model of ARDS, aerosol absorption into the bloodstream has been shown to be improved by addition of 10 cm $H_2O$ of positive end-expiratory pressure (PEEP), possibly as result of better alveolar recruitment.[24] However, in a later model, no difference between 0 cm $H_2O$ and 10 cm $H_2O$ of PEEP was demonstrated.[25] In patients requiring ventilator support for COPD exacerbation, setting the PEEP in a fashion that ameliorated intrinsic PEEP was shown to result in an improved response to the inhaled beta-agonist, salbutamol.[26]

As previously mentioned, humidification of inspired air results in expansion of hygroscopic particle diameter. This effect resulted in 40–50% decrease in aerosol delivery distal to the artificial airway in an in vitro model.[17] Some experts therefore recommend to turn off the ventilator-associated heated humidifier during therapy. This action must be balanced against the risk of respiratory mucosal damage, bronchospasm, and mucus impaction due to insufflation of the circuit with cold and dry air. Moreover, shutting down the heated humidifier may not immediately result in the anticipated increase in distal aerosol deposition since enough time is required to allow washout of residual water condensate from the ventilator circuit and the aerosol spacer chamber. This optimal time period is not currently known.[27] Nonetheless, a report based on *in vivo* data suggests that the reported degree of delivery impairment that is a result of circuit humidification may be overestimated.[28] When using a nebulizer device for delivery (also see section on nebulizers), incorporating the nebulizer into the "dry side" of the heated humidifier may provide better delivery results while allowing continuous heating and humidification of the inspired air.[17]

Many ICUs use heat and moisture exchanger (HME) as an adjunct or an alternative for a heated humidifier. Currently, the effect of HME devices on aerosol delivery is poorly defined.[29] However, experts recommend removing the HME during therapy as it represents a physical barrier to particle delivery.[12] Similarly, exchange of the particulate air filter on the expiratory ventilation limb should be considered following each individual treatment cycle to prevent filter clogging and airflow obstruction.[30]

### Type of Airway Access

The artificial airway often represents the point of highest resistance to flow across the ventilator circuit due to its relatively narrow caliber. Higher resistance results in higher flow rate which in turn results in more turbulence and less laminar flow. Hence, theoretically, greater diameter of the artificial airway should induce greater aerosol delivery distal to the artificial circuit, independent of delivery device and drug type. This rule however is likely more relevant to pediatric patient populations. In adults, nebulized aerosol loss was not significantly different when compared between 7.0 mm and 9.0 mm endotracheal tubes (ETTs).[31] Although tracheostomy tubes are shorter and tend to retain less medication than ETT, they also possess a significant curve that promotes aerosol impaction. Similarly, a right-angled swivel connector and/or the incorporation of a suction catheter adaptor between the Y-piece and the artificial airway may hamper laminar flow. Application of in-line connectors may bypass this potential problem.[32] Like ETT, tracheostomy tubes can accommodate both pMDI and nebulizer devices. During aerosol delivery via a tracheostomy tube, the inner cannula should preferably be removed thus increasing the effective airway diameter. However, when patients have fenestrated tracheostomy tubes, the fenestrations should be closed by insertion of a nonfenestrated inner cannula. In spontaneously breathing patients with tracheostomy tube in place, delivery via a T-piece has been shown to be more efficient than via a tracheostomy mask or via positioning the nebulizer in direct alignment with the tracheostomy port.[33]

## AEROSOL DELIVERY DEVICES AND THEIR INTEGRATION INTO THE VENTILATOR CIRCUIT

Currently available delivery apparatus commonly used in the ICU are pMDI and different types of nebulizers. Use of dry powder inhalers (DPIs) in patients requiring mechanical ventilation is hampered by deleterious effect of air heating and humidification on the powdered aerosol particles.[34] Furthermore, technical difficulties in introduction of powdered aerosolized particles into the ventilator circuit require further research and standardization before any recommendations regarding routine use of DPI in mechanically ventilated patients can be made. The use of soft mist inhalers in patients requiring mechanical ventilation remains a focus of ongoing research.[35] A great bulk of literature explored the utility of different delivery devices in multiple setups for promoting adequate nominal dose delivery of aerosolized drugs into the respiratory system of ventilator-dependent patients. Reports vary with respect to definitions of effective delivered dose and aerosol retention in the artificial circuit. This variability is accounted for a multitude of factors, such as differences in model systems (artificial ventilator and lung model, animal model, or human based), delivery devices, device incorporation into the ventilator circuit, of the studied aerosolized medication, means to measure pulmonary drug delivery, and, in human studies, different patient populations.

Choosing an optimal system requires consideration of many factors. These include drug formulations available via pharmacy, ventilator brand, direct drug and device costs, as well as indirect expenses such as disinfection costs and costs related to adverse effects of therapy. In contrast to pMDI, nebulizer systems require meticulous cleaning and disinfection after each use due to the risk of bacterial colonization and predisposition of patients to nosocomial upper and lower respiratory tract infections. Devices that require breach or interruption of the ventilator circuit predispose the patient to the consequences of intermittent cessation of ventilation and oxygenation as well as contamination of the circuit. Newer generation adapters, spacers, and holding chambers that are installed in-line with the ventilator tubing and remain in place between treatments may provide a partial solution for this problem.

Examples of commercially available pMDI adapters and various nebulizers are shown in Figures 1A to C and 2A to E. Table 2 provides suggested algorithms for standardized incorporation and operation of pMDI, jet nebulizer, and vibrating mesh nebulizer in ventilator-dependent patients.

## Pressurized Metered-Dose Inhalers

A typical pMDI consists of a meter-valved canister connected to an actuator that is designed to be used by a spontaneously breathing patient. Hence, an adapter device is required to allow instillation of pMDI-contained drug from the canister into the ventilator circuit. As illustrated

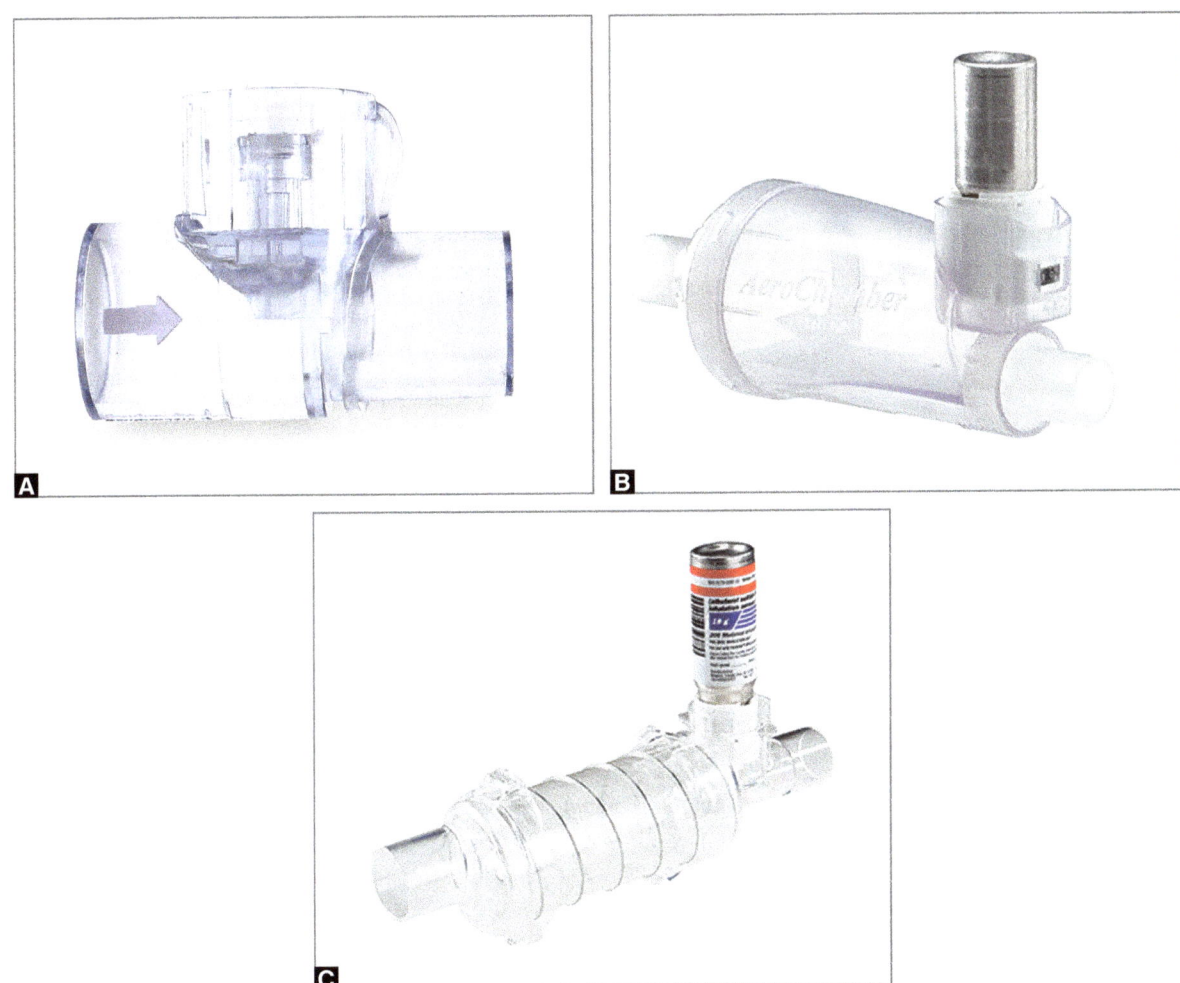

**Figs. 1A to C:** Ventilator adaptors for pressurized metered-dose inhaler (pMDI) application. All adaptors can accommodate canister with or without actuation counter. Arrows mark the direction of flow toward the patient. (A) SMDIA-1000™ MDI in-line adaptor (Reproduced with permission from Southmedic®). (B) AeroChamber Mini™ in-line holding chamber (Monaghan®). (C) AeroVent Plus™ collapsible holding chamber (Monaghan®).

**Table 2:** Suggested algorithm for optimal aerosol delivery.

Preparatory tasks common to all procedures:
- Verify medication order, including type, dose, and frequency
- Review patient's chart to obtain pertinent medical-, nursing-, and respiratory care-related information
- Sanitize hands and wear gloves. Don other protective equipment as necessary
- Identify patient using two identifiers
- Verify expiration date on the canister or drug sachet
- Explain the procedure to the patient and/or family member as appropriate
- Place patient in a sitting or semi-seated position, unless contraindicated
- Assess patient mental status, heart rate, respiratory rate, and skin color. Auscultate to the patient's chest
- If appropriate, turn off, but do not disconnect, the heated humidifier for a prespecified amount of time, based on local protocol
- Adjust ventilator settings, if patient condition permitting:
  - Achieve tidal volume of $\geq 500$ mL, while maintaining a plateau pressure of $\leq 30$ cm $H_2O$
  - Set duty cycle to 0.30–0.50 as tolerated and/or inspiratory flow to 15–40 L/min as tolerated. Ensure intrinsic PEEP does not develop
  - Do not change set PEEP and $FIO_2$
- Suction the airways.

*Pressurized metered-dose inhaler*
- Shake the pMDI vigorously
- Prime the pMDI by releasing several actuations into room air if necessary
- Attach pMDI canister to the spacer chamber adapter and place in ventilator circuit about 15 cm from the Y-piece
- If relevant, remove the HME and ensure there is no leak in the circuit
- Actuate pMDI in coordination with the inspiratory phase of the ventilator
- Allow at 30–60 seconds to elapse between actuations until full dose is delivered
- Detach pMDI canister from the adapter

*Jet nebulizer*
- Fill a volume of 4–6 mL of drug suspension into the nebulizer chamber
- Fill the manufacturer-recommended volume of drug suspension into the nebulizer chamber, keeping the nebulizer in an upright position
- Attach the nebulizer to the ventilator circuit. Possible locations along the circuit depend on local protocol and include:
  - "Dry side" of the heated humidifier; and
  - On the inspiratory limb, 40 cm proximal to the Y-piece
- Turn off continuous flow or flow-by during nebulizer operation
- If relevant, remove the HME and ensure there is no leak in the circuit
- Use the ventilator if it meets nebulizer flow requirement or an external source to apply gas flow to the nebulizer according to manufacturer recommendations (usually between 2 L/min and 8 L/min)
- If necessary, adjust minute ventilation to accommodate the added flow
- Allow enough delivery time and tap the nebulizer periodically
- Remove the nebulizer from the circuit
- Revert to original ventilator settings if changed for aerosol delivery
- Rinse and dry nebulizer according to manufacturer recommendations

*Vibrating mesh nebulizer*
- Assemble nebulizer and, if indicated, perform functionality testing prior to use. Avoid touching the mesh
- Fill the manufacturer-recommended volume of drug suspension into the nebulizer chamber, keeping the nebulizer in an upright position
- Attach the nebulizer to the ventilator circuit. Possible locations along the circuit depend on local protocol and drug administered:
  - "Dry side" of the heated humidifier
  - At a distance of 45 cm proximal to the Y-piece
  - At the ETT
- If relevant, remove the HME and ensure there is no leak in the circuit
- Turn on the nebulizer and allow enough delivery time
- Remove the nebulizer from the circuit
  - Clean the nebulizer according to manufacturer recommendations

Postprocedure tasks common to all procedures:
- Reconnect the HME and/or turn on the heated humidifier unit
- Monitor patient for adverse response
- Document medication administration
- Change the expiratory limb particulate air filter

(ETT: endotracheal tube; $FIO_2$: fraction of inspired oxygen; HME: heat and moisture exchanger; PEEP: positive end-expiratory pressure; pMDI: pressurized metered-dose inhaler)

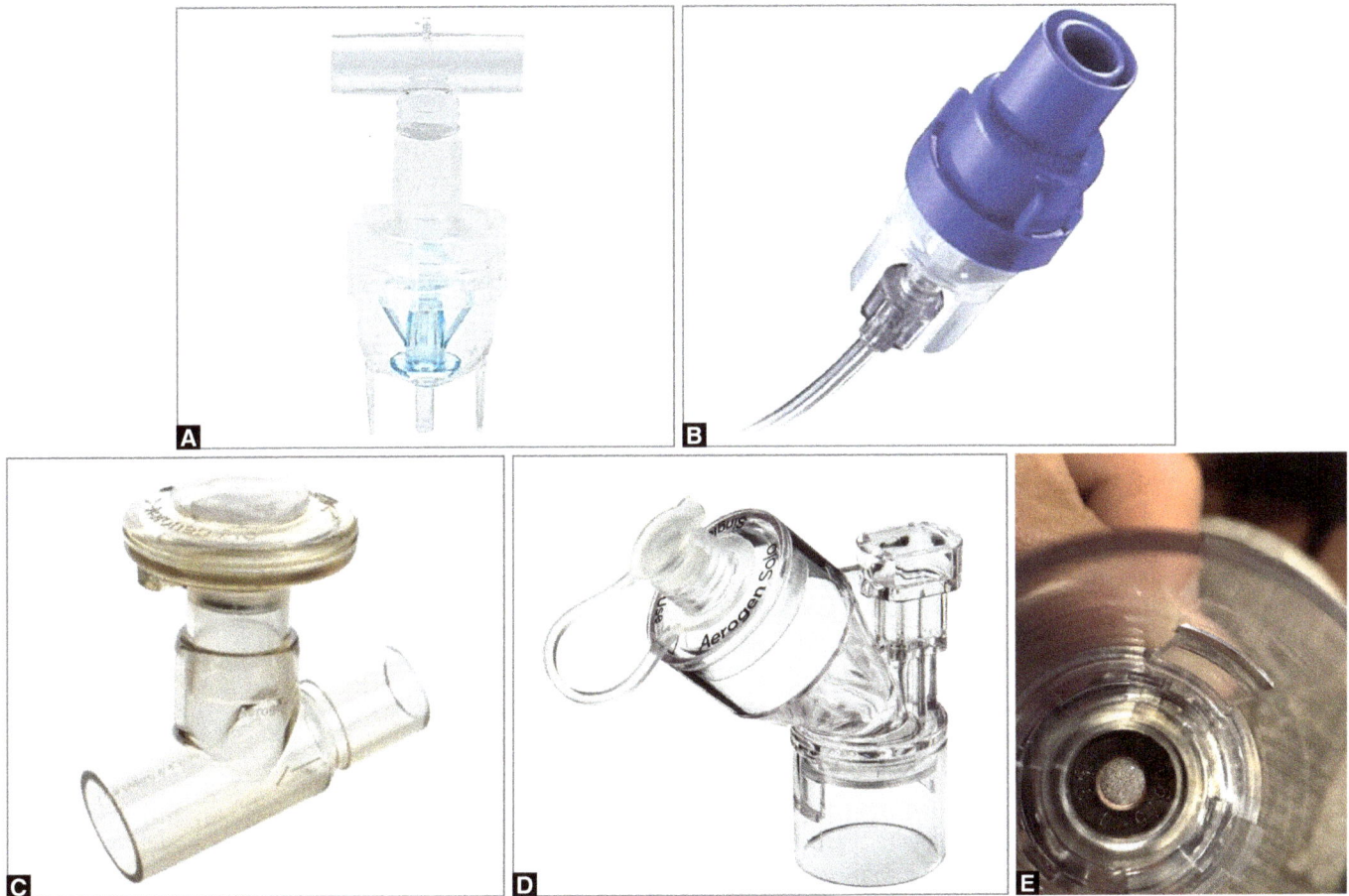

**Figs. 2A to E:** Ventilator-compatible nebulizers. (A) AirLife Misty Max 10™ disposable in-line jet nebulizer (Vyaire Medical®). (B) Sidestream disposable jet nebulizer (Philips Respironics®). (C) Aerogen Solo™ in-line vibrating mesh nebulizer (Aerogen®). (D, E) Aerogen Pro™ vibrating mesh nebulizer (Aerogen®) with a close-up on the mesh.

in Figures 1A to C, adapters are available as in-line uni- or bi-directional actuators.[36] In ventilator-supported patients with COPD, addition of spacer or valved holding chamber to the adapter was shown to result in a favorable effect on airway resistance indices.[37] Regardless of the chosen adapter device, strict administration technique needs to be maintained to assure effective pMDI drug delivery.[38,39] One *in vitro* study has demonstrated that positioning a holding chamber pMDI adapter 15 cm from the circuit Y-piece achieves best results in terms of medication delivery distal to the ETT (Fig. 3A).[17] pMDIs require vigorous shaking prior to use in order to mix the contents of the canister. In addition, prior to first use or if several days have elapsed between uses, pMDI should be primed by releasing several actuations into ambient air. Moreover, timing of pMDI actuations with the inspiratory phase of ventilation may improve distal drug delivery by up to 35%.[40] Maximal bronchodilator effect of short-acting beta-agonist delivered by pMDI with an in-line holder chamber adapter was shown to be reached at a dose of 400 µg, which is equivalent to approximately four pMDI actuations.[41] A time interval of 30–60 seconds should be allowed between actuations. The higher cost of some pMDI formulations, may be counterbalanced by their reproducible therapeutic effect, relatively short treatment time of 10–15 minutes, lack of need for a meticulous disinfection process, and potentially lower relative risk for ventilator-associated respiratory tract infection as these devices allow maintenance of circuit integrity.[42]

## Nebulizers

Nebulizers convert medications in liquid and suspension form into aerosol form. Currently available nebulizers in common use in ICUs include vibrating mesh, jet, and ultrasonic nebulizers. Much of the currently available data pertain to jet and vibrating mesh nebulizers, both of which will be the focus of this chapter. Ultrasonic nebulizers apply high-frequency vibrations to the surface of the medication solution resulting in breaking and aerosolization of droplets off the surface of the fluid. Although initially appealing, commercially available ultrasonic nebulizers have been shown to be relatively inefficient due to relatively large particle size with MMAD in the vicinity of 5 μm, high residual volumes, possible degeneration of heat-sensitive formulations, and limited ability to aerosolize viscous solutions.[17,43] In addition, they are relatively expensive and bulky.

Nebulizers can operate continuously throughout the respiratory cycle or intermittently during inspiration only. Intermittent drug delivery is appealing due to minimal potential aerosol loss during expiration.[44] Nevertheless, this modality requires separate tubing to ensure flow of inspiratory air from the ventilator to the nebulizer while also dictating longer treatment times.[45] There is significant variability between different groups of nebulizers and between different nebulizer brands within the same group.[46,47] Hence, attention to manufacturer recommendations regarding flow rates, volume of drug suspension, and operating pressure is crucial for optimal operation and drug delivery.

Newer-generation ventilators have built-in nebulization systems that may potentially improve functionality and synchronization with the respiratory cycle.[48] Furthermore, by use of dual-channel infusion pump that continuously creates a drug suspension in saline, these nebulizers can be used for prolonged aerosol delivery.[49] Finally, effective medication deposition within the pulmonary system is dependent on nebulizer position along the ventilator circuit. While too proximal of a placement on the inspiratory limb leads to significant drug deposition in the artificial tubing, too distal of a placement will result in drug loss into the expiratory limb.

### Jet Nebulizer

Jet nebulizers use high-velocity flow of compressed air or oxygen driven through a narrow opening into a reservoir containing the drug suspension. The shearing force of the jet of gas results in breakage and aerosolization of the suspension into 3–5 μm diameter particles.[50] These particles are in turn drawn by a pressure gradient up a capillary that is immersed in the drug suspension (Venturi and Bernoulli effects) and from there into the ventilator circuit. For optimal performance, jet nebulizers require an additional inflow at a range of 2–8 LPM, as specified by the manufacturer.

Jet nebulizers are relatively inexpensive and simple to operate and have been in the market for the longest time, all of which make them an attractive option for delivering drugs that cannot be delivered by pMDI. Their major limitations include a requirement for additional tubing and compressed gas source, inconsistent particle size leading to inconsistent dosing, and entrainment of additional gas flow into the ventilator system, which may adversely affect the preset tidal volume and flow rate or require adjustments of the ventilator settings in order to accommodate the increase in flow.[50] Another drawback is medication retainment of approximately 50% of the nominal dose,[18] which requires compensation in the form of higher suspension volumes, which in turn, results in longer treatment times. Other limitations, such as considerable noise production, bulky structure, and meticulous cleaning requirements have been addressed by manufacturers in newer-generation devices. Based on in vitro data, it is recommended to incorporate the jet nebulizer on the inspiratory limb proximal to the heated humidifier, between the ventilator unit and the heated humidifier (Fig. 3B)[17] or 30–40 cm proximal to the Y-piece.[31,46]

### Vibrating Mesh Nebulizer

Harnessing vibrations of a piezoelectric crystal, the drug suspension in the vibrating mesh nebulizer chamber is forced at very high frequency through a micropore mesh. Size of the micropores determines particle MMAD and particles less than 5 μm in diameter are achievable. Other benefits of mesh nebulizers include small residual volumes in the range of 3–10%,[18] shorter treatment times when compared with jet nebulizers, and higher respirable fraction allowing more efficient drug delivery into the lungs, possibly allowing dose reduction.[51] Newer generation breath-synchronized ventilator-compatible vibrating mesh nebulizers may further optimize drug delivery in ventilator-dependent patients.[52] Main shortcomings of mesh nebulizers include significantly higher costs, inability to aerosolize viscous drug suspensions due to mesh clogging, and a complex disinfection process. Available data suggests that optimal positioning of a vibrating mesh nebulizer is between the ventilator and the heated humidifier (Figs. 3C and D).[17,53] Incorporation of a vibrating mesh nebulizer at the ETT or 45 cm from the Y-piece was also shown to result in satisfactory lung deposition,[21] possibly allowing some degree of flexibility.

## AEROSOLIZED DRUGS AND THEIR USE IN VENTILATOR-SUPPORTED PATIENTS

The milieu of drug formulations available in aerosolized form or pMDI is constantly growing and new indications

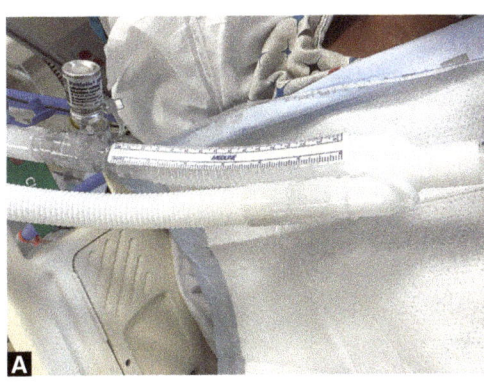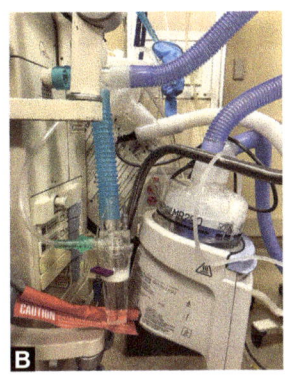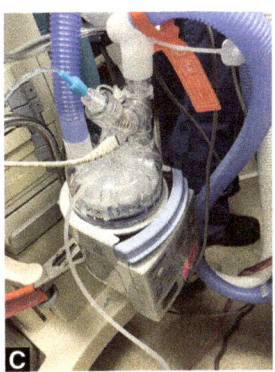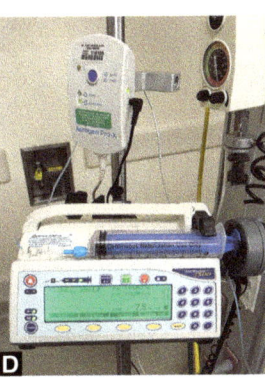

**Figs. 3A to D:** Device integration into the ventilator circuit. (A) SMDIA-1000™ MDI in-line adaptor (Southmedic®) integrated into the inspiratory limb at 15 cm proximal to the Y-connector. (B) MiniHEART™ continuous jet nebulizer (Westmed®) positioned between the ventilator and the heated humidifier. (C) Aerogen Solo™ vibrating mesh nebulizer (Aerogen®) positioned between the ventilator and the heated humidifier. (D) Aerogen Pro-X™ controller attached to a continuous nebulization tube set system (Aerogen®).

for aerosolized therapy are constantly investigated. Drugs can be delivered into the respiratory system for the purpose of localized action in the airways or lung parenchyma or for systemic absorption into the blood stream. In the section below, we discuss major groups of drugs commonly delivered in aerosolized form in the adult ICU.

## Bronchodilators

Aerosolized bronchodilators include mainly short- and long-acting beta2-agonists and muscarinic antagonists. This class of medications is frequently employed in ventilator-dependent patients with obstructive lung disease, such as asthma or COPD. Other indications for bronchodilator therapy are less established. In general, beta2-agonists therapy has been demonstrated to have favorable effect on certain outcomes such as wheezing, work of breathing, and measures of airway resistance; however, core outcomes, including overall duration of ventilator dependence, length of stay in the ICU, and mortality remain unaffected. In the subpopulation of obstructed patients with dynamic hyperinflation and intrinsic PEEP, administration of a short-acting beta2-agonist has been shown to improve airway resistance as well as hemodynamics.[26] The maximal therapeutic effect for albuterol sulfate was shown to be reached after four pMDI actuations or the equivalent of 400 μg[41] and 2.5 mg by nebulizer.[38,54] In ventilator-dependent patients with COPD, the bronchodilator effect of albuterol sulfate has been shown to last up to 2–3 hours.[54] This finding dictates a relatively frequent dosing schedule of every 3–6 hours in order to achieve persistent therapeutic effect over time. There are no comparison studies to support one beta2-agonist over another. Furthermore, beta2-agonsits were clearly shown to induce tachycardia and certain types of supraventricular and ventricular arrhythmia.[38] Hence, the potential harm of frequent administration of beta2-agonists should be carefully balanced against their potential benefit, especially in the elderly patients with known heart disease, patients with prior history of arrhythmia, or patients with other conditions which predispose to arrhythmia. The additive effect of muscarinic antagonists over beta2-agonists was shown to affect mainly measures of airway resistance in patients with respiratory failure due to COPD.[55,56] The evidence regarding use of long-acting bronchodilators, such as salmeterol or formoterol, in ventilator-supported patients is anecdotal.[56]

Suggested dosing regimens for commonly available short- and long-acting bronchodilators are provided in Table 3.

## Corticosteroids

The role of inhaled corticosteroids in ventilator-supported patients has yet been clearly defined. It is reasonable to assume that in most ICUs, treatment with systemic corticosteroids will be standard of care for patients with obstructive lung disease and respiratory failure. Therefore, the overall benefit of additional relatively small dose of corticosteroids via the inhaled route is questionable. Furthermore, inhaled corticosteroids have been associated with increased risk of pneumonia in nonventilated COPD patients,[57] placing further concern over their utility in critically ill patients with COPD exacerbation. Moreover, COPD in itself is an established risk factor for ventilator-associated pneumonia.[58] Currently, these data, in combination with the relatively high cost of inhaled

**Table 3:** Common bronchodilator formulations and dosing for mechanically ventilated patients.

| Class | Drug | Common indications | Delivery device | Suggested dose | Common adverse effects (>10%) | Serious adverse effects | Pregnancy category |
|---|---|---|---|---|---|---|---|
| Short-acting beta2-agonist | Albuterol/salbutamol | Asthma COPD Bronchospasm Dynamic hyperinflation | pMDI 90–100 µg/actuation with spacer or holding chamber | 4–6 actuations* every 3–6 h | Agitation, tremor, rhinitis, bronchospasm, pharyngitis, increased serum glucose, nausea, throat irritation | Anaphylaxis, cardiac arrhythmia, angina pectoris, hypokalemia, hypotension, acidosis | C |
| | | | Nebulizer solution 0.63–2.5 mg/3 mL | 1.25–2.5 mg every 4–8 h | | | C |
| | Terbutaline | Asthma COPD Bronchospasm Dynamic hyperinflation | pMDI 500 µg/actuation with spacer or holding chamber | 1–2 actuations* every 3–6 h | Agitation, tremor, hypokalemia, hyperglycemia | Anaphylaxis, cardiac arrhythmia, angina pectoris, hypokalemia, hypotension, acidosis | C |
| | | | Nebulizer solution 5 mg/2 mL | 1.25–2.5 mg every 4–8 h | | | C |
| Long-acting beta2-agonist | Formoterol | COPD | pMDI 5–10 µg/actuation with spacer or holding chamber | 3–4 actuations* up to every 4–6 h | | Anaphylaxis, angioedema, arrhythmia, angina pectoris, hypokalemia, hypotension, acidosis | C |
| | Fenoterol | COPD | pMDI 100 µg/actuation with spacer or holding chamber | 3–4 actuations* up to every 4–6 h | | Cardiac arrhythmia, angina pectoris, hypokalemia, hypotension, acidosis | C |
| Short-acting muscarinic antagonist | Ipratropium bromide | Asthma COPD Bronchospasm Dynamic hyperinflation | pMDI 17–18 µg/actuation with spacer or holding chamber | 4–6 actuations* every 3–6 h | Bronchitis, bronchospasm, sinusitis, urinary tract infection | Anaphylaxis, angioedema, glaucoma, hypotension, laryngospasm, urinary retention | B |
| | | | Nebulizer solution 0.02% | 0.5 mg every 6–8 h | | | B |

*Allow 30–60 seconds between each actuation.
(COPD: chronic obstructive pulmonary disease; pMDI: pressurized metered-dose inhaler)

corticosteroid formulations, diminish the attractiveness of this class of medications in ventilator-dependent patients.

## Antibiotics

Improvements in drug formulation led to the development of antibiotic drug suspensions for the purpose of aerosolized delivery, that are not as irritative to the airways as older formulations. As such, in ventilator-supported patients all aerosolized antibiotics are to be delivered via a nebulizer. Current data suggest that jet nebulizers appear less effective than vibrating mesh nebulizers for optimal nebulization of this class of drugs.[44] The bulk of current evidence supporting the use of inhaled antibiotics is coming from studies performed in spontaneously breathing noncritically ill patients, specifically those with CF and other forms of bronchiectasis. Major inhaled antibiotic formulations are aminoglycoside antibiotics and colistin. These formulations were designed for treatment of patients infected with multidrug resistant Gram-negative bacteria, such as *Pseudomonas* and *Acinetobacter*. Additional antibiotics available in aerosolizable form include ceftazidime, cefotaxime, vancomycin, amphotericin B, and aztreonam.

Current evidence for inhaled antibiotic use in addition or as an alternative to systemic antibiotics in ventilator-supported patients with respiratory tract infection do not demonstrate a therapeutic advantage.[59] Nevertheless, most currently available studies are plagued by relatively small patient cohorts and nonstandardized drug delivery protocols. Future results of larger trials using newer-generation delivery devices and/or formulations and incorporating standardized aerosol delivery protocols may provide clarity on this subject. Therefore, current guidelines either reserve treatment with aerosolized antibiotics for patients with ventilator-associated pneumonia not responsive to systemic antibiotics,[60] or recommend avoiding their use at present.[61] Accordingly, none of the currently available inhaled antibiotic formulations are currently approved by the US Food and Drug Administration or the European Medicines Agency for treatment of hospital-acquired or ventilator-associated pneumonia and their use in this patient population is considered off-label.

## Prostanoids

In patients with ARDS, inhaled pulmonary vasodilators have been demonstrated to reduce measures of pulmonary vascular resistance and right ventricular overload, resulting in improved right ventricular function, ventilation-perfusion mismatch, and oxygenation. Administration of these medications via the inhaled route also minimize systemic side effects, such as systemic vasodilation.[62,63] Nevertheless, these agents have yet to show impact on core outcomes of patients with ARDS, such as ventilator-free days, length of stay in the ICU, and mortality. Formulations currently available in aersolizable form for continuous nebulization include epoprostenol (prostaglandin $I_2$ analogue) and alprostadil (prostaglandin $E_1$ analogue). A commercially available system for continuous nebulization is shown in Figure 3D. Nebulized iloprost and treprostinil, both prostaglandin $I_2$ analogues, can be given intermittently, however the dosing interval in mechanically ventilated patients has yet been determined. Evidence in support of epoprostenol or alprostadil in ventilator-supported patients with refractory hypoxemia comes mainly from observational studies employing various dosing and administration protocols. In comparison to inhaled nitric oxide (iNO), continuous nebulization of either epoprostenol or alprostadil has been shown to be noninferior in terms of improving oxygenation and hemodynamic measures.[64-66] In the United States, epoprostenol and alprostadil formulations are also less expensive than iNO, providing another rationale for their use. Delivery via a vibrating mesh nebulizer positioned at the vicinity (either proximal or distal) to the heated humidifier seem to be most efficient to optimize delivered dose.[53]

## AEROSOLIZED THERAPY IN PATIENTS RECEIVING NONINVASIVE VENTILATION

Noninvasive positive pressure ventilation (NIPPV) is considered first-line therapy in certain patients with respiratory failure such as those with COPD exacerbation, decompensated heart failure, and pneumonia in the immunocompromised. NIPPV use in asthma is also rapidly gaining acceptance.[67] The most commonly used modes of NIPPV include bilevel and continuous positive airway pressure. The NIPPV interface significantly differs from that of invasive mechanical ventilation and includes a tight-fitting mask, single circuit limb, and a leak port which serves as an exhalation route. This leak port is an important source of aerosol loss into the environment. A heated humidifier can also be fitted into the NIPPV circuit if required. Critical care ventilators are able to deliver NIPPV. Similar to invasive mechanical ventilation circuits, these often utilize a dual-limb circuit comprised of separate inspiratory and expiratory routes. Aerosol delivery with this setup is the same as with invasive mechanical ventilation. All forms of delivery devices available for ventilator-supported patients can be used for administration of aerosolized medications in patients on NIPPV.

The therapeutic effect of aerosolized medications in patients on NIPPV has not been sufficiently studied. There is some evidence to support improved aerosol deposition when using NIPPV. In a study in children with CF, NIPPV augmented radiolabeled aerosol pulmonary deposition without an increase in particle impaction in proximal airways.[68] Likewise, in a prospective, randomized emergency department-based study, patients receiving nebulization via NIPPV achieved improvement in peak expiratory flow compared with nebulization alone.[69] Another study found that the use of NIPPV augmented the effect of aerosolized bronchodilators, with higher inspiratory pressures resulting in greater effect in a dose-dependent manner.[70] Although these results suggest an improvement in clinical variables, they do not definitively demonstrate improved aerosol delivery to the lungs since NIPPV alone, independent of nebulization, has a bronchodilatory effect.[71]

There are additional practical concerns to consider when administering aerosols via NIPPV. Administration with a full facial mask or helmet should be avoided to avoid contact between the aerosolized medication and the patient's eyes.[72] Data from in vitro studies demonstrate that vibrating mesh nebulizer may be superior to other nebulizers for more distal drug delivery.[73,74] Inspiratory synchronization may also enhance distal drug delivery.[73]

To avoid drug loss via the leak port, the optimal position of a nebulizer appears to be between the exhalation port and the mask.[75] Delivery with pMDI may be superior to nebulizer if the exhalation port is incorporated into the mask.[76] The effect of specific ventilator settings on distal drug delivery is likely minor in NIPPV due to the significant role of patient effort. Although, there is no data to support turning off the humidifier for optimal distal drug delivery, it is likely that particle size is increased with humidification and heating of the NIPPV system as happens in invasive ventilation systems. Finally, since some NIPPV settings use a nasal mask or pillows. In this setting and based on the degree of work of breathing imparted by the patient, the oral route may be considered for optimal delivery of aerosol.

## AEROSOLIZED THERAPY IN PATIENTS RECEIVING HIGH-FLOW NASAL CANNULA

High-flow nasal cannula (HFNC) allows delivery of humidified and heated supplemental oxygen to patients with various forms of respiratory failure. Whereas traditional nasal cannula can deliver flows of 2–6 LPM with variable fraction of inspired oxygen ($FIO_2$), HFNC is able to deliver flows of 20–60 LPM with an $FIO_2$ between 21% and 100%. The circuit is heated (up to 37°C) and humidified prior to delivering air to the nasal interface. Therapeutic doses of aerosol can be delivered through an HFNC setup; however, the manner in which aerosol is delivered through the HFNC system can greatly impact the delivery of aerosolized medications. In general, nasal aerosol inhalation in spontaneously breathing patients using traditional cannula has been shown to be prone to reduced efficacy of medication delivery due to turbulent nasopharyngeal flows.[77,78]

Delivery of the aerosol through heated and humidified nasal circuits that deliver a high flow of gas via the nasopharynx may result in increased impaction and aerosol loss in the circuit and the upper airways. This is enhanced by humidification and heating, both of which result in increases in particle size. These liabilities may be partially overcome by newer-generation systems that allow separation of high flow oxygen into one nostril and the aerosol into the other.[72]

### Effect of Flow Rates and Respiratory Rates

High-flow nasal cannula has flow-dependent physiologic effects on respiratory illness and high flows are well tolerated by patients. As a result, flow rates in patients with respiratory distress are typically started between 40 LPM and 60 LPM. Deposition rates of aerosolized medications are reduced by higher flow rates, likely as a result of turbulence. In an anatomic model, delivered medication dose decreased by approximately 50% when flow rate of 60 LPM was compared to 30 LPM.[79] This relationship remained consistent independent of respiratory rate, whether normal or tachypneic. The absolute value of delivered drug dose was shown to be higher when the model simulated tachypnea. Overall, the use of nebulizer in line with HFNC delivers clinically relevant doses between 6% and 10% of the nominal dose assuming closed mouth nebulization.[80]

### Effect of Nebulizer Position and Type

Both jet nebulizers and vibrating mesh nebulizers can be incorporated into the HFNC circuit; the nebulizer may be placed proximal or distal to the humidification chamber, or immediately proximal to the nasal cannula. Between 11% and 32% of the nebulized dose can be delivered to the nasal cannula outlet when the nebulizer was placed proximal to the humidification chamber.[81,82] A lower delivery ratio has been recorded when the nebulizer was placed immediately proximal to the nasal cannula.[81,83] No significant difference in efficacy was observed between jet and vibrating mesh nebulizers when placed prior to the humidification chamber.[81] Though HFNC remains a promising delivery device for aerosol therapy, more evidence is required before drawing clear conclusions about its efficacy in aerosol delivery.

## CONCLUSION

Administration of aerosolized medications is commonplace in ICUs worldwide. However, optimal drug delivery by the inhaled route to the ventilator-dependent patient requires thorough understanding of the pathophysiology of the patient's respiratory condition, technical system requirements, advantages, and limitations of each delivery system, and pharmacological properties of the administered medication. Furthermore, multidisciplinary team approach that includes physicians, nurses, respiratory therapists, and clinical pharmacologists is crucial to ensure implementation of evidence-based protocols for optimal administration of aerosolized medications to mechanically-ventilated patients. Structured training and continued education of the staff engaged in delivery of patient care is equally important. As the horizons of aerosolized drug delivery continue to expand, future studies will better delineate the optimal interplay between newer-generation delivery devices, ventilator settings, drug formulation, pharmacodynamics, and specific patient-related factors in order to allow tailoring the right therapy to the right patient using optimal delivery conditions.

## SALIENT POINTS

- Mechanically ventilated patients differ significantly from spontaneously breathing patients in terms of aerosol delivery due to lack of patient effort and interposition of the ventilator circuit.
- The strategy of drug delivery should be individually tailored based on the patient's underlying pathophysiology as well as characteristics of delivered drug and delivery device.
- Standardized protocols of aerosol delivery promote consistent dosing and reproducible drug effect.
- In comparison to metered dose inhalers and jet nebulizers, vibrating mesh nebulizers may promote more efficient drug delivery in mechanically and noninvasively ventilated patients.
- Efficacy of bronchodilators and prostanoids in mechanically ventilated patients is relatively well established.
- High-flow nasal cannula remains a promising delivery device of aerosol therapy; however, there is not sufficient evidence to draw conclusions about its efficacy.

## REFERENCES

1. Ehrmann S, Roche-Campo F, Bodet-Contentin L, et al. Aerosol therapy in intensive and intermediate care units: prospective observation of 2808 critically ill patients. Intensive Care Med. 2016;42(2):192-201.
2. Fink JB, Dhand R, Grychowski J, et al. Reconciling in vitro and in vivo measurements of aerosol delivery from a metered-dose inhaler during mechanical ventilation and defining efficiency-enhancing factors. Am J Respir Crit Care Med. 1999;159(1):63-8.
3. Lourenco RV, Cotromanes E. Clinical aerosols. I. Characterization of aerosols and their diagnostic uses. Arch Intern Med. 1982;142(12):2163-72.
4. Majoral C, Fleming J, Conway J, et al. Controlled, parametric, individualized, 2D and 3D imaging measurements of aerosol deposition in the respiratory tract of healthy human volunteers: in vivo data analysis. J Aerosol Med Pulm Drug Deliv. 2014;27(5):349-62.
5. Thomas SH, O'Doherty MJ, Fidler HM, et al. Pulmonary deposition of a nebulised aerosol during mechanical ventilation. Thorax. 1993;48(2):154-9.
6. Labiris NR, Dolovich MB. Pulmonary drug delivery. Part I: physiological factors affecting therapeutic effectiveness of aerosolized medications. Br J Clin Pharmacol. 2003;56(6):588-99.
7. Pavia D, Thomson ML, Clarke SW, et al. Effect of lung function and mode of inhalation on penetration of aerosol into the human lung. Thorax. 1977;32(2):194-7.
8. Graham DR, Chamberlain MJ, Hutton L, et al. Inhaled particle deposition and body habitus. Br J Ind Med. 1990;47(1):38-43.
9. Dal Negro RW, Micheletto C, Tognella S. Use of aerosols in bronchiectasis patients. Monaldi Arch Chest Dis. 2011;75(3):185-93.
10. Baskin MI, Abd AG, Ilowite JS. Regional deposition of aerosolized pentamidine. Effects of body position and breathing pattern. Ann Intern Med. 1990;113(9):677-83.
11. Ferrari F, Goldstein I, Nieszkowszka A, et al. Lack of lung tissue and systemic accumulation after consecutive daily aerosols of amikacin in ventilated piglets with healthy lungs. Anesthesiology. 2003;98(4):1016-9.
12. Dhand R. How should aerosols be delivered during invasive mechanical ventilation? Respir Care. 2017;62(10):1343-67.
13. Rees PJ, Clark TJ, Moren F. The importance of particle size in response to inhaled bronchodilators. Eur J Respir Dis Suppl. 1982;119:73-8.
14. Zanen P, Go LT, Lammers JW. Optimal particle size for beta 2 agonist and anticholinergic aerosols in patients with severe airflow obstruction. Thorax. 1996;51(10):977-80.
15. Johnson MA, Newman SP, Bloom R, et al. Delivery of albuterol and ipratropium bromide from two nebulizer systems in chronic stable asthma. Efficacy and pulmonary deposition. Chest. 1989;96(1):6-10.
16. Swift DL. Aerosols and humidity therapy. Generation and respiratory deposition of therapeutic aerosols. Am Rev Respir Dis. 1980;122(5 Pt 2):71-7.
17. Ari A, Atalay OT, Harwood R, et al. Influence of nebulizer type, position, and bias flow on aerosol drug delivery in simulated pediatric and adult lung models during mechanical ventilation. Respir Care. 2010;55(7):845-51.
18. Dugernier J, Ehrmann S, Sottiaux T, et al. Aerosol delivery during invasive mechanical ventilation: a systematic review. Crit Care. 2017;21(1):264.
19. Dugernier J, Reychler G, Wittebole X, et al. Aerosol delivery with two ventilation modes during mechanical ventilation: a randomized study. Ann Intensive Care. 2016;6(1):73.
20. Fink JB, Dhand R, Duarte AG, et al. Aerosol delivery from a metered-dose inhaler during mechanical ventilation. An in vitro model. Am J Respir Crit Care Med. 1996;154(2 Pt 1):382-7.
21. Dugernier J, Wittebole X, Roeseler J, et al. Influence of inspiratory flow pattern and nebulizer position on aerosol delivery with a vibrating-mesh nebulizer during invasive mechanical ventilation: an in vitro analysis. J Aerosol Med Pulm Drug Deliv. 2015;28(3):229-36.
22. Dolovich MA. Influence of inspiratory flow rate, particle size, and airway caliber on aerosolized drug delivery to the lung. Respir Care. 2000;45(6):597-608.
23. Hess DR, Dillman C, Kacmarek RM. In vitro evaluation of aerosol bronchodilator delivery during mechanical ventilation: pressure-control vs. volume control ventilation. Intensive Care Med. 2003;29(7):1145-50.

24. Barrowcliffe MP, Zanelli GD, Jones JG. Pulmonary clearance of radiotracers after positive end-expiratory pressure or acute lung injury. J Appl Physiol. 1989;66(1):288-94.
25. Vecellio L, Guerin C, Grimbert D, et al. In vitro study and semiempirical model for aerosol delivery control during mechanical ventilation. Intensive Care Med. 2005;31(6):871-6.
26. Tzoufi M, Mentzelopoulos SD, Roussos C, et al. The effects of nebulized salbutamol, external positive end-expiratory pressure, and their combination on respiratory mechanics, hemodynamics, and gas exchange in mechanically ventilated chronic obstructive pulmonary disease patients. Anesth Analg. 2005;101(3):843-50.
27. Lin H-L, Fink JB, Zhou Y, et al. Influence of moisture accumulation in inline spacer on delivery of aerosol using metered-dose inhaler during mechanical ventilation. Respir Care. 2009;54(10):1336-41.
28. Moustafa IOF, Ali MRA-A, Al Hallag M, et al. Lung deposition and systemic bioavailability of different aerosol devices with and without humidification in mechanically ventilated patients. Heart Lung. 2017;46(6):464-7.
29. Ari A, Alwadeai KS, Fink JB. Effects of heat and moisture exchangers and exhaled humidity on aerosol deposition in a simulated ventilator-dependent adult lung model. Respir Care. 2017;62(5):538-43.
30. Dhanani J, Fraser JF, Chan H-K, et al. Fundamentals of aerosol therapy in critical care. Crit Care. 2016;20(1):269.
31. O'Riordan TG, Greco MJ, Perry RJ, et al. Nebulizer function during mechanical ventilation. Am Rev Respir Dis. 1992;145(5):1117-2.
32. Longest PW, Azimi M, Golshahi L, et al. Improving aerosol drug delivery during invasive mechanical ventilation with redesigned components. Respir Care. 2014;59(5):686-98.
33. Ari A, Fink JB. Inhalation therapy in patients with tracheostomy: a guide to clinicians. Expert Rev Respir Med. 2017;11(3):201-8.
34. Jashnani RN, Byron PR, Dalby RN. Testing of dry powder aerosol formulations in different environmental conditions. Int J Pharm. 1995;113(1):123-30.
35. Dellweg D, Wachtel H, Hohn E, et al. In vitro validation of a Respimat(R) adapter for delivery of inhaled bronchodilators during mechanical ventilation. J Aerosol Med Pulm Drug Deliv. 2011;24(6):285-92.
36. Dhand R. Inhalation therapy with metered-dose inhalers and dry powder inhalers in mechanically ventilated patients. Respir Care. 2005;50(10):1331-5.
37. Dhand R, Jubran A, Tobin MJ. Bronchodilator delivery by metered-dose inhaler in ventilator-supported patients. Am J Respir Crit Care Med. 1995;151(6):1827-33.
38. Manthous CA, Hall JB, Schmidt GA, et al. Metered-dose inhaler versus nebulized albuterol in mechanically ventilated patients. Am Rev Respir Dis. 1993;148(6 Pt 1):1567-70.
39. Dhand R, Tobin MJ. Inhaled bronchodilator therapy in mechanically ventilated patients. Am J Respir Crit Care Med. 1997;156(1):3-10.
40. Diot P, Morra L, Smaldone GC. Albuterol delivery in a model of mechanical ventilation. Comparison of metered-dose inhaler and nebulizer efficiency. Am J Respir Crit Care Med. 1995;152(4 Pt 1):1391-4.
41. Dhand R, Duarte AG, Jubran A, et al. Dose-response to bronchodilator delivered by metered-dose inhaler in ventilator-supported patients. Am J Respir Crit Care Med. 1996;154(2 Pt 1):388-93.
42. Kallet RH. Adjunct therapies during mechanical ventilation: airway clearance techniques, therapeutic aerosols, and gases. Respir Care. 2013;58(6):1053-73.
43. Watts AB, McConville JT, Williams RO. Current therapies and technological advances in aqueous aerosol drug delivery. Drug Dev Ind Pharm. 2008;34(9):913-22.
44. Miller DD, Amin MM, Palmer LB, et al. Aerosol delivery and modern mechanical ventilation: in vitro/in vivo evaluation. Am J Respir Crit Care Med. 2003;168(10):1205-9.
45. Wan G-H, Lin H-L, Fink JB, et al. In vitro evaluation of aerosol delivery by different nebulization modes in pediatric and adult mechanical ventilators. Respir Care. 2014;59(10):1494-500.
46. O'Doherty MJ, Thomas SH, Page CJ, et al. Delivery of a nebulized aerosol to a lung model during mechanical ventilation. Effect of ventilator settings and nebulizer type, position, and volume of fill. Am Rev Respir Dis. 1992;146(2):383-8.
47. Berlinski A, Willis JR. Albuterol delivery by 4 different nebulizers placed in 4 different positions in a pediatric ventilator in vitro model. Respir Care. 2013;58(7):1124-33.
48. Ehrmann S, Lyazidi A, Louis B, et al. Ventilator-integrated jet nebulization systems: tidal volume control and efficiency of synchronization. Respir Care. 2014;59(10):1508-16.
49. Siobal MS, Kallet RH, Pittet J-F, et al. Description and evaluation of a delivery system for aerosolized prostacyclin. Respir Care. 2003;48(8):742-53.
50. Hess D, Fisher D, Williams P, et al. Medication nebulizer performance. Effects of diluent volume, nebulizer flow, and nebulizer brand. Chest. 1996;110(2):498-505.
51. Waldrep JC, Dhand R. Advanced nebulizer designs employing vibrating mesh/aperture plate technologies for aerosol generation. Curr Drug Deliv. 2008;5(2):114-9.
52. Dhand R, Sohal H. Pulmonary drug delivery system for inhalation therapy in mechanically ventilated patients. Expert Rev Med Devices. 2008;5(1):9-18.
53. Anderson AC, Dubosky MN, Fiorino KA, et al. The effect of nebulizer position on aerosolized epoprostenol delivery in an adult lung model. Respir Care. 2017;62(11):1387-95.
54. Duarte AG, Momii K, Bidani A. Bronchodilator therapy with metered-dose inhaler and spacer versus nebulizer in mechanically ventilated patients: comparison of magnitude and duration of response. Respir Care. 2000;45(7):817-23.
55. Fernandez A, Munoz J, de la Calle B, et al. Comparison of one versus two bronchodilators in ventilated COPD patients. Intensive Care Med. 1994;20(3):199-202.
56. Guerin C, Chevre A, Dessirier P, et al. Inhaled fenoterol-ipratropium bromide in mechanically ventilated patients with chronic obstructive pulmonary disease. Am J Respir Crit Care Med. 1999;159(4 Pt 1):1036-42.
57. Ernst P, Gonzalez AV, Brassard P, et al. Inhaled corticosteroid use in chronic obstructive pulmonary disease and the risk of hospitalization for pneumonia. Am J Respir Crit Care Med. 2007;176(2):162-6.

58. Tejerina E, Frutos-Vivar F, Restrepo MI, et al. Incidence, risk factors, and outcome of ventilator-associated pneumonia. J Crit Care. 2006;21(1):56-65.
59. Sole-Lleonart C, Rouby J-J, Blot S, et al. Nebulization of antiinfective agents in invasively mechanically ventilated adults: A systematic review and meta-analysis. Anesthesiology. 2017;126(5):890-908.
60. Kalil AC, Metersky ML, Klompas M, et al. Management of adults with hospital-acquired and ventilator-associated pneumonia: 2016 Clinical Practice Guidelines by the Infectious Diseases Society of America and the American Thoracic Society. Clin Infect Dis. 2016;63(5):e61-111.
61. Rello J, Sole-Lleonart C, Rouby J-J, et al. Use of nebulized antimicrobials for the treatment of respiratory infections in invasively mechanically ventilated adults: a position paper from the European Society of Clinical Microbiology and Infectious Diseases. Clin Microbiol Infect. 2017;23(9):629-39.
62. Haraldsson A, Kieler-Jensen N, Ricksten SE. Inhaled prostacyclin for treatment of pulmonary hypertension after cardiac surgery or heart transplantation: a pharmacodynamic study. J Cardiothorac Vasc Anesth. 1996;10(7):864-8.
63. Meyer J, Theilmeier G, Van Aken H, et al. Inhaled prostaglandin E1 for treatment of acute lung injury in severe multiple organ failure. Anesth Analg. 1998;86(4):753-8.
64. Walmrath D, Schneider T, Schermuly R, et al. Direct comparison of inhaled nitric oxide and aerosolized prostacyclin in acute respiratory distress syndrome. Am J Respir Crit Care Med. 1996;153(3):991-6.
65. Domenighetti G, Stricker H, Waldispuehl B. Nebulized prostacyclin (PGI2) in acute respiratory distress syndrome: impact of primary (pulmonary injury) and secondary (extrapulmonary injury) disease on gas exchange response. Crit Care Med. 2001;29(1):57-62.
66. Torbic H, Szumita PM, Anger KE, et al. Inhaled epoprostenol vs inhaled nitric oxide for refractory hypoxemia in critically ill patients. J Crit Care. 2013;28(5):844-8.
67. Nanchal R, Kumar G, Majumdar T, et al. Utilization of mechanical ventilation for asthma exacerbations: analysis of a national database. Respir Care. 2014;59(5):644-53.
68. Fauroux B, Itti E, Pigeot J, et al. Optimization of aerosol deposition by pressure support in children with cystic fibrosis: an experimental and clinical study. Am J Respir Crit Care Med. 2000;162(6):2265-71.
69. Pollack CV, Fleisch KB, Dowsey K. Treatment of acute bronchospasm with beta-adrenergic agonist aerosols delivered by a nasal bilevel positive airway pressure circuit. Ann Emerg Med. 1995;26(5):552-7.
70. Brandao DC, Lima VM, Filho VG, et al. Reversal of bronchial obstruction with bi-level positive airway pressure and nebulization in patients with acute asthma. J Asthma. 2009;46(4):356-61.
71. Galindo-Filho VC, Brandao DC, Ferreira R de CS, et al. Noninvasive ventilation coupled with nebulization during asthma crises: a randomized controlled trial. Respir Care. 2013;58(2):241-9.
72. Hess DR. Aerosol therapy during noninvasive ventilation or high-flow nasal cannula. Respir Care. 2015;60(6):880-3.
73. Michotte J-B, Jossen E, Roeseler J, et al. In vitro comparison of five nebulizers during noninvasive ventilation: analysis of inhaled and lost doses. J Aerosol Med Pulm Drug Deliv. 2014;27(6):430-40.
74. Galindo-Filho VC, Ramos ME, Rattes CS, et al. Radioaerosol pulmonary deposition using mesh and jet nebulizers during noninvasive ventilation in healthy subjects. Respir Care. 2015;60(9):1238-46.
75. Sutherasan Y, Ball L, Raimondo P, et al. Effects of ventilator settings, nebulizer and exhalation port position on albuterol delivery during non-invasive ventilation: an in-vitro study. BMC Pulm Med. 2017;17(1):9.
76. Branconnier MP, Hess DR. Albuterol delivery during noninvasive ventilation. Respir Care. 2005;50(12):1649-53.
77. Usmani OS, Biddiscombe MF, Barnes PJ. Regional lung deposition and bronchodilator response as a function of beta2-agonist particle size. Am J Respir Crit Care Med. 2005;172(12):1497-504.
78. Heyder J, Gebhart J, Rudolf G, et al. Deposition of particles in the human respiratory tract in the size range 0.005-15 μm. J Aerosol Sci. 1986;17(5):811-25.
79. Golshahi L, Longest PW, Azimi M, et al. Intermittent aerosol delivery to the lungs during high-flow nasal cannula therapy. Respir Care. 2014;59(10):1476-86.
80. Dolovich MB, Ahrens RC, Hess DR, et al. Device selection and outcomes of aerosol therapy: Evidence-based guidelines: American College of Chest Physicians/American College of Asthma, Allergy, and Immunology. Chest. 2005;127(1):335-71.
81. Réminiac F, Vecellio L, Heuzé-Vourc'hN, et al. Aerosol Therapy in Adults Receiving High Flow Nasal Cannula Oxygen Therapy. J Aerosol Med Pulm Drug Deliv. 2016;29(2):134-41.
82. Bhashyam AR, Wolf MT, Marcinkowski AL, et al. Aerosol delivery through nasal cannulas: an in vitro study. J Aerosol Med Pulm Drug Deliv. 2008;21(2):181-8.
83. Perry SA, Kesser KC, Geller DE, et al. Influences of cannula size and flow rate on aerosol drug delivery through the Vapotherm humidified high-flow nasal cannula system. Pediatr Crit Care Med. 2013;14(5):e250-6.

# CHAPTER 19

# Extracorporeal Membrane Oxygenation

*Nirvik Pal, Patricia A Nicolato, Sarah L Wachter*

## INTRODUCTION

Extracorporeal membrane oxygenation (ECMO) is essentially cardiopulmonary bypass (CPB) with technical modifications to permit a longer duration of safe implementation.[1-5] As a principal, CPB is designed for the conduct of cardiac or lung surgeries in an operating room whereas the ECMO is used for recovery from heart and/or lung injury in intensive care unit (ICU). CPB uses an open reservoir, requires complete anticoagulation with activated clotting time (ACT) greater than 600 seconds, uses autotransfusion, and (usually) an in-line arterial filter in anesthetized patients. ECMO does not require an open reservoir, requires a lesser degree of anticoagulation (ACT around 180 seconds), requires neither autotransfusion nor an arterial filter, and is typically provided to unanesthetized patients.

## HISTORY

Historically invention of CPB leads to evolution of ECMO.[1] Dr John Gibbon invented the CPB machine which was successfully used in 1953 during repair of an atrial septal defect in an 18-year old. Cardiac surgeon Dr Walton Lillehei further developed this technology for heart surgeries. DeWall developed the bubble oxygenator and in 1957 Kammermeyer invented the silicon membrane oxygenator. This would withstand the hydrostatic pressure and still permit gas exchange. Dr Robert H Bartlett (Father of modern ECMO) and Drinker went on to design the first ECMO machine in 1972 first clinically used for 36 hours in a 2-year old infant with cardiac failure following the Mustard procedure for transposition of great arteries. They recognized the fact that unlike a CPB circuit used during surgery, which has multiple points of stagnation and therefore requires full anticoagulation, ECMO circuits have much less stagnation and require lesser anticoagulation. They also developed partial thromboplastin time (PTT)—guided algorithms for ECMO. In 1975, Dr Bartlett moved on to the ECMO technology to care for neonates with respiratory distress syndrome. In USA in 1983, only three medical centers were using ECMO on a regular basis: University of Michigan, University of Pittsburgh, and Virginia Commonwealth University, Richmond. In 1989 the Extracorporeal Life Support Organization (ELSO) was formed. As of 2016 there were more than 460 centers worldwide that were members of ELSO (Figure 1 showing ECMO runs). The inaugural edition of ELSO's "Red Book" was published in 1992. Currently it is on the 5th edition in 2016.

## INDICATIONS[4-15]

Extracorporeal membrane oxygenation comes in a variety of configurations and designs specific to the need of the patient and the etiology. As per ELSO (Table 1), broadly there are two indications, refractory hypoxemia which may present with distributive or cardiogenic shock and refractory hypercapnia with or without hypoxemia. Depending on the presentation of the patient, either a venoarterial (VA),[16] venovenous (VV)[17] or extracorporeal carbon dioxide removal ($ECCO_2R$) may be planned.

The use of clinical ECMO has been growing worldwide (Fig. 1) since its introduction in the 1990s.[1] It is not uncommon to have patient to be placed on EMCO emergently. Careful assessment for suitability for an ECMO prior to placement is imperative. Over the last three decades, as usage of ECMO has increased, and our understanding of outcomes has improved. Careful patient selection and timely institution of ECMO is the key to successful outcome (Tables 1 and 2). The ELSO registry classifies the assessment for suitability of ECMO as "indication", "consideration" and "contraindication". On similar principles the ECMO net, CESAR (Conventional ventilatory support vs extracorporeal

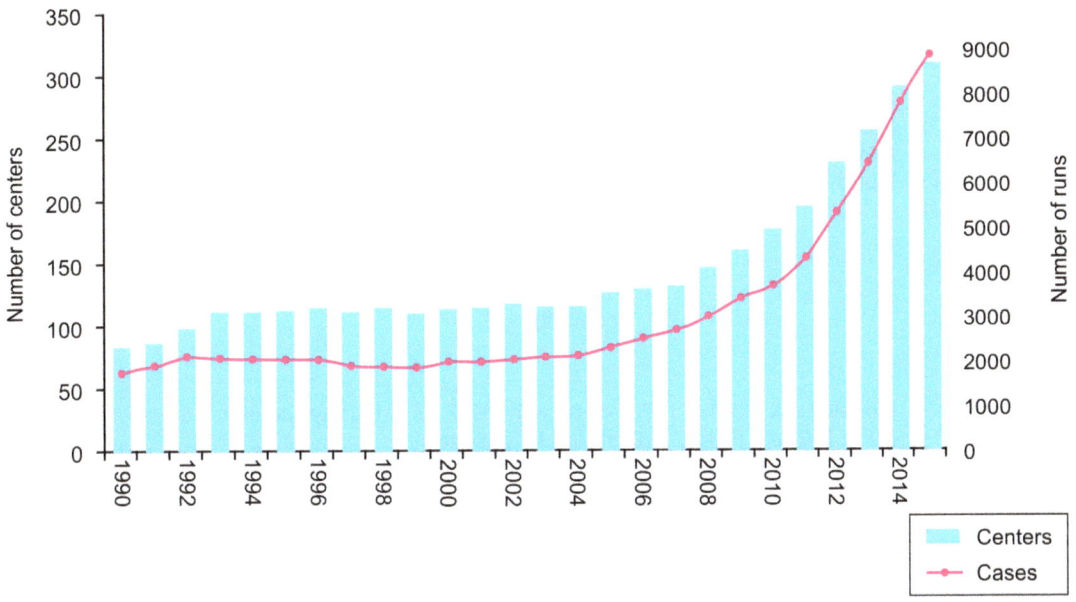

**Fig. 1:** Global trends in extracorporeal membrane oxygenation (ECMO) utilization over the years.
*Source:* Adapted with permission from 'ELSO Red Book'.

| Table 1: Indications for ECMO. |
|---|
| • *Respiratory* <br> – $PaO_2/FiO_2 < 80$ mm Hg on $FiO_2 > 90\%$ <br> – $PaCO_2 > 80$ mm Hg <br> – Inability to achieve $P_{plateau} < 30$ cmH$_2$O <br> – Severe air leak syndrome leading to reduced ventilation <br> • *Cardiac* <br> – Need for cardiorespiratory support (otherwise VAD) <br> – Malperfusion from low cardiac output syndrome (LCOS) with hypotension <br> – Myocarditis <br> – Myocardial infarction <br> – Peripartum cardiomyopathy <br> – Decompensated chronic heart failure <br> • *Distributive shock* <br> – Sepsis <br> • *Cardiopulmonary resuscitation* <br> – Whenever reversible event with excellent CPR, may consider ECMO |
| (ECMO: extracorporeal membrane oxygenation; FiO$_2$: fraction of inspired oxygen; PaO$_2$: partial pressure of oxygen; PaCO$_2$: partial pressure of carbon dioxide; VAD: ventricular assist device). |

| Table 2: Contraindications for ECMO. |
|---|
| • *Respiratory:* <br> – ≥7 days on mechanical ventilation with FiO$_2$ of 90% and $P_{plateau}$ pressure > 30 cmH$_2$O <br> – Absolute neutrophil count > 400/cu cm <br> • *Cardiac:* <br> – *Absolute:* <br>   - Unsalvageable heart in a non-transplant or VAD patient <br>   - Prolonged CPR with no tissue perfusion <br>   - Chronic multi-organ dysfunction including emphysema, cirrhosis, renal failure <br> – *Relative:* <br>   - Patient has contraindication for anticoagulation <br>   - Advanced age <br>   - Obese (difficult to attain perfusion with cannula sizes) <br> • *CPR Contraindications:* <br> – Unsuccessful CPR, considered no ROSC for 5 to 30 minutes (although may be indicated if adequate perfusion with appropriate metabolic support attained) <br> • *Neurologic:* <br> – Recent or expanding intracranial hemorrhage <br> – Unable to receive anticoagulation secondary to intracranial process. |
| (CPR: cardiopulmonary resuscitation; ECMO: extracorporeal membrane oxygenation; FiO$_2$: fraction of inspired oxygen; ROSC: return of spontaneous circulation; VAD: ventricular assist device). |

membrane oxygenation for severe adult respiratory failure) trial, EOLIA (rescue lung injury in severe acute respiratory distress syndrome) trial classifies patient assessment for ECMO (Table 3). The ELSO registry uses a "Murray score" for classification of acute respiratory distress syndrome (ARDS). Although now dated, the Murray score is still used and applied (Table 4). Another newer score often utilized for assessing prognosis or suitability of ECMO is the **S**urvival **A**fter **V**eno-arterial **E**CMO (SAVE) score (Table 5).[18]

## PATHOPHYSIOLOGY OF GAS EXCHANGE[1]

The goal of ECMO is to ensure the patient receives adequate oxygenation so as to maintain an aerobic respiration at the tissue level. In other words, at the cardiopulmonary level, this is ensuring that the ratio of $DO_2/VO_2$ stays above 1,

**Table 3:** Scoring based indication for VV-ECMO.

| Clinical group reference | ELSO | ECMO | CESAR | EOLIA |
|---|---|---|---|---|
| Indication to ECMO | • Mortality risk > 80%<br>• P/F < 80 with FiO$_2$ > 0.90<br>• Murray score of 3–4 | • OI > 30<br>• P/F < 70 with PEEP ≥ 15 cmH$_2$O for patients in an ECMO center<br>• pH < 7.25 × ≥ 2 hours<br>• Hemodynamic instability | • Potentially reversible respiratory failure<br>• Murray score ≥ 3.0<br>• pH < 7.20 despite optimum conventional treatment | • P/F < 50 with FiO$_2$ > 0.8 × > 3 hours<br>• P/F < 80 with FiO$_2$ > 0.8 for > 6 hours<br>• pH < 7.25 for > 6 hours (RR increased to 35/min) with MV settings adjusted to keep P$_{plateau}$ < 32 cmH$_2$O |
| Consideration for ECMO | • Mortality risk > 50%<br>• P/F < 150 with FiO$_2$ > 0.90<br>• Murray score 2–3 | P/F < 100 with PEEP ≥ 10 cmH$_2$O for patients awaiting transfer to ECMO center | Murray score ≥ 2.5 | |
| Contraindication for ECMO | • Incompatible with normal life<br>• Preexisting conditions affecting QoL (e.g. ESRD, CNS status)<br>• Age<br>• Futility: Too sick<br>• On conventional therapy for too long (MV > 7 days) | • Intracranial bleeding<br>• Other C/I for anticoagulation<br>• Poor prognosis of underlying disease<br>• MV > 7 days | • Peak inspiratory pressure > 30 cmH$_2$O<br>• FiO$_2$ > 0.8<br>• Ventilation > 7 days<br>• Intracranial bleeding<br>• Contraindication to anticoagulation<br>• Contraindication to continuation of active treatment | • MV ≥ 7 days<br>• Age, 18 years<br>• Pregnancy<br>• BMI > 45 kg/sq m<br>• Chronic respiratory insufficiency treated with long duration oxygen or respiratory assistance<br>• Previous h/o HIT<br>• Malignancy with fatal prognosis within 5 years<br>• Patient moribund<br>• SAPS II > 90<br>• Nondrug induced coma after cardiac arrest<br>• Irreversible CNS pathology<br>• ECMO cannulation not possible |

(BMI: body mass index; CESAR: conventional ventilatory support vs. extracorporeal membrane oxygenation for severe adult respiratory failure; CNS: central nervous system; C/I: confidence interval; ECMO: extracorporeal membrane oxygenation; ELSO: Extracorporeal Life Support Organization; EOLIA: extracorporeal membrane oxygenation for severe acute respiratory distress syndrome; ESRD: end-stage renal disease; FiO$_2$: fraction of inspired oxygen; HIT: heparin-induced thrombocytopenia; MV: mechanical ventilation; OI: oxygenation index; P/F: PaO$_2$/FiO$_2$; PaO$_2$: partial pressure of oxygen; PEEP: positive end-expiratory pressure; QoL: quality of life; RR: respiratory rate; SAPS; Simplified Acute Physiology Score; VV: vevovenous).

*Source:* Adapted with permission from ELSO "Red Book".

where DO$_2$ stands for delivery of oxygen and VO$_2$ stands for consumption of oxygen. DO$_2$ is the content of oxygen (CaO$_2$) in blood multiplied by the cardiac output (CO). Content of oxygen may be calculated as:

$$CaO_2 = (1.34 \times Hb \times SpO_2) + (PaO_2 \times 0.003)$$

Therefore DO$_2$ would be CO times the content of oxygen in arterial blood (CaO$_2$):

$$DO_2 = CaO_2 \times CO$$

Assuming hemoglobin (Hb) of 15 g/dL and a saturation of 100%, a normal person will have about 20 mL/dL of oxygen content. Usually the normal CO is about 4.5–5 L/min, which yields a delivery of oxygen of about 100 mL/min at the tissue level. If body surface area taken into account, it would translate to about 500–600 mL/min/m$^2$.

Consumption of oxygen (VO$_2$) is a measure of metabolism. As long as aerobic metabolism is maintained,

| Table 4: Murray score calculation table. | | | | | |
|---|---|---|---|---|---|
| | Scores | | | | |
| Parameters | 0 | 1 | 2 | 3 | 4 |
| PaO$_2$/FiO$_2$ | >300 | 225–299 | 175–225 | 100–174 | <100 |
| CXR (number of infiltrated quadrants) | 0 | 1 | 2 | 3 | 4 |
| PEEP (cmH$_2$O) | <5 | 6–8 | 9–11 | 12–14 | >15 |
| Compliance (cu cm/ cmH$_2$O) | >80 | 60–79 | 40–59 | 20–39 | <19 |

(CXR: chest X-ray; FiO$_2$: fraction of inspired oxygen; PaO$_2$: partial pressure of oxygen; PEEP: positive end-expiratory pressure).

| Table 5: SAVE Score (The Survival after veno-arterial ECMO score). | |
|---|---|
| Variable | Score |
| *Diagnosis* | |
| Myocarditis | +3 |
| Refractory VT/VF | +2 |
| Post heart or lung transplantation | +3 |
| Congenital heart disease | –3 |
| Other diagnosis | 0 |
| *Age (years)* | |
| 18–38 | +7 |
| 39–52 | +4 |
| 53–62 | +3 |
| ≥63 | 0 |
| *Weight (kg)* | |
| ≤65 | 1 |
| 65–89 | 2 |
| ≥90 | 0 |
| *Cardiac* | |
| Pulse pressure pre-ECMO ≤20 mmHg[1] | –2 |
| Diastolic BP pre-ECMO ≥40 mmHg[1] | +3 |
| Pre-ECMO cardiac arrest | –2 |
| *Respiratory* | |
| Peak inspiratory pressure ≤20 cmH$_2$O | +3 |
| Intubation duration pre-ECMO (hrs) | |
| ≤10 | 0 |
| 11–29 | –2 |
| ≥30 | –4 |
| *Renal* | |
| Acute renal failure[2] | –3 |
| Chronic renal failure[3] | –6 |
| HCO$_3$ pre-ECMO ≤15 mmol/L[4] | –3 |
| *Other organ failures pre-ECMO* | |
| Central nervous system dysfunction[5] | –3 |
| Liver failure[6] | –3 |
| Total score | –35 to 17 |

Survival prediction: Total score >5, survival 75%; total score 1 to 5, survival 58%; total score –4 to 0, survival 42%; total score –9 to –5, survival 30%; ≤ –10, survival 18%
[1]Worst value within 6 hours prior to cannulation.
[2]Creatinine levels > 133 micromol/L (5mg/dl)
[3]Kidney damage or eGFR <60ml/min/1.73 sq meter for >/= 3 months
[4]Worst value before cannulation
[5]Neuroblastoma, stroke, encephalopathy, cerebral embolism, seizure, epileptic syndrome
[6]Bilirubin > 33 micromol/L or elevation of serum ALT/AST > 70 IU/L at ECLS cannulation
All values prior to cannulation
(ALT: alanine aminotransferase; AST: aspartate aminotransferase; BP: blood pressure; CNS: central nervous system; ECLS: extracorporeal life support, eGFR: estimated glomerular filtration rate; VF: ventricular fibrillation; VT: ventricular tachycardia).

*Source:* http://www.save-score.com/

the quantity of $CO_2$ produced is equal to $O_2$ consumed. Typically, $VO_2$ at resting states are:
- Adult = 3 mL/kg/min
- Child = 4 mL/kg/min
- Neonate = 5 mL/kg/min

As a law of nature, the human homeostasis is tuned to maintain a $DO_2/VO_2$ ratio of 5:1. This is better understood by calculating the ratio of content of oxygen on the arterial side ($CaO_2$) to the venous return ($CvO_2$). Assuming the Hb to be 15 g/dL, oxygen saturation on arterial side to be 100% and on venous side to be 80%, the net $O_2$ consumption is only 20%, thereby meaning a ratio of delivery to consumption of 5:1. In other words, out of the four molecules of $O_2$ attached to Hb molecule only about one gets utilized and the remaining three remain in reserve!

During conditions when the $DO_2/VO_2$ ratio starts to downtrend to about 2:1, anaerobic metabolism sets in leading to lactic acidosis. This may happen for any of four reasons: failure of the pump (cardiac failure) leading to reduced CO and hence delivery ($DO_2$); reduced Hb from anemia or shock leading to reduced content of oxygen ($CaO_2$); poor gas exchange (lung injury) leading to reduced uptake and desaturation (low $DO_2$) and increased metabolic demand from conditions such as sepsis leading to increased demand and high $VO_2$. ECMO therapy is titrated to maintain the ratio of $DO_2/VO_2$ to more than 2:1 to avoid anaerobic respiration until there is recovery from the primary mechanism of insult. Conceptually, pump flow rate (PFR) and CO ratio of 1 would mean the whole CO is circulating through ECMO; if it is close to 0 would mean no blood is flowing through ECMO. Of note, PFR should never be 0 in VA-ECMO in order to avoid circuit thrombosis.

With an ECMO "membrane lung" $CO_2$ diffusion (clearance) is determined by the rate of counter current flow of fresh gas also known as "sweep speed". With sweep speed to blood flow at ratio of 1:1, clearance of $CO_2$ will be the same $O_2$ uptake, but it will be much faster with a greater sweep speed such as 8:1.

## TYPES AND BASIC PRINCIPLES OF EXTRACORPOREAL MEMBRANE OXYGENATION

As noted earlier, ECMO may be classified in four types: VV,[17] VA,[16] hybrid and $ECCO_2R$. The VA ECMO may further be subdivided into peripheral and central depending on cannulation sites (Flowchart 1, Figs. 2 to 4). In VV ECMO the cannulas may be located at any two major veins like femoral vein, superior vena cava (SVC) and inferior vena cava (IVC), or may be a "double-barrel" cannula placed in a single (usually internal jugular) vein (IJV). A *hybrid* ECMO is one where initial cannulation start with either VA or VV and then another cannula placed in an artery or vein either to increase oxygenation in proximal aorta (Harlequin effect) or to offload the left ventricle (Flowcharts 1 and 2, Fig. 5). Hence, this ECMO becomes a VA-V or VV-A also known as "one-and-half ECMO".[19-22]

### Conduct of VA-Extracorporeal Membrane Oxygenation[1]

- Suggested cannulas of choice are mentioned in Tables 6 and 7.
- Estimate metabolic rate and CO (flow) needed. Adults, children, neonate 3, 4, 5 mL/kg/min respectively. An adult septic patient may need 5 instead of 3 mL/kg/min. Usually 4.5–5 L/min are required to supply 300 mL $O_2$/min.
- Estimate venous drainage cannula size. With larger cannulas one may initiate with complete bypass and nonpulsatile flow, then reduce flow rate to achieve arterial line pulse contour to about 10–15 mm Hg. Try to titrate down the vasoactive medications so as to promote left ventricular (LV) healing from reduced afterload. In case LV has no function, a left atrial drainage may be needed.
- Assess $O_2$ kinetics in 6–12 hours after institution of ECMO. Target a goal of $DO_2/VO_2 > 3:1$. Adequate sedation with or without paralysis, ensuring Hb between 12 g/dL and 14 g/dL, keeping the arterial saturation >90% and venous saturation >65%. A minimum flow of about 1,500 mL/min needs to be maintained to avoid

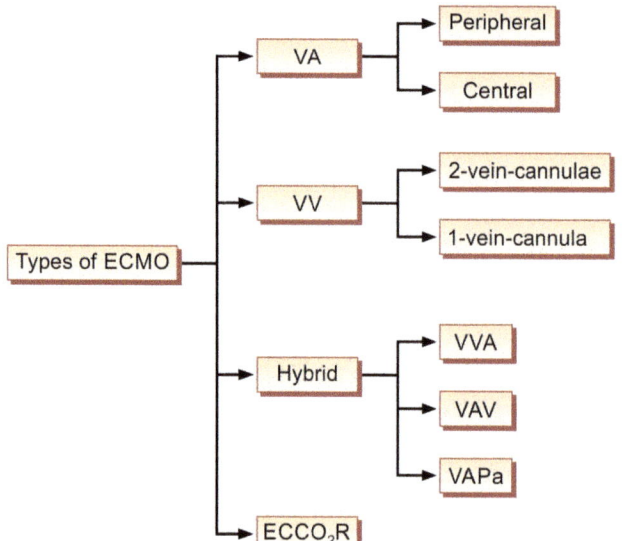

**Flowchart 1:** Types of ECMO as per cannulation sites.

(ECMO: extracorporeal membrane oxygenation; $ECCO_2R$: extracorporeal carbon dioxide removal; VA: vevoarterial; VAPa: venovenous pulmonary artery; VAV: venoarterial venous; VV: vevovenous; VVA: vevovenous arterial).

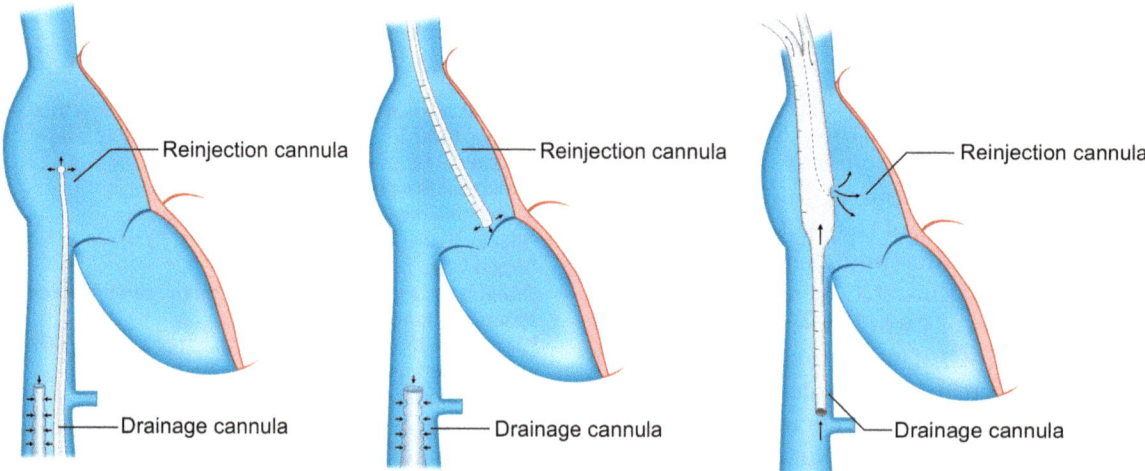

**Fig. 2:** Vevovenous extracorporeal membrane oxygenation (VV-ECMO) cannulations.
*Source:* Banfi C, Siegenthaler N, Brunner ME, et al. Veno-venous extracorpeal membrane oxygenation: cannulation techniques. J Thorac Dis. 2016;8(12):3762-73.

# Chapter 19
## Extracorporeal Membrane Oxygenation

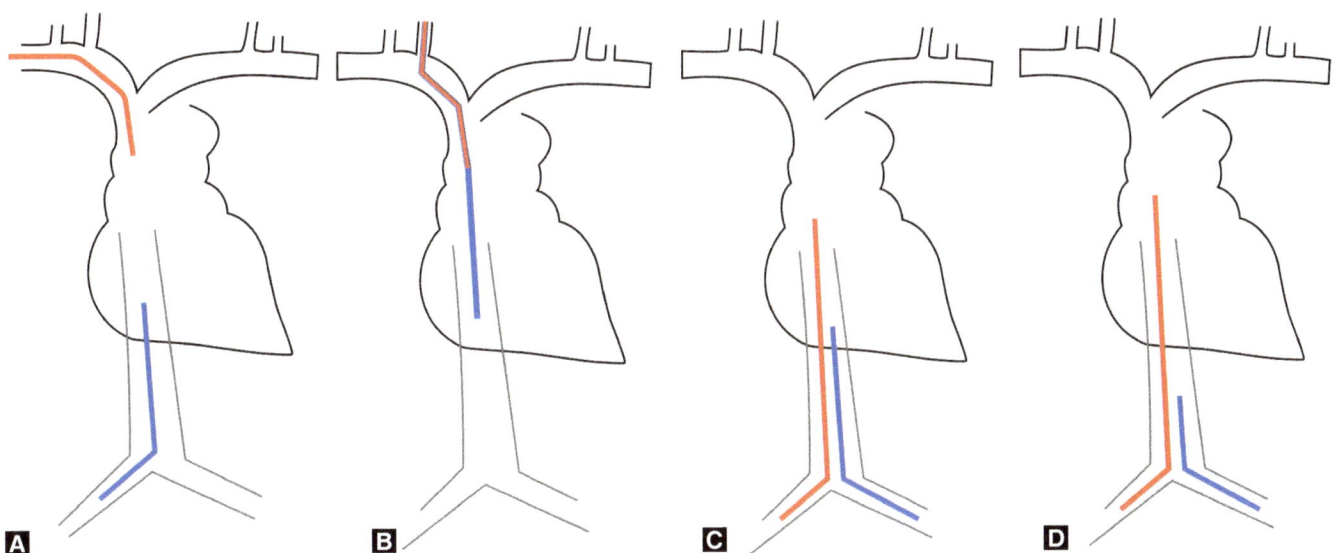

**Figs. 3A to D:** Vevovenous extracorporeal membrane oxygenation (VV-ECMO) cannulations: (A) Subclavian vein-femoral vein cannulation; (B) double lumen internal jugular vein cannulation; (C) femoral vein-femoral vein cannulation with both cannulas in right atrium; (D) femoral vein-femoral vein cannulas with drainage cannula in common iliac vein.

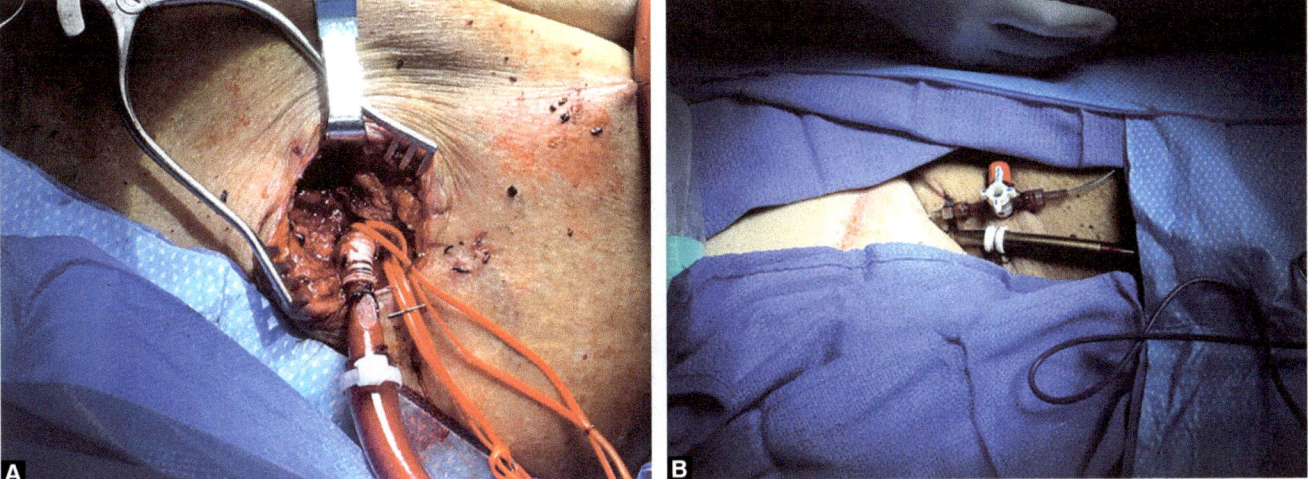

**Figs. 4A and B:** Right subclavian artery cannula with graft (A) and simultaneous left femoral vein cannula (B) in same patient.

clotting or circuit-backflow. Recording a plot of $DO_2$ and $VO_2$ may be helpful.
- Monitor recovery of heart function by reducing the flow and observing the pulse contour. Venous saturation should remain above 65%. Transesophageal echocardiography may be very helpful to guide therapy. If satisfactory LV recovery ensured, proceed to weaning and decannulation.

## Conduct of VV-Extracorporeal Membrane Oxygenation[1,23]

- Suggested cannulas are mentioned in Tables 6 and 7.
- Estimate metabolic rate and CO (flow) as above. Plan for a complete CPB support.
- Estimate the maximal venous drainage. Adjust the ventilator settings to lung protective strategy with

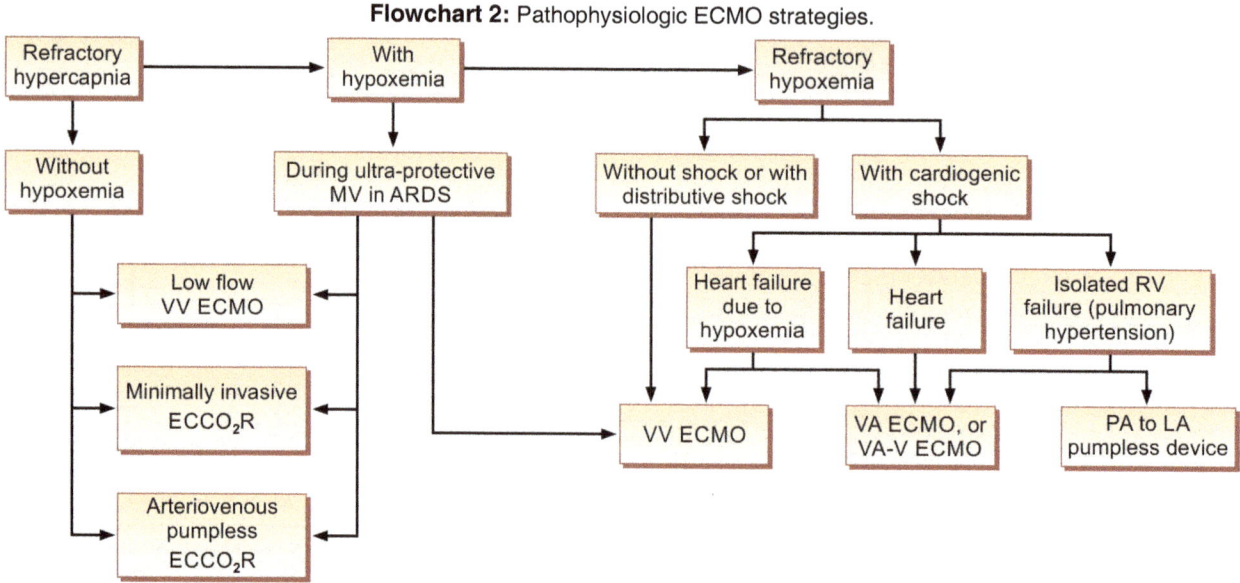

**Flowchart 2:** Pathophysiologic ECMO strategies.

(ARDS: acute respiratory distress syndrome; ECMO: extracorporeal membrane oxygenation; ECCO$_2$R: extracorporeal carbon dioxide removal; LA: left atrium; MV: mechanical ventilation; PA: pulmonary artery; RV: right ventricular; VA: vevoarterial; VV: vevovenous).

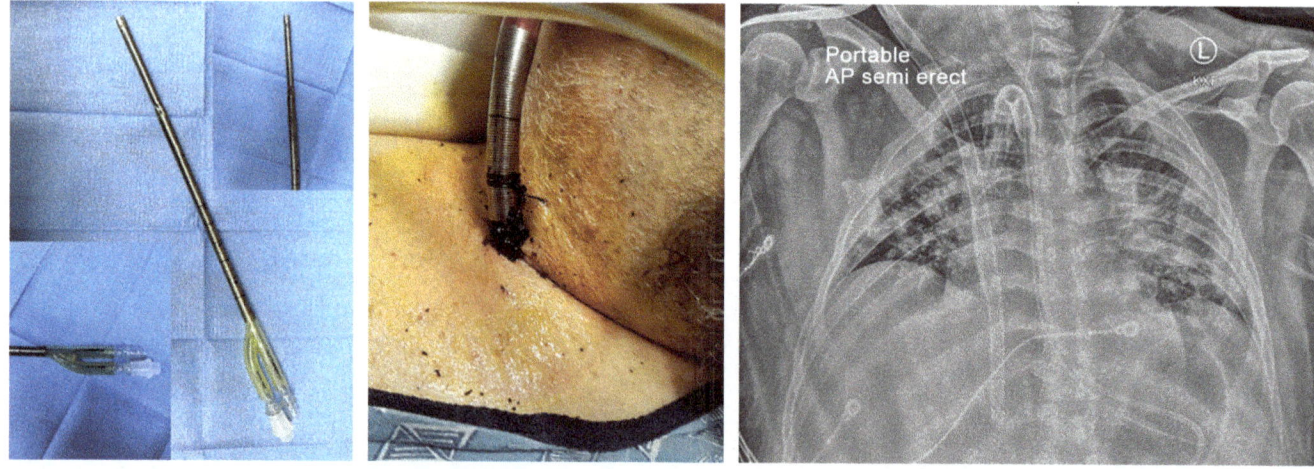

**Fig. 5:** Right internal jugular neck cannulation for vevovenous extracorporeal membrane oxygenation (VV-ECMO; center) showing Avalon catheter on left and chest X-ray on right.

reduced tidal volume, high positive end-expiratory pressure (PEEP), low fraction of inspired oxygen (FiO$_2$). Try tapering vasoactive drugs to reduce afterload on the heart. Titrate the sweep speed to maintain PaCO$_2$ at about 40 mm Hg.
- Assess O$_2$ kinetics at 6–12 hours. Maintain DO$_2$/VO$_2$ > 3:1. If the ratio starts trending down, despite adequate Hb and adequate sedation and muscle relaxation, suspect that venous drainage may be inadequate for the patient. A transesophageal echocardiogram may help assess cardiac function. Maintain a graphic plot of DO$_2$ and VO$_2$.
- When arterial saturation remains >95% and venous saturation remains >70%, reduce the flow. Maintain sweep to keep PaCO$_2$ at 40 mm Hg. If lung function will permit, attempt to wean off the flows and decannulate.

## MANAGEMENT OF EXTRACORPOREAL MEMBRANE OXYGENATION

### Hemodynamic[7,24,25]

Central VA-ECMO provides better *hemodynamic support* than peripheral VA-ECMO. Most frequently central VA-ECMO is implemented during cardiac surgical cases with sternotomy and difficulty weaning from CPB. Initiation of ECMO may be less orderly and less well-controlled when initiated as part of extracorporeal cardiopulmonary resuscitation (EC-CPR). Peripheral ECMO is often the *quickest* way of establishing extracorporeal life support.

Several unique hemodynamic issues may be encountered in peripheral ECMO.
- *Harlequin syndrome:* As the heart function starts to recover and ejects blood (Fig. 6), partially desaturated blood from the native lung starts to perfuse the right hemisphere of brain and right arm through the innominate artery. In order to detect this, it is important to compare right and left arm arterial oxygen saturation simultaneously. If this persists due to cardiac recovery preceding lung recovery, placement of a cannula from the arterial (oxygenated) side of ECMO to the right atrium, therefore creating a VA-V ECMO also called "one and a half" ECMO might help.
- *LV afterload*: With peripheral VA-ECMO, on the other hand, with poor cardiac function the retrograde flow from the peripheral circulation may increase afterload sufficiently to delay cardiac recovery even further. This

**Table 6A:** Variety of cannulas.

| Manufacturer | Size (Fr) | Length (cm) | Pressure gradient At 4 L/min mm Hg | Features |
|---|---|---|---|---|
| Avalon elite | 20–31 | 31 | 110 (31 Fr return) 30 (31 Fr drainage) | Kink-resistant material, wire-reinforced Radio-opaque Deflectable inner membrane Distal and proximal drainage ports |
| Novaport | 18–24 | 27 | N/A | Kink-resistant Wire-reinforced Heparin coated |
| OriGen | 23–32 | 20–30 | 140 (13 Fr return) 30 (13 Fr drainage) | Wire-reinforced Separate infusion and drainage ports |

**Table 6B:** Cannula sizes.

| Patient Weight (Kg) | Atrial cannula (Fr) | Aortic cannula (Fr) | Anticipated flows (L/min) |
|---|---|---|---|
| <10 | 14–28 | 10–16 | 1–2 |
| 10–20 | 20–36 | 14–20 | 3–4 |
| 21–40 | 24–46 | 18–21 | 4–6 |
| 41–60 | 28–50 | 20–24 | 6–8 |
| >60 | 36–52 | 22–24 | 8–10 |

[Fr: French (size)].

**Table 7:** Suggested cannula sizes.

| ECMO configuration | Cannula size (Fr) | Cannula length (cm) | Cannula tip position | Blood flow (L/min) | Recirculation | Hemodynamic support | Lower limb ischemia |
|---|---|---|---|---|---|---|---|
| Femoral-jugular VV-ECMO | Inflow: 23–29 Outflow: 15–23 | Inflow: 38–68 Outflow: 15–23 | Inflow: Hepatic IVC Outflow: Right atrium | 2–7 | ++ | No | No |
| Femoral-femoral VV-ECMO | Inflow: 23–29 Outflow: 23–29 | Inflow: 38–68 Outflow: 55–68 | Inflow: Hepatic IVC Outflow: Right atrium | 2–4 | +++ | No | No |
| Dual lumen cannula VV-ECMO | 23–31 | 31 | Inflow: Hepatic IVC and SVC Outflow: Right atrium | 2–5 | + | No | No |
| Femoral-femoral-jugular VA-V ECMO | Inflow: 23–29 V-outflow: 15–23 A-outflow: 15–19 | Inflow: 38–68 V-Outflow: 15–23 A-Outflow: 15 | Inflow: Hepatic IVC Outflow: Right atrium and femoral artery | 2–7 | ++ | Yes | Yes |

[ECMO; extracorporeal membrane oxygenation; Fr: French (size); IVC: inferior vena cava; SVC: superior vena cava; VV: venovenous].

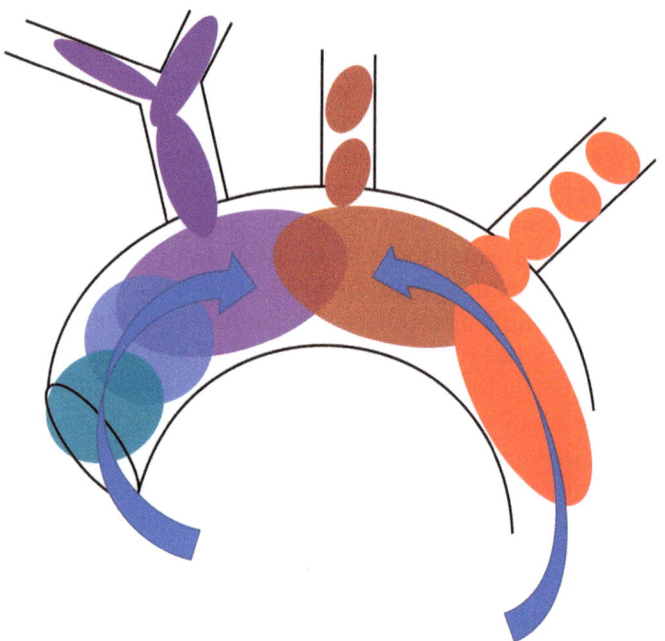

**Fig. 6:** Harlequin syndrome: Flow competition happening from recovering ventricle ejecting deoxygenated blood and ECMO pushing out oxygenated blood into the aortic arch. This may lead to delivery of deoxygenated blood to the brain.

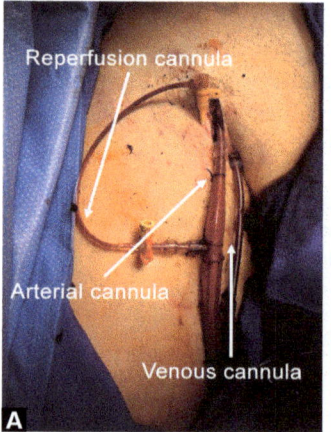 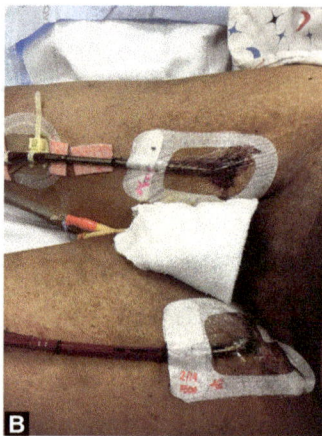

**Figs. 7A and B:** (A) Left femoral artery and left vein cannulation for vevoarterial extracorporeal membrane oxygenation (VA-ECMO) with reperfusion cannula in left femoral artery. (B) Right femoral vein and left femoral artery cannulation for VA-ECMO without reperfusion cannula.

may be identified on echocardiogram with a much dilated left atrium. Other than escalating inotropes to help the LV, management of this situation may be achieved by offloading the LV by:
- Placing a cannula in the pulmonary artery or LV to vent or drain blood to the venous side of the ECMO, so creating a "one and a half" ECMO or a VA-V ECMO.
- Placing a transaortic axial device (Impella pump), "temporary LVAD".
- Creation of interatrial septostomy to create a left to right shunt.

• *Limb ischemia*: This may be encountered in VA-ECMO with peripheral cannulation. Large bore arterial cannulae placed in the femoral artery may impair the distal blood flow. To overcome this, a small reperfusion cannula (Figs. 7A and B) from the arterial side of the ECMO may be placed distal to the arterial cannulation site.

## Anticoagulation[1,2,26,27]

Maintaining adequate anticoagulation in these patients is a major challenge. Most ECMO-related complications arise from either hemorrhage or circuit clotting.

• *Agents*:
  - *Heparin*: The most commonly used anticoagulant for ECMO is unfractionated heparin (UFH). Heparin acts through antithrombin III (ATIII) and tissue factor pathway inhibitor (TFPI). About 70% of anticoagulation by heparin may be attributed to antithrombin and 30% to TFPI. Heparin catalyzes the bonding between antithrombin III and thrombin, preventing activation of the intrinsic pathway. Antithrombin inhibits all serine proteases (except factor VIIA and protein C) including factor Xa (FXa). Heparin undergoes hepatic metabolism, renal excretion, has a plasma half-life of 30–60 minutes and is reversible by protamine. Occasionally, "heparin resistance" may be encountered in which despite the addition of extra heparin the ACT will not increase. This happens due to consumption of AT III. Treatment for this condition has traditionally been fresh frozen plasma (FFP), there being about 1 unit of AT III per mL of FFP. Nowadays, AT III concentrates are available in both pooled form (Thrombate) and recombinant form (ATryn).
  - For cannulation a bolus of heparin is given usually between 50 units/kg and 100 units/kg, thereafter maintained at 10–15 units/kg/hour to 40–60 units/kg/hour maximum to maintain a protocolized goal driven activated partial prothrombin time (aPTT) or ACT. Some suggested guidelines are mentioned hereby, but a lot of variation is observed amongst different institutions.

- A major side effect seen in patients with prior exposure to heparin is heparin induced thrombotic thrombocytopenia (HITT). In this condition exogenous heparin causes formation of antibodies IgG against platelet factor 4-heparin complex on the platelet surface. Clinical suspicion of HITT is made by "4Ts", timing (5–14 days), thrombocytopenia (<50% drop), thrombosis and the exclusion of other causes (fourth "T"). Diagnosis requires confirmation with serotonin release assay (SRA). Treatment requires that all forms of heparin be discontinued with substitution of a direct thrombin inhibitor.
- *Bivaluridin*: Bivaluridin is the most commonly used direct thrombin inhibitor. Advantages are no risk of HITT, plasma half-life is about 25 minutes, metabolized by plasma esterases, and only 20% is excreted renal, titrated to PTT (50-60 seconds) and ACT. The usual maintenance dose is 0.045–0.48 mg/kg/h. Major limitation is that it is not as cost-effective as heparin. Other clinically used alternatives are argatroban.
- Monitoring:
  - *Activated clotting time*: In a worldwide survey by ELSO, 97% of ECMO center were monitoring coagulation with ACTs. ACT measures the whole blood clotting time in seconds. Despite the variability in celite versus kaolin cartridge and manufacturer, the ACT is usually maintained at about 200 seconds.
  - *Activated partial thromboplastin time (aPTT)*: The aPTT measures the intrinsic and final common pathway. Adults may be managed using an algorithm-based titration of heparin to achieve a desired aPTT. Neonates and young children are more challenging as these patients may have a reduced baseline antithrombin and other clotting factors due to an immature liver. Also in critically ill patients, aPTT may be falsely reduced due to high F VIII or may be falsely increased due to high C-reactive protein (CRP).
  - *Anti-factor Xa (anti-FXa)*: Multiple trials have shown that anti-FXa provides a more reliable measure of anticoagulation than aPTT in neonates and young children. In an ELSO survey about 65% ECMO centers mentioned using anti-FXa for anticoagulation titration. It depends on AT III activity and falsely elevated or reduced numbers should be expected in conditions like blood transfusions, excess hemolysis, or addition of supplemental AT III. Hence it may be best to be guided by two means of monitoring rather than just one, like both ACT and anti-FXa. Therapeutic levels range between 0.3 IU/mL and 0.7 IU/mL. Suggested titration algorithms are mentioned in Tables 8A to D.

**Table 8A:** Anticoagulation parameters.

| Antifactor Xa goal range (units/mL) | Antifactor Xa level (units/mL) | UNFH rate change | ACT goal range (seconds) |
|---|---|---|---|
| | <0.3 | Increase 10–20% | Increase 10–20 seconds |
| 0.3–0.5 | 0.3–0.5 | No change | No change |
| | >0.5 | Decrease 10–20% | Decrease 10–20 seconds |
| | <0.4 | Increase 10–20% | Increase 10–20 seconds |
| 0.4–0.6 | 0.4–0.6 | No change | No change |
| | >0.6 | Decrease 10–20 seconds | Decrease 10–20 seconds |
| | <0.5 | Increase 10–20% | Increase 10–20 seconds |
| 0.5–0.7 | 0.5–0.7 | No change | No change |
| | >0.7 | Decrease 10–20 seconds | Decrease 10–20 seconds |

(ACT: activated clotting time; UNFH: unfractionated heparin)
*Source:* Adapted with permission from 'ELSO Red Book'.

**Table 8B:** Anticoagulation laboratory frequency.

| Anticoagulation lab | Guideline |
|---|---|
| ACT | Q1h–2h |
| aPTT | Q6h–12h |
| Anti-factor Xa Assay | Q6h |
| Platelets | Q6h–12h |
| INR | Q6h–12h |
| Fibrinogen | Q12h–24h |
| CBC | Q6h–12h |
| Antithrombin level | Daily-PRN |
| Thromboelastography | Daily-PRN for bleeding or clotting complications |

(ACT: activated clotting time; aPTT: activated partial thromboplastin time; CBC: complete blood count).
*Source:* Adapted with permission from 'ELSO Red Book'.

**Table 8C:** Clinical approach to anticoagulation.

| Abnormality | Approach |
|---|---|
| R > 10 min (low clotting factor) or CT (extem) > 100 sec | Administer FFP or PCC |
| MA <54 mm or MCF <45 mm and abnormal fibrinogen level (decreased platelet function or count) | Administer platelet concentrate |
| Low fibrinogen at functional fibrinogen (<150 mg/dL) test or FIBTEM (<6 mm) test | Administer cryoprecipitate/fibrinogen concentrate Usually associated with a prolonged R time, so treat prolonged R time with FFP first, and if the angle is still low, then administer cryoprecipitate as above |
| EPL >15% or LY30 >7.5% and CI ≤CLI30 <85% | Consider treatment with antifibrinolytic for primary fibrinolysis |

(CI: confidence interval; CLI: clot lysis index. CT; computed tomography; EPL: estimated percent lysis; FFP: fresh frozen plasma; FIBTEM: fibrin-based extrinsically activated test with tissue factor and the platelet inhibitor cytochalasin D; MA: maximal amplitude: MCF: maximum clot formation; PCC: prothrombin complex concentrate).
*Source:* Adapted with permission from 'ELSO Red Book'.

**Table 8D:** Anticoagulation guidelines.

| Anticoagulation lab | Guidelines |
|---|---|
| Platelets | Maintain between 80,000–100,000 μL |
| INR | FFP transfusion to maintain INR < 2 |
| Fibrinogen | Cryoprecipitate to keep fibrinogen > 100 mg/dL, or |
| | >150 mg/dL if bleeding or prior surgical intervention |
| Hematocrit | PRBCs to maintain hematocrit >30% (consider higher goal for neonatal and children with cyanotic congenital heart disease or lower goal for stable, adult patients) |
| Antithrombin | >50–80% (>0.5–0.8 U/mL), consider AT replacement if on maximum dose of UNFH and unable to obtain therapeutic antifactor Xa assay |

(FFP: fresh frozen plasma; INR: international normalized ratio; PRBC: packed red blood cells; UNFH: unfractionated heparin).
*Source:* Adapted with permission from 'ELSO Red Book'.

- *Thromboelastogram (TEG):* In addition to the above, advanced coagulation monitoring may be accomplished using TEG or rotational thromboelastmetry (ROTEM).

## Other Systematic Management

- *Central nervous system (CNS):*[28] Since ECMO patients are generally critically ill to start with, irrespective of the etiology, most will benefit from a period of sedation for up to 48 hours be maintained until some stability achieved on ECMO. Since intracerebral hemorrhage is a feared severe complication and baseline cerebral function may not have been assessed prior to initiation of ECMO, most centers will wean sedation promptly in order to perform a CNS exam.
- *Ventilation:*[29,30] Regardless of disease states and type of ECMO, lung protective strategies with reduced tidal volume, PEEP and low $FiO_2$ are advised to facilitate lung recovery.
- *Endocrine:* In these critically ill patients, blood glucose control may be problematic. Mostly all over the world nontight control is followed with blood sugars between 120 mg/dL and 180 mg/dL. It is still debated whether thyroid hormone replacement has a role to play in recovery of overall metabolism.
- *Kidney:* Acute or chronic kidney dysfunction is common in these patients. Renal replacement therapy may be needed.
- *Nutrition:* Adequate nutrition is essential for recovery. In most cases postpyloric enteral feeding is preferred.
- *Infection:*[31] These patients are at increased risk for infection due to exposed cannulation sites and immunocompromised from critical illness. Regular dressing changes are advised. Infections are initially treated with broad spectrum antibiotics pending results of cultures.
- *Hematologic:* Generally, the hematocrit will be maintained at a minimum of 30% to ensure adequate oxygen carrying capacity.
- *Physical therapy:* Since these patients are often sedated and paralyzed, precautions must be taken to prevent bed sores be taken. Patient turns and other movements require great care so as not to dislodge cannulas.

## TROUBLESHOOTING DURING CONDUCT OF EXTRACORPOREAL MEMBRANE OXYGENATION[23]

During the conduct of ECMO, multiple challenges may surface. Common day-to-day issues and their management are mentioned in Table 9. Most of these may be managed by intervention at the patient-level or the ECMO-level.

## Table 9: Common problems and interventions in conduct of ECMO.[23]

| Problem | | Where and what to do |
|---|---|---|
| Hypoxemia | Machine | Consider to increase ECMO flow/RPMs |
| | Patient | Consider a volume challenge if flows are reduced suddenly, increase $FiO_2$, increase PEEP, reduce metabolic demand (add sedation, cooling, muscle relaxation) |
| Hypercarbia | Machine | Increase sweep speed |
| | Patient | Reduce demand (add sedation, cooling, muscle relaxation) |
| Reduced flow on ECMO circuit | Machine | Increase ECMO flow/RPMs |
| | Patient | Physical obstruction: Assess for patient position changes; Hypovolemia; Consider change in line position |
| "Line chatter" vibration of ECMO tubing | Machine | Reduce ECMO flow/RPMs |
| | Patient | Consider volume challenge, rule out physical obstruction: Assess for patient position changes |
| High outflow line pressure | Machine | Reduce ECMO flow/RPMs |
| | Patient | No intervention |
| High pre-ECMO $SpO_2$ | Machine | Rule out possible recirculation: Ensure systemic $SpO_2$ is lower, reassess cannula positioning and manipulation |
| | Patient | Improving heart/lung function, or blood transfusion |
| Low pre-ECMO $SpO_2$ | Machine | Increase ECMO flow |
| | Patient | Increase cardiac output, transfuse blood, reduce patient $O_2$ demand, consider/address low $ScvO_2$ |
| High negative-pressure in inflow line | Machine | Reduce ECMO flow/RPMs |
| | Patient | Volume challenge, physical obstruction: Assess patient positioning |
| High transmembrane pressure | Machine | Consider membrane (oxygenator) change |
| | Patient | Increase anticoagulation, ensure no hypercoagulation/membrane clots |

(ECMO: extracorporeal membrane oxygenation; $FiO_2$: fraction of inspired oxygen; PEEP: positive end-expiratory pressure; RPM: revolutions per minute; $ScvO_2$: central venous oxygen saturation).

## WEANING[24,32]

The plan for weaning should be instituted the day ECMO is initiated. Weaning plans will differ depending on the primary problem (heart vs lung failure), and on the form of ECMO (VA vs VV; Flowcharts 3 and 4 respectively). Laboratory values to be followed typically include serial lactate, arterial blood gases (ABG), and venous blood gases. Neurologic status, ventilation parameters, and echocardiography will be assessed during weaning. If patient tolerates minimal support (Table 10), weaning and decannulation may be performed. VV ECMO can be discontinued in the intensive care unit (ICU) but with central cannulation for VA ECMO, decannulation will most often be performed in the operating room.

## COMPLICATIONS[33,34]

Extracorporeal membrane oxygenation is not a benign procedure. There is potential for multiple complications (Fig. 8). Often these are divided into "device related" or "patient related" (Table 11). Acute kidney injury is the most prevalent patient related complication. Due to the obligatory anticoagulation, bleeding and hemorrhagic complications are fairly common too. Infection is also relatively common, particularly when ECMO has been initiated under emergency circumstances.

## HOW I DO IT—BY DR P NICOLATO

### Protocol for Placement of Femoral VA Extracorporeal Membrane Oxygenation Cannulation

- Review consults for indications. A quick evaluation includes age <70 years. Body mass index (BMI) < 40 in VA cases, however pure respiratory cases with larger BMIs seem to do well if you can place the cannulas. Make an assessment of etiology, as it needs to be a reversible cause. Once you have determined the patient

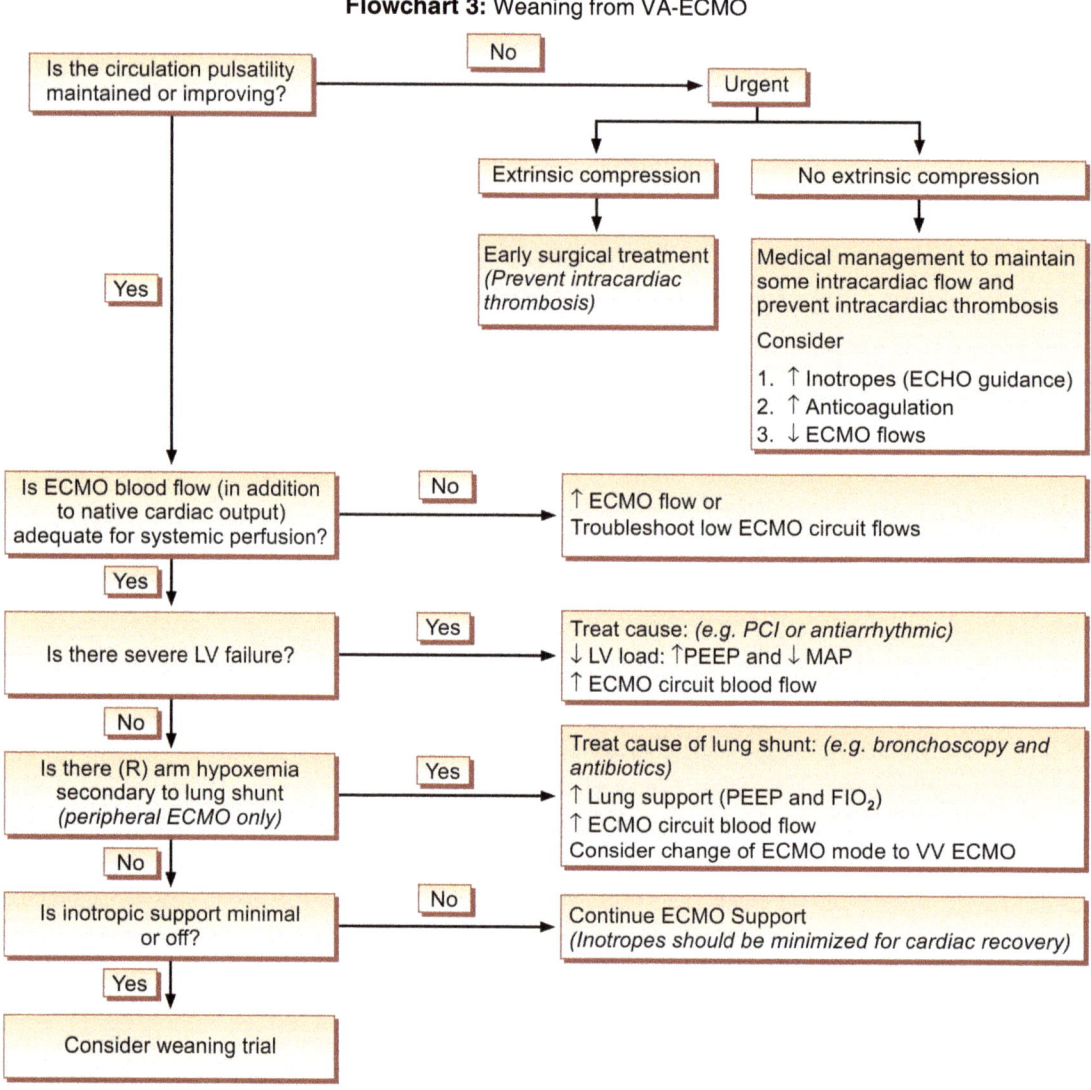

**Flowchart 3:** Weaning from VA-ECMO

(ECHO: echocardiography; ECMO: extracorporeal membrane oxygenation; FiO2: fraction of inspired oxygen; LV: left ventricle; MAP: mean arterial pressure; PEEP: positive end-expiratory pressure; VA: vevoarterial; VV: vevovenous).
*Source:* "ELSO Red Book" with permission.

is a possible candidate, do a more in-depth review of the case to determine if the patient is a candidate. For example, does the patient have coagulopathy or any areas of bleeding, does the patient have more than moderate aortic insufficiency, aortic dissection, pulmonary hypertension or any other absolute contraindication. Notify the perfusion department to bring the equipment and cannulas to bedside. It is helpful to inform them of your plan so they bring the appropriate cannulas.

- Place wires in the femoral vessels. There are two types of introducer kits, make sure you use the right length wire for each.
  - Pic A for arterial and Pic V for venous. The difference is the length of the wire. Both sets of dilators go up to 16 French.
  - Now is the optimal time to place a wire down the femoral arterial side for a reperfusion cannula to the lower extremity.
- Once the wires are in, assess the need to give 10,000 units of heparin. If you have already given it for a previous procedure then you need an ACT of 200 seconds.
- Take your time dilating the vessels, i.e. leave each dilator in place for about 5 seconds. This helps with ease of cannulation. If you notice the wire gets bent, it is easier

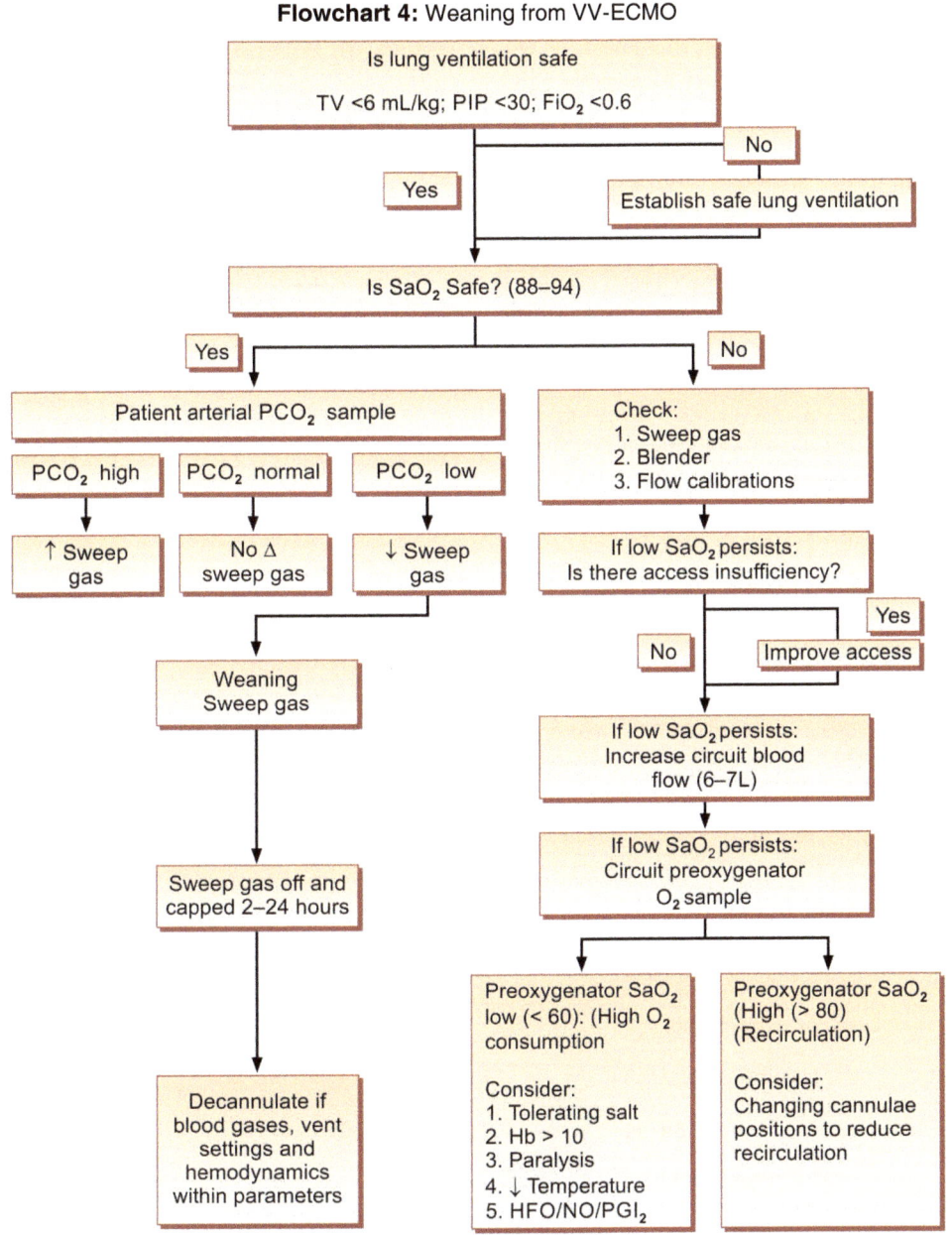

**Flowchart 4:** Weaning from VV-ECMO

(ECMO: extracorporeal membrane oxygenation; FiO₂: fraction of inspired oxygen; HFO: high frequency oscillation; NO: nitric oxide; PGI₂: prostacyclin; PCO₂: partial pressure of carbon dioxide; SaO₂: oxygen saturation; TV: tidal volume; VV: vevovenous).
*Source:* "ELSO Red Book" with permission.

to replace the wire than to try to cannulate over a bent wire.
- By the time you are finished dilating the vessels, the heparin will be circulated and then proceed with cannulation.
- Next, cut the circuit lines and secure to the table. When the perfusionist hands off the lines, clamp securely and cut the lines from the packing. It is very important to not entrain air in the lines. Any bubbles will stop the pump unless your bubble detector has been disarmed.
- Place both cannulas without removing the dilator and wire. When you are ready to connect to the circuit, pull the dilator and wire out of one cannula, clamp securely, then immediately connect to the appropriate line. Check for air and then unclamp the line. Repeat the same steps with the second cannula. If you pull

the dilator and wire out and clamp for a short amount of time the cannula will form clot. If this happens you will have to open the cannula and try to remove clots. I have used a wire to do this and it is very cumbersome with significant blood loss. To avoid this, remember to connect to the circuit immediately after removing the dilator.

- Make sure the arterial side is connected to the arterial forward flow on the pump. When connecting to the

**Table 10:** Target following minimal support parameters for 24 hours as per weaning protocol.

| VA ECMO weaning parameters: | VV ECMO weaning parameters: |
|---|---|
| • LVEF ≥25% | • $FiO_2$ < 50% (reduce to 21% keeping $spO_2$ > 90%) |
| • MAP ≥60 mm Hg | • Flow 3–4 LPM |
| • Pump flow 1–1.5 LPM | • Sweep < 1 LPM |
| • Echo $VTI_{AV}$ ≥ 12 cm | • PEEP 10–14 $cmH_2O$ |
| • Lateral E' MV ≥6 cm/sec | • RR 5–7 breath/min |
| | • TV 4 mL/kg |
| | • PIP <30 mm Hg and $P_{plateau}$<25 mm Hg |

(ECMO: extracorporeal membrane oxygenation; $FiO_2$: fraction of inspired oxygen; LVEF: left ventricular ejection fraction; MAP: mean arterial pressure; MV: mechanical ventilation; PEEP: positive end-expiratory pressure; PIP: peak airway pressure; RR: respiratory rate; $spO_2$: peripheral capillary oxygen saturation; TV: tidal volume; VA: vevoarterial; VTI: velocity time integral; VV: vevovenous).

**Table 11:** Complications associated with ECMO.

| Device related | Patient related |
|---|---|
| • Tubing rupture or disconnection<br>• Pump malfunction<br>• Cannula dislodgement<br>• Air embolism from entrainment | • CNS<br>  – Intracranial hemorrhage<br>  – Leg ischemia in peripheral ECMO<br>  – Temperature dysregulation<br>• Infectious<br>  – Sepsis<br>  – Bacteremia<br>  – Decubitus ulcer<br>• End-organ damage<br>  – Acute kidney injury<br>  – Splanchnic hypoperfusion<br>  – GI bleeding with perforation or ulceration<br>  – Liver failure<br>• Anticoagulation<br>  – Coagulopathy versus inadequate anticoagulation<br>  – Hemodilution<br>  – Factor consumption<br>  – Thrombocytopenia |

(CNS: central nervous system; ECMO: extracorporeal membrane oxygenation; GI: gastrointestinal).

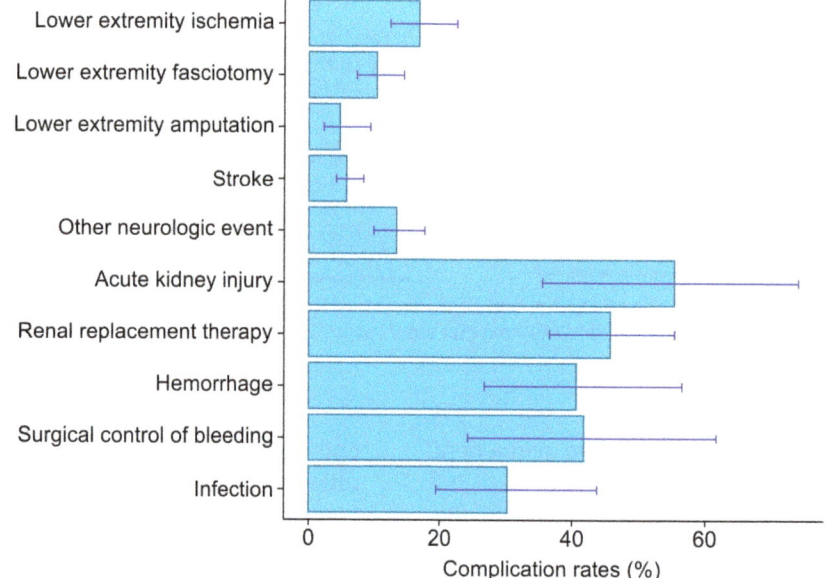

**Fig. 8:** Incidence of complications on ECMO.
Reproduced with permission from Elsevier.
*Source:* Cheng R, Hachamovitch R, Kittleson M, et al. Complications of extracorporeal membrane oxygenation for treatment of cardiogenic shock and cardiac arrest: a meta-analysis of 1,866 adult patients. Ann Thorac Surg. 2014;97:610-6.

pump, if you have two operators, one should control the clamp, gently open to fill the pump tubing with blood when putting the two together. There cannot be any air. If there is only one operator, perfusion will drip in saline to displace any air in the connection. Let the perfusionist know if you wish to do it this way so they are prepared.
- Repeat on the venous side.
- Make sure all clamps are off and go on bypass slowly. Before ramping up flow wait for the blood to complete the circuit.
- Remember that you are taking out about 500–700 cc of blood abruptly and giving a large bolus of cold saline. Now is a good time to assess blood pressure (BP) and give 500 cc of albumin or blood. The pumps are flow dependent, and need volume not inotropes or vasopressors to increase flow from the pump. Monitor venous pump saturation for goal over 60–65.
- Next place your reperfusion cannula (5 or 6 French catheter) over the wire that should be in place. Deair and connect to connector.
- To splice into the circuit, you will come off bypass, clamp distal and proximal to connector and connect to reperfusion cannula. Again, be careful the connectors are secure and that you do not entrain air.
- Once on bypass remember that you need to optimize the ventilator to match the right hand sat or right radial ABG.
- Manage BP by mean arterial pressure (MAP) optimally greater then 60, usually fresh a myocardial infarction (MI) in cardiogenic shock 70–80s should be adequate. At this time, usually inotropes and vasopressors can be titrated down rapidly to allow for the system to equilibrate.
- Secure lines to the patient and the bed.
- Anticoagulation, most commonly heparin is started when PTT drifts down to less than 100 seconds. Then titrate per protocol to manage PTT 60–80 seconds.

## Protocol for Placement of Femoral VV Extracorporeal Membrane Oxygenation Cannulation

The protocol for placing the VV ECMO circuit is similar except that wires are placed in both femoral veins.
- When choosing cannulas, the inflow cannula to the patient with the oxygenated blood should be positioned in the right atrium and the venous outflow cannula from the patient should be below the diaphragm. You can place the cannulas next to each other so you can estimate how far in to place each cannula. Also, you should confirm positioning with an X-ray or these can be placed with fluoroscopy.
- Give anticoagulation after wires are in place and prior to placing the cannulas.
- Once the cannulas are in place, remember to remove one dilator and wire and connect to the circuit immediately after, and followed by the second cannula.
- Remember to check the lines for air before taking clamps off.
- Remember to go on bypass slowly, and wait for the blood to complete the circuit before ramping up flow.
- Often you will need to give volume at this time, preferable albumin or blood.
- Adjust inotropes, vasopressors, and ventilator settings.
- Start anticoagulation when the PTT drops below 100 seconds and maintain between 60 seconds and 80 seconds.
- Secure lines to the patient and the bed.

## SALIENT POINTS

- Extracorporeal membrane oxygenation is an established means to provide temporary mechanical support in cardiopulmonary failure.
- Despite the potential benefits, there are major side-effects and complications.
- For optimal results, careful patient selection weighing in benefits versus risks is necessary as every clinical scenario is different.
- Experienced centers with dedicated ECMO teams have shown to outperform centers managing occasional ECMO.

## REFERENCES

1. Brogan TV, Lequier L, Lorusso R, et al. ELSO Guidelines for Cardiopulmonary Extracorporeal Life Support Extracorporeal Life Support Organization. Extracorporeal Life Support: The ELSO Red Book, 5th edition. Michigan: ELSO; 2017.
2. Esper SA. Extracorporeal Membrane Oxygenation. Adv Anesth. 2017;35(1):119-43.
3. White A, Fan E. What is ECMO? Am J Respir Crit Care Med. 2016;193(6):P9-10.
4. Ostadal P, Rokyta R, Kruger A, et al. Extracorporeal membrane oxygenation in the therapy of cardiogenic shock (ECMO-CS): rationale and design of the multicenter randomized trial. Eur J Heart Fail. 2017;19(Suppl 2):124-7.
5. Rousse N, Juthier F, Pincon C, et al. ECMO as a bridge to decision: Recovery, VAD, or heart transplantation? Int J Cardiol. 2015;187: 620-7.
6. Mosier JM, Kelsey M, Raz Y, et al. Extracorporeal membrane oxygenation (ECMO) for critically ill adults in the emergency department: history, current applications, and future directions. Crit Care. 2015;19:431.

7. Meuwese CL, Ramjankhan FZ, Braithwaite SA, et al. Extracorporeal life support in cardiogenic shock: indications and management in current practice. Neth Heart J. 2018;26(2):58-66.
8. Hayanga JW, Shigermura N, Aboagya JK, et al. ECMO Support in Lung Transplantation: A Contemporary Analysis of Hospital Charges in the United States. Ann Thorac Surg. 2017;104(3):1033-9.
9. ANZ ECMO Influenza Investigators, Davies A, Jones D, et al. Extracorporeal Membrane Oxygenation for 2009 Influenza A (H1N1) Acute Respiratory Distress Syndrome. JAMA. 2009;302(17):1888-95.
10. Aissaoui N, Luyt CE, Leprince P, et al. Predictors of successful extracorporeal membrane oxygenation (ECMO) weaning after assistance for refractory cardiogenic shock. Intensive Care Med. 2011;37(11):1738-45.
11. Hilder M, Herbstreit F, Adamzik M, et al. Comparison of mortality prediction models in acute respiratory distress syndrome undergoing extracorporeal membrane oxygenation and development of a novel prediction score: the PREdiction of Survival on ECMO Therapy-Score (PRESET-Score). Crit Care. 2017;21(1):301.
12. Muller G, Flecher E, Lebreton G, et al. The ENCOURAGE mortality risk score and analysis of long-term outcomes after VA-ECMO for acute myocardial infarction with cardiogenic shock. Intensive Care Med. 2016;42(3):370-8.
13. Peigh G, Cavarocchi N, Keith SW, et al. Simple new risk score model for adult cardiac extracorporeal membrane oxygenation: simple cardiac ECMO score. J Surg Res. 2015;198(2):273-9.
14. Chen CY, Tsai J, Hsu TY, et al. ECMO Used in a Refractory Ventricular Tachycardia and Ventricular Fibrillation Patient: A National Case-Control Study. Medicine (Baltimore). 2016;95(13):e3204.
15. Tonna JE, Johnson NJ, Greenwood J, et al. Practice characteristics of Emergency Department extracorporeal cardiopulmonary resuscitation (eCPR) programs in the United States: The current state of the art of Emergency Department extracorporeal membrane oxygenation (ED ECMO). Resuscitation. 2016;107:38-46.
16. Banfi C, Pozzi M, Brunner ME, et al. Veno-arterial extracorporeal membrane oxygenation: an overview of different cannulation techniques. J Thorac Dis. 2016;8(9):E875-E885.
17. Banfi C, Pozzi M, Siegenthaler N, et al. Veno-venous extracorporeal membrane oxygenation: cannulation techniques. J Thorac Dis. 2016;8(12):3762-73.
18. ELSO. (2017). SAVE SCORE. The SAVE Score has been developed by ELSO and The Department of Intensive Care at The Alfred Hospital, Melbourne. It is designed to assist prediction of survival for adult patients undergoing extracorporeal membrane oxygenation for refractory cardiogenic shock. It should not be considered a substitute for clinical assessment. [online] Available from http://www.save-score.com/.
19. Pavlushkov E, Berman M, Valchanov K. Cannulation techniques for extracorporeal life support. Ann Transl Med. 2017;5(4):70.
20. Jayaraman AL, Cormican D, Shah P, et al. Cannulation strategies in adult veno-arterial and veno-venous extracorporeal membrane oxygenation: Techniques, limitations, and special considerations. Ann Card Anaesth. 2017;20(Supplement):S11-S18.
21. Kanji HD, Chouldechova A, Harvey C, et al. Safety and Outcomes of Mobile ECMO Using a Bicaval Dual-Stage Venous Catheter. ASAIO J. 2017;63(3):351-5.
22. Lehle K, Phillipp A, Müller T, et al. Flow dynamics of different adult ECMO systems: a clinical evaluation. Artif Organs. 2014;38(5):391-8.
23. Fierro MA, Daneshmand MA, Bartz RR. Perioperative Management of the Adult Patient on Venovenous Extracorporeal Membrane Oxygenation Requiring Noncardiac Surgery. Anesthesiology. 2018;128(1):181-201.
24. Le Gall A, Follin A, Cholley B, et al. Veno-arterial-ECMO in the intensive care unit: From technical aspects to clinical practice. Anaesth Crit Care Pain Med. 2018;37(3):259-68.
25. Gu K, Zhang Y, Gao B, et al. Hemodynamic Differences Between Central ECMO and Peripheral ECMO: A Primary CFD Study. Med Sci Monit. 2016;22:717-26.
26. Raffini L. Anticoagulation with VADs and ECMO: walking the tightrope. Hematology Am Soc Hematol Educ Program. 2017;2017(1):674-80.
27. Bolliger D, Zenklusen U, Tanaka KA. Point-of-care coagulation management algorithms during ECMO support: are we there yet? Minerva Anestesiol. 2016;82(9):1000-9.
28. Langer T, Santini A, Bottino N, et al. "Awake" extracorporeal membrane oxygenation (ECMO): pathophysiology, technical considerations, and clinical pioneering. Crit Care. 2016;20(1):150.
29. Serpa Neto A, Schmidt M, Azevedo LC, et al. Associations between ventilator settings during extracorporeal membrane oxygenation for refractory hypoxemia and outcome in patients with acute respiratory distress syndrome: a pooled individual patient data analysis: Mechanical ventilation during ECMO. Intensive Care Med. 2016;42(11):1672-84.
30. Camporota L, Nicoletti E, Malafronte M, et al. International survey on the management of mechanical ventilation during ECMO in adults with severe respiratory failure. Minerva Anestesiol. 2015;81(11):1170-83.
31. Trudzinski FC, Schlotthauer U, Kamp A, et al. Clinical implications of Mycobacterium chimaera detection in thermoregulatory devices used for extracorporeal membrane oxygenation (ECMO), Germany, 2015 to 2016. Euro Surveill. 2016;21(46).
32. Pappalardo F, Pieri M, Arnaez Corada B, et al. Timing and Strategy for Weaning From Venoarterial ECMO are Complex Issues. J Cardiothorac Vasc Anesth. 2015;29(4):906-11.
33. Lamb KM, Hirose H. Vascular Complications in Extracoporeal Membrane Oxygenation. Crit Care Clin. 2017;33(4):813-24.
34. Millar JE, Fanning JP, McDonald CI, et al. The inflammatory response to extracorporeal membrane oxygenation (ECMO): a review of the pathophysiology. Crit Care. 2016;20(1):387.

# CHAPTER 20

# Extracorporeal Membrane Carbon Dioxide Removal

*Pramod K Guru, Anjali Agarwal, Devang Sanghavi*

## INTRODUCTION

The evolution of modern critical care practice is based on invention and application of mechanical ventilatory (MV) support for patients with respiratory failure. MV support has undoubtedly saved scores of patients' lives over the years. However, there is still an unmet need to help and improve the outcomes of patients with both acute and chronic respiratory failure. There are many reasons, but these are mostly limited to the failure to achieve the intended physiologic goals of ventilation and oxygenations, and the adverse consequences of positive-pressure mechanical ventilation. Many strategies have been tried to circumvent the negative consequences of positive-pressure ventilations. One such strategy is the application of extracorporeal membrane oxygenation (ECMO) in the management of respiratory failure. ECMO has the capabilities to take over of lung function by assisting in both oxygenation and ventilation. There are many forms of ECMO systems, and extracorporeal carbon dioxide removal ($ECCO_2R$) is one of them. Over the past decade, the technical advancement and clinical experience in application of the technology has led to growing interest in $ECCO_2R$ for management of acute respiratory failure secondary to varied etiology. The chapter will describe the basic differences of the various available systems, summarize the scientific literature in clinical applications, and appraise future challenges.

## EXTRACORPOREAL PRINCIPLES AND TYPES

The ECMO is based on the principle of blood oxygenation and decarboxylation outside the body, thereby reducing the intrinsic lung functions. The principle of extracorporeal support of heart and lung function is credited to the development of heart-lung bypass machine by Dr Gibbon in 1953. However, the physiological idea of separation of oxygenation and ventilation was first championed in 1978 by Gattinoni et al. The principle of "Apneic oxygenation" is based on the assumptions that removal of the carbon dioxide ($CO_2$) by extracorporeal means reduces the lung function and facilitates the oxygenation of alveoli by supplemental oxygenation.[1,2]

### Circuit and Physiology

Essential features of all forms of ECMO system consist of drainage of the deoxygenated venous blood from the venous compartment of the body, exchange of gases through the semipermeable membrane lung, and return of the oxygenated and decarboxylated blood to the either venous or arterial compartment (Fig. 1). When the blood is returned to the venous compartment, the configuration is called venovenous ECMO (VV-ECMO), and when it is returned to arterial compartment, it is called venoarterial ECMO (VA-ECMO). In VV-ECMO, the extracorporeal circuit is in-series with the native cardiopulmonary circuit, whereas in VA-ECMO it works in-parallel. While VV-ECMO only supports the respiratory system, VA-ECMO has the capability to support both the cardiac and respiratory systems. Currently the membrane lungs for gas exchange are exclusively made of polymethylpentene (PMP) or siloxane.[3] The mesh-like design of the membrane is responsible for increase in the surface area for membrane-to-blood contact and gas exchange efficiency. The diffusion gradient for exchange of gas is produced across the semipermeable membrane by the flow of deoxygenated blood and the sweep gas (air mixture with high $O_2$ content but little or no $CO_2$) side by side. Anticoagulation with heparin or other available agents is needed to prevent thrombus formation and smooth functioning of the extracorporeal circuit in all the available devices.

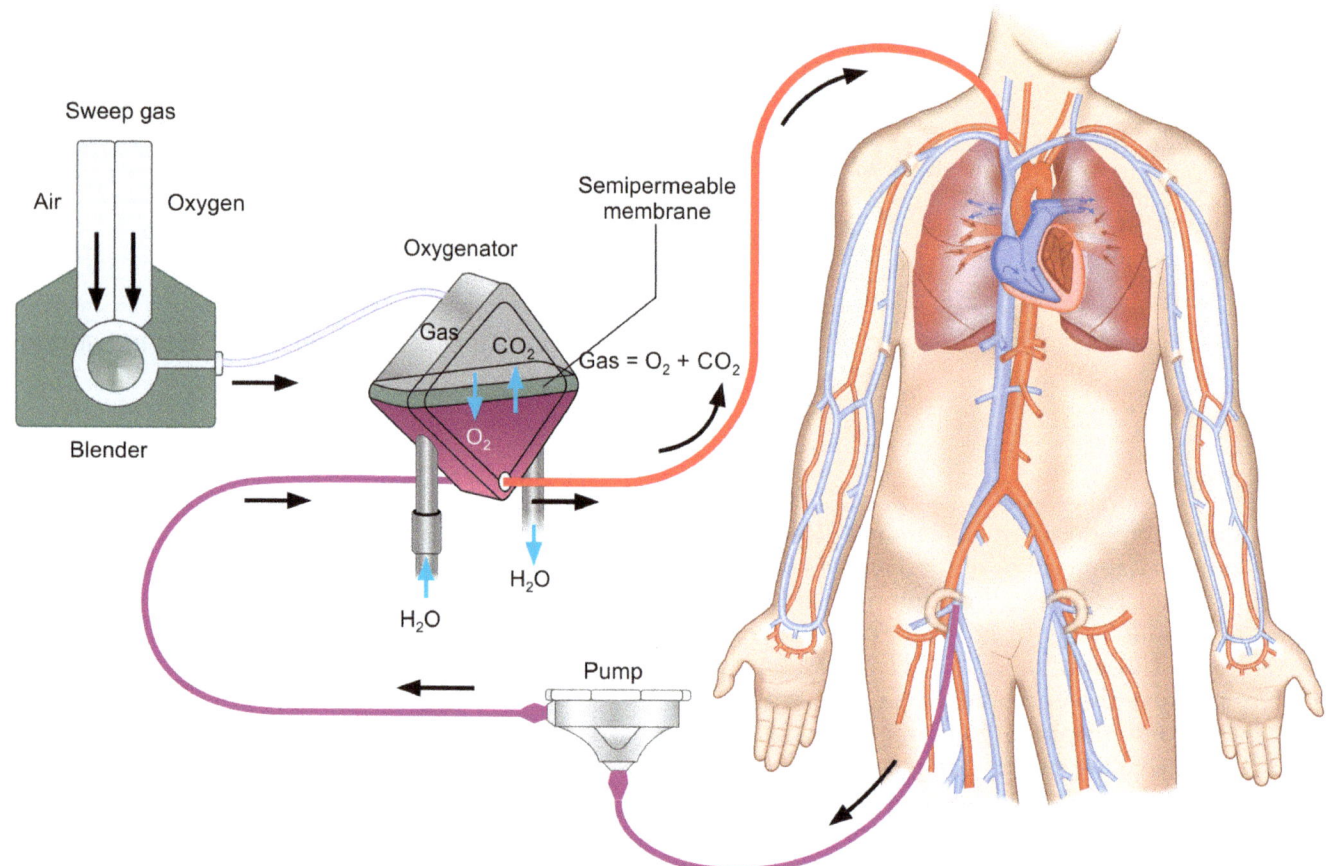

**Fig. 1:** Extracorporeal circuit configuration. The circuit configuration shows a femoral vein drainage cannula (extending into the junction of inferior vena cava and right atrium) with deoxygenated blood (purple colored) and an internal jugular vein return cannula (extending into the junction of superior vena cava and right atrium) with oxygenated blood (pink colored) for the two-site approach (also called femoroatrial or cavoatrial approach) to venovenous extracorporeal membrane oxygenation (ECMO) cannulation.

Extracorporeal $CO_2$ removal is a *modified* form of VV-ECMO, which is aimed primarily for decarboxylation ($CO_2$ removal) with a reduced amount of extracorporeal blood flow (range from 200 mL/min to 1,500 mL/min). The goal of $ECCO_2R$ is to decrease the $PaCO_2$ to allow reduction in work of breathing and the level of support of mechanical ventilation. As a result of reduced blood flow needs secondary to sole focus on decarboxylation, lead to the need to have smaller vascular catheters (12–14 French) as compared to the conventional extracorporeal circuit. Table 1 outlines the major differences between the systems. While the basic circuit principle remains the same, the system has been divided into multiple modes depending upon the type of pumps and other external features. There are four types of commercially available products for $ECCO_2R$ removal, such as (1) Pumpless system, (2) Pump system, (3) Gas exchange catheters, and (4) Respiratory dialysis. $ECCO_2R$ systems vary in relation to their technology, gas exchange ability, and application characteristics.

## Arteriovenous Pumpless System

Arteriovenous (AV) pumpless system, also called AV system, is the oldest system available in market. The circuit configuration consists of an arterial cannula, mostly in femoral artery, a membrane oxygenator for decarboxylation, and a return cannula in venous system (unilateral or contralateral femoral vein). Blood flow in the circuit is dependent on the systemic pressure, and requires a minimum mean arterial pressure (MAP) greater than 60 mm Hg for efficient function. The utilization of this simplified system in clinical practice certainly achieved the intended goal as reported by multiple studies.[4] However, the system has been out of favor due to the need for inotropic support, inability to use in hemodynamically compromised patients, and the need for arterial cannulation with risk of injury and limb ischemia. The prototype of AV system is interventional lung assist (iLa; NovaLung), with its use well described in the study by Florchinger et al.[5]

**Table 1:** Differences between various forms of extracorporeal therapy.

|  | VV-ECCO$_2$R | AV-ECCO$_2$R | VV-ECMO | VA-ECMO |
|---|---|---|---|---|
| Extracorporeal blood flow rate | 0.3–1.5 L/min | 0.3–1.5 L/min | 3–7 L/min | 3–7 L/min |
| Arterial cannulation | No | Yes | No | Yes |
| Catheter diameter | Small | Small | Large | Large |
| Pump in the circuit | Yes | No | Yes | No |
| Need for anticoagulation | Minimal | Minimal | Maximal | Maximal |
| Gas exchange | Mainly CO$_2$ removal | Mainly CO$_2$ removal | Both CO$_2$ removal and oxygenation | Oxygenation, CO$_2$ removal and circulatory support |
| Cardiorespiratory support | Hypercapnic respiratory failure | Hypercapnic respiratory failure | Hypoxic and hypercapnic respiratory failure | Support both failed cardiac and respiratory system |
| Ventilation | Yes | Yes | Yes | Yes |
| Oxygenation | Minimal | Nil | Excellent | Excellent |
| Risk of complications | Minimal | Intermediate | Intermediate | Maximal |

(VV-ECCO$_2$R: veno-venous extracorporeal carbon dioxide removal; AV-ECCO$_2$R: atrio-venous extracorporeal carbon dioxide removal; VV-ECMO: veno-venous extracorporeal membrane oxygenation; VA-ECMO: veno-atrial extracorporeal membrane oxygenation).

## Venovenous Pump System

In the venovenous (VV) system, there is an integrated pump (either centrifugal or roller pumps) in the circuit to drain the blood from the patient for gas exchange. Addition of the pump not only circumvents the dependence on systemic arterial pressure, but also reduces the risk of limb ischemia by avoiding arteriotomy. There is a conceptual similarity between VV-ECO$_2$R and dialysis with respect to use of cannulas and in cannulation technique. The new generation systems provide better control of the blood flow and give an opportunity for step up for oxygenation in the same circuit. The commercially available products come in two forms: single console with integrated pump and oxygenator or separated pump and oxygenator. Most of the recently published studies of ECCO$_2$R are on the VV system. Vascular access for VV system is most often achieved via a single or dual lumen catheter in the internal jugular or femoral veins (preferred sites) depending on system and the desired blood flow rate. Commercial available systems vary not only in sizes but also membrane surface area and blood flow rates (Table 2).[6]

One of the prominent limitation of both the AV and VV system for ECCO$_2$R is the amount of CO$_2$ removal per a given time frame per a given blood flow. CO$_2$ is carried in the blood mostly as carbonic acid (85%), minor fraction is bound to proteins (10%), and only 5% in solution. Physiologically most of the CO$_2$ in blood is in the bicarbonate form (also called wet form), which needs to be dissociated for exchange via the membrane. This is because, only the dissolved or dry CO$_2$ (which constitutes only one-third of total CO$_2$) in blood is available for exchange via the membrane oxygenator. The chemical conversion reaction of bicarbonate to free CO$_2$ is in contrast to that of dissociation of oxygen and hemoglobin. It follows linear kinetics principle, and does not become saturated. This is why CO$_2$ diffusion from the blood is more efficient (x20 faster) than O$_2$. The CO$_2$ clearance from the blood relies on many factors such as blood CO$_2$ content, pH and hemoglobin; gradient of CO$_2$ across the membrane, membrane surface area and efficiency, the sweep gas flow rate and the blood flow rate.[7]

Carbon dioxide removal follows a biphasic pattern with initial rapid (dissolved CO$_2$) followed by steady state (liberated from bicarbonate).[8] Available ECCO$_2$R systems are capable of removing up to 25% of daily CO$_2$ production to allow at least 50% reduction in minute ventilation.[9] To optimize the CO$_2$ clearance for maximal effect, many newer devices with unique strategies have been developed recently.

## Gas Exchange Catheters

The primary principle of these catheters is to increase the dissociation of bicarbonate in the blood, and achieve the CO$_2$ removal in vivo. Some of the catheters are also designed to improve oxygenation. Intravenocaval oxygenator and CO$_2$ removal device (IVOX) is the first catheter experimented in animals.[10] Some of the limitations of the earlier versions of catheters have been bypassed by the newer balloon-based or impeller-based design. However, they are not yet ready for prime time for day to day care of patients.

| Table 2: Commercially available system characteristics. | | | | | |
|---|---|---|---|---|---|
| Type | System name | Trade name | Catheter size (Fr) | Membrane surface area (m²) | Blood flow rates (mL/min) |
| Venovenous (VV) | iLA activve MiniLung petite kit | NovaLung | 18 | 0.32 | 100–800 |
| VV | Prismalung | Baxter | 13–14 | 0.32 | <450 |
| VV | Hemolung respiratory assist system | Alung | 15.5 | 0.59 | 350–550 |
| VV | iLA activve MiniLung kit and NovaLung XLung kit | NovaLung | 18–24 | 0.65 | 350–2,400 |
| Arteriovenous (AV) pumpless | iLA membrane ventilator | NovaLung | 13–21 | 1.3 | 100–1,500 |
| VV | iLA activve iLA kit | NovaLung | 18–24 | 1.3 | 500–4,500 |
| VV | Diapact | B. Braun | 13 | 1.35–1.8 | 200–500 |
| VV | ProLung | Estor | 13.5 | 1.8 | <450 |

*Source:* Modified with permission from Reference 6.

## Respiratory Dialysis

Respiratory dialysis utilizes the principle of conventional dialysis for renal failure to remove the $CO_2$ in form of pure bicarbonate. A membrane lung is integrated into a continuous renal replacement circuit to achieve the goal. Regional blood acidification to increase the bioavailability of $CO_2$ by dissociation of bicarbonate ion in the blood is an attractive method.[11,12] However, the current setup is associated with significant electrolyte and acid-base disturbances in real world practice. Respiratory dialysis still remains in experimental stage, even though it holds a great promise for future.

The efficiency of $ECCO_2R$ devices varies widely, and is compared by the amount of $CO_2$ removed per minute and per 100 mL of blood flow. Knowing the efficiency of each system is of paramount importance as it determines the rate of the blood flow and size of the catheter required for adequate $CO_2$ removal in a given clinical scenario. Factors which affect the efficiency of the devices include optimal catheter site, extent of recirculation in the circuit, and individual patient factors such as body mass index (BMI) and intra-abdominal hypertension. Future research will clarify the some of the questions surrounding these topics.

## UNMET NEEDS: PROBLEMS IN RELATION TO THE CURRENT STANDARD OF CARE

### Mechanical Ventilation

Acute respiratory distress syndrome (ARDS) remains one of the biggest challenges to conquer in clinical practice of critical care medicine. In the recently concluded LUNG SAFE trial, ARDS constituted approximately 23% of the entire need for mechanical ventilation across the globe. On classifying the ARDS patients according to the Berlin definition, the researcher found that most of the patients fall into the category of moderate ARDS. There is a graded relationship between severity and mortality: 35%, 40%, and 46% for mild, moderate, and severe ARDS, respectively.[13] Unfortunately, there is no pharmacologic cure available for ARDS patients. The management is based on the support of the failed respiratory system with help of MV; and possible prevention and treatment of the underlying cause of ARDS. The MV strategies responsible for reducing mortality in ARDS patients are primarily aimed at limiting tidal volume and plateau pressure [TV of 6 mL/kg of predicted body weight (PBW), and Pplat of <30 cm $H_2O$]. However, this low tidal volume ventilation use is not universal despite the perceived and proven benefits. One of the barrier to apply low tidal volume MV strategies in ARDS patient is development of hypercapnia and it is antecedent complications.[14] Hypercapnia complicates about 14% ARDS patients managed on the basis of ARDSNet protocol with an aim to lower the respiratory rate.[15]

Chronic obstructive pulmonary disease (COPD) is the fourth leading cause of death worldwide, and expected to rise one position up by 2030. Most of the mortality and morbidity associated with COPD are attributed to the acute exacerbation leading to primarily hypercapnic respiratory failure. Noninvasive mechanical ventilation (NIV) is the current standard of care for acute respiratory failure due to COPD. However, NIV is failed in significant proportion

(25–30%) of patients, and there by needing MV support.[16] MV is not only associated with increased mortality (30–40%) in this group of patients, but also associated with failed weaning, prolonged hospital stay, and increased cost.[17]

The MV is not an innocuous support system. It is associated with multitude of problems including trauma to airways, risk of ventilator-induced injury, and the need for sedation and analgesics for synchrony. In the ideal world, the injured lung should not be subjected to further damage rather it needs rest and time to recovery.

## Hypercapnia: Friend or Foe?

Permissive hypercapnia is regarded as an acceptable consequence of low tidal volume ventilation. Not only it helps to achieve the targeted oxygenation goals, but also is claimed to reduce inflammations in the lungs. However, data suggests that acidosis related to rising $CO_2$ is not without its adverse consequences. Mortality odds progressively increase in patients managed with mechanical ventilator starting with a partial pressure of carbon dioxide ($PCO_2$) level above 50. Hypercapnia is also not welcome in patients with elevated intracranial pressure due to risk of increase cerebral blood flow. Persistent hypercapnia is associated with worsening of right ventricular function, resultant hemodynamic compromises and arrhythmias. It is also associated with worsening inflammations and immune paralysis. Overall there is a need to circumvent the challenges related to the hypercapnia in clinical practice.

## CLINICAL APPLICATION OF EXTRACORPOREAL $CO_2$ REMOVAL

### Acute Respiratory Distress Syndrome

The challenge of ARDS care stems in the absence of definitive therapy. The direct and indirect insult to the lung results in widespread alveolar and capillary damage. The clinical phenotypes differ as the lung pass through the different stages, e.g. exudative, proliferative and fibrotic stage of ARDS. The basic problems of oxygenation and ventilation are primarily due to the ventilation/perfusion (V/Q) mismatch. And, the poor outcome in these patients is mostly related to development of ventilator-induced lung injury (VILI). The principle of $ECCO_2R$ was first applied in clinical care of ARDS back in 1970. The aim was to protect the lungs from the adverse consequences of the VILI. The limited initial success dampened the enthusiasm for widespread application. Though, recently there are renewed interests in its application. In the absence of definitive treatment for ARDS, the only supportive measures which provide mortality benefit are low tidal volume and low plateau pressure MV strategies. $ECCO_2R$ technology by avoiding the hypercapnia eases the lung rest, and facilitates low minute ventilation goals. The available studies vary in their conclusion regarding the benefits. In the systematic review of older available randomized controlled trial (RCT) and observational studies, $ECCO_2R$ is not associated with mortality benefits in ARDS patients. In the recently concluded studies, the duration of ventilatory support is shown to be less in $ECCO_2R$ supported ARDS patients. However, there is no reduction in intensive care unit (ICU) stay or organ failure days. The complication rates vary widely among the published reports.[18] A definitive trial with focus on patient-centered outcomes is need of the time given the claimed benefits of the technology.

While a tidal volume of 6 mL/kg PBW is the current standard of care for ARDS patients, both animal and human studies suggest that further reduction in tidal volume could help these patients by provision of greater lung protection. The proposed ultraprotective ventilatory strategy (tidal volume <4 mL/kg PBW) also puts the patient at risk for the deleterious effect of hypercapnia. $ECCO_2R$ technology has been shown to facilitate the implementation of these ultraprotective ventilatory strategies in multiple studies.[19] Post hoc analysis of a small randomized control trial involving AV system in ARDS patient showed the benefits of low tidal volume (3 mL/kg PBW vs 6 mL/kg PBW). Multiple ongoing feasibility and safety trials in ARDS patients will help the medical community to take educated decision about the role of this promising technology.

### Chronic Obstructive Pulmonary Disease

The characteristics of acute respiratory failure in COPD patients are increased small airway resistance and increased expiratory time. The physiological manifestation of the process is characterized by the dynamic hyperinflation and increased intrinsic positive end-expiratory pressure. The hypercapnic acute exacerbation predisposes and begins a vicious cycle of increased ventilatory demand, increased production and decreased clearance of $CO_2$, and ultimately V/Q mismatch and muscle fatigue. The rapid removal of retained $CO_2$ by $ECCO_2R$ has the potential to break this cycle and help the COPD patients to restore the baseline status quickly. Also, the ability to reduce the minute ventilation can help to decrease the intrinsic positive end-expiratory pressure and volume, and improvement in dead space ventilation. The reduction of minute ventilation is helpful to avoid the intubation in nonintubated, and early extubation in already intubated patients. There are plenty of feasibility studies of ECCO$_2$R to demonstrate the physiological benefits such as reduction in PCO$_2$, improvement in acidosis and hemodynamics available in both in animals and human.

There is no large RCT published in management of COPD patient to advocate universal applications.[17,20] Available case reports, series and prospective studies are small in numbers, and have contradictory results. Nevertheless, the principal ways ECCO$_2$R has been in use in clinical practice are mainly to avoid intubation, facilitate lung protective MV and weaning of MV in acute exacerbation of COPD. Two recent reviews have nicely summarized all the past and the upcoming studies of ECCO$_2$R in COPD. The rational and the benefits of ECCO$_2$R in prevention of intubation and facilitation of extubation from invasive mechanical ventilation in patients with acute hypercapnic and hypoxemic respiratory failure in COPD patients and severe status asthmaticus are compelling, but need further research for widespread application.

### Lung Transplant

A large proportion of patients waiting for lung transplant could not make into the transplant list due to hypercapnic failure, deconditioning and many other factors. The ease of use and physiological benefits of ECCO$_2$R has the potential to help these patients in pretransplant period as a bridging therapy.[21,22] Use of ECCO$_2$R as a bridge to lung transplant in small group of 20 patients has shown to be beneficial in terms of achieving physiological goals and ultimate excellent patient-centered outcomes such as transplantation (95%) and hospital survival (75%).[22]

## CHALLENGES OF THE CURRENT DEVICES AND METHODS

The major challenges can be broadly classified into three groups:
1. *Patient-related challenges*: Bleeding related to vascular access and anticoagulation, hemolysis, heparin-induced thrombocytopenia.
2. *Circuit and catheter-related challenges*: Vascular injury, vascular occlusion, thrombosis, hematoma, aneurysm, bleeding from the cannula site, kinking/displacement of the cannulas, infections.
3. *Mechanical challenges*: Air embolism, formation of clots, malfunctioning or failure of pump, oxygenator or heat exchange malfunctions.

The characteristic complications associated with arterial catheterization for the AV system ECCO$_2$R technique are distal limb ischemia, compartment syndrome, and pseudoaneurysm formations.[23] Although these complications can also occur with VV system, these incidences are significantly less in the VV system.[24] Bleeding complications remain the most difficult task to manage in patients on extracorporeal supports including ECCO$_2$R. Several factors related to patients, circuit, and treatment may lead to an increased risk of hemorrhage.[6] The mortality and morbidity associated with bleeding have improved significantly in past years. However, optimization hemostasis balance to achieve desired outcome is a priority for the ECMO community.

## CONCLUSION

Extracorporeal CO$_2$ removal in the care of acute respiratory failure is a promising form extracorporeal therapy. It has been used both as an adjunct and as an alternative to conventional respiratory supportive system in patients with persistent hypercapnia. The indications, patient, and device selections remain in developmental stages. Carefully conducted research, gathering of clinical data and sharing of experience will help to clarify the current barriers and future safe and widespread applications.

## SALIENT POINTS

- An optimal management strategy for hypercapnic respiratory failure remains elusive.
- Both the prevention and treatment of mechanical ventilator induced lung injury are a daunting task for physicians in the ICU.
- The primary focus of ECCO$_2$R, a modified form of extracorporeal support, is to remove CO$_2$ from patients with minimal effect on oxygenation in a less invasive manner as compared to traditional extracorporeal methods.
- Extracorporeal CO$_2$ removal principle has facilitated the application of both protective and ultraprotective mechanical ventilation strategies in patients with severe ARDS.
- Extracorporeal CO$_2$ removal is an encouraging form of extracorporeal therapy to avoid intubation, and shorten the MV need in patients with acute exacerbation of COPD.
- Both technological advances and clinical experiences in the application of ECCO$_2$R technology have been associated with improvements in side effects.

- There is a need for additional research and clinical data to promote ECCO$_2$R as standard of care.
- Future studies should focus on patient-centered benefits of ECCO$_2$R as compared to the time-tested advantages and disadvantages of mechanical ventilation.

## REFERENCES

1. Kolobow T, Gattinoni L, Tomlinson T, et al. An alternative to breathing. J Thorac Cardiovasc Surg. 1978;75:261-6.
2. Kolobow T, Pesenti A, Solca ME, et al. A new approach to the prevention and treatment of acute pulmonary insufficiency. Int J Artif Organs. 1980;3:86-93.
3. Horton S, Thuys C, Bennett M, et al. Experience with the Jostra Rotaflow and QuadroxD oxygenator for ECMO. Perfusion. 2004;19:17-23.
4. Cove ME, MacLaren G, Federspiel WJ, et al. Bench to bedside review: extracorporeal carbon dioxide removal, past present and future. Crit Care. 2012;16:232.
5. Florchinger B, Philipp A, Klose A, et al. Pumpless extracorporeal lung assist: a 10-year institutional experience. Ann Thorac Surg. 2008;86:410-7; discussion 7.
6. Boyle AJ, Sklar MC, McNamee JJ, et al. Extracorporeal carbon dioxide removal for lowering the risk of mechanical ventilation: research questions and clinical potential for the future. Lancet Respir Med. 2018;6:874-84.
7. Park M, Costa EL, Maciel AT, et al. Determinants of oxygen and carbon dioxide transfer during extracorporeal membrane oxygenation in an experimental model of multiple organ dysfunction syndrome. PLoS One. 2013;8:e54954.
8. Muller T, Lubnow M, Philipp A, et al. Extracorporeal pumpless interventional lung assist in clinical practice: determinants of efficacy. Eur Respir J. 2009;33:551-8.
9. Fanelli V, Ranieri MV, Mancebo J, et al. Feasibility and safety of low-flow extracorporeal carbon dioxide removal to facilitate ultra-protective ventilation in patients with moderate acute respiratory distress syndrome. Crit Care. 2016;20:36.
10. Cox CS Jr, Zwischenberger JB, Kurusz M. Development and current status of a new intracorporeal membrane oxygenator (IVOX). Perfusion. 1991;6:291-6.
11. Zanella A, Mangili P, Giani M, et al. Extracorporeal carbon dioxide removal through ventilation of acidified dialysate: an experimental study. J Heart Lung Transplant. 2014;33:536-41.
12. Zanella A, Mangili P, Redaelli S, et al. Regional blood acidification enhances extracorporeal carbon dioxide removal: a 48-hour animal study. Anesthesiology. 2014;120:416-24.
13. Bellani G, Laffey JG, Pham T, et al. Epidemiology, patterns of care, and mortality for patients with acute respiratory distress syndrome in intensive care units in 50 countries. JAMA. 2016;315:788-800.
14. Rubenfeld GD, Cooper C, Carter G, et al. Barriers to providing lung-protective ventilation to patients with acute lung injury. Crit Care Med. 2004;32:1289-93.
15. Kregenow DA, Rubenfeld GD, Hudson LD, et al. Hypercapnic acidosis and mortality in acute lung injury. Crit Care Med. 2006;34:1-7.
16. Hoo GW, Hakimian N, Santiago SM. Hypercapnic respiratory failure in COPD patients: response to therapy. Chest. 2000;117:169-77.
17. Barrett NA, Camporota L. The evolving role and practical application of extracorporeal carbon dioxide removal in critical care. Crit Care Resusc. 2017;19:62-7.
18. Morelli A, Del Sorbo L, Pesenti A, et al. Extracorporeal carbon dioxide removal (ECCO$_2$R) in patients with acute respiratory failure. Intensive Care Med. 2017;43:519-30.
19. Terragni PP, Del Sorbo L, Mascia L, et al. Tidal volume lower than 6 ml/kg enhances lung protection: role of extracorporeal carbon dioxide removal. Anesthesiology. 2009;111:826-35.
20. Pettenuzzo T, Fan E, Del Sorbo L. Extracorporeal carbon dioxide removal in acute exacerbations of chronic obstructive pulmonary disease. Ann Transl Med. 2018;6:31.
21. Burns J, Cooper E, Salt G, et al. Retrospective observational review of percutaneous cannulation for extracorporeal membrane oxygenation. ASAIO J. 2016;62:325-8.
22. Schellongowski P, Riss K, Staudinger T, et al. Extracorporeal CO$_2$ removal as bridge to lung transplantation in life-threatening hypercapnia. Transpl Int. 2015;28:297-304.
23. Kluge S, Braune SA, Engel M, et al. Avoiding invasive mechanical ventilation by extracorporeal carbon dioxide removal in patients failing noninvasive ventilation. Intensive Care Med. 2012;38:1632-9.
24. Bein T, Weber-Carstens S, Goldmann A, et al. Lower tidal volume strategy (approximately 3 ml/kg) combined with extracorporeal CO$_2$ removal versus 'conventional' protective ventilation (6 ml/kg) in severe ARDS: the prospective randomized Xtravent-study. Intensive Care Med. 2013;39:847-56.

CHAPTER 21

# High Frequency Oscillatory Ventilation

*Albert Phan Nguyen, Ulrich H Schmidt*

## INTRODUCTION

Mechanical ventilation (MV) has been instrumental in providing life sustaining treatment for patients with various causes of respiratory failure. The concept of positive pressure ventilation (IPPV) began in the 1950s during the polio epidemic and was pioneered by the anesthesiologist Bjorn Ibsen. During this period, approximately 1,500 medical students were used to provide greater than 1,65,000 hours of manual ventilation. This led to a 47% reduction in deaths attributed to polio. What had started with simple "hand-bag" ventilation has evolved into complex systems relying on microprocessors to deliver targeted flow, pressure, and volume. Despite MV's ability to save lives, severe side effects have been identified.[1]

Ventilator induced lung injury is a broad category of pulmonary trauma caused by the use of mechanical ventilation. Ventilation at excessive volumes can lead to barotrauma due to overdistention of lung resulting in air leaks. Atelectrauma results from repetitive opening and closing of the alveoli that result in epithelial sloughing, development of hyaline membranes, and pulmonary edema. MV can induce the production and release of cytokines and inflammatory mediators resulting in biotrauma. Recognizing the complications associated IPPV has led to using lower tidal volume and positive end expiratory pressure (PEEP) to prevent lung injury from overdistention and atelectrauma.[2] In certain instances, such as severe acute respiratory distress syndrome (ARDS), conventional mechanical ventilation cannot be optimized to match the patient's lung pathology without causing further injury. In these circumstances, unconventional ventilation such as high frequency oscillatory ventilation (HFOV), have been utilized.

## PRINCIPLES AND CLINICAL APPLICATIONS

High frequency oscillatory ventilation was first described in 1972 as a mechanical means of providing oxygenation and ventilation without thoracic cage excursion. Its clinical application in the pediatric population was first described in 1983 and in the adult population in 1997.[3,4] The attractiveness of this mode of ventilation came from its potential to reduce ventilator-induced lung injury by ventilating below anatomic dead space and avoidance of cyclical alveolar collapse.

### Indications

In the adult population, HFOV had been used primarily as a rescue mode of ventilation for patients with refractory ARDS. HFOV has also been used in the treatment of ARDS in the pediatric population and was demonstrated to improve oxygenation and decrease adverse events such as barotrauma. HFOV's ability to ventilate at low tidal volumes and mean airway pressure has been utilized in the management of pediatric patients with pneumothorax, mediastinal emphysema, and pulmonary interstitial emphysema. HFOV has been successfully implemented in pediatric patients with asthma and bronchiolitis without causing air trapping or barotrauma. In neonates, HFOV has been indicated for bronchopulmonary dysplasia.

### Initiation of HFOV

High frequency oscillatory ventilation utilizes an oscillatory pump and large membrane diaphragms to generate sinusoidal pressures around a set airway pressure (Paw).[5] The Paw is generally set 5 cmH$_2$O above the patient's peak airway pressure that was recorded on conventional mechanical ventilation (CMV). While the set pressure is higher, it is not fully transmitted to the bronchi. The impedance in the endotracheal tube can reduce the Paw by as much as 16% by the time the pressure reaches the trachea. The inspiratory-expiratory ratio is another important parameter that regulates the pressure delivery to the lung and should be set initially at 1:3. The tidal volume is set to deliver between 1 and 3 mL/Kg of ideal body weight. This is accomplished by manipulating the oscillation frequency (3–10 Hz) and amplitude pressure. The mechanism of HFOV allows gas exchange to continuously occur between the upper and lower inflection points of the pressure–volume loop curve. This is thought to prevent alveoli injury by not subjecting it to cyclical opening and closing that occurs with CMV.[6]

High frequency oscillatory ventilation depends on a continuous flow termed a bias flow to deliver fresh gas and remove carbon dioxide. It should initially be set to 25 L/min and increased as needed. It is different from CMV in two ways; first, it delivers tidal volumes below anatomic dead space, and second, both inspiration and expiration are active processes.

The gas flow distribution that allows for gas exchange to take place is dependent on 7 different mechanisms. Bulk convention, which is important in CMV, plays a smaller role in HFOV in gas exchange at the proximal alveoli. Asymmetric velocity profiles rely on the skewing of the inspiratory profile and symmetric expiratory profile. At airway bifurcations, it allows the inner airway walls to move gas toward the alveoli and outer walls to gas away. Taylor dispersion is the movement of oxygen gas by a fast moving central jet deep into the bronchial tree. Pendelluft effect facilitates gas movement between lung areas due to compliance and time constant differences. Airway turbulence in the large vessels enhances gas mixing. Molecular diffusion at the alveolar capillary membrane facilitates localized gas exchange. Oxygen uptake by gas mixing from cardiac oscillation has been another mechanism proposed for gas exchange associated with HFOV.[7] These mechanisms are illustrated in Figure 1.

## Managing Hypoxemia

After initiation of HFOV, the Paw, breathing frequency, amplitude, $FiO_2$, inspiratory-expiratory ratio, and bias flow can be adjusted to optimize gas exchange. The Paw is an important parameter to improve oxygenation. Its optimization can recruit lung volume and reduce alveoli overdistention. Increasing the $FiO_2$ can further improve oxygenation.

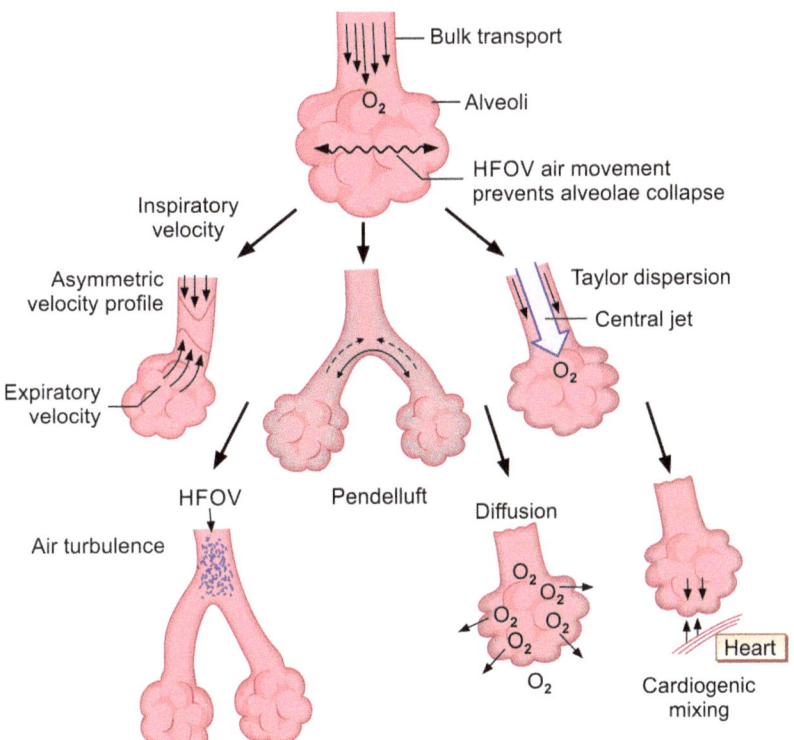

**Fig. 1:** Different mechanisms for gas flow distribution during HFOV.

### Managing Hypercarbia

Carbon dioxide removal is facilitated by increasing the inspiratory-expiratory ratio and increasing the bias flow. The oscillation frequency should be decreased to facilitate carbon dioxide removal and deflating the endotracheal tube cuff can further improve respiratory waste removal.[8-10]

### Weaning from HFOV

Consideration for weaning from HFOV occurs when the patient is able to maintain $SaO_2$ more than or equal to 88% on $FiO_2$ less than 0.5 and the mPaw has been decreased to 24 $cmH_2O$ or less. Meeting these criteria, HFOV is switched to a conventional ventilation using pressure-control mode. The pressure is adjusted to target a tidal volume of 6–8 cc/kg of ideal body weight and an initial PEEP of 10 $cmH_2O$. Ideally, the peak inspiratory pressure should be similar to the mPaw before discontinuation of HFOV.[10]

### HFOV and Hemodynamics

When optimized, HFOV has comparable effects to CMV on organ blood flow, right atrial pressure, and cardiac output. The parameter with the highest influence on hemodynamic alterations is the Paw. Set too high, it can cause overdistention of the lung and cause a reduction in venous return, which may lead to decrease in cardiac output and cerebral perfusion. Severe paroxysmal sinus bradycardia has also been reported when the use of HFOV lead to overdistention of the alveoli. In the premature neonate population, HFOV induced lung injury can also lead to the development of ischemic-hemorrhagic brain injury. Otherwise, HFOV's effects on cerebral circulation has been similar to that of CMV.[9]

## ADVANTAGES AND DISADVANTAGES OF HFOV

High frequency oscillatory ventilation has numerous proposed advantages. As mentioned previously, the continuous pressure oscillation allows for gas exchange to take place in the ideal portion of the pressure–volume loop curve. The continuous pressure keeps the alveoli open, reduces sheer stress, and formation of biotrauma. The lower tidal volumes generated allows for safer ventilation of small and heterogenous lungs in patients with ARDS. The high set Paw is thought to have a larger margin of safety in recruiting lung segments without overdistention because of minimal cyclic stretch. Compared to CMV, the shorter inspiratory time is thought to create a more homogenous ventilation. Lastly, the proposed benefit of HFOV is the active expiration process that prevents gas trapping and improved carbon dioxide clearance.[11,12]

There are known risks and disadvantages associated with the use of this unconventional mode of ventilation. In CMV, spontaneous breathing is tolerated and sedation is kept to a minimum and none if possible. In HFOV, spontaneous breathing is not well tolerated due to patient discomfort. Heavy sedation is required and in some cases paralysis is necessary. A poorly set Paw can distend the lungs and impede venous return causing hemodynamic instability. The ventilator is a noisy machine and can obstruct the clinician's ability to perform physical exams that can diagnose endotracheal tube dislodgement, pneumothorax, or other pathologic lung findings. Another disadvantage of HFOV compared to CMV is the lack of a transport ventilator HFOV capability making it difficult to coordinate patient movement intra and interhospital.[4,9]

## HFOV IN ADULT AND PEDIATRIC POPULATION

In 1997, the first adult case series in the use of HFOV for ARDS was published.[4] This garnered enthusiasm as the authors showed that 76% of their patients on HFOV for severe ARDS had significant improved $PaO_2/FiO_2$ ratio and a 30-day survival of 47%. Further excitement for the use of HFOV occurred with the completion of the Multicenter Oscillatory Ventilation for ARDS trial in 2001. This multicenter randomized control trial compared HFOV to conventional mechanical ventilation for patients in ARDS as defined by a $PaO_2/FiO_2$ less than or equal to 200 mm Hg on a PEEP of 10 $cmH_2O$ or greater. With HFOV, improvement in $PaO_2/FiO_2$ occurred at 16 hours compared to CMV. In the HFOV group had a 30-day mortality of 37% compared to the CMV group of 52%. An increase in the number of ventilator-free patients at 30 days was also seen in the HFOV group.[10]

Despite early studies suggesting that HFOV may be beneficial in the adult population, subsequent studies have essentially led to discarding this mode of ventilation. In a study comparing prone conventional ventilated patients to prone-HFOV patients demonstrated statistically similar improvements in $Pa/FiO_2$ ratios. Measuring bronchial washings from both groups showed that the prone-HFOV group had higher IL-8 and neutrophil production than the conventional ventilation group. This suggested that patients on HFOV were being subjected to cyclical alveoli opening and closing and possibly overstretching.[13] In sheep models using adult sized endotracheal tubes, HFOV was found to transmit high oscillating pressures to the airway and alveoli were found to be overdistended and injured from the rapid pressure swings.[14] Concerning was that the adult sized endotracheal tubes did not attenuate the transmitted pressures like that of the smaller pediatric endotracheal tubes. HFOV was also suggested to exacerbate right ventricular dysfunction in patients with ARDS. Using transesophageal echocardiography, right ventricular function was measured by measuring the ratio right ventricular end-diastolic area (RVEDA) to left ventricular end-diastolic area (LVEDA). It was found that the standard set Paw could worsen the RVEDA:LVEDA ratio by up to 40% and reduce cardiac output leading to end organ failure.[15] The two large multicenter studies published in 2013, OSCAR and OSCILLATE demonstrated nonsuperiority and even harm in using HFOV as compared to conventional mechanical ventilation. The results of these two studies significantly reduced the use of this unconventional mode of ventilation.[16,17]

HFOV has been utilized in the pediatric patient population since the 1980s. It has been successful in the management of patients with pulmonary interstitial emphysema, persistent pulmonary hypertension, meconium aspiration, and congenital diaphgramatic hernia. A random, multicenter trial suggested that HFOV demonstrated superiority in oxygenation compared to conventional mechanical ventilation and lower incidence of barotrauma.[18] Mortality, however, was similar between the two groups. A recent Cochrane analysis on the use of HFOV in patients with respiratory distress syndrome concluded that the mode of ventilation conferred a small protection against chronic lung disease. The study did not, however, find a mortality difference between HFOV and CMV. Currently, HFOV remains in use for the treatment of severe hypoxemia in the pediatric population.[19]

## SALIENT POINTS

- HFOV generates rapid and repetitive small tidal volumes to keep cyclical opening and closing of alveoli minimized.
- In HFOV, the peak airway, breathing frequency, amplitude, $FiO_2$, I:E ratio, and bias flow can be adjusted to improve gas exchange.
- There are seven different mechanisms for gas exchange and occur at different areas in the bronchial tree.
- Poorly set HFOV can impair cardiopulmonary function and cerebrovascular integrity.
- HFOV requires heavy sedation for patient tolerance.

## REFERENCES

1. Slutsky AS. History of mechanical ventilation. From vesalius to ventilator-induced lung injury. Am J Respir Crit Care Med. 2015;191(10):1106-15.
2. Slutsky AS, Ranieri VM. Ventilator-Induced Lung Injury. N Engl J Med. 2013;369(22):2126-36.
3. Dorkin HL, Stark AR, Werthammer JW, et al. Respiratory system impedance from 4 to 40 Hz in paralyzed intubated infants with respiratory disease. J Clin Invest. 1983;72(3):903-10.
4. Fort P, Farmer C, Westerman J, et al. High-frequency oscillatory ventilation for adult respiratory distress syndrome—A pilot study. Crit Care Med. 1997;25(6):937-47.
5. Facchin F, Fan E. Airway pressure release ventilation and high-frequency oscillatory ventilation: Potential strategies to treat severe hypoxemia and prevent ventilator-induced lung injury. Respir Care. 2015;60(10):1509-21.
6. Nguyen AP, Schmidt UH, MacIntire NR. Should high-frequency ventilation in the adult be abandoned? Respir Care. 2016;61(6):791-800.
7. Chang HK. Mechanisms of gas transport during ventilation by high-frequency oscillation. J Appl Physiol Respir Environ Exerc Physiol. 1984;56(3):553-63.
8. Riphagen S, Bohn D. High frequency oscillatory ventilation. Intensive Care Med. 1999;25:1459-62.
9. Bouchut JC, Godard J, Claris O. High-frequency oscillatory ventilation. Anesthesiology. 2004;100(4):1007-12.
10. Derdak S, Mehta S, Stewart TE, et al. Multicenter Oscillatory Ventilation for Acute Respiratory Distress Syndrome Trial (MOAT) Study Investigators. High-frequency oscillatory ventilation for acute respiratory distress syndrome in adults: A randomized, controlled trial. Am J Respir Crit Care Med. 2002;166(6):801-8.
11. Ali S, Ferguson ND. High-frequency oscillatory ventilation in ALI/ARDS. Crit Care Clin. 2011;27(3):487-99.
12. Guo R, Fan E. Beyond low tidal volumes: Ventilating the patient with acute respiratory distress syndrome. Clin Chest Med. 2014;35(4):729-41.
13. Papazian L, Gainnier M, Marin V, et al. Comparison of prone positioning and high-frequency oscillatory ventilation in patients with acute respiratory distress syndrome. Crit Care Med. 2005;33(10):2162-71
14. Imai Y, Kawano T, Miyasaka K, et al. Inflammatory chemical mediators during conventional ventilation and during high frequency oscillatory ventilation. Am J Respir Crit Care Med. 1994;150(6 Pt I):1550-4.
15. Guervilly C, Forel JM, Hraiech S, et al. Right ventricular function during high-frequency oscillatory ventilation in adults with acute respiratory distress syndrome. Crit Care Med. 2012;40(5):1539-45.
16. Young D, Lamb SE, Shah S, et al. High-frequency oscillation for acute respiratory distress syndrome. N Engl J Med. 2013;368(9):806-13.
17. Ferguson ND, Cook DJ, Guyatt GH, et al. OSCILLATE Trial Investigators; Canadian Critical Care Trials Group. High-frequency oscillation in early acute respiratory distress syndrome. N Engl J Med. 2013;368(9):795-805.
18. Arnold JH, Hanson JH, Toro-Figuero LO, et al. Prospective, randomized comparison of high-frequency oscillatory ventilation and conventional mechanical ventilation in pediatric respiratory failure. Crit Care Med. 1994;22(10):1530-9.
19. Sud S, Sud M, Friedrich JO, et al. High-frequency oscillatory ventilation versus conventional ventilation for acute respiratory distress syndrome. Cochrane Database Syst Rev. 2016;4:CD004085.

# CHAPTER 22

# Domiciliary and Palliative Ventilation

Saurabh Vig

## INTRODUCTION

A patient requiring short-term ventilator support with an acute illness is managed in an intensive care unit (ICU) or a high dependency unit (HDU) under trained medical and nursing staff; on the other hand, patients requiring long-term ventilator requirements are preferably managed at home with support of family members and thus have specific areas of concern for their management.

The number of patients requiring ventilator assistance and being discharged for care at home has increased in the past few decades. The increase in domiciliary ventilation could be explained by:
- Advances in medicine and technology have increased the survival rates of critically ill patients.
- Increased emphasis on reducing the cost of medical care with focus on early discharge and care of patients with long-term special needs at a low-cost setting, which can be provided at patients home.
- Availability of simple and versatile ventilator equipment for home use.
- Introduction of noninvasive modes of ventilation like noninvasive ventilation (NIV) and continuous positive airway pressure (CPAP), which provide better patient comfort thus increasing patient compliance to long-term ventilator protocols.

### Definition of Long-term Ventilator-Assisted Patients[1]

Long-term ventilator-assisted patients are defined by the American College of Chest Physicians (ACCP) as individuals requiring mechanical ventilation for at least 6 hours per day for 21 days or more.

Long-term ventilator-assisted patients can be described under two groups: (1) those recovering from an acute illness and unable to maintain adequate ventilation for prolonged periods, and (2) those with chronic progressive cardiopulmonary disorders.

### Goals of Domiciliary or Palliative Ventilation

Each patient may require different levels of supportive care; the overall aim is to bring the patient to a level of maximum functional independence with minimal need of supportive care. To achieve this, various aspects of basic goal of long-term domiciliary or palliative ventilation are:[1]
- Improving physical and physiological level of function
- Reducing morbidity
- Reducing hospitalizations
- Extending life
- Providing cost-effective care.

## PATIENT SELECTION FOR DOMICILIARY VENTILATION

Conditions requiring long-term or home-based ventilation are summarized in Table 1. Patient selection for home-based ventilation is done taking three aspects into consideration:[1-3]
1. Disease process and clinical stability
2. Psychological evaluation of patient and family
3. Financial considerations.

### Disease Process and Clinical Stability

The need for home-based ventilation may be due to three disease processes:
1. Patients recovering from acute illnesses and acute respiratory failure with failure of weaning from ventilator. For example, recovering from acute respiratory distress syndrome (ARDS) or severe

**Table 1:** Common conditions requiring long-term ventilation.

| Types of disorders | Conditions |
|---|---|
| Respiratory disorders | • Obstructive sleep apnea<br>• COPD<br>• Complications of acute lung injury<br>• Complications of infectious pneumonias<br>• Pulmonary fibrotic diseases |
| Skeletal disorders | • Kyphoscoliosis<br>• Thoracic wall deformities |
| Neuromuscular disorders | • Amyotrophic lateral sclerosis<br>• Guillain-Barré syndrome<br>• Muscular dystrophy<br>• Myasthenia gravis<br>• Polio and post-polio sequelae<br>• Spinal muscular atrophy<br>• Congenital childhood hypotonia<br>• Myotonic dystrophy |
| Central nervous system disorders | • Cerebrovascular disorders<br>• Disorders of control of breathing<br>• Spinal cord traumatic injuries |

(COPD: chronic obstructive pulmonary disease)

pneumonia with superimposed malnutrition, heart disease, or systemic infection, thus leading to repeated failures of weaning from ventilator.
2. Patients with chronic respiratory or neuromuscular disorders requiring mechanical ventilation for some part of the day (e.g. ventilatory support at night). For example, chronic obstructive pulmonary disease (COPD), obstructive sleep apnea, kyphoscoliosis, and progressive neuromuscular disorders.
3. Patients with complete loss of respiratory function, thus requiring continuous ventilator support. For example, respiratory muscle failure due to high spinal cord injury, end-stage neuromuscular disorders, or end-stage interstitial lung diseases.

## Psychological Evaluation of Patient and Family

The ability of the caregivers and the patient to handle the physical and emotional challenges of home-based ventilation should be assessed before planning for home-based ventilation and care. Family members must be counseled about the patient's prognosis and the anticipated challenges in taking care of a ventilated patient at home. A motivated and counseled caregiver team is essential for the success of home-based ventilation.

## Financial Considerations

Despite the fact that home-based care of a patient on long-term ventilation is economically cheaper as compared to care in an ICU or HDU, managing patient at home still posts significant costs for the family. Cost burden of the ventilator hardware and other ancillary equipment should be discussed with the family before planning home-based ventilation for a patient.

## SETTING UP THE HARDWARE—VENTILATOR SELECTION

Positive-pressure ventilator is the most commonly used device for providing ventilatory support for the homecare. Reliability, safety, and user friendly interface are major concerns while purchasing a home ventilator. Ventilators available for home care can be classified into first and second generation (Table 2).[1]

For patients on long-term ventilation backup, ventilatory support must be available in case of electrical failure or equipment malfunction. If a patient can maintain spontaneous ventilation for 4 or more consecutive hours, a manual resuscitator will be sufficient as a backup ventilation device. For patients who are totally dependent on ventilatory support or those who live far from medical support, a second mechanical ventilator is necessary as a backup. Those patients who require supplemental oxygen also should have an oxygen cylinder as a backup.

## Modalities of Ventilation in Home-based Ventilation[1,4-6]

- *Invasive mode:* Positive-pressure ventilation
- *Noninvasive mode:* NIV, nasal CPAP, bilevel positive airway pressure (BI-PAP)
- *Rarely used methods:* Negative-pressure ventilation, noninvasive devices, and diaphragm pacing.

### Positive-pressure Ventilation

Positive-pressure ventilation is usually administered as an invasive mode of ventilation. Ventilation is delivered via a tracheostomy tube attached to a first- or second-generation portable ventilator. This mode of ventilation is used in patients who are ventilator dependent, i.e. with persistent symptomatic hypoventilation and in patients who do not tolerate NIV or do not meet the selection criteria for NIV.

A patient with no spontaneous respiratory drive and complete dependence on ventilator will benefit from mandatory ventilator settings like volume-controlled

| Table 2: Classification of home-based ventilators. | |
|---|---|
| First-generation ventilators | Second-generation ventilators |
| No longer manufactured. Older versions still being used | Currently manufactured and used |
| Easy to operate, piston driven | Microprocessor controlled, piston driven ventilators |
| Modes—VC-CMV, VC-IMV | Additional functions like SIMV, patient triggering, and PEEP delivery available |
| Operate from a 115–120 Volt AC electrical outlet | May be patient or time triggered, pressure or volume targeted, pressure volume or flow time cycled |
| For example, LP-6 Plus, LP-10, LP-20 (Puritan Bennett Covidien Ltd) Lifecare PLV 100, and PLV 102 (Phillips Respironics) | For example, Achieva, Achieva PS, and PSO2 (Covidien-Nellcor Puritan Bennett, Boulder, Colo.) iVent (VersaMed/GE Healthcare) |

(PEEP: positive end-expiratory pressure; SIMV: synchronized intermittent mandatory ventilation; VC-CMV: volume-controlled continuous mandatory ventilation, VC-IMV: volume-controlled intermittent mandatory ventilation)

continuous mandatory ventilation/volume-controlled intermittent mandatory ventilation (VC-CMV/VC-IMV). Patient triggered modes like synchronized intermittent mandatory ventilation (SIMV) can be used in patient spontaneous efforts or partially dependent on ventilator.

Long-term invasive positive-pressure ventilation may lead to specific airway related mechanical complications like pharyngeal, laryngeal, or tracheal injury. Other mechanical complications include granuloma formation, tracheal fistula, or stenosis, etc. Pulmonary complications like ventilator-associated pneumonia are another cause of concern in these patients. Also, loss of speech and problems in deglutition and feeding lead to poor quality of life for the patient.

### Noninvasive Ventilation

To avoid problems associated with invasive positive-pressure ventilation, NIV or negative-pressure ventilation can be used as alternatives for home-based ventilation.

Noninvasive ventilation was introduced in the 1940s as a method of ventilation in cases of acute respiratory failure. In the recent times, the uses of NIV have expanded. There is robust evidence advocating the use of NIV in exacerbation of COPD, cardiogenic pulmonary edema, neuromuscular disorders leading to respiratory failure, obstructive sleep apnea, etc.

Noninvasive ventilation may alter the natural history of a condition and palliate symptoms; this has led to its use in conditions where it was not used previously, e.g. amyotrophic lateral sclerosis (ALS)/motor neuron disorders. Recent literature shows that use of NIV in progressive neuromuscular disorders without significant bulbar involvement may lead to improvement in symptoms and increase the quality of life.

In a palliative setting, there are two ways of administering NIV—*(a) strictly palliative approach (b) palliative and probably curative approach.*

- The strictly palliative approach: It may be used in—(1) patient in terminal phase of chronic respiratory failure who has already had NIV at home and has been given a do not tracheotomize order; and (2) patient with end-stage acute respiratory failure who has not had any experience with home-based ventilation.
- The palliative and probably curative approach: It is mainly intended to avoid intubation in patients who have refused intubation or have DNI (do not intubate orders).

Noninvasive ventilation can also be used to aid extubation as a postextubation supportive therapy.

### Negative-pressure Ventilation

The technique of negative-pressure ventilation aims to mimic the physiological process of chest expansion by creating a negative-pressure gradient to aid in air entry. Negative-pressure ventilation may be given through specialized devices such as an iron lung (tank ventilator), the cuirass, and the body suit or jacket ventilator.

Negative-pressure ventilation does not require any specialized invasive airway device, thus the patient can eat and speak with ease. Also, long-term complications of positive-pressure ventilation are avoided.

Negative-pressure ventilation as a long-term mode of ventilation is used less often than invasive ventilation or NIV. However, it may be used in neuromuscular diseases, spinal cord injuries, chest wall disorders, central hypoventilation syndromes, or for night time use in COPD patients.

Some contraindications to the use of negative-pressure ventilation are excessive secretions, decreased pulmonary compliance, increased airway resistance, risk of aspiration, etc.

## Other Devices and Techniques[1]

### Diaphragmatic Pacing

This is a therapeutic intervention where the phrenic nerve is electrically stimulated through surgically implanted phrenic electrodes connected to an implanted receiver.

It may be used in children with high spinal cord injuries or central hypoventilation who cannot use other noninvasive methods to assist ventilation. Its uses are limited due to invasive procedure of electrode implantation and high costs.

### Rocking Bed and Pneumobelt

Both these devices work on the principle of rhythmically moving the abdominal contents and the diaphragm to aid in breathing. Rocking bed is a motorized bed on which the patient is placed supine; this bed moved in the longitudinal plane from Trendelenburg to reverse Trendelenburg position through an arc of 40–60°.

Pneumobelt is an inflatable bladder placed between the umbilicus and the pubic arch, used by the patient in the sitting position. This device inflates and deflates to push the abdominal contents up and down and aid in expiration and inspiration.

Both these devices are obsolete and may be used as an alternative form of ventilation.

## Supportive Equipment

Other than ventilator, a variety of other equipment will be required to ventilate a patient at home. These are summarized in the Table 3.

**Table 3:** Ancillary equipment needed for home care of a ventilated patient.

List of equipment to be available for domiciliary ventilated patient

| | |
|---|---|
| Mechanical ventilator related equipment | • Circuits (disposable or nondisposable)<br>• Humidifier, heater, and heat-moisture exchanger<br>• Manual resuscitation bag<br>• Tracheostomy attachments<br>• Patient monitor<br>• Test lung for ventilator |
| Airway management equipment | • Suction machine and suction catheters<br>• Latex gloves<br>• Backup tracheostomy tubes<br>• Tracheostomy care kits<br>• Speaking valve for tracheostomy |
| Oxygen administration equipment | • E-cylinder backup<br>• Oxygen tubing |
| Disinfectant solution | • Vinegar/water 1:3<br>• Quaternary ammonium compound |
| Miscellaneous | • Nebulizer for aerosolized medications<br>• Spacers for metered-dose inhaler medications |

## PREPARATION FOR DISCHARGE AT HOME[1,3]

After selection of a patient and assessing readiness of the family for home-based care, adequate preparation needs to be done to ensure safe and optimal care of the patient at home. Ideally, a multidisciplinary team consisting of the primary caregiver, home-care professionals involved in nursing care, and medical follow-up of the patient should formulate the plan of discharging patient on ventilator to home-care setting. The major aspects which should be taken into consideration while planning discharge of patient for home-based ventilation.

### Geographic Home Assessment

A team of professionals is needed to assess the feasibility of patient's home for proper care. The team should look into the space available to accommodate the ventilator equipment and availability of proper electrical connections to power the equipment. Proper arrangements should be made to ensure seamless purchase and setting up of hardware like ventilators and suction equipment at home.

### Family Education

At least three caregivers should be selected, with one being trained at a high enough level to be able to train and instruct other caregivers. Components of caregiver education include operating domiciliary ventilators, disinfection of equipment, tracheostomy care, suctioning, physiotherapy, bowel and bladder care, bathing, and nutrition of the patient.

Caregiver is also taught to recognize signs and symptoms of respiratory infections, emergency ventilation using manual resuscitator, and a protocol for contact in case of emergency. Before discharging the patient and placing the patient solely under home care, it is advisable that the trained caregivers spend at least 24–48 hours taking care of the patient in hospital under the watchful eyes of nursing and medical staff. In this way, practical aspects of handling the patient and other equipment may be streamlined to ensure a hassle free transfer to home care.

## Speaking with a Tracheostomy Tube[7-9]

A tracheotomized patient inspires and expires through the tracheostomy tube. The expiratory breath exits through the tracheostomy tube and does not pass through the larynx and vocal cords. Thus, the ability to produce a subglottic pressure of 2 $cmH_2O$ with the expiratory breath is lost, leading to loss of vocalization.

Loss of speech is a significant cause of psychological distress and poor sense of wellbeing among patients on long-term invasive ventilation. Efforts must be made to restore the function of speech in tracheotomized patients to improve patient's quality of life.

Approaches to restore speech in tracheotomized patient are summarized in Table 4 and are briefly discussed further. Any of these techniques may be used to train a patient on long-term ventilation to articulate and speak, thus improving the quality of life of the patient.

### Talking Tracheostomy Tubes

These tubes consist of a specialized gas line with thumb occlusion port. This gas line is connected to a gas source. The gas flow through the specialized gas line exits above the cuff in the upper airway, thus generating the required pressure for vocal cord resonance and voice generation. These tubes allow generation of voice with the tracheostomy cuff inflated, thus in practice decoupling speech and breathing. These tubes are mostly used in ventilated patients and are seldom required in a patient breathing spontaneously on tracheostomy tube. A spontaneously breathing patient with risk of aspiration may require these tubes. Advantage with these tubes is that cuff is not deflated, thus there is no loss of ventilation and no risk of aspiration. Drawback is that a low quality whispering sound is produced and an assistant is needed to control the accessory gas flow through the tube, e.g. Pitt speaking tracheostomy tube.

### Cuff Down with Speaking Valve

A deflated cuff or a cuff-less tube allows the expiratory gases to escape from the upper airway thus helping in voice generation. A speaking valve (e.g. Passy Muir valve) is a one-way valve designed to allow air entry through it and prevents exit of air. A speaking valve attached to the proximal end of the tracheostomy tube between the tube and the ventilator thus allows air entry but stops exit of air from the tube. Air thus exits around the deflated cuff into the upper airway. This method allows voice generation during expiratory phase of breath cycle.

### Cuff Down without Speaking Valve

Voice generation in a mechanically ventilated patient with deflated tracheostomy cuff (without speaking one way valve), is possible by doing a few changes in ventilator setting to overcome the inspiratory gas leak and generate some resistance to avoid exit of gases from tracheostomy tube during exhalation. These changes are—(1) use of longer inspiratory time to overcome inspiratory gas leak and (2) use of positive end-expiratory pressure (PEEP) to bypass expiratory gases to the upper airway.

### Cuff Down with Finger Occlusion

A spontaneously breathing patient with no risk of aspiration can easily be trained to articulate by deflating the tracheostomy tube cuff and occluding the tube by his/her finger during expiration to deviate expiratory gases to the upper airway and thus generating voice.

## Expiratory Muscle Aids and Secretion Clearance[1,10]

Clearance of respiratory secretions is of utmost importance in a patient on long-term ventilation. Retained or pooled secretions can lead to aspiration, recurrent respiratory infections, and increased morbidity and mortality.

Adequate respiratory muscle strength is essential for coughing out and clearing secretions. A minimum vital capacity of 1.5 liters and a minimum peak expiratory flow rate of 3 liters/second need to be generated in order to generate effective cough to clear out secretions. Most patients on long-term ventilation have neuromuscular disorders leading to muscle weakness, thus cannot produce effective cough.

Secretion clearance may be relatively straightforward in a tracheotomized patient with help of suction catheters

**Table 4:** Approaches to restore speech in a tracheotomized patient.

| Type of ventilation in patient having tracheostomy tube | Options to restore speech |
| --- | --- |
| Patient on mechanical ventilation | • Talking tracheostomy tubes<br>• Cuff down technique with speaking valve<br>• Cuff down technique without speaking valve |
| Spontaneously breathing patient | • Talking tracheostomy tubes<br>• Cuff down technique with speaking valve<br>• Cuff down technique with finger occlusion |

and automated suction devices; however, patients on noninvasive ventilator support require specialized techniques to effectively clear out secretions.

A number of techniques and specialized devices may be used in a patient on invasive or noninvasive ventilation to aid secretion clearance. These may be listed as:
- Assisted coughing
- High frequency mechanical oscillation
- Mechanical insufflation-exsufflation.

### Assisted Coughing

This technique aims to increase the expiratory gas flow by applications of thrusts or compression on the anterior chest wall during expiration. This technique requires a coordinated effort between the patient and the caregiver; patient is instructed to take a deep breath nearing inspiratory capacity, as the patient passively expires the caregiver gives anterior chest wall compressions or anterior abdominal thrusts. A well-coordinated effort can increase the expiratory flow rate up to 5 liters/sec, thus dislodging and clearing secretions. This technique should not be performed on a patient with full stomach, is contraindicated in patient with osteoporosis, and may not be effective in scoliotic or obese patient.

### High Frequency Mechanical Oscillation

In this technique, rapid pressure pulses are applied to the chest and the upper airway with the help of a wearable vest connected to an external machine producing rapid pressure pulses. Vibrations are produced via series of pressure pulses by the external air compressor connected to the vest; this vest delivers these pressure pulses to the chest wall, thus producing mechanical oscillations of the chest wall and dislodging secretions for clearance. A number of vests are commercially available for home-based use. For example, The Vest® Airway Clearance System and The Monarch™ Airway Clearance System (registered trademark of Hill-Rom Services, Inc.)[11,12] are shown in Figures 1 and 2. The working of these two airway clearance systems is summarized in Table 5.

### Mechanical Insufflations-Exsufflation

This technique involves inflating the patient's lungs manually via a face mask or tracheotomy tube and then providing a forced expiration. The basic premise behind this technique is rapid switch between positive pressure breath and decrease to subatmospheric pressure during forced expiration which dislodges and clears secretions. Commercially available insufflator–exsufflator (JH

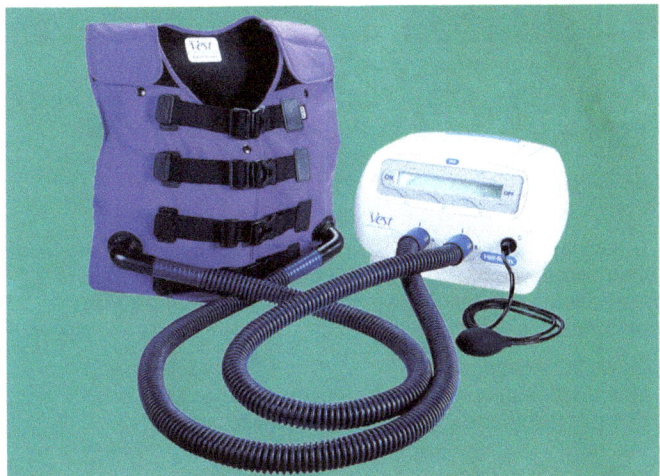

**Fig. 1:** The Vest® Airway Clearance System (registered trademark of Hill-Rom Services, Inc.). © 2019 Hill-Rom Services, Inc. *Source:* Reprinted with permission. All rights reserved.

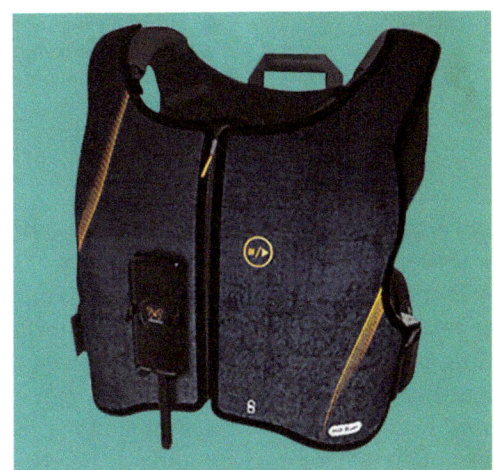

**Fig. 2:** The Monarch™ Airway Clearance System (registered trademark of Hill-Rom Services, Inc.). © 2019 Hill-Rom Services, Inc. *Source:* Reprinted with permission. All rights reserved.

Emerson Co., Cambridge, Mass) allows better patient caregiver coordination. This technique is usually reserved for use in patients for whom manually assisted coughing has been inadequate in clearing secretions. Use of this technique is contraindicated in patients predisposed to barotrauma e.g. bullous emphysema.

### Care of Ventilator Equipment and Disinfection Techniques[10,13]

Disinfection and decontamination of ventilator equipment is important to prevent infections and improve patient outcomes. Disinfection of home based ventilation

**Table 5:** Equipment to aid in secretion clearance.[12,13]

| The Vest® Airway Clearance System | The Monarch® Airway Clearance System |
|---|---|
| Based on high frequency chest wall oscillation (HFCWO) to dislodge mucous from bronchial walls | Based on same principle (HFCWO), but comes with advanced features |
| Consists of a jacket connected with tubing connected to a machine which generates oscillations | Consists of a jacket containing eight magnetic pulmonary oscillating discs (PODs) |
| Gives better secretion clearance than conventional chest physiotherapy without the need to change posture during the procedure | The PODs oscillate and provide a targeted kinetic energy to the lungs |
| The vest is connected via tubing to external frequency generator, thus patient immobilized during therapy | Not connected to a fixed energy generator, thus allows patient to move freely during therapy |
| | Enabled with Wi-Fi and Bluetooth connectivity, thus easier for patient and physician to access information and set therapeutic goals |

equipment is an important part of patient care at home and needs to be thoroughly taught to all caregivers.

Basic hygiene practices like washing hands before and after touching patients, and use of unsterile gloves in handling patient should be used by every caregiver. Equipment like ventilator tubings, suction catheter, and other reusable equipment related disinfection procedures need to be taught to the caregivers and practiced diligently.

### Ventilator Circuit Disinfection

Circuit needs to be changed only when only when it is nonfunctional or visibly soiled with secretions and blood. In general, rates of ventilator-associated pneumonia are lesser in the home care setting than acute care setting. The following steps can be followed for circuit cleaning and disinfection:
- First step is to disassemble the equipment and rinse with tap water.
- Mixture of lukewarm water and mild detergent can be used to remove visible foreign matter.
- After rinsing thoroughly with tap water, the equipment is now dipped in for 10–15 minutes in disinfectant solutions.
- White vinegar mixed with distilled water (acetic acid content of 1.25%), activated glutaraldehydes, and quaternary ammonium compounds are effective disinfectants which can be used at home.
- After taking out from disinfectant solution, equipment is thoroughly rinsed and dried.

Ideally, a patient should have at least three circuits: one in use, second being disinfected, and third disinfected dried and packed

## FOLLOW-UP AND EVALUATION

After setting up supplies and equipment at home, a dry run should be conducted to ensure their proper functioning. While transferring patient to home, the home care team must be present to alleviate minor concerns of patient and family and to formulate a follow-up plan.

In the initial phase of home care, the involvement of home care team will be more and they may have to attend to the patient on daily basis. Once the patient and the family are settled in a routine, follow-up is usually done on monthly basis. In between follow-ups, the caregiver team may be contacted on an emergency basis as and when required. Evaluations during home visits may include patient assessment parameters such as bedside pulmonary function studies, vital signs, and pulse oximetry.

## CONCLUSION

Home-based ventilation or palliative ventilation for long-term ventilated patient is aimed to improve the quality of life of the patient. With increased longevity and improved care of the critically ill patient, the number of patients requiring long-term ventilation is increasing. Thus, primary caregivers need to be updated on the criteria for patient selection and the multipronged approach involving family members, respiratory therapists, and home care team to seamlessly transfer patient to home-based ventilator care. The success of home-based ventilation will reduce case load on acute care facilities, bring down patient care costs, and improve quality of life of the patient.

## SALIENT POINTS

- Long-term ventilator-assisted patients are defined by the ACCP as individuals requiring mechanical ventilation for at least 6 hours per day for 21 days or more.
- These patients can be described under two groups: (1) those recovering from an acute illness and (2) those with chronic progressive cardiopulmonary disorders.
- Basic goals of home-based or palliative ventilation are reducing morbidity, providing cost effective care, and improving patient's quality of life.

- Setting up mechanical ventilation at home requires a team approach, and careful education, training, and motivation of family members is crucial for the success of home-based ventilation.
- Main modalities of home-based ventilation are NIV and positive-pressure ventilation via tracheostomy tube.
- Home-based ventilators are classified into first and second generation with second-generation ventilators being more advanced and offer both patient triggered and mandatory modes of ventilation.
- Speech therapy is an important aspect of care in a patient on long-term ventilation. A tracheotomized patient who is able to speak has a better quality of life and improved sense of wellbeing.
- Other aspects of home care of a ventilated patient are nutrition, prevention, and treatment of respiratory complications, care of the ventilator equipment, etc.

## REFERENCES

1. Cairo J. Pilbeam's Mechanical Ventilation, 6th edition. St. Louis: Elsevier; 2015. pp. 415-39.
2. Laub M, Midgren B. Survival of patients on home mechanical ventilation: a nationwide prospective study. Resp Med. 2007;101(6):1074-8.
3. Polkey MI, Lyall RA, Davidson AC, et al. Ethical and clinical issues in the use of home non-invasive mechanical ventilation for the palliation of breathlessness in motor neuron disease. Thorax. 1999;54(4):367-71.
4. Perrin C, Jullien V, Duval Y, et al. Noninvasive ventilation in palliative care and near the end of life. Revue des Maladies Respiratoires. 2008;25(10):1227-36.
5. Sakakihara Y, Kubota M, Kim S, et al. Long-term ventilator support in patients with Werdnig–Hoffmann disease. Pediatr Int. 2000;42(4):359-63.
6. Gale NK, Jawad M, Dave C, et al. Adapting to domiciliary non-invasive ventilation in chronic obstructive pulmonary disease: a qualitative interview study. Pall Med. 2015;29(3):268-77.
7. Hess DR. Facilitating speech in the patient with a tracheostomy. Resp Care. 2005;50(4):519-25.
8. Passy V, Baydur A, Prentice W, et al. Passy-Muir tracheostomy speaking valve on ventilator-dependent patients. Laryngoscope. 1993;103(6):653-8.
9. Ten Hoorn S, Elbers PW, Girbes AR, et al. Communicating with conscious and mechanically ventilated critically ill patients: a systematic review. Crit Care. 2016;20(1):333.
10. McGoldrick M. Preventing infections in patients using respiratory therapy equipment in the home. Home Healthcare Now. 2010;28(4):212-20.
11. The Vest® Airway Clearance System - Acute Care Model 205. [online] Available from: https://www.hill-rom.com/usa/Products/Category/Respiratory-Care/The-Vest-205-Acute-Care/ [Last Accessed April 2019].
12. The Monarch® Airway Clearance System. [online] Available from: https://www.hill-rom.com/usa/Products/Category/Respiratory-Care/monarch-airway-clearance-system/ [Last Accessed April 2019].
13. American Thoracic Society. Statement on home care for patients with respiratory disorders. Am J Resp Crit Care Med. 2005;171:1443.

# SECTION 2

# Fluids and Electrolytes

23. Body Fluid Homeostasis
24. Intravenous Fluids
25. Approach to the Patient with Hypovolemia
26. Fluid Therapy for Specific Clinical Conditions
27. Approach to the Patient with Hyponatremia and Hypernatremia
28. Approach to the Patient with Hypokalemia and Hyperkalemia
29. Approach to the Patient with Hypocalcemia and Hypercalcemia
30. Approach to the Patient with Hypophosphatemia and Hyperphosphatemia
31. Approach to the Patient with Hypomagnesemia and Hypermagnesemia

# CHAPTER 23

# Body Fluid Homeostasis

*Anumeha Bhagat*

## INTRODUCTION

One of the major "big idea" or core concept in science and specifically physiological science is the idea of homeostasis. The concept was originally proposed in the 17th century by Claude Bernard as the constancy of the internal environment. Fifty years later, Walter Bradford Cannon introduced the term "homeostasis".[1]

The live human system can be considered relatively independent of the surrounding environment because the internal environment sort of shields the body from outside influences. Thus for a normal healthy existence of any individual, the constant conditions of internal environment which primarily include the fluids circulating in the body should remain undisturbed. Any disturbance of the factors which together maintain the constancy of the internal environment will lead to derangements of the normal physiological processes. Regulation of the composition and volume of the body fluids is fundamental to physiology and complete understanding of these principles is fundamental for application of theory into practice.

In 2007, in a meeting of a group of 21 biologists from a range of disciplines, homeostasis was identified as a core concept in science. The concept has been widely explained by physiologists as one of the initial concepts to be understood by the undergraduate medical students. In 2009, the American Association of Medical Colleges identified the ability to apply knowledge about homeostasis as one of the core competencies.[2]

## DAILY WATER FLUX IN THE BODY

For an adequate water balance in the body, the intake should be equivalent to the output of water. Everyday approximately 2,100 mL of water is added as a result of ingestion of liquids and another 200 mL as a result of water in food and that produced during oxidation of carbohydrates. However, ingestion of liquids is highly variable and subject to differ from person to person. It is also variable for time of the day, different days, different climate, habits, physical activity, etc.

In an adult human (on an average) there is water output from the body via kidney as urine output (1,400 mL/day), evaporation from respiratory tract (350 mL/day) and transpiration through skin (350 mL/day). The latter two are termed as insensible loss. Water is also lost via sweating (100 mL/day to 1–2 L/day) and small amount is lost through feces (100 mL/day). However, here also water losses through the kidney can be highly variable from 5L/day to 20L/day determined by the variability of intake or affected by ions such as sodium, potassium, and chloride. In case of burns when the cornified layer of skin is no longer present, to regulate the water loss severe dehydration can result.[3]

A normal healthy adult man of 70 kg requires 2,500 mL of water per day containing 30 mM of sodium and 15–20 mM of potassium.

## BODY FLUID COMPARTMENTS

The fluid that one ingests is distributed in the body. In a 70 kg man, the total body fluid is 42 L (60% of body weight). Twenty percent of body weight goes into the extracellular fluid (ECF) and 40% is in the intracellular fluid (ICF). This distribution of total body fluid to various body fluid compartments is determined by the quantity, concentration, and movement between compartments of water, plasma proteins, electrolytes mainly sodium.

In a 70 kg man, the ICF constitutes two-third of total body water (TBW) (28 L) and ECF constitutes one-third of TBW (14 L). This includes interstitial fluid (ISF) and plasma volume (PV). ISF is calculated by subtracting PV from ECF volume. It is approximately 11 L. Intravascular fluid (IVF)

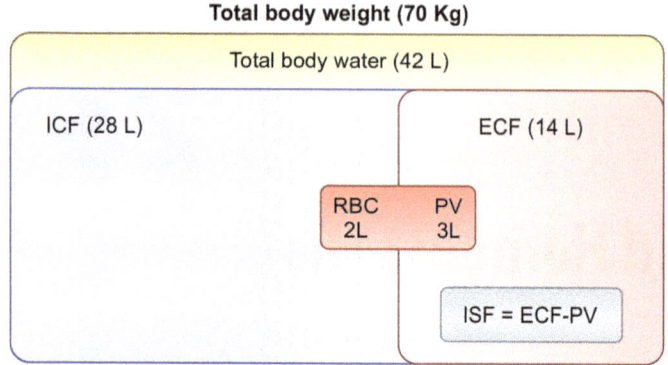

**Fig. 1:** Distribution of body fluid.
(ECF: extracellular fluid; ICF: intracellular fluid; PV: plasma volume; RBC: red blood cell)

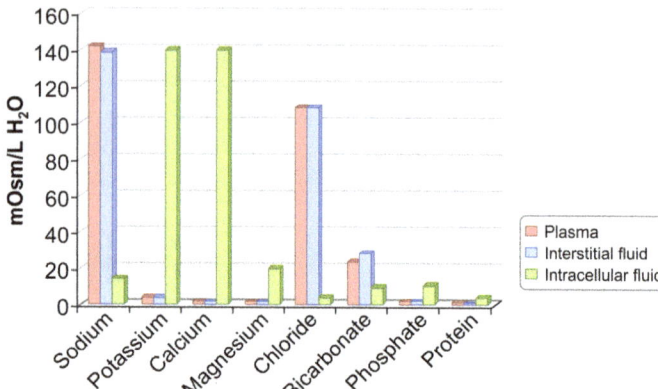

**Fig. 2:** Osmolar substances in plasma, interstitial fluid and intracellular fluid.

is 5 L of which 3 L is plasma and 2 L is red blood cell (RBC) volume (Fig. 1).

However, this conceptualization of the body as an interconnected group of anatomical spaces between which fluid distributes itself is a very simplified concept, far away from the complexity in which fluid is distributed dynamically over time.

The fluid in ECF is distributed into PV and ISF. The PV undergoes changes when intravascular boluses of fluid are given. The ISF is composed of proteoglycans, collagen fibers, water, and has a gel-like consistency. An infusion of sodium mainly distributes to the ECF. ECF volume is regulated primarily by sodium balance and water balance regulates ICF volume.

## Composition of Body Fluid Compartments

Two solutions of different ionic concentrations separated by a semipermeable membrane will obtain equal ionic concentration on both sides of the membrane in due course of time. This is a result of the process of diffusion in which substance move from area of higher concentration to area of lower concentration across a semipermeable membrane.

However, if there is an impermeable solute in one of the solutions then the ionic concentrations of both the solutions do not equalize, this is called Donnan effect. The equilibrium that results is a balance between the electrostatic forces and the osmotic forces affecting the ions.

The ICF proteins which are fixed intracellular negative charges, lead to unequal distribution of ions on both sides of the cell membrane. Due to this effect, the concentration of positively charged ions is slightly more in comparison to negatively charged ions in the ISF.[4]

However, for all practical purposes the ionic concentration in the ISF and in plasma is considered to be about equal. The concentration of protein and electrolytes in ICF and ECF is markedly different (Fig. 2).

Sodium which is the primary determinant of tonicity and osmolality is predominantly distributed in the ECF. ICF concentration of sodium is very miniscule. The plasma colloidal oncotic pressure is determined by the plasma proteins albumin and globulin. This maintains adequate PV. Albumin due to its large size does not easily pass across capillaries into ISF. The protein gradient maintains the properties of the circulating PV and ISF volume.

## Principles Governing Movement of Water between Intracellular Fluid and Interstitial Fluid

### Osmosis

It is defined as movement of water between two compartments separated by a semipermeable membrane and having different solute concentrations. Water diffuses to the side of the membrane where concentration of osmotically active solutes is greatest. Osmotic pressure is defined as the pressure needed to exactly oppose the movement of water down a solute concentration gradient. Osmotic pressure is proportional to the number of molecules of the solute and not its molecular weight.

### Osmolarity and Osmolality

The osmotic concentration of solution in osmoles per liter of solution is called osmolarity. Osmolality is a measurement of the number of osmotically active particles per kilogram of solvent. Osmolarity is affected by change in temperature, pressure as well as change in water content; and its value may be slightly less than osmolality. Since body fluids are dilute solutions, the two terms, i.e. osmolarity and osmolality can be used synonymously because of small ionic differences. Since it is difficult to express body fluid quantities in kilogram, so for all calculation purposes osmolarity is the preferred unit. Osmolality is measured in laboratory by freezing point depression osmometer or vapor pressure depression osmometer; while osmolarity is calculated at bedside from laboratory values (serum sodium, blood glucose and blood urea) measured in solution. Freezing point of normal human plasma is -0.54°C corresponding to osmolality of 290 (275–300) mOsmol/kg. Formula for osmolarity

$$\text{Osmolarity} = (\text{Serum Na}^+ \times 2) + \text{Blood Glucose} + \text{Blood Urea}$$

[All values are in mOsm/L]

Conditions like hypernatremia, hyperglycemia, and uremia increase serum osmolality.

### Tonicity

Osmolality of a solution relative to plasma is termed as tonicity. Solutions that have same osmolality as plasma are iso-osmotic, those with greater osmolality are hypertonic, and those with lesser osmolality are hypotonic.

The 0.9% saline is isotonic, 5% dextrose solution is slightly hypotonic when infused but since dextrose is metabolized so it becomes significant hypotonic fluid.

## Principles Governing Movement of Water between Plasma and Interstitial Fluid

### Colloid Oncotic Pressure

The pore size of normal capillary endothelium is 6.5 nm. The capillaries are freely permeable to small molecules and electrolytes but not to large protein molecules. Plasma proteins exert a colloidal oncotic pressure of 25 mm Hg or 1.2 mOsmol/kg.

Starling's forces exist at the capillary where the exchange of fluid between intravascular compartment and the ISF take place. The net fluid movement is proportional to the difference between the hydrostatic pressure gradient and the osmotic pressure gradient across the capillary wall.[3]

Net filtration pressure (NFP) = Pc - Pif - ∏p + ∏if
Pc: Capillary hydrostatic pressure
Pif: Interstitial fluid hydrostatic pressure
∏p: Plasma colloidal osmotic pressure
∏if: Interstitial fluid colloidal osmotic pressure

- *Filtration rate = NFP* multiplied by the filtration coefficient
- *Filtration coefficient (Kf)* is a product of surface area times the hydraulic conductivity of membrane

## MEASUREMENT OF BODY FLUID SPACES

There are various methods for measurement of body fluid spaces.

### Indicator Dilution Principle

The volume of fluid compartment in the body can be measured by putting a known quantity of an indicator/tracer substance in that compartment, allowing it to disperse evenly throughout the compartment, and then calculating the dilution obtained of that substance. This method is based on the principle of conservation of mass according to which the total mass of a substance after evenly mixing with the fluids in a compartment will be equal to the total mass injected into the compartment as depicted in Figure 3.[3]

Tracers used for determining volume of different body fluid compartments are shown in Table 1.

Properties of an ideal indicator are:
- It should be nontoxic.
- It should be distributed exclusively in the volume to be measured.

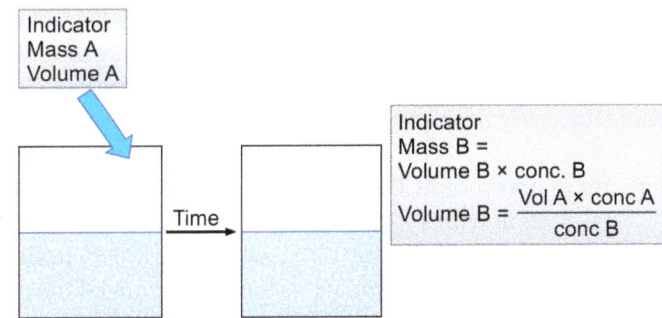

**Fig. 3:** Diagrammatic representation of indicator dilution principal.

**Table 1:** Tracers used for determining volume of body fluid compartments.

| Volume | Indicator |
| --- | --- |
| Total body water (TBW) | $^3H_2O$, $^2H_2O$, antipyrine |
| Extracellular fluid (ECF) | $^{22}$Na, $^{125}$I-iodothalamate, thoisulfate, inulin, mannitol, sucrose |
| Intracellular fluid (ICF) | Calculated as TBW-ECF |
| Plasma volume (PV) | $^{125}$I-albumin, Evans blue dye |
| Blood volume (BV) | $^{51}$Cr labeled RBCs, [Calculated as BV = PV/(1-Hematocrit)] |
| Interstitial fluid | ECF-PV |

- It should be evenly and rapidly distributed in that volume.
- It should not undergo metabolism during the time of equilibration.
- Other indicator properties that have important bearing over the choice of an indicator are availability, ease of preparation, purity, sampling procedure, technique of analysis, and cost.

### Total Body Water

A decrease of 15% can be life threatening. Several factors affect the state of hydration, e.g. physical activity, feeding status, meal composition, fluid intake, environmental temperature and humidity, menstrual cycle, etc.

Most accurate measurement is by weighing organs and the whole human cadavers and then desiccating to constant weight. However, such data is very limited and on severely diseased patients, and therefore not applicable to healthy humans.

### Extracellular Fluid

The indicator in this case should be a substance that disperses in the plasma and ISF but does not readily permeate the cell membrane. These substances disperse in 30–60 minutes. Sodium and insulin also partially diffuse into the cell in small quantities, so measurements of ECF using these are termed as sodium space or inulin space.

Since limits of the ECF space are ill defined, it is difficult to measure ECF volume. The lymphatic system is in continuation with ECF and cannot be separated from it. Tracers/indicators enter the CSF slowly due to blood-brain barrier. Similarly, equilibration is slow with synovial fluid, aqueous humor, dense connective tissue, cartilage, and bone. The ECF is most accurately measured by inulin.

### Plasma Volume

It is measured by using dyes that bind to plasma proteins.

### Intracellular Fluid

It cannot be measured directly because it is difficult to sample it, as substances that equilibrate in it also equilibrate in plasma. Its volume can be derived by subtracting PV from ECF.

## Anthropometric Measurements of Body Fluids

Based on the relationship of body fluid volume to size of the subject, various equations have been developed to predict body fluid volumes from anthropometric data. TBW can be predicted from gender, age, weight, and height or from body surface area or body mass index.

However, such predictions are only accurate for a population which is similar to the reference population. So, these values based on these predictions might not be correct for an ethnically diverse population.

In the operation theatre when body fluid compartments need to be measured, it is important that these procedures are simple, the time of surgery should be more than the mixing time of the tracer if dilution principle is used, and tracer should have rapid elimination rate so that repeated measurements can be made.[5]

## Bioelectrical Impedance Analysis

When an electrical current is applied, the conductivity and dielectric properties of various biological tissues is different. For bioelectrical impedance analysis (BIA) measurement, the assumption is that the body behaves like a uniform isotropic conductor of electricity and it is assumed to be a single cylinder. However, both these assumptions are incorrect. Since the limbs are much thinner than the trunk, the former will dominate the obtained estimate. BIA measurements are more useful in community studies on healthy people. In the intensive care unit (ICU) or operation theater (OR), the presence of stray capacitances also might lead to faulty estimates.[5]

## Bioimpedance Spectroscopy

It is a development of BIA in which a single frequency is replaced by a multifrequency approach. In the bioimpedance spectroscopy (BIS) model for the body, the intracellular compartment is considered to be a resistance which is in series with the cell membrane acting as a capacitor, both of which are in parallel with the extracellular resistance. Low frequency current will flow through the extracellular water because of the membrane capacitance. High frequency current can flow freely through TBW.[5]

# REGULATION OF EXTRACELLULAR FLUID COMPOSITION AND VOLUME

Regulation of the composition and volume of each fluid compartment is done by complex interplay of reflexes mediated by sympathetic nervous system, renal mechanisms, and humoral factors such as vasopressin (ADH), natriuretic peptides, and the renin angiotensin aldosterone system.

## Regulation of Tonicity

### Effect of Changes in Plasma Osmolality on Vasopressin Secretion

Normal plasma osmolality is between 280 mOsm and 295 mOsm. The total body osmolality is directly proportional to the total body sodium plus total body potassium divided by TBW.

Change in body fluid osmolality can occur when the amount of electrolytes and amount of water intake/output from the body is disproportionate. Therefore, tonicity is regulated by ADH secretion and thirst mechanism.

An increase in the effective osmotic pressure of plasma leads to increase in ADH secretion and activation of thirst mechanism.

Vasopressin secretion leads to water retention and activation of thirst mechanism leads to water ingestion, both of which lead to dilution of ECF and thereby decreasing the osmotic pressure. Secretion of ADH is maximally inhibited at 285 mOsm and stimulated at higher values.

### Mechanism of Action of Vasopressin

Vasopressin hormone acts on the collecting ducts of the kidney by binding to V2 receptors. V2 receptor is a G protein coupled receptor and binding of ADH leads to stimulation of G protein which leads to rise in cyclic adenosine monophosphate (cAMP) levels. Activation of this second messenger pathway leads to insertion of aquaporin 2(AQP-2) water channels into the apical/luminal membrane of the principal cells of collecting duct. This leads to increased transfer of water from the lumen to the interstitium. The urine volume decreases and it becomes concentrated. Retention of water in excess of solute leads to decrease in effective osmotic pressure of ECF.

Half-life of circulating ADH is approximately 18 minutes and it is rapidly inactivated in the liver and kidney. Secretion of ADH is regulated by osmoreceptors present outside the blood-brain barrier in the circumventricular organs mainly in the organum vasculosum of lamina terminalis (OVLT). Osmolality changes of just 1% can bring significant changes in ADH secretion.

Although both thirst mechanism and ADH secretion are simulated by increase in effective osmotic pressure/change in ECF volume; but the pathways mediating either of these responses are separate.

Conditions in which sensation of thirst is diminished and may lead to dehydration are:
- Direct damage to diencephalon
- Depressed consciousness
- Psychosis
- Hypothalamic disease
- Lesions of anterior communicating artery.

### Effect of Changes in Plasma Volume on Vasopressin Secretion

A decrease in ECF volume stimulates ADH secretion and an increase in ECF volume decreased ADH secretion. In the vascular system, there are low- and high-pressure stretch receptors.

Low-pressure receptors are present in the great veins, right and left atria, and pulmonary vessels. High-pressure receptors are baroreceptors present in the carotid sinus and arch of aorta.

The low-pressure receptors, which monitor the fullness of the vascular system by sensing, moderate decrease in blood volume (by decreasing central venous pressure without having effect on arterial pressure). The low-pressure receptors are the primary mediators of volume effect on ADH secretion. When they get stimulated, impulses pass via the vagus nerve to the nucleus of tractus solitarius (NTS). The NTS inhibits the caudal ventrolateral medulla (CVLM) and there is a direct excitatory pathway from the CVLM to the hypothalamus (Flowchart 1).

Angiotensin II reinforces this response acting on the circumventricular organs. Other stimuli that can lead to increased ADH secretion are pain, emotion, stress, exercise, nausea and vomiting, standing, drugs (carbamazepine, clofibrate), and angiotensin II.

Integrated mechanism for regulation of tonicity is shown in Flowchart 2.

**Flowchart 1:** Mechanism of action of low-pressure receptors.

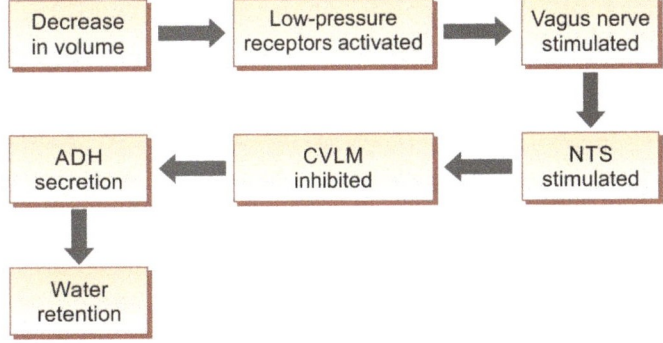

(ADH: antidiuretic hormone; CVLM: caudal ventrolateral medulla; NTS: nucleus tractus solitaries)

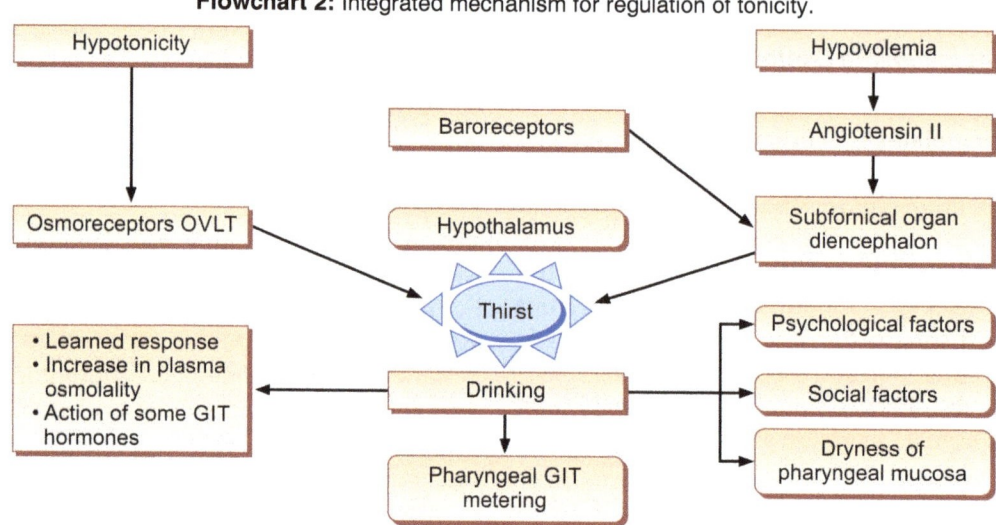

Flowchart 2: Integrated mechanism for regulation of tonicity.

(GIT: gastrointestinal; OVLT: organum vasculosum lamina terminalis)

## Clinical Aspect of Vasopressin

### Diabetes Insipidus

It is a condition resulting from deficiency of ADH. When the disease is in hypothalamic nuclei, hypothalamic hypophyseal tract, or posterior pituitary it is termed central diabetes insipidus and when the problem is due to renal pathology it is termed nephrogenic diabetes insipidus. The primary causes for occurrence of diabetes insipidus are hypothalamic neoplasia (30%), post-traumatic (30%), idiopathic (30%), and vascular lesions (10%). Secondary causes are mutation in gene for V2 receptor (an X-linked recessive disorder) and mutation in gene for AQP-2 receptor (an autosomal recessive disorder)

### Syndrome of Inappropriate Antidiuretic Hormone Secretion

In this condition, there is inappropriately high ADH secretion relative to serum osmolality, blood volume, and blood pressure. There is retention of water which leads to low plasma osmolality but urine is more hyperosmotic than expected on the basis of low plasma osmolality. Causes of syndrome of inappropriate ADH secretion (SIADH) include infections and neoplasm of the brain, antitumor drugs, carcinoma lung, etc.

### Regulation of ECF Volume

Extracellular fluid volume is determined by the total amount of osmotically active solutes in ECF. Since sodium and chloride are the most abundant osmotically active

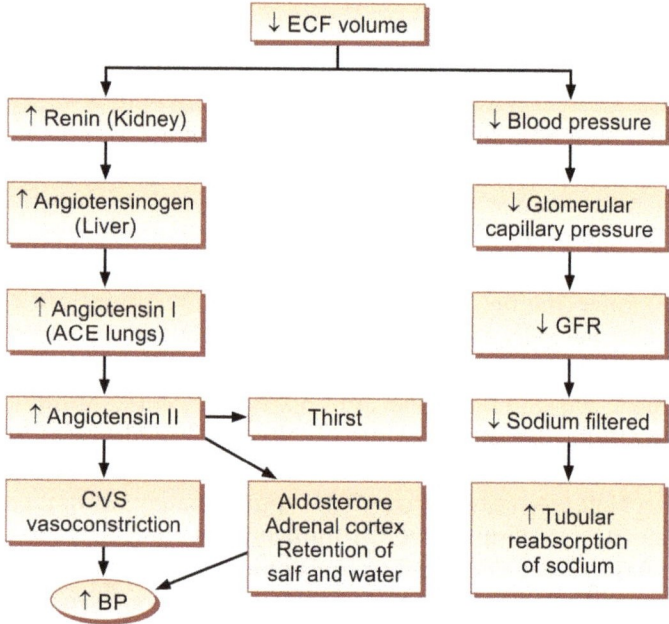

Flowchart 3: Mechanisms activated by decrease in extracellular fluid (ECF) volume.

(ACE: angiotensin converting enzyme; BP: blood pressure; CVS: cardiovascular system; GFR: glomerular filtration rate)

solutes in ECF and as changes in chloride are mainly secondary to changes in sodium, the amount of sodium in the ECF is the most important determinant of ECF volume. So, the regulation of sodium balance is the primary mechanism for maintaining ECF volume.[6]

Flowchart 3 explains mechanisms activated by decrease in ECF volume.

## Role of Other Hormones

### Atrial Natriuretic Peptide

Stretch on the atria leads to release of atrial natriuretic peptide (ANP) from the atria. This acts on renal tubules to increase sodium excretion and glomerular filtration rate, inhibits renin secretion and inhibits renal vasoconstriction, inhibits aldosterone synthesis, vasodilation, and shift of fluid from the IVF to the ISF.

### Brain Natriuretic Peptide

Brain natriuretic peptide (BNP), initially thought to be released from brain, is primarily a cardiac hormone in humans. It is secreted by left ventricle in response to increased cardiac volume or arterial pressure. Its functions are similar to ANP, and it acts as a part of central mechanism for control of blood volume, blood pressure, electrolytes, and body fluid homeostasis. BNP also mediates the salt wasting and hyponatremia seen in patients who have subarachnoid hemorrhage.

## Fluid Losses during Surgery and Trauma and the Concept of Third Space

Surgical procedures lead to an increased interstitial water load. Coupled with this, there is also an inevitable fluid shift from intravascular space to interstitial space due to the porous nature of capillary endothelial wall. Surgery and trauma lead to enhancement of this extravasation of body fluids. Due to increased capillary permeability, more fluid escapes to the interstitium. The ECV includes plasma, interstitial space, and small amounts of transcellular fluids such as gastrointestinal fluids, cerebrospinal fluids, ocular fluid, and synovial fluid. Blood loss constitutes a significant fluid loss during major operations. Loss of blood causes a change in the colloid osmotic pressure.

Loss of fluid to the interstitial space is an inevitable phenomenon which consists mainly of small molecules leaving through an intact vascular barrier. Due to surgery or trauma, this loss can occur in large amounts and lead to accumulation within the interstitial space or the "functional ECV". The lymphatic system is not able to remove all of this when it is overloaded due to excessive fluid load or cessation of urine output.

Fluid within this hypothetical third space is considered to be "nonfunctional" body fluid separated from the interstitial space. Losses to these spaces are no longer in equilibrium with the ECF and therefore nonfunctional.

## Disturbances of Volume

### Hypovolemia

Hypovolemia is defined as a depletion of effective circulating volume. It can be absolute hypovolemia resulting from losses from the body or relative hypovolemia resulting from fluid sequestration within the body (Table 2). Expansion of ECF volume results in decrease in effective circulating volume. This can happen in conditions such as sepsis, liver disease, and anaphylaxis. Due to anesthesia, sympathetic reflexes are blunted which results in absolute or relative hypovolemia. Volatile and intravenous anesthetic agents also lead to vasodilatation further contributing to relative hypovolemia. Blockage of efferent sympathetic vasomotor signals in spinal or epidural anesthesia also produces relative hypovolemia.[7]

### Edema

Accumulation of fluid within the body is clinically evident as edema. Various causes of edema are:
- Hydrostatic pressure effect: Cardiac failure, renal failure, neurogenic pulmonary edema, fluid overload
- Reduced oncotic pressure: Cirrhosis, preeclampsia, nephrotic syndrome, malnutrition, critical illness

**Table 2:** Causes of hypovolemia.

| | |
|---|---|
| *Absolute hypovolemia* | |
| GIT | Hemorrhage |
| | Emesis |
| | Diarrhea |
| | Fistula |
| | Tube drainage |
| Renal | Diabetes insipidus |
| | Osmotic diuresis |
| Skin | Large exudative lesions |
| | Burns |
| Trauma | Long bone fracture |
| | Hemothorax |
| | Ruptured spleen |
| Surgical | Blood loss |
| *Relative hypovolemia* | |
| Internal fluid shift | Third space loss |
| | Nephrotic syndrome |
| | Cirrhosis |
| Capillary leak | Anaphylaxis |
| | Sepsis |
| Sequestration | Intestinal obstruction |
| | Peritonitis |

(GIT: gastrointestinal tract)

- Increased capillary permeability: Sepsis, burns, brain injury, reperfusion injury, acute lung injury.

## SALIENT POINTS

- In a 70 kg man, the ICF constitutes two-third of TBW (28 L), and ECF constitutes one-third of TBW (14 L). This includes ISF and PV. ISF is calculated by subtracting PV from ECF volume. It is approximately 11 L. IVF is 5 L of which 3L is plasma and 2L is RBC volume.
- There are various methods for measurement of body fluid spaces. These include indicator dilution method, anthropometric methods, BIA, and BIS.
- Normal plasma osmolality is between 280 mOsm and 295 mOsm. The total body osmolality is directly proportional to the total body sodium plus total body potassium divided by TBW.
- An increase in the effective osmotic pressure of plasma leads to increase in ADH secretion and activation of thirst mechanism. The pathway mediating thirst mechanism is separate from the pathway mediating the secretion of ADH.
- The low-pressure receptors monitor the fullness of the vascular system by sensing moderate decrease in blood volume which decreases central venous pressure without decreasing arterial pressure.
- The regulation of sodium balance is the primary mechanism for maintaining ECF volume.
- Fluid within the hypothetical third space is considered to be "nonfunctional" body fluid separated from the interstitial space. Losses to these spaces are no longer in equilibrium with the ECF and therefore nonfunctional.

## REFERENCES

1. Michael J. Conceptual assessment in the biological sciences: a National Science Foundation-sponsored workshop. Adv Physiol Educ. 2007;31:389-91.
2. Modell H, Cliff W, Michael J, et al. A physiologist's view of homeostasis. Adv Physiol Educ. 2015;39(4):259-66.
3. In: Guyton AC, Hall JE (Eds). Textbook of Medical Physiology, 23rd edition. Philadelphia: WB Saunders Company; 2011.
4. In: Barrett KE, Barman SM, Boitano S, Brooks HL (Eds). Ganong's Review of Medical Physiology, 12th Edition. New Delhi: Tata McGraw-Hill; 2010.
5. In: Hahn RG, Prough DS, Svensen CH (Eds). Perioperative Fluid Therapy. New York, USA: Informa Health Care; 2007.
6. In: Hemmings H, Hopkins P (Eds). Foundations of Anesthesia. Basic and Clinical Sciences. London, UK: Harcourt Publishers Limited; 1999.
7. In: Hemmings HC, Egan TD (Eds). Pharmacology and Physiology for Anaestheisa. Foundations and Clinical Applications. Philadelphia: Elsevier Saunders; 2013.

# CHAPTER 24

# Intravenous Fluids

*Nilanchal Chakraborty, Addy Yh Tan*

## INTRODUCTION

Fluid therapy dates back to the time of British cholera epidemic in 1830s when there was little understanding about physiology of cholera. William O'Shaughnessy, a young Edinburgh Chemistry graduate postulated that cure of cholera was dependent on restoring the natural specific gravity of the blood and restoring deficient saline. On hearing this analysis, Thomas Latta injected 6 pints of hypotonic solution containing saline and sodium bicarbonate into an elderly woman with cholera, which restored circulating volume transiently. 30 years after the Crimean War, it was recognized that danger of blood loss can be mitigated with fluid infusion to compensate lost vascular content regardless of its erythrocyte content as long as the infused fluid is not directly injurious. Gum acacia was one of the first colloid solutions. It was difficult to manufacture and may result in agglutinated red cells and caused serious reactions. Dextran, produced from sucrose was first recognized as a potential plasma substitutes in 1944 and then clinical products were created by partial hydrolysis and fractionation of dextran molecule. Over the years, various types of fluids were produced with the primary function of being a plasma volume expander.

## CLASSIFICATION OF FLUIDS

In 1861, a Scottish chemist, Thomas Graham, who is lauded as the father of colloid classified fluids based on the ability to diffuse across parchment membrane to crystalloid and colloids. Crystalloids are inorganic compounds that dissociate into ions when mixed with water. Colloids (originated from the Greek word for glue, kolla) are homogeneous fluids made up of nonsoluble large molecular size substance that are dispersed throughout a second substance usually an electrolyte-based solvent. Tables 1 and 2 describe the composition of different crystalloids and colloids in practice.

## Osmotic Properties of Fluids

The movement of fluids when given intravenously will depend on the osmolality of the fluid. Osmolality refers to the total solute concentration of a fluid. Water will move from one fluid compartment with a lower osmolality to another fluid compartment with a higher osmolality that is separated by a semipermeable membrane via the process of osmosis. An isotonic intravenous fluid, e.g. balanced salt solution, has the same osmolality as the serum and extracellular space. Since there is no difference in osmolality between the intravenous fluid and the extracellular fluid, there will be no osmotic pressure gradient driving the movement of water. However, fluid shifts will still occur due to dynamic movement of solutes and difference in hydrostatic pressure. Hence, fluid will still be redistributed between the various compartments depending on the solute composition and fluid status of the patient. A hypotonic solution, e.g. Ringer's lactate solution, has a lower osmolality than serum, hence it has the potential to drive fluid into compartments, e.g. intracranial compartment. On the other hand, a hypertonic fluid, e.g. 3% NaCl solution is able to draw fluid out from a compartment. Hence 3% NaCl solution is used to treat raised intracranial pressure.

## CRYSTALLOIDS

Crystalloid solutions are considered by many to be as the first-line resuscitation fluid regardless of their propensity to cause significant interstitial edema because of its wide availability and cost effectiveness.
- 0.9% NaCl solution

## Section 2
## Fluids and Electrolytes

**Table 1:** Characteristics of common crystalloid solutions compared to plasma.

|  | Plasma | 0.9% saline | Ringer's lactate | Sterofundin® | Plasma-Lyte® | Premix solution (0.33% Saline, 5% dextrose) |
|---|---|---|---|---|---|---|
| Sodium (mmol/L) | 135–145 | 154 | 130 | 145 | 140 | 56 |
| Potassium (mmol/L) | 3.5–5 | 0 | 4 | 4 | 5 | 20 |
| Magnesium (mmol/L) | 0.8–1 | 0 | 0 | 1 | 1.5 | 0 |
| Calcium (mmol/L) | 2.2–2.6 |  | 3 | 2.5 | 0 | 0 |
| Chloride (mmol/L) | 98–106 | 154 | 109 | 127 | 98 | 76 |
| Acetate (mmol/L) | 0 | 0 | 0 | 24 | 27 | 0 |
| Gluconate (mmol/L) | 0 | 0 | 0 | 0 | 23 | 0 |
| Lactate (mmol/L) | 0 | 0 | 29 | 0 | 0 | 0 |
| Malate (mmol/L) | 0 | 0 | 0 | 5 | 0 | 0 |
| eSID (mEq/L) | 42 | 0 | 27 | 25.5 | 50 | 0 |
| Theoretical osmolarity (mOsmol/L) | 291 | 308 | 278 | 309 | 295 | 405 |
| Actual Osmolarity (mOsmol/kg H$_2$O) | 287 | 286 | 256 | Not stated | 271 | 0 |
| pH | 7.35–7.45 | 4.5–7 | 5–7 | 5.1–5.9 | 4–8 | 3.5–6.5 |
| Common adverse effect/limitations | – | Hyperchloraemic metabolic acidosis | Worsen cerebral oedema | Metabolic alkalosis | Metabolic alkalosis | Ineffective plasma expander |

**Table 2:** Electrolyte composition (mmol/L) of commonly available colloids.

|  | Albumin 5% | Albumin 20% | Gelofusine® | Voluven® (waxy maize HES 6% 130/0.4) | Volulyte® (waxy maize HES 6% 130/0.4) |
|---|---|---|---|---|---|
| Sodium (mmol/L) | 154 | 154 | 154 | 154 | 137 |
| Potassium (mmol/L) | 0 | 0 | 0 | 0 | 4 |
| Chloride (mmol/L) | 154 | 154 | 120 | 154 | 110 |
| Calcium (mmol/L) | 0 | 0 | 0.4 | 0 | 0 |
| Magnesium (mmol/L) | 0 | 0 | 0 | 0 | 1.5 |
| Bicarbonate (mmol/L) | 0 | 0 | 0 | 0 | 0 |
| Lactate (mmol/L) | 0 | 0 | 0 | 0 | 0 |
| Acetate (mmol/L) | 0 | 0 | 0 | 0 | 34 |
| Malate (mmol/L) | 0 | 0 | 0 | 0 | 0 |
| Duration of action (hours) | 12 | 12 | 12–24 | 24 | 24 |
| Oncotic pressure (mm Hg) | 20 | 70 | 35 | 30 | 30 |
| Common adverse effect/limitations | No benefit shown as plasma expander. Viral transmission. Adverse immunological effect. Increased mortality in patients with traumatic brain injury. | No benefit shown as plasma expander. Viral transmission. Adverse immunological effect. Increased mortality in patients with traumatic brain injury. | Anaphylactic reaction. | Acute kidney injury in critically ill patients. Impairs platelet function. Increase mortality. | Acute kidney injury in critically ill patients. Impairs platelet function. Increase mortality. |

(HES: hydroxyethyl starch)

- Lactated Ringer's (Hartmann) solution
- Balanced salt solutions
- Dextrose containing fluid
- Isotonic bicarbonate solution.

## 0.9% Sodium Chloride Solution

0.9% NaCl solution is one of the most widely used crystalloid solutions; it is commonly called normal saline. The concentration of sodium and chloride is 154 mmol/L. The term "normal saline" had been erroneously bestowed because of its tonicity but it is neither a balanced nor a normal physiologic solution. Its tonicity is slightly higher than plasma and has the same concentration of Na$^+$ and Cl$^-$ which is higher than that of plasma. As sodium and chloride ions have an overall osmotic coefficient of 0.926, the effective osmolality is 287 mOsmol/kg which is similar to plasma osmolality (iso-osmolar).[1] The 0.9% NaCl solution has a pH of 4.5-7, far lower than plasma or water. This low pH appears to be related to the polyvinyl chloride packaging containers, exposure to atmosphere, and the electrolytes. However, the propensity of 0.9% NaCl solution to cause metabolic acidosis is not related to the intrinsic pH of the solution but due to its supraphysiologic chloride concentration which when given in large amount, reduces the strong ion difference (SID) in the blood.[2] 0.9% NaCl solution has the propensity to increase the plasma concentration of sodium and chloride. However, the physiologic plasma concentration of chloride is about 100 mmol/L which is significantly lower than sodium, which is 145 mmol/L. This will confer a greater concentration gradient for chloride to increase when exposed to 0.9% NaCl solution resulting in a higher increase in the plasma concentration for chloride than sodium, leading to a narrowing of SID, directing the body homeostatic system to generate more hydrogen ions, causing metabolic acidosis.

Studies have shown that 0.9% NaCl in comparison to balanced salt solution causes the mean renal artery flow velocity and renal cortical tissue perfusion to be reduced in healthy volunteers due to its hyperchloremic properties.[3] 0.9% NaCl solution is conventionally regarded as the default choice of fluid for patients who have renal impairment because it is potassium free. But, multiple studies have shown that when compared to potassium containing lactated Ringer's solution, 0.9% NaCl results in increasing the risk of hyperkalemia when administered to renal transplant patients.[4]

## Lactated Ringer's (Hartmann) Solution

The lactated Ringer's solution was developed to provide fluids which mimics the composition of normal body fluids. Sydney Ringer first conducted experiments *in vitro* and highlighted the effect of other nonsodium inorganic chloride salts on cardiac contractility. Alexis Hartmann made modifications to Ringer's solution by including sodium lactate to buffer against effect of acidity. The low-chloride content in this solution makes way for other anions in making the SID to be 27-29 mEq/L, which is nearer to plasma. Hartmann's solution has a pH of 6.5 with osmolality less than 280 mOsmol/kg. However, Hartmann's solution has a osmolality of only 254 mOsmol/kg *in vitro* due to partial ionization of its components making it a hypotonic solution. This would be less appropriate to be used in cases of traumatic brain injury or cerebral edema. Many would avoid the use of Hartmann's solution in patients with hyperkalemia because of the small amount of potassium it contains. However, as mentioned above, there are studies which had shown that it does not increase the serum potassium concentration.[4] The presence of calcium can reverse the effects of citrated anticoagulants in blood products resulting in clots.

The lactate content in this solution may potentially cause hyperlactatemia especially in the presence of liver dysfunction but no data has demonstrated this. Unlike hyperlactatemia caused by anaerobic metabolism, lactate when given as a salt (as in Hartmann's solution) is lower propensity to result in metabolic acidosis because the strong anion influence is balanced by the presence of cations.[5] Furthermore, lactate is readily metabolized by the liver. However, it is prudent to avoid using Hartmann's solution in situations of severe liver dysfunction.

## Balanced Salt Solutions

Balanced salt solutions are used to denote crystalloid solutions with solute compositions which mimic that of plasma. Balanced salt solutions contain a lower concentration of chloride but with a more physiologic osmolality. Different anions like acetate, gluconate, and malate are added in place of chloride to maintain electrical neutrality. These anions will be metabolized by the liver to carbon dioxide as the immediate end product which ultimately results in increase in bicarbonate concentration.

The higher concentration of chloride in the 0.9% NaCl has the potential to cause acute kidney injury associated with the retention of Na$^+$. Increased Cl$^-$ content in the blood from supraphysiologic crystalloid infusion leads to decreased proximal tubular Cl$^-$ reabsorption causing a higher delivery of Cl$^-$. As more Cl$^-$ enter into macula densa, this will result in the release of adenosine, leading to vasoconstriction of the afferent arteriolar vasculature. The increased resistance will decrease the renal blood flow and glomerular filtration rate with the consequence of a reduction in urine production and Na+ retention. Despite clinical studies showing the adverse effect of infusing large volume of 0.9% NaCl solution, clinical relevance is yet to be proven.[6]

Sodium acetate had been used during hemodialysis in place of bicarbonate because of the incompatibility between bicarbonate with calcium or magnesium. Previous studies have shown that sodium acetate solution can correct blood pH in cases of metabolic acidosis.[7,8] Acetate containing balanced solution stabilizes pH more rapidly than lactate. Acetate quickly converts to bicarbonate in equimolar quantity, which means 1 mmol of acetate contributes to 1 mmol of bicarbonate. The metabolism of acetate is not entirely hepatic in nature and is less affected in severe shock, unlike lactate. However, studies had suggested that hemodynamic instability from vasodilation and negative inotropic effect is associated with high-dose renal replacement therapy and acetate.[9,10]

The physiological impact of gluconate is still not clear and 80% of gluconate is eliminated via kidney in unchanged form. Animal studies had shown that rest of the gluconate is converted to glucose. Many studies also showed gluconate only acts as osmotic diuretic.[11] The effects of malate are less well documented than those of acetate. At pH of 7.4, malate remains as a divalent anion (malate$^{2-}$), so for every molecule of malate oxidized, two molecules of bicarbonate are produced. The resultant alkalinizing effect is significantly slower than that of acetate.

These bicarbonate precursors ultimately enter citric acid cycle, which consumes H+ ion. Consumption of H+ ion is equivalent to generation of $HCO_3^{2-}$ ion.

Plasma-Lyte® and Sterofundin® are two most popular balanced solutions in the market with composition close to plasma. Both are considered balanced although they differ in their composition significantly.

1. *Sterofundin®:* Sterofundin® contains magnesium, calcium, and potassium as cation; acetate and malate as anions. Sterofundin® does not contain gluconate but has a higher chloride (127 mmol/L) concentration than plasma content.
2. *Plasma-Lyte® 148:* The numeric "148" in Plasma-Lyte® 148 is derived from the sum of each of Plasma-Lyte® 148 cationic concentration. [(Na) 140 mEq + (K) 5 mEq + (Mg) 3 mEq = 148 mEq]. Plasma-Lyte® contains chloride, gluconate, and acetate salts of sodium along with magnesium and potassium. Depending on the country of manufacture its pH varies from 6.5 to 8 and is supplied in a polyvinyl chloride bag. Its caloric content is 16 kcal/L. Plasma-Lyte® has an osmolarity of 280–296 mOsm/L. Hypersensitivity or anaphylactoid reactions have been reported with Plasma-Lyte® solutions. The absence of calcium and alkalinizing effect of Plasma-Lyte® may precipitate hypocalcemia in patients receiving Plasma-Lyte® as the only fluid. Due to its alkalinizing effect of balanced salt solution, renal elimination of acidic drugs such as aspirin and barbiturate, lithium may increase. On the other hand, renal elimination of alkaline drugs such as quinidine, dextroamphetamine, and sympathomimetics may be decreased.

According to the studies published thus far, balanced salt solutions are associated with less morbidity compared to 0.9% NaCl solution in the perioperative setting, although there is currently lack of adequate evidence.[12] Studies had suggested that the use of Plasma-Lyte® in diabetic ketoacidosis was associated with rapid improvement of metabolic acidosis.[13] When Plasma-Lyte® was used for patients undergoing hepatic resection, patients were noted to have lower levels of lactate, bilirubin, and prothrombin time. Studies comparing 0.9% sodium chloride solution, Hartmann's solution, and Plasma-Lyte® in postrenal transplant patients showed Plasma-Lyte® in having the best metabolic profile.[14]

Balanced salt solutions generally incur a higher cost as opposed to the use of conventional solutions; it is associated with less morbidity when compared to 0.9% NaCl solution. But interestingly acetate and gluconate are not normal anions present in plasma in normal physiological conditions. A recent study has tried to compare effects of Plasma-Lyte® with 0.9% NaCl solution in resuscitation of ICU patients. Although only less than 2 L of fluids were used, no difference in adverse renal outcome or increased mortality could be demonstrated.[15]

## Dextrose-containing Fluids

Dextrose-containing fluids are commercially available in various concentration ranging from 5% to 50%. 5% dextrose solution contains 50 g of dextrose per liter of solution. 5% dextrose is also available mixed with various concentrations of sodium chloride (0.33–0.9%) as well as potassium chloride. 1 g of dextrose provides 3.4 kcal of energy. Hence, 1 L of 5% dextrose provides 170 kcal. 5% dextrose is hypo-osmolar (253 mmol/L) and it provides only electrolyte free water upon complete metabolism of dextrose. Hence, electrolyte free dextrose solutions can worsen neurologic outcome by increasing intracranial pressure and cerebral ischemia. Hence, its use should be avoided for patients with traumatic brain injury or with brain pathology that predispose to cerebral edema.[16]

When 1,000 mL of dextrose solution is administered, it redistributes according to the composition of body fluids in intracellular and extracellular compartments. Hence, only 80 mL stays in the intravascular compartment after redistribution, making it an ineffective plasma expander. However, it is still useful as a fluid for hydration purpose.

### Isotonic Bicarbonate Solution

150 mmol of sodium bicarbonate (8.4%) when added to 1 L of 5% dextrose solution can be constituted to form isotonic bicarbonate solution which contains 1.3 g of bicarbonate in each 100 mL of solution. Studies have shown rapid infusion of any hypertonic solution like 20% mannitol and hypertonic saline may increase serum potassium. Hence, clinicians are still divided regarding the use of 8.4% sodium bicarbonate solution for hyperkalemia. However, slow infusion of isotonic bicarbonate solution has been found to be useful in cases of hypercalcemia and hyperchloremic metabolic acidosis.

## COLLOIDS

A colloid fluid contains substance with a high molecular weight and confined in the intravascular compartment, exerting oncotic pressure. Colloidal molecules do not cross semipermeable capillary membrane; hence they have higher tendency to be confined within the intravascular space, acting as intravascular volume expander, and maintaining oncotic pressure.

The advantage of colloids, as compared to crystalloids, is less volume will be needed to achieve the same clinical outcome. The volume of crystalloid to be given is conventionally described as three times the volume of blood loss. However, equivalent volume of colloids can be given for the replacement of blood loss.

Colloids can be classified as natural and artificial:
- *Natural colloid*: Human albumin
- *Artificial colloid*: Gelatin, dextran, hydroxyethyl starch (HES)

Two molecular weights are quoted to classify the different colloidal fluids.
1. Number average molecular weight (Mn) which reflects oncotic pressure and weight average molecular weight (Mw), which better reflects the viscosity.[17]
2. Albumin is usually mono-dispersed as the molecular weight for all the molecules are the same (Mw = Mn). But artificial colloids are polydispersed as there is a range in the molecular weight.

### Human Albumin

Albumin is the main natural colloid constituting 50–60% of plasma protein. Albumin has a molecular weight of 66.5 kDa and it is a single polypeptide chain of 585 amino acids. It is synthesized in the liver and secreted into the blood stream. 42% of secreted albumin remains in the intravascular compartment and it undergoes transcapillary exchange between intra and extravascular compartments with the help of transporter alpondin. Albumin has the following functions:[18]
- Maintenance of intravascular oncotic pressure
- Binding agent for calcium, hydrophobic organic anion, fatty acids, bilirubin, hematin, and drugs
- Metabolism of endogenous lipids and eicosanoids and other compounds, e.g. disulfiram
- Plasma buffer
- Anti-oxidant

The half-life of human albumin is 20 days and it has a physiological pH. But the albumin fluid is prepared by alcoholic precipitation pooled from multiple human plasma sources. It is pasteurized for at least 10 hours at 60°C and is considered to be of minimal risk in transmitting infectious disease. Albumins are prepared in 0.9% NaCl solution. Human albumin fluids are available in hypo-oncotic (4%), iso-oncotic (5%), or hyper-oncotic (20–25%) preparations. Iso-oncotic albumin leads to 80% of initial volume expansion whereas hyper-oncotic albumin can result in 200–400% initial increase in volume. This effect only persists for 16–24 hours, although half-life of albumin ranges from 16 to 21 days. Under physiologic condition, albumin synthesis is balanced by metabolism resulting in an equilibrium. 10% of plasma albumin content is metabolized per day. 60% of albumin stays in the extravascular space determined by transcapillary escape rate, which is determined by many disease conditions (e.g. major surgery, trauma, infection, sepsis, and shock, etc.). The main factors governing albumin production is oncotic pressure in the extravascular space of the liver. During sepsis, trauma or major surgery, redistribution of albumin due to capillary leak and catabolism cause hypoalbuminemia. Hence, after transfusion of albumin, up to 75% of transfused albumin can migrate to extravascular space after 2 days.[19]

Human albumin has no adverse effects on coagulation compared to other synthetic colloids when used for volume replacement. The SAFE trial, which is a randomized, double-blinded trial on 7,000 patients, compared volume replacement with 0.9% NaCl versus 4% human albumin. No significant benefit was found in either mortality or intensive care unit (ICU) stay. Post-hoc analysis of trauma subgroup suggested patients with traumatic brain injury were associated with higher mortality when albumin was used.[20] In patients undergoing living related liver transplant, albumin is still the fluid of choice, however, no large scale prospective trial has yet proven the benefits of human albumin when compared to other synthetic colloids. Hypoalbuminemia is associated with higher risk of a mortality and morbidity in critically ill patients. A randomized controlled trial on patients with severe sepsis, compared the use of hyper-oncotic (20%) albumin with crystalloid solution to achieve serum albumin more than 30 g/L, did not demonstrate any difference in 28-day mortality. There was also no difference in requirement of total fluid volume.[21] Though the albumin group achieved higher mean arterial pressure values in first 7 days, there were no difference in ICU stay or degree of organ dysfunction. FEAST study also did not demonstrate any advantages in using albumin as resuscitation fluid.[22]

## Dextran

Dextrans are highly branched polysaccharide molecules, produced by dextransucrase from bacterium leuconostoc mesenteroides (B512 strain). Dextran is available as dextran 40 and dextran 70 preparation. Dextran 70 (molecular weight of 70 kDa) is mainly used for volume resuscitation and is available as a 6% preparation. Whereas dextran 40 (molecular weight of 40 kDa) is mainly used to improve blood flow to the microcirculation and is available as a 10% solution. Dextran leads to 100–150% increase in volume expansion and effect lasts up to 3–5 hours.[23] Dextran 40 improves microcirculation both by hemodilution as well as by reducing erythrocyte aggregation. The kidneys play major role in excretion of dextran molecules, but the larger molecules tend to stay in the circulation for days. Infusion of dextrans is associated with several adverse effects like anaphylactic reactions, platelets dysfunction and increased risk of fibrinolysis, interferes with cross matching of blood and precipitates renal failure.[23]

## Gelatin

The use of gelatin in human studies was started in 1915. Gelatins are derived from hydrolysis of animal connective tissue. Gelatin fluids of high molecular weight has the tendency to solidify if stored at low temperature. Hence, the weight-average molecular weight of the currently available preparations is kept below 35 kDa. This reduces the exerted oncotic pressure and duration of action as a plasma expander.

Three types of gelatin solutions are available:
1. Succinylated or modified fluid gelatins (e.g. Gelofusine®, Plasmagel®, Plasmion®)
2. Urea-crosslinked gelatins (e.g. Polygeline®)
3. Oxypolygelatins (e.g. Gelifundol®).

Succinylated gelatin (Gelofusine®) has a chloride content of 120 mmol/L and calcium content of 0.4 mmol/L. This is beneficial for high volume resuscitation and is compatible with blood products. It is nonpyogenic and preservative free with a shelf-life of 3 years when stored at temperature less than 30°C. The increase in plasma volume after administration of succinylated gelatin is equal to or 10% less than the volume infused. Other gelatin-based fluids have different calcium content and physical properties compared to Gelofusine®. The short plasma half-life of gelatin is due to its low molecular weight and it is excreted by the kidneys. The effect of plasma expansion is about 4 hours.[24]

Gelatin-based fluids are cheaper compared to other colloids and albumin. However, acute kidney injury had been reported after gelatin infusion, and their use in renal failure must be carried out with caution.[25] Gelatin may cause anaphylactoid reactions. Its effects on coagulation are similar to other colloids but of lower magnitude. A decrease in activity of von Willebrand factor has also been observed.

## Hydroxyethyl Starch

Hydroxyethyl starches are procured from maize or potato starch, amylopectin. The rate at which amylopectin is broken down is reduced by substituting the hydroxyl radicals in positions C2, C3, and C6. Substitutions at the C2 and C6 position occurred most frequently. A lower ratio of C2 and C6 substitution will have a lesser effect on blood coagulation. Greater molar substitution (MS) will result in higher tendency to worsen blood coagulation.[26] This modification makes HES more likely to be stored in reticular connective tissues, spleen, skin, liver, kidneys, and it potentially may lead to osmotic nephrosis, which are shown in animal studies. Three numbers are used to describe HES (e.g. 6% HES 130/0.4)—the first number shows concentration of the fluid, the second is the molecular weight (MW) in kDa, and the third represents MS.

Concentration (6% vs. 10%) usually influences initial volume effect and volume effect of hyperoncotic (10%) HES exceeds infused volume (about 145%). Larger molecules stay longer in the intravascular compartment while molecules below 45–60 kDa are excreted by the kidneys.

The medium size molecules are excreted in bile and feces. Some fraction gets accumulated in reticuloendothelial system.[23]

With a higher degree of substitution, degradation is slower and it remains longer is the intravascular compartment. Molar substitution is the average number of hydroxyethyl residues per glucose subunit.

Hydroxyethyl starch will effectively expand the intravascular volume up to 100%. 5% albumin has a similar effect of volume expansion and it can persist for 8–12 hours. HES reduces von Willebrand factor and Factor VIII levels. HES also impairs platelet function, prolongs partial thromboplastin time. It is associated with anaphylactoid reaction and pruritus due to its accumulation in skin. HES with high molecular weight has been associated with acute kidney injury especially in critically ill patients with known history of chronic kidney disease.[27]

Third-generation HES (6% HES 130/0.4) has lower risk of affecting the coagulation. Studies have shown that with the use of 6% HES (130/0.4) for resuscitation, less volume is needed to reach hemodynamic stability when compared with 0.9% NaCl solution.[28] CHEST trial showed patients resuscitated with HES compared to 0.9% NaCl solution has a higher risk of requiring renal replacement therapy.[29] The 6S trial has shown that there is an increased risk of death at 90 days if HES 130/0.42 is used for resuscitation compared to Ringer's lactate group. The same study group has also concluded that patients receiving 6% HES had more severe bleeding compared to the other group.[30] Hence, the use of HES fluids for resuscitation had fallen out of favor especially for septic shock patients.

## SALIENT POINTS

- Crystalloids should be used as the first-line resuscitation fluid of choice.
- Avoid using solutions that contain high chloride content, e.g. 0.9% NaCl solution.
- Use of balanced salt solution is associated with less morbidity.
- Colloids may be used for its volume sparing effect.
- Hydroxyethyl starch and dextran-based fluids should be avoided because of the potential adverse effect.
- Albumin-based fluids may be beneficial in specific indications but to be avoided in patients with traumatic brain injury.

## REFERENCES

1. Guidet B, Soni N, Della Rocca G, et al. A balanced view of balanced solutions. Crit Care. 2010;14(5):325.
2. Moritz ML, Ayus JC. Maintenance intravenous fluids in acutely Ill patients. N Engl J Med. 2015;373(14):1350-60.
3. Chowdhury AH, Cox EF, Francis ST, et al. A randomized, controlled, double-blind crossover study on the effects of 2-L infusions of 0.9% saline and plasma-lyte® 148 on renal blood flow velocity and renal cortical tissue perfusion in healthy volunteers. Ann Surg. 2012;256(1):18-24.
4. O'Malley CM, Frumento RJ, Hardy MA, et al. A randomized, double-blind comparison of lactated Ringer's solution and 0.9% NaCl during renal transplantation. Anesth Analg. 2005;100(5):1518-24.
5. Kraut JA, Madias NE. Lactic acidosis. N Engl J Med. 2014;371(24):2309-19.
6. Ince C, Groeneveld AB. The case for 0.9% NaCl: is the undefendable, defensible? Kidney Int. 2014;86(6):1087-95.
7. McCague A, Dermendjieva M, Hutchinson R, et al. Sodium acetate infusion in critically Ill trauma patients for hyperchloremic acidosis. Scand J Trauma Resusc Emerg Med. 2011;19:24.
8. Ekblad H, Kero P. Sodium acetate infusion to correct acidosis in premature infants. Am J Dis Child. 1986;140(1):9-10.
9. Thaha M, Yogiantoro M, Soewanto, et al. Correlation between intradialytic hypotension in patients undergoing routine hemodialysis and use of acetate compared in bicarbonate dialysate. Acta Med Indones. 2005;37(3):145-8.
10. Schrander-vd Meer AM, ter Wee PM, Kan G, et al. Improved cardiovascular variables during acetate free biofiltration. Clin Nephrol. 1999;51(5):304-9.
11. Reddy S, Weinberg L, Young P. Crystalloid fluid therapy. Crit Care. 2016;20:59.
12. Padhi S, Bullock I, Li L, et al. National Institute for Health and Care Excellence (NICE) Guideline Development Group. Intravenous fluid therapy for adults in hospital: Summary of NICE guidance. BMJ. 2013;347:f7073.
13. Chua HR, Venkatesh B, Stachowski E, et al. Plasma-Lyte 148 vs 0.9% saline for fluid resuscitation in diabetic ketoacidosis. J Crit Care. 2012;27(2):138-45.
14. Weinberg L, Collins N, Van Mourik K, et al. Plasma-Lyte 148: A clinical review. World J Crit Care Med. 2016;5(4):235-50.
15. Young P, Bailey M, Beasley R, et al. SPLIT Investigators; ANZICS CTG. Effect of a buffered crystalloid solution vs saline on acute kidney injury among patients in the intensive care unit. The SPLIT randomized clinical trial. JAMA. 2015;314(16):1701-10.
16. Tommasino C, Picozzi V. Volume and electrolyte management. Best Pract Res Clin Anaesthesiol. 2007;21(4):497-516.
17. Huskisson L. Intravenous volume replacement: Which fluid and why? Arch Dis Child. 1992;67(5):649-53.
18. Nicholson JP, Wolmarans MR, Park GR. The role of albumin in critical illness. Br J Anaesth. 2000;85(4):599-610.
19. Boldt J. Use of albumin: an update. Br J Anaesth. 2010;104(3):276-84.
20. Finfer S, Bellomo R, Boyce N, et al. SAFE Study Investigators. A comparison of albumin and saline for fluid resuscitation in the intensive care unit. N Engl J Med. 2004;350(22):2247-56.
21. Caironi P, Tognoni G, Masson S, et al. ALBIOS Study Investigators. Albumin replacement in patients with severe sepsis or septic shock. N Engl J Med. 2014;370(15):1412-21.

22. Maitland K, Kiguli S, Opoka RO, et al. FEAST Trial Group. Mortality after fluid bolus in African children with severe infection. N Engl J Med. 2011;364(26):2483-95.
23. Niemi TT, Miyashita R, Yamakage M. Colloid solutions: a clinical update. J Anesth. 2010;24(6):913-25.
24. Klotz U, Kroemer H. Clinical pharmacokinetic considerations in the use of plasma expanders. Clin Pharmacokinet. 1987;12(2):123-35.
25. Saw MM, Chandler B, Ho KM. Benefits and risks of using gelatin solution as a plasma expander for perioperative and critically ill patients: a meta-analysis. Anaesth Intensive Care. 2012;40(1):17-32.
26. von Roten I, Madjdpour C, Frascarolo P, et al. Molar substitution and C2/C6 ratio of hydroxyethyl starch: influence on blood coagulation. Br J Anaesth. 2006;96(4):455-63.
27. Treib J, Baron JF, Grauer MT, et al. An international view of hydroxyethyl starches. Intensive Care Med. 1999;25(3):258-68.
28. Guidet B, Martinet O, Boulain T, et al. Assessment of hemodynamic efficacy and safety of 6% hydroxyethyl starch 130/0.4 vs. 0.9% NaCl fluid replacement in patients with severe sepsis: The CRYSTMAS study. Crit Care. 2012;16(3):R94.
29. Myburgh JA, Finfer S, Bellomo R, et al. CHEST Investigators; Australian and New Zealand Intensive Care Society Clinical Trials Group. Hydroxyethyl starch or saline for fluid resuscitation in intensive care. N Engl J Med. 2012;367(20):1901-11.
30. Perner A, Haase N, Guttormsen AB, et al. 6S Trial Group; Scandinavian Critical Care Trials Group. Hydroxyethyl starch 130/0.42 versus Ringer's acetate in severe sepsis. N Engl J Med. 2012;367(2):124-34.

# CHAPTER 25

# Approach to the Patient with Hypovolemia

*Tom Carmeliet, Robert Wise, Jan Van der Mullen, Manu Malbrain*

## INTRODUCTION

One of the most challenging tasks for the intensive care clinician is the accurate assessment of patients' intravascular volume status. Correct assessment of the fluid status is of outmost importance because both hypovolemia and hypervolemia are associated with increased morbidity and mortality.[1,2]

The assessment is made up of diverse clinical signs, laboratory investigations and a wide range of hemodynamic and other monitoring systems. Many different techniques and devices are available to assist the clinician, but understanding the limitations and clinical applicability of these tools is vital. This chapter includes the current literature regarding the assessment of hypovolemia in the intensive care unit (ICU), starting with definitions and pathophysiological implications related to hypovolemia.

## CASE

A 19-year-old woman with no significant past history was admitted to the burn unit after suffering flame burns (41% total body surface area, TBSA). In this case we will try to identify the best monitoring tool to assess the volemic status during the different phases of shock and we will try to provide answers to the four basic but crucial questions that need to be addressed in order to avoid harm: (1) When should I start giving fluids; (2) when should I stop giving fluids; (3) when should I start removing fluid and finally; (4) when should I stop fluid removal?

The patient was electively intubated and mechanically ventilated in the emergency department where a radial arterial line (A-line) and two peripheral lines were placed. She received maintenance fluids (ready-from-the-shelve maintenance solution Glucion 5%) at a rate of 84 mL/hr. Clinical examination showed an increased capillary refill time of 4 seconds and her extremities were cold. Her initial assessment showed a mean arterial blood pressure (MAP) of 55 mm Hg with a heart rate at 115 bpm and resuscitation fluids (Plasmalyte) are given at 200 mL/hr. An increased lactate of 2.9 mmol/L prompts the placement of a central venous catheter (CVC), with and initial central venous pressure (CVP) of 6 mm Hg. Despite resuscitation with a 500 mL bolus of fluid over 30 minutes, as well as an increased infusion of 220 mL/hr, there was an inadequate effect on MAP (remained at 53 mm Hg). The pulse pressure variation (PPV), obtained via the Philips IntelliVue monitor, was 21% and lactate further increased to 3.4, while the CVP was 10 mm Hg. At this time, the passive leg raising test (PLR) resulted in an increased MAP and a decreased PPV. A further fluid bolus of 500 mL over 30 minutes was given and resuscitation fluids were increased to 275 mL/hr. However, PPV remained high at 23% and lactate further increased to 4.1 mmol/L. Another bolus of 500 mL over 30 minutes was given but with an inadequate effect on hemodynamics. A non-calibrated continuous cardiac output (CCO) monitor was then connected to the A-line (PulsioFlex, Getinge) confirming the high PPV of 22% and a low CCI 2.4 L/min/m². A further 500 mL bolus of Plasmalyte was given over 30 min and resuscitation fluids were increased to 350 mL/hr. Around that time, albumin 20% was commenced at 20 mL/hr. The PPV dropped transiently to 6% while lactate decreased to 2.5 mmol/L. The urine output started to decrease. Approximately eight hours after admission, a PPV rise to 31% is observed and lactate also increases 4.2 mmol/L with a corresponding drop in CCI 1.9 L/min/m². An additional bolus of 500 mL/30 min was administered and resuscitation fluids were increased to 440 mL/hr together with albumin 20% at 30 mL/hr. The effect was marginal and calibrated CCO (obtained via transpulmonary thermodilution with PiCCO, Getinge) showed a CI of 1.7 L/min/m², other derived parameters demonstrate a low global ejection fraction (GEF) of 13%, an extremely low global end-diastolic volume index (GEDVI) of 350 mL/m$^2$, and a normal extravascular lung water (EVLWI) of 7 mL/PBW. The PPV was still high at 33% with a MAP of 51 mm Hg and an apparent normal CVP of 13 mm Hg. Ventilation was maintained in BIPAP mode with an IPAP of 25 cm H$_2$O, PEEP of 7 cm H$_2$O, and a P/F ratio of 250. More intravenous boluses of 500 mL was given over 30 min and resuscitation fluids were increased to 550 mL/hr. Finally, evolution overnight is favorable with an increase in CI from 1.7 to 2.6 L/min/m$^2$, GEDVI from 350 to 646 mL/m$^2$, and EVLWI from 7 to 9 mL/kg PBW, while PPV dropped from 40 to 5%. Lactate returned to normal (1.5 mmol/L). Meanwhile the CVP decreased from 13 to 8 mm Hg with filling, confirming the inaccuracy of CVP in this scenario, and the opposite changes between barometric and volumetric preload indicators. The following day maintenance fluids were kept at 84 mL/hr while resuscitation fluids were de-escalated to Plasmalyte at 137 mL/hr and albumin at 27 mL/hr. The concomitant use of norepinephrine 0.3 ug/kg/min and dobutamine 3 ug/kg/min occurred. Between days 2 and 5 the CI increased to 5.7 L/min/m$^2$, GEDVI to 905 mL/m$^2$, EVLWI to 12 mL/kg PBW, and PPV again increased to 19%. The patient remained tachycardic at 125 bpm with a normal MAP of approximately 70 mm Hg. The CVP was 15 mm Hg with an increased intra-abdominal pressure (IAP) noted at 13 mm Hg. Norepinephrine and dobutamine were stopped on day 4. The patient was still hypothermic, acidotic and coagulopathic during wound care. This is a typical therapeutic dilemma but we decided to give fluids because: PPV was high and PLR was positive. The GEDVI of 905 was relatively low (in relation to a GEF of 20%), despite the increased CVP and higher EVLWI (IVCCI was almost 50%).

On Day 5, however, respiratory function deteriorated and P/F ratio dropped below 200. Transthoracic echocardiography showed a dilated right ventricle (R/L ratio around 1/1) with tricuspid regurgitation 3-4/4 and calculated pulmonary artery pressures of 44 + CVP (around 60–70 mm Hg), with septal dyskinesia and D-shaping of the left ventricle. A CT-angiogram on day 6 excluded pulmonary embolism but confirmed secondary ARDS with typical zones of ventilated, recruitable and collapsed lung units. On day 7 EVLWI increased to 16 ml/PBW (pulmonary vascular permeability index rose maximal to 2.5) and P/F ratio dropped to 98 (despite aggressive ventilation with IPAP 30 and PEEP 8). Lungs were recruited and driving pressures reduced to 16. Inhaled NO was started at 5 ppm and increased up to 20 ppm overnight. Simultaneously PAL therapy was started (this is a sequential combination of PEEP set at the level of IAP, hyperoncotic albumin 20% and furosemide). After initiation of deresuscitation, chest X-ray, EVLWI and P/F ratio all improved and further weaning from the ventilator could occur.

## DEFINITIONS

### Hypovolemia

Hypovolemia is the term used to describe a patient with insufficient intravascular volume. It does not refer to total body fluid, but rather refers solely to the intravascular compartment. Total body fluid comprises approximately 60% of the body weight of men and 50% for women.[3] Blood volume can be estimated according to Gilcher's rule of fives at 70 mL/kg for men and 65 mL/kg for women.[4] Blood loss is frequently followed by recruitment of interstitial fluid from compartments distant to the central compartment. Vasoconstriction of the splanchnic mesenteric vasculature is one of the first physiologic responses.[5] Sodium and water retention results from activation of the renin-angiotensin-aldosterone system (RAAs) which replenishes the interstitial reserves and maintains trans-capillary perfusion.[6] As a result, the body may lose up to 30% of blood volume before hypovolemia becomes clinically apparent.[7] Therefore, undiagnosed hypovolemia may be present long before clinical signs and symptoms occur. Hypovolemia can also occur in edematous patients, where total body water in increased, but intravascular volume is reduced (e.g. eclamptic patients). Finally, some patients are fluid responsive, but not necessarily hypovolemic. Even the most basic of paradigms, such as the description of early sepsis and distributive shock being a hypovolemic state needing aggressive fluid resuscitation, has recently been called into question,[8] with data suggesting improved outcomes with less or even no administered intravenous fluid.[8,9] Greater focus on the health and function of the microcirculation and the endothelial glycocalyx, potential new treatment paradigms calling for less fluids, and earlier vasopressor use have become the focus.[8,10-12] These elements make accurate assessment of fluid status in the critically ill a challenging task.

### Fluid Balance

Daily fluid balance is the difference between all fluids given to a patient during a 24-hour period and their combined output. As a consequence, daily fluid balance can be negative, neutral or positive. The daily fluid balance does not usually include insensible losses, unless the patient is being cared for on an ICU bed that can weigh the patient.[13] Caution should be exercised when using daily weight as muscle and tissue loss cannot be easily measured.

## Cumulative Fluid Balance

The cumulative fluid balance is the sum of fluid accumulated over a set period. Usually the first week of ICU stay is taken into account for prognostication.[13]

## Fluid Loss

Fluid loss is defined as a negative fluid balance, regardless of intravascular status. Fluid gain is the opposite of fluid loss.

## Dehydration

Defined as excessive loss of body water, dehydration has a wide range of etiologies, including gastrointestinal loss of fluid (vomiting or diarrhea), heat exposure, prolonged vigorous exercise, kidney disease and medication (e.g. diuretics). A drop in weight might be an indication of dehydration, though regular weight monitoring is often difficult in ICU. The percentage of fluid loss is defined by dividing the cumulative fluid balance in liters by the patient's baseline body weight and multiplying by 100%. Dehydration is defined by a minimum value of 5% fluid loss. Dehydration is considered mild (5–7.5%), moderate (7.5–10%), while loss of over 10% is considered severe.[14] Overhydration or fluid overload at any stage is the opposite and is defined by a minimum value of 10% fluid accumulation. As already mentioned, fluid overload is also associated with worse outcomes.

## Fluid Responsiveness

Fluid responsiveness describes the situation in which a patient will increase their stroke volume and/or cardiac output (or their surrogates) in response to fluid administration. A minimum increase in cardiac output of 15% is most often used for this definition.[15] It is important to realize that a patient can be fluid responsive regardless of the (intravascular) fluid status (hypovolemia, euvolemia, or hypervolemia). This concept is based on the Frank-Starling principle, where an increase in preload causes further stretch on cardiac myofilaments, resulting in improved contractility (steep part of the slope), limited by a maximum ability to stretch and contract (upper flat part of the curve). When preload is maximized, further stretch will not result in increased contractility. Fluid responsiveness, however, does not provide the clinician with exact information on the intravascular status of the patient. It simply suggests a likely increase in cardiac output should a bolus of intravenous fluid be administered.

## Shock

Vincent et al. described *shock* as "the clinical expression of circulatory failure that results in inadequate cellular oxygen utilization, resulting in an imbalance between oxygen delivery and oxygen consumption".[16] Four categories can be distinguished: (1) hypovolemic (internal and/or external fluid loss); (2) cardiogenic (i.e. acute coronary (3) syndrome with myocardial infarction, cardiomyopathy), obstructive (i.e. cardiac tamponade, tension pneumothorax, pulmonary embolism); and (4) distributive (i.e. severe sepsis, anaphylaxis).[16] A further in-depth analysis of the different states of shock is beyond the scope of this chapter.

## ETIOLOGY OF HYPOVOLEMIA

As mentioned before, the etiology of hypovolemia can be diverse. Although it may commonly be the result of bleeding, there are often other causes in critically ill patients, such as loss of vascular integrity and fluid leakage into the interstitial compartment. Increased loss of fluid (i.e. diarrhea, vomiting) that exceeds the replenishment capabilities will inevitably lead to hypovolemia, and should be considered since fluids such as stool and vomitus are often not quantified and included in fluid balance calculations. Redistribution of fluids into the interstitial compartment, and into the pleural and peritoneal compartment, occurs in sepsis, severe inflammation (e.g. pancreatitis, burns) and anaphylaxis. An inability to take in fluids (e.g. during coma) will exhaust fluid reserves until overt hypovolemia is established.

## CONSEQUENCES OF HYPOVOLEMIA

Intravascular fluids are needed to transport nutrients, the most important of which is oxygen. Diminished oxygen delivery results in cellular dysfunction and eventually multi-organ failure (MOF). Compensatory mechanisms permit some organs to maintain a degree of functionality (auto-regulation) with a reduced oxygen supply, but a persistently low perfusion pressure following loss of circulatory blood volume in excess of 30% will eventually result in MOF and death.[17]

## APPROACH TO HYPOVOLEMIC PATIENT

### Clinical Assessment

A thorough history and physical examination is important in the initial assessment of the volume status of patients. Emphasis should be placed on considering overt and occult fluid loss (bleeding, vomiting, diarrhea) or reduced fluid intake. The type of fluid the patient is receiving is also of great importance. Some fluids may actually contribute to dehydration rather than rehydration (e.g. coffee, black tea, stimulants or several popular lemonades). The presence of thirst may indicate dehydration and hypovolemia but is neither sensitive nor specific. This is because of the role that plasma osmolality plays in thirst. For example, many osmotic disturbances (e.g. hyperglycemia), electrolyte disturbances (e.g. hypernatremia), pathologies (xerostomia, stomatitis, heart failure) or commonly used medications (anticholinergics, tricyclic antidepressants, proton pump inhibitors) can trigger a sensation of thirst.[18]

Physical examination should focus on signs of dehydration. Vital signs such as blood pressure (including all aspects, namely mean arterial pressure, systolic and diastolic pressures, and pulse pressure), pulse rate, presence of orthostatic hypotension, or tachycardia are useful indicators. They are, however, dependent on the type and amount of fluid loss. Capillary refill time (normally less than 2 seconds), skin turgor, presence of dry mucosae, the temperature of extremities, and difference between central and peripheral temperature, together with skin perfusion (color, mottling) may be useful although often difficult to interpret because of several confounding factors in critically ill patients.[19] Weighing ICU patients may be of value although this has practical limitations. Box 1 summarizes the clinical signs of hypovolemia.

Urine output is monitoring is accepted as standard of care, but is influenced by many variables. It cannot be used as the only clinical assessment of hypovolemia because of many associated confounding issues in critically ill patients.[20] A more specific sign of hypovolemia in the critically ill, is an abrupt decrease in blood pressure after initiation of mechanical ventilation or when performing a recruitment maneuver.[16] Two main pathophysiological reasons have been proposed for this observation. Firstly, positive intrathoracic pressure causes a decrease in venous return resulting in reduced preload and thus decreased cardiac output. Hypovolemic patients do not tolerate the decrease in venous return as well as euvolemic patients. Secondly, sedative-induced vasodilation is more pronounced in these patients. These effects are more pronounced with the use of high positive end-expiratory pressure (PEEP) or the presence of auto-PEEP.

It is clear that none of these clinical signs and symptoms alone can provide the clinician with the correct information on intravascular fluid status. They require integration into a broader assessment of volume status.[20]

## Laboratory Biomarkers

Even laboratory results, although providing useful information, cannot provide independent markers of volume status. There are no single biomarkers to assess hypovolemia. Some point-of-care tests are of value (e.g. arterial blood gas analysis, lactate, etc.). Box 2 summarizes the laboratory biomarkers that may be useful in hypovolemia.

### Arterial Blood Gas

Although there are currently no published data on the relationship between hypovolemia and hemoglobin, it is widely accepted that hypovolemia will cause hemoglobin and hematocrit to rise due to hemoconcentration. However, this process is subject to confounders such as pre-existing or new anemia, or the toxic medullary effect

---

**Box 1:** Clinical signs of hypovolemia.

- Body weight ↓
- Fluid balance ↓
- Cumulative FB ↓
- Absence of pitting edema
- Decreased skin turgor
- Absence of 2nd and 3rd space fluid accumulation
- JVP normal and HJR absent
- Capillary refill time (>2 sec) ↑
- No orthopnea or platydeoxia
- Dry mucosa, thirst
- Mottled skin (livedo reticularis), peripheral cyanosis
- Central to peripheral temperature difference ↑
- Drop in urine output ↓ < 0.5 mL/kg/hr

(FB: fluid balance; HJR: hepatojugular reflex; JVP: jugular venous pressure).

---

**Box 2:** Laboratory biomarkers for hypovolemia.

- Lactate ↑ S(c)vO$_2$ ↓
- Albumin leak index ↑ (ratio urine albumin/urine creatinine)
- Hemoconcentration: hemoglobin ↑
- Total protein ↑ and albumin ↑
- Serum Na ↑
- CLI ↑ = ↓ (ratio serum CRP/serum albumin)
- Serum osmolality ↑, COP ↑
- BNP and NT-pro-BNP ↓
- (In) activation RAAS
- Urine electrolytes: Na ↓ osm ↑

(BNP: brain natriuretic peptide; CLI: capillary leak index; COP: colloid oncotic pressure; CRP: C-reactive protein; Na: sodium; RAAS: renin angiotensin aldosterone system; ScvO$_2$: mixed central venous oxygen saturation).

of severe infection. Bedside arterial blood gas analysis allows for easy measurement of hemoglobin and hematocrit. Hemoconcentration may contribute towards oxygen imbalance and eventually end-organ failure.[21] Point-of-care blood gas analysis provides information on arterial lactate levels that may be helpful when combined with base deficit, and central venous or mixed venous oxygen saturation.[22]

## Renal Function

Hypovolemia can significantly influence renal function, although the effects of temporary decreased renal perfusion appears to depend predominantly on the condition of pre-existing renal physiology. An elevated serum urea over creatinine ratio above 20–50 may indicate hypovolemia. However, when pre-existent kidney function is normal, creatinine levels may remain within normal limits. On the other hand, proximal gastro-intestinal bleeding can elevate serum urea due to digestion of red blood cells without kidney injury (this may be occult in nature, or overt bleeding with evidence of hypovolemia).

## Electrolytes

Plasma sodium levels are of specific interest in volume regulation. They can also be measured by point-of-care tests in combination with arterial blood gas analysis and are strongly associated with volume status. Widespread baroreceptors sense hypovolemia and activate secretion of antidiuretic hormone by the posterior pituitary gland (arginine vasopressin). Antidiuretic hormone induces net retention of water, resulting in dilutional hyponatremia. This hyponatremia is augmented when patients are given hypotonic fluids to replace losses.[23] Of note, not every patient with hyponatremia will be hypovolemic, and not every hypovolemic patient develops hyponatremia. If a net fluid loss is not replaced, sodium will rise resulting in hypernatremia. Sodium values are also confounded by medication (e.g. tricyclic antidepressants, diuretics—especially thiazides or indapamide and spironolactone), the type of fluid loss, adrenal activity, and choice of replacement fluid. Determining the exact cause of low sodium levels can be very difficult in critically ill patients, and is often multifactorial. Detailed investigation and physical examination may help in appropriate management of these patients.

## Renin Angiotensin Aldosterone System

Renal hypoperfusion occurring as a consequence of hypovolemia is sensed by renal baroreceptors in the juxtaglomerular apparatus, which in turn activate the RAAS resulting in aldosterone secretion and sodium and water retention. Although plasma renin activity and plasma-aldosterone levels have closely linked to volume status, measurement of these hormones or their activity is impractical and not feasible in most ICUs patients.[6]

## Plasma Osmolality

Plasma osmolality ($P_{osm}$) has previously been considered the perfect biomarker for hydration status, as it reflects intracellular osmolality and operates in very narrow ranges (normal value of approximately 285–295 mOsm/kg in healthy, well-hydrated individuals). This hypothesis has been under pressure in recent years.[25,26] Acute changes in extra-cellular fluid status will rapidly alter $P_{osm}$. The degree that $P_{osm}$ increases depends on the type of fluid lost (e.g. diarrhea, or vomitus, or sweat, etc.). When the extracellular hypovolemia persists, maintenance of fluid homeostasis is attempted by recruiting intracellular fluid as explained previously. A new equilibrium will therefore develop, causing the $P_{osm}$ to shift back to its normal value as much as possible. This is why $P_{osm}$ does not readily reflect chronic hypovolemia. Secondly, $P_{osm}$ is influenced by several factors, the most important of which is elevation of the non-soluble fraction of the extra-cellular compartment, namely elevated concentrations of serum lipids or proteins. Many medications (e.g. diuretics, mannitol) influence the $P_{osm}$ and should be considered during evaluation of volume status.

## Plasma Colloid Oncotic Pressure

Plasma colloid oncotic pressure (COP) normally ranges between 20 and 25 mm Hg and is an important determinant in the development of edema and the regulation of fluid exchange.[27] COP tends to decrease with age, is lower in females, and also in patients confined to bed rest. COP may increase in dehydrated patients and is related to left ventricular filling pressure, and thus may be a useful biomarker for the differential diagnosis of pulmonary edema (hydrostatic vs. hyperpermeability). COP is increased in hydrostatic edema and is associated with increased left ventricular end-diastolic pressure (LVEDP), whereas in hyperpermeability edema, COP is usually decreased.

## Urinalysis

Urine output decreases in states of hypovolemia, largely initiated through water and sodium retention as discussed previously. This decrease is not necessarily a sign of kidney dysfunction, but rather of maximum physiological reaction (activation of the RAAS) of a normal kidney.[28] A urinary sodium less than 100 mEq/24 hr strongly suggests hypovolemia.[28] However, this is of no use in determining volume status at the bedside or when immediate therapeutic interventions are needed. Urine output measurement in combination with urine electrolyte assessment remains very important when attempting to evaluate immediate changes.[24] They are cheap and easy to obtain, and contain much more information than most clinicians suspect. Decreased urinary sodium excretion is probably evident long before changes in vital signs occur, and are most likely evidence of an adequate response to hypovolemia leading to increased aldosterone activity.[28] The response of both serum and fractional urinary excretion of sodium to the administration of normal saline (1–2 L/day for 2 days) is of particular interest. If serum sodium increases by greater than 5 mmol/L and fractional urinary excretion of sodium increases by less than 0.5% then it is highly suggestive of hypovolemic hyponatremia.[23] However, it should be remembered that urine sampling should only be performed a minimum of 6 hours after the last dose of diuretics. An alternative is to check the fractional excretion of urea.

## Imaging and Hemodynamic Monitoring Techniques

Box 3 summarizes the different imaging techniques that can be useful in hypovolemia.

### Chest X-ray

Assessing volume status on a chest X-ray in the critically ill is very difficult due to highly variable signs that are neither sensitive nor specific. Furthermore, the absence of typical radiological signs for hypervolemia (e.g. Kerley B-lines, prominent vascular hili, pleural effusion) does not imply hypovolemia, nor are there signs typical of hypovolemia. Chest X-ray is therefore of no use in detecting hypovolemia in critically ill patients.[29]

### Ultrasound Assessment

There are numerous advantages to bedside ultrasound. It is readily available, easy to use and accurate. It gives real-time direct, non-invasive or minimally invasive images of organs, vessels and other clinically relevant structures.[30] M-mode and Doppler can generate dynamic measurements that guide efficient therapy at the bedside. Some authors suggest it is close to the ideal hemodynamic monitoring system.[31] However, it is operator dependent and measures should be taken to minimize inter-observer variability. Ultrasound has grown to be an important clinical tool for practicing intensivists and emergency physicians and may turn out to be the stethoscope of the intensivist in the 21st century.[32-35]

### Venous Collapsibility Index

During the respiratory cycle, inferior vena cava (IVC) diameter changes due to negative and positive intrathoracic pressure. Measuring the change in diameter provides an index that correlates with a patient's volume status (Figs. 1A and B).[32,36] There is growing evidence suggesting that IVC is not only valid in spontaneously breathing patients, but also in those receiving mandatory positive pressure ventilation, which has been previously debated.[32] The effect of PEEP appears to be negligible. In ventilated patients, the maximum and minimum IVC diameters are measured to calculate the IVC collapsibility index (IVCCI), rather than inspiratory and expiratory values alone. An alternative to measuring the IVC is to use the superior vena cava (SVC) or the subclavian vein which has also been correlated successfully to hemodynamics.[36] Even in inexperienced hands, the IVC is easily accessible with ultrasound, with acceptable accuracy and reproducibility after minimal training.[37,38] However, IVC measurement also has important limitations, including technical (e.g. limited visualization in surgical and obese patients) and implementation-related (i.e. requirement for new equipment, limited number of trained sonographers, incomplete understanding of relationships to existing invasive hemodynamic monitoring devices).[32,35,36] As with every tool, the physician using it determines the utility. Despite the above, controversy remains regarding utility of IVC measurement. IVC measurement in combination with passive leg raising (as will be discussed further), has been shown to be a good predictor of fluid responsiveness.[31,39-42]

### Transthoracic Cardiac Ultrasound

Another interesting point-of-care noninvasive examination is transthoracic echocardiography (TTE). TTE can rapidly assess systolic and diastolic function of the ventricles, loading conditions (pre-and afterload), valve function and morphology, and great vessel anatomy at the bedside.

---

**Box 3:** Radiologic and imaging signs of hypovolemia.

- Normal chest X-ray, absence of Kerley-B lines, no pleural effusion
- Abdominal US: no ascites
- TTE: low E/e', LVOT VTI variations ↑
- IVCCI ↑ > 50% (IVC ↑ < 1.5 cm)
- Left atrium volume ↓
- Normal lung US: no B-lines

(IVC: inferior vena cava; IVCCI: inferior vena cava collapsibility index; LVOT: left ventricular outflow tract; TTE: transthoracic echocardiography; US: ultrasound; VTI: velocity time integral).

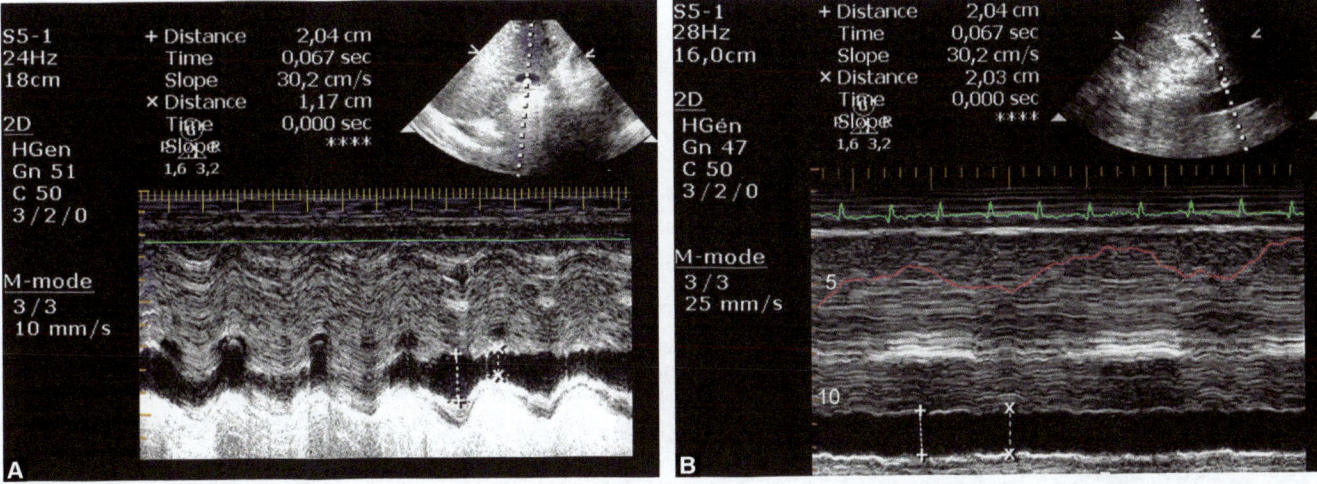

**Figs. 1A and B:** Calculation of the inferior vena collapsibility index. (A) Patient in early phase of septic shock that was fluid responsive. The inferior vena collapsibility index (IVCCI) was more than 50%. Adapted from Vermeiren et al. with permission;[48] (B) Patient in late phase of septic shock, before starting de-resuscitation, that was fluid unresponsive. The inferior vena collapsibility index (IVCCI) was negligible (around 0%).

Its value has been reported by several studies (Figs. 2A to H).[43] Although intensive training is needed to fully utilize echocardiography, the non-cardiologist intensivist can be trained to gather valuable and reproducible information. Studies show that TTE based information can immediately influence management in as much as 40% of patients and also provides clinically important information to an additional 48%.[44] One study reported that non-cardiologists could be trained to estimate left ventricular (LV) function with as little as 6 hours of training.[45] Transthoracic echocardiography may be difficult in the ICU, particularly on those who have abdominal or thoracic dressings, external devices that cannot be displaced (e.g. left ventricular assist devices, thorax drainage systems), difficult body constitution, limited cooperation, or hyperinflated lungs (COPD, positive pressure ventilation, high PEEP).

### Transesophageal Cardiac Ultrasound

Transesophageal echocardiography (TEE) is another, more invasive technique to visualize the heart and is increasingly being used in the intensive care population because many patients are already sedated and mechanically ventilated. TEE enables better visualization of the heart, particularly posterior structures. This results in a better assessment of global function, preload, afterload, and fluid responsiveness. TEE is also less limited by difficult visualization than TTE and although it requires more preparation, good quality images are potentially easier to obtain. Miniature TEE probes have been developed in recent years, minimizing the risk of trauma and diminishing the need for sedation and analgesia associated with this technique. These probes can be left in place for up to 72 hours and are useful in hemodynamic monitoring,[46] but visualization is not as good as normal TEE and are less helpful in diagnosing structural problems.[47]

### Volumetric Assessment

Even in perfect circumstances, volumetric assessment of the heart via echocardiography is often challenging. In the ICU, circumstances are frequently even more difficult.[48] Right ventricular end-diastolic volume (RVEDV), left ventricular end-diastolic volume (LVEDV) and global end-diastolic volume (GEDV) are all measurements that can indicate hypovolemia when low. The latter will be discussed further when reviewing transpulmonary thermodilution techniques. Still the subject of debate, normal dimensions of the heart chambers often rely on "eyeballing" assessments. Normal LVEDV is greater than RVEDV and the septum bulges slightly in the right ventricle. As a result, right ventricle end-diastolic diameter (RVEDD) is around 0.6–0.8 of LVEDD. Fluid overload is suggested if these are reversed.[48] Normal left ventricular end diastolic area (LVEDA) is between 10 cm$^2$ and 20 cm$^2$. A LVEDA less than 10 cm$^2$ signifies hypovolemia and an area more than 20 cm$^2$ is suggestive of volume overload.

### Esophageal Doppler Monitoring

Esophageal doppler monitoring (EDM) probes have a unidirectional echo-Doppler that can be directed to the

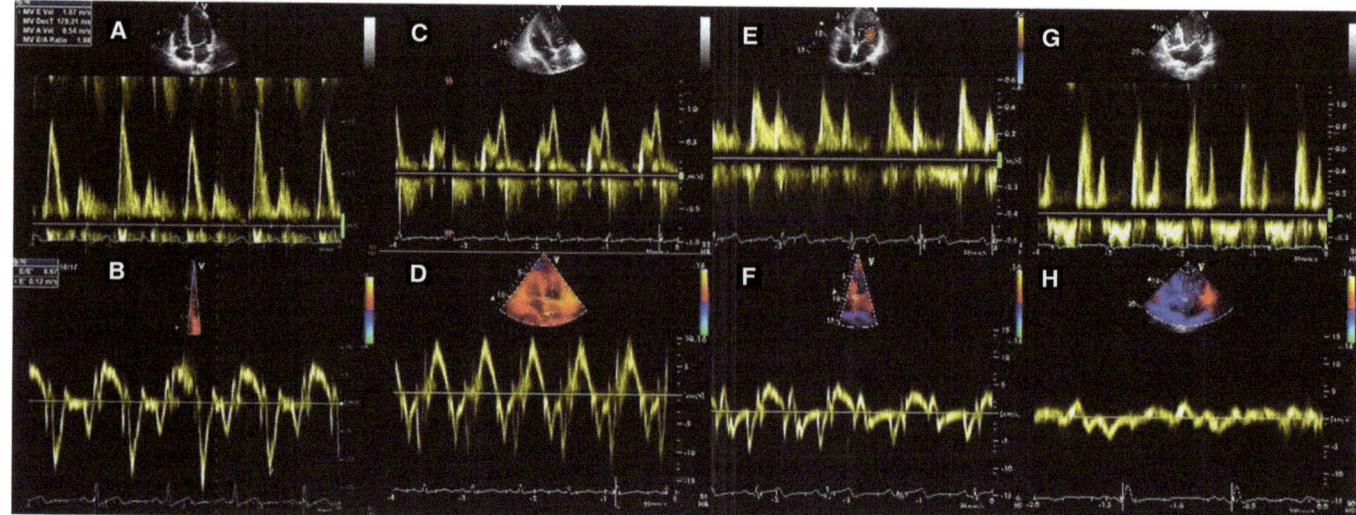

**Figs. 2A to H:** Diastolic function in reality. (A and B) Respectively show the mitral inflow velocity and e' in a 23-year-old man with normal left atrial pressure (LAP). E/A = 1.5, e' = 12 cm/s and E/e' = 8.67; (C and D) Show the mitral inflow velocity and e' respectively, in a patient with delayed relaxation (diastolic dysfunction grade 1) in a 68-year-old female suffering from hypertensive left ventricular hypertrophy. E/A = 0.53, e' = 9 cm/s and E/e' = 7.8; (E and F) Show the mitral inflow velocity and e' respectively, in a patient with pseudo normalized mitral inflow pattern (diastolic dysfunction grade 2). E/A = 1.34, e' = 4.5 cm/s and E/e' = 13.3. One can easily observe the contribution of the e' to allow discrimination between normal and pseudo normal inflow velocities; (G and H) Show the mitral inflow velocity and e' respectively, in a patient with restrictive inflow pattern due to cardiac amyloidosis. E = 110 cm/s, E/A = 2.2, e' = 3.3 cm/s and E/e' = 33. The pulmonary artery occlusion pressure (PAOP) can be estimated from E/e' with the following formula: PAOP = 1.24 × (E/e') + 1.9 mm Hg.
*Source:* Adapted from Vermeiren et al. with permission.[48]

descending aorta to measure blood flow in real time and has shown a decent correlation with pulmonary artery catheter (PAC) and transesophageal echocardiography.[49,50] The main limitation is the size of the probe, often causing discomfort resulting in movement, loss of Doppler signal and need for additional sedation and analgesia.[35,51] Adding to these limitations is the fact that several pathologies, especially aortic disease, have an important influence on the measurements, strongly limiting the popularity of EDM in ICU.

### Hemodynamic Monitoring

Hemodynamic monitoring techniques to assess hypovolemia consist of barometric preload parameters (central venous and pulmonary artery occlusion pressure), volumetric preload measurements (right ventricular and global end-diastolic volume, extravascular lung water), functional hemodynamic variables (stroke volume and pulse pressure variation) and different tests to predict fluid responsiveness (passive leg raising and end-expiratory occlusion tests). Box 4 summarizes the different hemodynamic parameters that can be useful in hypovolemia.

### Central Venous Pressure

The central venous pressure (CVP) was previously the primary parameter for assessing volume status, but is no longer used for this purpose. High CVP would indicate hypervolemia, low CVP hypovolemia and fluid responsiveness. However, a large number of studies have shown no correlation between cardiac output (CO), fluid responsiveness and CVP due to a large number of possible confounders. Stroke volume (SV) will only increase if the heart fibers have the right length, a phenomenon known as the Frank-Starling law (discussed previously).[52] Stroke volume and CO are dependent on venous return, right ventricular compliance, peripheral venous tone,

---

**Box 4:** Hemodynamic parameters in hypovolemia.

- MAP (< 55 mm Hg)↓, HR ↑ = ↓
- CVP ↓, PAOP ↓
- GEF/GEDVI (<680) ↓
- RVEF/RVEDVI (<80) ↓
- Presence of FR (CI increase > 15%)
- PPV ↑, SVV ↑, SPV ↑, Δdown ↑ (> 12–15%)
- Positive PLR (CI increase > 10%)
- Positive EOT (CI increase > 5%)

(CI: cardiac index; CVP: central venous pressure; EOT: end-expiratory occlusion; FR: fluid responsiveness; GEF: global ejection fraction; GEDVI: global end-diastolic volume index; HR: heart rate; MAP: mean arterial blood pressure; PAOP: pulmonary artery occlusion pressure; PLR: passive leg raising; PPV: pulse pressure variation; RVEF: right ventricular ejection fraction; RVEDVI: right ventricular end-diastolic volume index; SPV: systolic pressure variation; SVV: stroke volume variation).

underlying pulmonary vascular disease, intra-abdominal pressure and heart disease (valvular, ischemic, structural changes).[53] For example, patients with abdominal compartment syndrome, due to severe pancreatitis, will usually have high CVP due to the intra-abdominal hypertension, but are most likely to be hypovolemic due to interstitial fluid losses. These variables make CVP a weak indicator of volume status and fluid responsiveness. The likelihood that CVP can accurately predict fluid responsiveness is only 56%, making a single measurement as useful as a chance occurrence, such as flipping a coin.[54] It is also possible to have a low CVP and not be fluid responsive. If there is an intact sympathetic response, the CVP may fall in response to fluid administration due to loss of compensatory venoconstriction.[55] A low CVP will thus not be able to diagnose hypovolemia, nor accurately predict fluid responsiveness and management should never solely rely on the observation of high or low CVP. CVP trends may be marginally more reliable, but due to numerous confounders noted above, still remains doubtful in being able to accurately assess intravascular status. In cases of high CVP, one can calculate transmural CVP by taking into account the index of transmission for positive end-expiratory pressure (PEEP) as shown by Teboul et al.[56] or intra-abdominal pressure (IAP) as shown in Figure 3.[57]

### Pulmonary Artery Occlusion Pressure

In cardiac surgery, a pulmonary artery catheter (PAC or Swan-Ganz catheter) is sometimes used, where a catheter is placed via a central vein through the right atrium, ventricle and into the pulmonary artery. Ideally, the pulmonary artery occlusion pressure (PAOP) is related to LVEDV (preload) and thus a good parameter to assess volume status. However, studies have failed to demonstrate a good correlation between PAOP, volume status, and fluid responsiveness.[29,42,57,58] Some even suggested a negative effect on outcome for patients in which this catheter is placed due to many, potentially severe complications during placement and measurement. Consequently, PAOP is not routinely used in the assessment of volume status in critically ill patients.[59] It is used in some parts of the world to refine therapy in patients with known pulmonary hypertension (PHT) or to diagnose PHT when suspected.

### Volumetric Swan-Ganz

A pulmonary artery catheter can be used to diagnose hypovolemia, and is suspected when the right ventricular end-diastolic volume and its index (RVEDVI) and concomitant CO are all low. A RVEDVI below 80 mL/m²

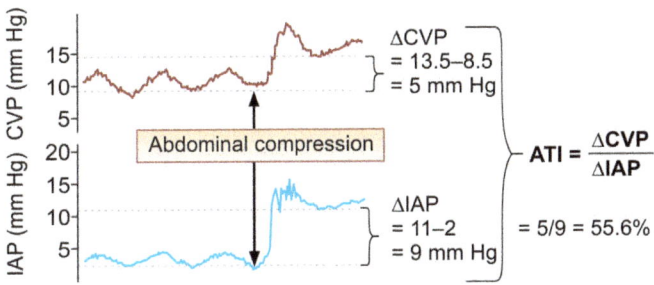

**Fig. 3:** Calculation of the abdomino-thoracic index of transmission and transmural central venous pressure at the bedside. Simultaneous central venous pressure (CVP) and intra-abdominal pressure (IAP) tracing before and during abdominal compression (e.g. by applying an abdominal velcro belt).

The abdomino-thoracic index of transmission (ATI) can be calculated as follows:

The change in end expiratory CVP ($\Delta CVP_{ee}$ = 13.8 – 8.5 mm Hg = 5 mm Hg) divided by the change in end expiratory IAP ($\Delta IAP_{ee}$ = 11 – 2 = 9 mm Hg) and expressed as a percentage. The abdomino-thoracic index (ATI) of transmission = $\Delta CVP / \Delta IAP$ = 5/9 = 55.6%. The transmural CVP ($CVP_{tm}$) can then be calculated as follows:

$$CVP_{tm} = CVP_{ee} - IAP_{ee} \times ATI$$

A simpler way to calculate $CVP_{tm}$ is to subtract half of the IAP from $CVP_{ee}$. (as average ATI is about 50%):

$$CVP_{tm} = CVP_{ee} - IAP/2$$

*Source:* Adapted from Malbrain et al. with permission.[57]

is suggestive of hypovolemia and can be confirmed with this technique.[60] This technique is limited by an invasive nature.[59]

### Transpulmonary Thermodilution

Cardiac output and cardiac index can also be estimated by transpulmonary thermodilution (TPTD), where several parameters can be calculated based on the degree of cooling of blood after a bolus of cold fluid is administered intravenously and passes through the pulmonary vascular bed. Other parameters calculated through this technique include global end-diastolic volume (GEDV) and its index (GEDVI), global ejection fraction (GEF), extravascular lung water (EVLW) and its index (EVLWI), and pulmonary vascular permeability (PVP). Transpulmonary thermodilution is now the standard of care in many ICUs.[61-63] Several different devices are available to perform this bedside technique and assist with diagnosis of hypovolemia. A low CI with low GEDV(I)/EVLW(I) and high PPV is pathognomonic for hypovolemia, whereas a high CI with low GEDV(I) is suggestive of a distributive problem requiring fluid administration (e.g. septic shock). In the latter, the EVLW(I) determines the amount and kind of fluid administered and the necessary

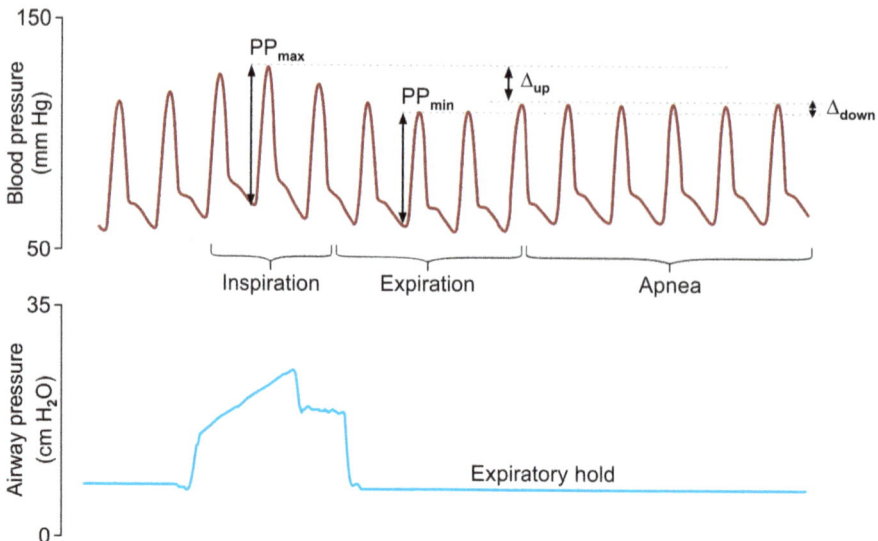

**Fig. 4:** Example of fluid unresponsiveness: Increased pulse pressure variation (PPV) and systolic pressure variations (SPV) in a patient with IAP of 18 mm Hg. The PPV can be calculated as $[(PP_{max} - PP_{min})/PP_{mean}] \times 100\,(\%)$. After an apnea test it becomes clear that the increased SPV and PPV seen on the monitor is mainly related to a $\Delta_{up}$ phenomenon as only a smaller portion is caused by $\Delta_{down}$. This means that the increased PPV and SPV are not necessarily correlated to fluid responsiveness and higher thresholds are probably needed.

adjunctive medication (e.g., vasopressor).[60] The limitations of this technique include the need for invasive procedures (insertion of a central venous line and arterial line) and no good nomograms exist with normal values in different patient populations.[53]

### Stroke Volume Variation and Pulse Pressure Variation

Normal breathing results in negative intrathoracic pressure on inspiration and positive intrathoracic pressure on exhalation. This in turn causes a decrease in systolic pressure on inspiration and an increase on exhalation. The opposite occurs in mechanically ventilated patients. Intrathoracic positive pressure decreases venous return and thus decreases right ventricular filling (preload), whereas left ventricular preload increases due to an increase in pulmonary vascular bed pressure. The difference between maximum and minimal systolic pressure is called pulse pressure variation. Stroke volume variation is calculated through pulse contour analysis and the area under the curve of the systolic portion of the arterial pressure curve.[64] PPV and SVV are higher in the hypovolemic patients making it useful to detect hypovolemia. However, there are some prerequisites to consider, including the need for a normal sinus rhythm, mechanical ventilation without spontaneous breathing, a tidal volume of at least 8 mL/kg, and the patient also needs to have a closed chest.[53] There must also be absence of right heart failure and intra-abdominal hypertension (IAP equal to or above 12 mm Hg).

SVV and PPV may be falsely increased if these conditions are not met. In those circumstances it may be better to calculate systolic pressure variation and to separate $\Delta_{up}$ from $\Delta_{down}$ as only the latter relates to fluid responsiveness (Fig. 4). Furthermore, PPV and SVV are validated to predict fluid-responsiveness rather than sensing hypovolemia. PPV is more reliable than SVV in this estimation because SVV requires a calculation while PPV is measured directly.[29,65]

### Passive Leg Raising Test

The PLR test assesses a patient's response to an intravenous fluid challenge of 150–200 mL (the estimated volume of the bolus of blood caused by raising the lower limbs), without expanding intravascular volume.[40,41] Correct execution of this procedure is vital for correct interpretation. A patient should be in the semi-recumbent position with the head up at 30–45°. The patient should then be switched to the PLR-position in which the legs are now 45° up (Fig. 5). A positive response is defined as an increase in stroke volume of 10%.[41,66] Alternatively, the left ventricle can be estimated visually or the left ventricle end-diastolic area index can be calculated during PLR, avoiding the need for an invasive blood pressure monitoring system.[67] This procedure has its own limitations, e.g. the adrenergic response from pain or stimulation during PLR may lead to false positive results. In patients with heart failure and dilated ventricles, the rapid filling effect experienced from the PLR will be eliminated or partially neutralized.

# Chapter 25
## Approach to the Patient with Hypovolemia

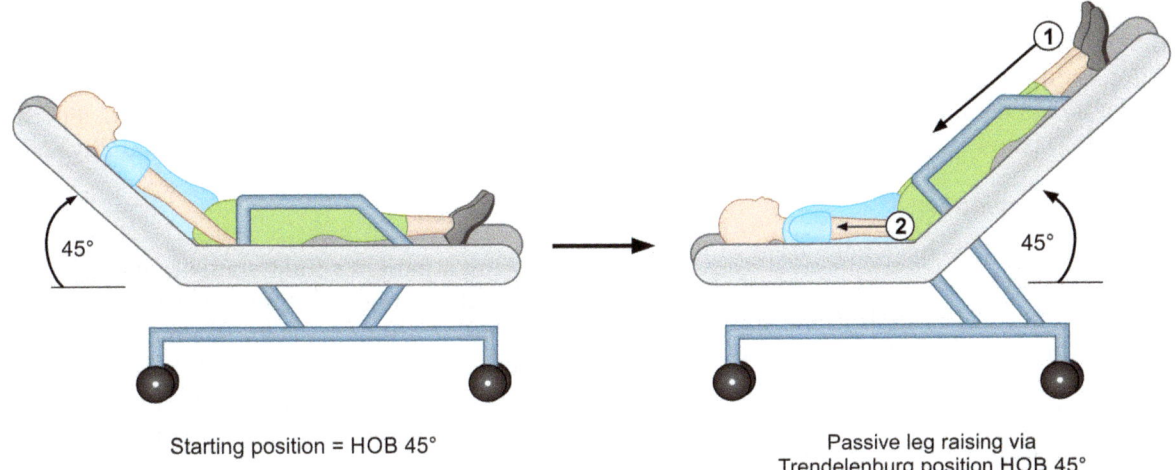

**Fig. 5:** The passive leg raising (PLR) test. In order to perform a correct PLR test, one should not touch the patient in order to avoid sympathetic activation. The PLR is performed by turning the bed from the starting position (head of bed elevation 30–45°) to the Trendelenburg position. The PLR test results in an autotransfusion effect via the increased venous return from the legs and the splanchnic mesenteric pool. Monitoring of stroke volume is required as a positive PLR test is defined by an increase in SV with at least 10%. See text for explanation.
*Source:* Adapted from Reference 79.

### End-Expiratory Occlusion Test

End-expiratory occlusion test (EOT) in mechanically ventilated patient causes continued positive intrathoracic pressure, increasing left ventricular preload. It has been demonstrated that an EOT of 15 seconds increases left ventricular preload sufficiently to increase pulse pressure and cardiac index by more than 5%, without the need for additional IV fluids.[68] This technique predicted fluid responsiveness with an accuracy that was similar to that seen with PLR and cardiac index and was better than that of pulse pressure to PLR. Thus, EOT has proven a useful alternative to techniques already discussed.[69] As mentioned before, fluid responsiveness does not always equate to hypovolemia (i.e. distributive shock) but can be strongly suggestive. Limitations for the EOT are comparable to other techniques using functional hemodynamics (as described above).

### Other Techniques

Box 5 summarizes the other parameters that can be useful in hypovolemia.

### Bioelectrical Impedance Analysis

Bioelectrical impedance analysis (BIA) uses electrical current to calculate body composition and volumes. Five different assumptions need to be made in order to be able to produce reliable measurements. Firstly, the procedure sees the body as a cylinder. Secondly, that cylinder consists of five smaller cylinders (torso being the central one with 2 arms and 2 legs counting for the other four). Thirdly, the body composition is considered to be homogeneous. Fourthly, the composition of the body cannot be altered, so the only variables are the volumes. Lastly, environmental changes do not have an influence on the measurements. These assumptions are rarely true in ICU patients (e.g. amputations, local edema, muscle wasting, etc.).[3,69-71] However, BIA seems promising as it can measure not only

---

**Box 5:** Assessment of organ dysfunction related to hypovolemia.

- EVLWI ↓ = ↑, PVPI ↓ = ↑
- P/F ratio ↓
- GIPS
- IAP ↑, APP ↓ (= MAP-IAP)
- RPP ↓ renal venous congestion
- AKI: biomarkers (N-GAL ↑, cystatin C ↑)
- CARS, polycompartment syndrome
- EIT: V/Q mismatch
- BIA: TBW ↓ ECW/ICW ratio ↓ = ↑ Volume excess = ↓
- Total CBV (technetium albumin) ↓
- Bioreactance: BVI ↓

(AKI: acute kidney injury; APP: abdominal perfusion pressure; BIA: bio-electrical impedance analysis; BVI: blood volume index; CARS: cardio-abdominal-renal syndrome; CBV: circulating blood volume; ECW: extracellular water; EIT: electrical impedance tomography; EVWLI: extravascular lung water index; GIPS: global increased permeability syndrome; IAP: intra-abdominal pressure; ICW: intracellular water; MAP: mean arterial blood pressure; P/F ratio: $pO_2$ over $FiO_2$ ratio; RPP: renal perfusion pressure; PVPI: pulmonary vascular; permeability index; TBW: total body water; V/Q: ventilation/perfusion).

total body water (TBW), but also extra- and intracellular water (ECW/ICW), the ECW/ICW ratio, and the presence of excess fluid volume.[3,72] Further studies are required before BIA can be recommended as a useful tool to detect dehydration in ICU patients.

### Isotope Dilution Techniques

Labeled solutes or isotopes have been used in research to determine total body water, most commonly hydrogen or oxygen isotopes (i.e. $D_2O$, $3H_2O$).[24] Tracer distribution occurs in all of the body fluid compartments, reaching an equilibrium after several hours and then measured in plasma or urine. Total body water (TBW) content can be determined based on the concentration measured.[25,73] There are some specific tracers that only get distributed in extra-cellular compartments that enable estimation of extra-cellular water (ECW) content. The difference between total body water and extra-cellular water content is an estimation of the intracellular water compartment. Although this is an exact and correct measurement of water distribution in different body fluid compartments, it is very exhaustive, requiring specific technical apparatus and carrying risk of adverse infusion reactions, and limiting its implementation in clinical practice.

### Sublingual Microcirculation

The microcirculation is the collection of the smallest blood vessels in the body and consists of the arterioles, capillaries, and venules. In recent years the microcirculation has attracted more attention because of the improved ability to study it.[74-76] Research has shown the essential role of these vessels, the most important being oxygen delivery.[77] Furthermore, the microcirculation is nearly always compromised in critically ill patients.[74,75] Standard care in septic and hypovolemic shock, such as abundant IV fluids and vasopressors, is guided by parameters of inadequate macrocirculation, such as mean arterial pressure (MAP) and lactic acid. This does not tell us what happens at the level of the microcirculation which seems to be critical in the development of shock. Currently, however, we have no technique to observe global microcirculation adequately in routine practice. In this setting, over-administration of fluids and vasoactive drugs may lead to impairment in the microcirculation, potentially causing harm to the patient. Monitoring the microcirculation is possible through the sublingual space.[78] Therapy should strive towards hemodynamic coherence: parallel improvement in the macro- and microcirculation. Hypovolemia may present itself as failure of the microcirculation, now visualized through these novel devices.[74,78] However, elucidating dysfunction of the microcirculation is sometimes difficult and does not always indicate hypovolemia (sepsis and obstructive flow being other causes). Furthermore, limitations include inter-observer variability and cost.

## CONCLUSION

Assessing a patient's fluid status remains a challenging task for all healthcare professionals, especially critically ill patients. Despite the elaborate monitoring techniques that are presently at our disposal, no single ideal method exists to assess and monitor hydration and volume status. Fluid status assessment still largely depends on interpretation of these techniques by the clinician and should, therefore, always be preceded by a thorough clinical examination. Understanding the mechanisms (and inherent limitations) behind each strategy is essential. Together with clinical findings, careful interpretation of laboratory results and specific attention to plasma sodium, COP and $P_{osm}$ is necessary. Twenty-four-hour urine collection and cumulative fluid balance are useful guides to ongoing fluid therapy, while simple urine indices are readily available and provide instant information. A daily chest X-ray for the purpose of volume assessment is not recommended, whereas daily ultrasound screening (IVC, cardiac ultrasound) by an experienced clinician has shown to directly influence fluid therapy.

When these non-invasive tools are insufficient, invasive monitoring should be implemented. Transpulmonary thermodilution with volumetric monitoring provides additional information in unstable ICU patients while the PAC can be helpful in obstructive shock, right heart failure or pulmonary hypertension. Future techniques and biomarkers will undoubtedly find their way into the ICU and change our approach to assessment of volume status in the critically ill.

### Case Revisit

This case demonstrates the different tools that can be used to assess hypovolemia. Starting with clinical examination and A-line, monitoring was soon escalated towards barometric preload, functional hemodynamics, passive leg raising, uncalibrated CO monitoring and finally calibrated CO and monitoring of organ function (EVLWI, IAP). This case also demonstrates the biphasic clinical course during shock, represented by the ebb and flow as well as the inability of traditional filling pressures to guide us through these different phases. This case also illustrates and provides answers to the four basic but crucial questions that need to be addressed in order to avoid harm: (1) When should I start giving fluids, (2) when should I stop giving fluids, (3) when should I start removing fluid, and finally 4) when should I stop fluid removal?

## SALIENT POINTS

- Hypovolemia can cause tissue and organ hypoperfusion and must be avoided
- The longer the duration of hypovolemia, the greater the end-organ damage
- Edematous (fluid overloaded) patients can also be hypovolemic intravascular
- We need to answer the four questions on fluid therapy: (1) When should I start giving fluids, (2) when should I stop giving fluids, (3) when should I start removing fluid, and finally (4) when should I stop fluid removal?
- Clinical signs of hypovolemia are unreliable and calculation of correct fluid balance is often cumbersome
- Radiological and imaging techniques can be helpful and point-of-care ultrasound has become the modern stethoscope
- Advanced (functional) hemodynamic and volumetric monitoring should be performed in unstable critically ill patients where intravascular volume status and presence or absence of fluid responsiveness are uncertain
- The role of biomarkers and laboratory parameters is not well validated and urine electrolytes deserve more attention
- Other less invasive techniques like bioreactance and bio-electrical impedance analysis seem promising
- Frequent re-assessment of volume status is warranted.

## ACKNOWLEDGMENTS

Parts of this chapter were previously published under the Open Access CC BY Licence 3.0.[79] Parts of this chapter were presented during the International Fluid Academy (IFA). The IFA is integrated within the not-for-profit charitable organization iMERiT, International Medical Education and Research Initiative, under Belgian law. The IFA website (http://www.fluidacademy.org) is now an official SMACC affiliated site (Social Media and Critical Care) and its content is based on the philosophy of FOAM (Free Open Access Medical education – #FOAMed). The site recently received the HONcode quality label for medical education (https://www.healthonnet.org/HONcode/Conduct.html?HONConduct519739).

## CONFLICTS OF INTEREST

Manu Malbrain is founding President of WSACS (The Abdominal Compartment Society) and current Treasurer, he is also member of the medical advisory Board of Getinge (Pulsion Medical Systems) and consults for ConvaTec, Acelity, Spiegelberg and Holtech Medical. Manu Malbrain is co-founder of the International Fluid Academy (IFA). The other authors have no possible conflicts of interest in relation to the content of this chapter.

## REFERENCES

1. Bellamy MC. Wet, dry or something else? Br J Anaesth. 2006;97(6):755-7.
2. Chappell D, Jacob M, Hofmann-Kiefer K, et al. A rational approach to perioperative fluid management. Anesthesiology. 2008;109(4):723-40.
3. Malbrain MLNG, Huygh J, Dabrowski W, et al. The use of bio-electrical impedance analysis (BIA) to guide fluid management, resuscitation and deresuscitation in critically ill patients: a bench-to-bedside review. Anaesthesiol Intensive Ther. 2014;46(5):381-91.
4. Nadler SB, Hidalgo JH, Bloch T. Prediction of blood volume in normal human adults. Surgery. 1962;51(2):224-32.
5. Miller TE, Raghunathan K, Gan TJ. State-of-the-art fluid management in the operating room. Best Pract Res Clin Anaesthesiol. 2014;28(3):261-73.
6. Jacob G, Robertson D, Mosqueda-Garcia R, et al. Hypovolemia in syncope and orthostatic intolerance role of the renin-angiotensin system. The American Journal of Medicine. 1997;103(2):128-33.
7. Duchesne JC, Kaplan LJ, Balogh ZJ, et al. Role of permissive hypotension, hypertonic resuscitation and the global increased permeability syndrome in patients with severe hemorrhage: adjuncts to damage control resuscitation to prevent intra-abdominal hypertension. Anaesthesiol Intensive Ther. 2015;47(2):143-55.
8. Marik P, Bellomo R. A rational approach to fluid therapy in sepsis. Br J Anaesth. 2016;116(3):339-49.
9. Hjortrup PB, Haase N, Bundgaard H, et al. Restricting volumes of resuscitation fluid in adults with septic shock after initial management: the CLASSIC randomised, parallel-group, multicentre feasibility trial. Intensive Care Medicine. 2016; 42(11):1695-705.
10. Myburgh JA, Mythen MG. Resuscitation fluids. N Engl J Med. 2013;369(25):2462-3.
11. Malbrain ML, Van Regenmortel N, Owczuk R. It is time to consider the four D's of fluid management. Anaesthesiol Intensive Ther. 2015;47 Spec No:1-5.
12. Malbrain MLNG, Van Regenmortel N, Saugel B, et al. Principles of fluid management and stewardship in septic shock: It is time to consider the four D's and the four phases of fluid therapy. Annals Intensive Care. 2018; 8:66.
13. Malbrain ML, Marik PE, Witters I, et al. Fluid overload, de-resuscitation, and outcomes in critically ill or injured patients: a systematic review with suggestions for clinical practice. Anaesthesiol Intensive Ther. 2014;46(5):361-80.

14. Pruvost I, Dubos F, Chazard E, et al. The value of body weight measurement to assess dehydration in children. PLoS One. 2013;8(1):e55063.
15. Marik PE, Monnet X, Teboul JL. Hemodynamic parameters to guide fluid therapy. Ann Intensive Care. 2011;1(1):1.
16. Vincent JL, De Backer D. Circulatory shock. N Engl J Med. 2013;369(18):1726-34.
17. Rossaint R, Bouillon B, Cerny V, et al. The European guideline on management of major bleeding and coagulopathy following trauma, fourth edition. London: Critical care. 2016;20:100.
18. Arai S, Stotts N, Puntillo K. Thirst in critically ill patients: from physiology to sensation. American journal of critical care : an official publication, American Association of Critical-Care Nurses. 2013;22(4):328-35.
19. Saugel B, Ringmaier S, Holzapfel K, et al. Physical examination, central venous pressure, and chest radiography for the prediction of transpulmonary thermodilution-derived hemodynamic parameters in critically ill patients: a prospective trial. J Crit Care. 2011;26(4):402-10.
20. Padhi S, Bullock I, Li L, et al. National Institute for H, Care Excellence Guideline Development G: Intravenous fluid therapy for adults in hospital: summary of NICE guidance. BMJ. 2013;347:f7073.
21. Van Beaumont W. Evaluation of hemoconcentration from hematocrit measurements. J Appl Physiol. 1972;32(5):712-3.
22. Perel A, Saugel B, Teboul JL, et al. The effects of advanced monitoring on hemodynamic management in critically ill patients: a pre and post questionnaire study. J Clin Monit Comput. 2015.
23. Liamis G, Filippatos TD, Elisaf MS. Correction of hypovolemia with crystalloid fluids: Individualizing infusion therapy. Postgrad Med. 2015;127(4):405-12.
24. Baron S, Courbebaisse M, Lepicard EM, et al. Assessment of hydration status in a large population. Br J Nutr. 2015;113(1):147-58.
25. Armstrong LE. Assessing hydration status: the elusive gold standard. J Am Coll Nutr. 2007;26(5 Suppl):575S-84S.
26. Perrier E, Rondeau P, Poupin M, et al. Relation between urinary hydration biomarkers and total fluid intake in healthy adults. European Journal of Clinical Nutrition. 2013;67(9):939-43.
27. Morissette MP. Colloid osmotic pressure: its measurement and clinical value. Can Med Assoc J. 1977;116(8):897-900.
28. Gattinoni L, Carlesso E. Supporting hemodynamics: what should we target? What treatments should we use? London: Critical care. 2013;17 Suppl 1:S4.
29. Kalantari K, Chang JN, Ronco C, et al. Assessment of intravascular volume status and volume responsiveness in critically ill patients. Kidney Int. 2013;83(6):1017-28.
30. Lichtenstein D, van Hooland S, Elbers P, et al. Ten good reasons to practice ultrasound in critical care. Anaesthesiol Intensive Ther. 2014;46(5):323-5.
31. Vincent JL, Rhodes A, Perel A, et al. Clinical review: Update on hemodynamic monitoring – a consensus of 16. Crit Care. 2011;15(4):229.
32. Stawicki SP, Adkins EJ, Eiferman DS, et al. Prospective evaluation of intravascular volume status in critically ill patients: does inferior vena cava collapsibility correlate with central venous pressure? The Journal of Trauma and Acute Care Surgery. 2014;76(4):956-63.
33. Moore CL. Does Ultrasound Improve Clinical Outcomes? Prove It. Crit Care Med. 2015;43(12):2682-3.
34. Moore CL, Copel JA. Point-of-care ultrasonography. The New England Journal of Medicine. 2011;364(8):749-57.
35. Kelly N, Esteve R, Papadimos TJ, et al. Clinician-performed ultrasound in hemodynamic and cardiac assessment: a synopsis of current indications and limitations. Eur J Trauma Emerg Surg. 2015;41(5):469-80.
36. Pasquero P, Albani S, Sitia E, et al. Inferior vena cava diameters and collapsibility index reveal early volume depletion in a blood donor model. Crit Ultrasound J. 2015;7(1):17.
37. Kent A, Bahner DP, Boulger CT, et al. Sonographic evaluation of intravascular volume status in the surgical intensive care unit: a prospective comparison of subclavian vein and inferior vena cava collapsibility index. The Journal of Surgical Research. 2013;184(1):561-6.
38. Stawicki SP, Braslow BM, Panebianco NL, et al. Intensivist use of hand-carried ultrasonography to measure IVC collapsibility in estimating intravascular volume status: correlations with CVP. J Am Coll Surg. 2009;209(1):55-61.
39. Monnet X, Marik PE, Teboul JL. Prediction of fluid responsiveness: an update. Ann Intensive Care. 2016;6(1):111.
40. Monnet X, Marik P, Teboul JL. Passive leg raising for predicting fluid responsiveness: a systematic review and meta-analysis. Intensive care medicine. 2016;42(12):1935-47.
41. Monnet X, Teboul JL. Passive leg raising: five rules, not a drop of fluid! Critical care (London, England) 2015;19:18.
42. Michard F, Teboul JL. Predicting fluid responsiveness in ICU patients: a critical analysis of the evidence. Chest. 2002;121(6):2000-8.
43. Poelaert JI, Schupfer G. Hemodynamic monitoring utilizing transesophageal echocardiography: the relationships among pressure, flow, and function. Chest. 2005;127(1):379-90.
44. Manasia AR, Nagaraj HM, Kodali RB, et al. Feasibility and potential clinical utility of goal-directed transthoracic echocardiography performed by noncardiologist intensivists using a small hand-carried device (SonoHeart) in critically ill patients. J Cardiothorac Vasc Anesth. 2005;19(2):155-9.
45. Melamed R, Sprenkle MD, Ulstad VK, et al. Assessment of left ventricular function by intensivists using hand-held echocardiography. Chest. 2009;135(6):1416-20.
46. Stec S, Zaborska B, Sikora-Frac M, et al. First experience with microprobe transoesophageal echocardiography in non-sedated adults undergoing atrial fibrillation ablation: feasibility study and comparison with intracardiac echocardiography. Europace. 2011;13(1):51-6.
47. Toole BJ, Slesnick TC, Kreeger J, et al. The Miniaturized Multiplane Micro-Transesophageal Echocardiographic Probe: A Comparative Evaluation of Its Accuracy and Image Quality. J Am Soc Echocardiogr. 2015;28(7):802-7.
48. Vermeiren GL, Malbrain ML, Walpot JM. Cardiac Ultrasonography in the critical care setting: a practical approach to asses cardiac function and preload for the "non-cardiologist". Anaesthesiol Intensive Ther. 2015;47 Spec No:89-104. doi: 10.5603/AIT.a2015.0074.

49. DiCorte CJ, Latham P, Greilich PE, et al. Esophageal Doppler monitor determinations of cardiac output and preload during cardiac operations. Ann Thorac Surg. 2000;69(6):1782-6.
50. Lichtenberger M, DeBehnke D, Crowe DT, et al. Comparison of esophageal Doppler monitor generated minute distance and cardiac output in a porcine model of ventricular fibrillation. Resuscitation. 1999;41(3):269-76.
51. Stawicki PS, Braslow B, Gracias VH. Exploring measurement biases associated with esophageal Doppler monitoring in critically ill patients in intensive care unit. Annals of Thoracic Medicine. 2007;2(4):148-53.
52. de Tombe PP, ter Keurs HE. Cardiac muscle mechanics: Sarcomere length matters. J Mol Cell Cardiol. 2016;91:148-50.
53. Hofkens PJ, Verrijcken A, Merveille K, et al. Common pitfalls and tips and tricks to get the most out of your transpulmonary thermodilution device: results of a survey and state-of-the-art review. Anaesthesiol Intensive Ther. 2015;47(2):89-116.
54. Marik PE, Cavallazzi R. Does the central venous pressure predict fluid responsiveness? An updated meta-analysis and a plea for some common sense. Crit Care Med. 2013;41(7):1774-81.
55. Marik PE, Baram M. Noninvasive hemodynamic monitoring in the intensive care unit. Critical Care Clinics. 2007;23(3):383-400.
56. Teboul JL, Pinsky MR. Estimating cardiac filling pressure in mechanically ventilated patients with hyperinflation. Crit Care Med. 2000;28(11):3631-6.
57. Malbrain ML, De Waele JJ, De Keulenaer BL. What every ICU clinician needs to know about the cardiovascular effects caused by abdominal hypertension. Anaesthesiol Intensive Ther. 2015;47(4):388-99.
58. Osman D, Ridel C, Ray P, et al. Cardiac filling pressures are not appropriate to predict hemodynamic response to volume challenge*. Crit Care Med. 2007;35(1):64-9.
59. Shah MR, Hasselblad V, Stevenson LW, et al. Impact of the pulmonary artery catheter in critically ill patients: meta-analysis of randomized clinical trials. Jama. 2005;294(13):1664-70.
60. De Backer D, Fagnoul D, Herpain A. The role of invasive techniques in cardiopulmonary evaluation. Curr Opin Crit Care. 2013;19(3):228-33.
61. Reuter DA, Huang C, Edrich T, et al. Cardiac output monitoring using indicator-dilution techniques: basics, limits, and perspectives. Anesth Analg. 2010;110(3):799-811.
62. Sakka SG, Ruhl CC, Pfeiffer UJ, et al. Assessment of cardiac preload and extravascular lung water by single transpulmonary thermodilution. Intensive Care Med. 2000;26(2):180-7.
63. Marx G, Schuerholz T, Sumpelmann R, et al. Comparison of cardiac output measurements by arterial trans-cardiopulmonary and pulmonary arterial thermodilution with direct Fick in septic shock. Eur J Anaesthesiol. 2005;22(2):129-34.
64. Morelot-Panzini C, Lefort Y, Derenne JP, et al. Simplified method to measure respiratory-related changes in arterial pulse pressure in patients receiving mechanical ventilation. Chest. 2003;124(2):665-70.
65. Marik PE, Cavallazzi R, Vasu T, et al. Dynamic changes in arterial waveform derived variables and fluid responsiveness in mechanically ventilated patients: a systematic review of the literature. Critical Care Medicine. 2009;37(9):2642-7.
66. Maizel J, Airapetian N, Lorne E, et al. Diagnosis of central hypovolemia by using passive leg raising. Intensive Care Med. 2007;33(7):1133-8.
67. Poelaert J. Assessment of loading conditions with cardiac ultrasound. A comprehensive review. Anaesthesiol Intensive Ther. 2015;47(5):464-70.
68. Monnet X, Osman D, Ridel C, et al. Predicting volume responsiveness by using the end-expiratory occlusion in mechanically ventilated intensive care unit patients. Crit Care Med. 2009;37(3):951-6.
69. Laher AE, Watermeyer MJ, Buchanan SK, et al. A review of hemodynamic monitoring techniques, methods and devices for the emergency physician. Am J Emerg Med. 2017;35(9):1335-47.
70. Kyle UG, Bosaeus I, De Lorenzo AD, et al. Bioelectrical impedance analysis-part II: utilization in clinical practice. Clin Nutr. 2004; 23(6):1430-53.
71. Kupersztych-Hagege E, Teboul JL, Artigas A, et al. Bioreactance is not reliable for estimating cardiac output and the effects of passive leg raising in critically ill patients. Br J Anaesth. 2013;111(6):961-6.
72. Samoni S, Vigo V, Resendiz LI, et al. Impact of hyperhydration on the mortality risk in critically ill patients admitted in intensive care units: comparison between bioelectrical impedance vector analysis and cumulative fluid balance recording. Critical care (London, England). 2016;20:95.
73. Armstrong LE. Hydration assessment techniques. Nutr Rev. 2005;63(6 Pt 2):S40-54.
74. Kara A, Akin S, Ince C. Monitoring microcirculation in critical illness. Curr Opin Crit Care. 2016;22(5):444-52.
75. Ince C. The microcirculation is the motor of sepsis. Crit Care. 2005;9 (Suppl 4):S13-9.
76. Gruartmoner G, Mesquida J, Ince C. Fluid therapy and the hypovolemic microcirculation. Curr Opin Crit Care. 2015;21(4):276-84.
77. De Backer D, Orbegozo Cortes D, Donadello K, et al. Pathophysiology of microcirculatory dysfunction and the pathogenesis of septic shock. Virulence. 2014;5(1):73-9.
78. Ince C. Hemodynamic coherence and the rationale for monitoring the microcirculation. Crit Care. 2015;19 Suppl 3:S8.
79. Van der Mullen J, Wise R, Vermeulen G, et al. Assessment of hypovolaemia in the critically ill. Anaesthesiol Intensive Ther. 2018;50(2):141-9.

# CHAPTER 26

# Fluid Therapy for Specific Clinical Conditions

*Ram Baalachandran, Rahul Nanchal*

## INTRODUCTION

Intravenous (IV) fluid therapy is one of the most common interventions in the critically ill. It represents the cornerstone for the treatment of hypoperfusion. The history of fluid resuscitation dates to the cholera pandemic in the 1830s (Fig. 1—patient dying of cholera). Jaehnichen first infused 6 oz of water into a cholera patient,[1] which resulted in improvement in the patient's pulse. The first written account of crystalloid resuscitation appeared in the Lancet in 1832 when Thomas Latta injected a sodium chloride solution into the veins of patients suffering from cholera. Despite many clinical trials and investigative efforts to determine appropriate fluid management for shock, this topic remains controversial. This chapter will deal with the various aspects of IV fluid resuscitation.

## PATHOPHYSIOLOGY

What is the primary goal of fluid therapy? In clinical practice, hypotension is a common trigger for initiating IV fluids. But maintaining normal systemic blood pressure should not be the primary goal. For example, in hemorrhage, maintaining blood pressure with crystalloids can be deleterious.[2] Thus, the primary objective for IV fluid resuscitation should be restoration of tissue perfusion by ensuring adequate oxygen delivery to the tissues. Achieving this requires an understanding of systemic hemodynamics and microcirculation (Flowchart 1).[3]

There are four vascular components, which affect tissue perfusion—(1) vascular Content (vC), (2) Blood Flow (BF), (3) vascular Tone (vT) and (4) vascular Barrier (vB).[3] vC refers to the blood volume or the volume containing red cells. This mainly refers to the intravascular volume and does not always correlate with total body volume. A classic example is the patient with heart failure or hypoalbuminemia, who may be hypervolemic but "intravascularly depleted" (low vC), hence resulting in poor tissue perfusion. There are not many bedside parameters that can accurately determine intravascular volume. In experimental settings, dilution techniques using indocyanine green have been used to calculate macrocirculatory volume (see details in chapter on *Body fluid homeostasis*). Handheld video

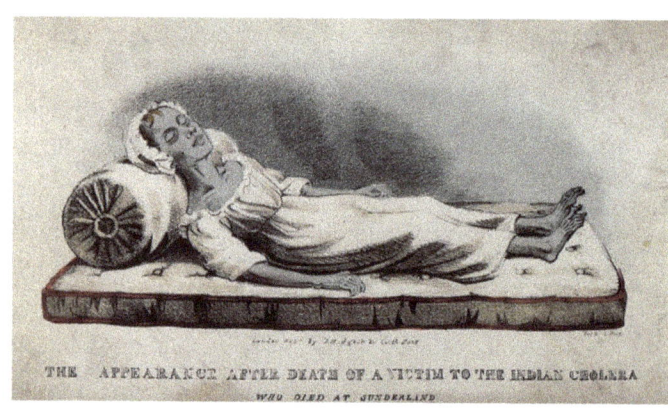

**Fig. 1:** A dead victim of cholera in 1832. "Colored lithograph by IWG". (*Credit:* Wellcome Collection; CC BY 4.0; *Source:* https://wellcomecollection.org/works/zpfky38b).

**Flowchart 1:** Goals of fluid therapy and actors which affect tissue perfusion.

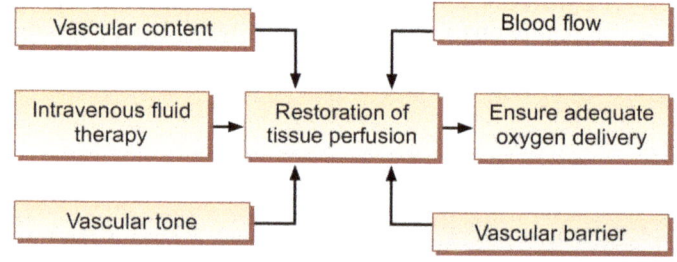

microscopy has been used to calculate capillary density and microcirculatory hematocrit, which can then be used to estimate microcirculatory volume.[3]

Vascular tone is an important determinant of perfusion pressure. Systemic vascular resistance is often used as a surrogate of vT. Surviving sepsis guidelines recommend a mean arterial pressure (MAP) greater than 65 mm Hg to maintain adequate organ BF.[4] In clinical practice, individualizing blood pressure targets, especially in patients who are chronically hypertensive, may benefit organ function.[5,6] Similarly, Thooft et al. demonstrated that increasing the MAP above 65 mm Hg resulted in improvements in microvascular function in some patients.[7]

"Leaky capillaries" is another problem encountered during fluid resuscitation. vB consists of the endothelial cell lining and the glycocalyx lining the inner surface of vessels.[3] They play an important role in maintaining and modulating fluid and solute transport across the vessels. At present, there is no bedside tool to assess vB function. Assessing vB can help determine the pathophysiology of shock and choose appropriate fluids. Some experts believe that colloid solution may be a better choice for resuscitation if vB is intact, but this remains controversial.[3]

Apart from adequate oxygen content in the intravascular volume, adequacy of systemic BF needs to be established for appropriate delivery of oxygen at the cellular level. Transport of oxygen is closely coupled with cardiac output which is a surrogate marker for BF at the systemic level. Venous and arterial tone determine driving pressure differences, which define flow in microcirculation.[8] Adequate BF is critical for matching oxygen demand with supply.

## Microvascular Blood Flow

Intensivists are often vexed with the problem of edema formation. Although edema formation can be insidious or rapid, resolution of edema is challenging and may take days. This can be partly explained by Starling forces which describe fluid shifts across capillaries.[9] Starling concluded that fluid flux across capillaries was contingent on the following factors:
- Intravascular colloid osmotic pressure (COP) due to macromolecules like plasma proteins ($\Pi_p$)
- Intravascular hydrostatic pressure due to pulsating BF ($P_c$)
- Interstitial fluid (ISF) COP ($\Pi_i$)
- Interstitial hydrostatic pressure ($P_i$)
- Staverman's osmotic reflection coefficient ($\sigma$) which represents the leakiness of the capillary wall to the specific solute.

Thus, this relationship can be reflected by the equation,
$J_v / A = * L_p \{(P_c - P_i) - \sigma (\Pi_p - \Pi_i)\}$

Where, $J_v$ is the volume filtration per endothelial area A. $L_p$ refers to hydraulic conductivity, which can be defined as the fluid flow per unit pressure gradient driving fluid across the barrier.

Usually, the interstitium has low COP and hydrostatic pressure. Also, the $\Delta P$ (difference between the capillary hydrostatic pressure and interstitial hydrostatic pressure) is rarely lower than the $\Delta \Pi$ or $\Delta COP$ (difference between the capillary COP and interstitial COP). Hence filtration occurs more readily than absorption. When the $\Delta P$ is lowered below the $\Delta \Pi$, absorption occurs transiently and stops when this is maintained for longer. This is especially true for the lung and subcutaneous tissues. There are three reasons for this observation. First, capillary filtration itself influences the ISF COP and second, the ISF COP near the fenestrations is usually lower than the ISF COP itself. This was shown in a synovial membrane model where changing $\Pi_i$ had much less effect on absorption than changing $\Pi_p$.[10] Also, the ISF hydrostatic pressure does not increase linearly with volume because it can accommodate more volume.[11] Considering there is minimal absorption in the downstream capillaries, lymphatic drainage plays an important role in maintaining ISF homeostasis.

The glycocalyx is a complex network of glycosaminoglycans and sialoglycoproteins lining the inner surface of the capillaries. They also line the entrance of the intercellular cleft and most fenestrations. Thus, they play a major role in determining the permeability of the capillaries. It is the subglycocalyx COP that is more relevant than the ISF COP in determining fluid transport across vessels. The COP in subglycocalyx is very low for various reasons including the structure of the intercellular clefts.[11]

There are two kinds of pathways for fluid flux across the vessels—(1) the "small pore" pathway (0.4 nm in diameter) and (2) "large pore" (22.5 nm in diameter). Under normal conditions, the small pores contribute to 95% of the filtration coefficient of capillaries in skeletal muscle.[12] During mild inflammation, the number of large pore increases significantly thus contributing to the "leaky capillaries" (Figs. 2A and B).

During hypotensive stress, around 500 mL fluid can be absorbed from the interstitial space to maintain plasma volume. On the other hand, edema is formed mainly due to altered Startling forces, altered permeability, and impaired lymphatic drainage.[13]

## Volume or Preload Responsiveness

It has been shown that only 40–72% of the critically ill respond to fluids by a significant increase in cardiac

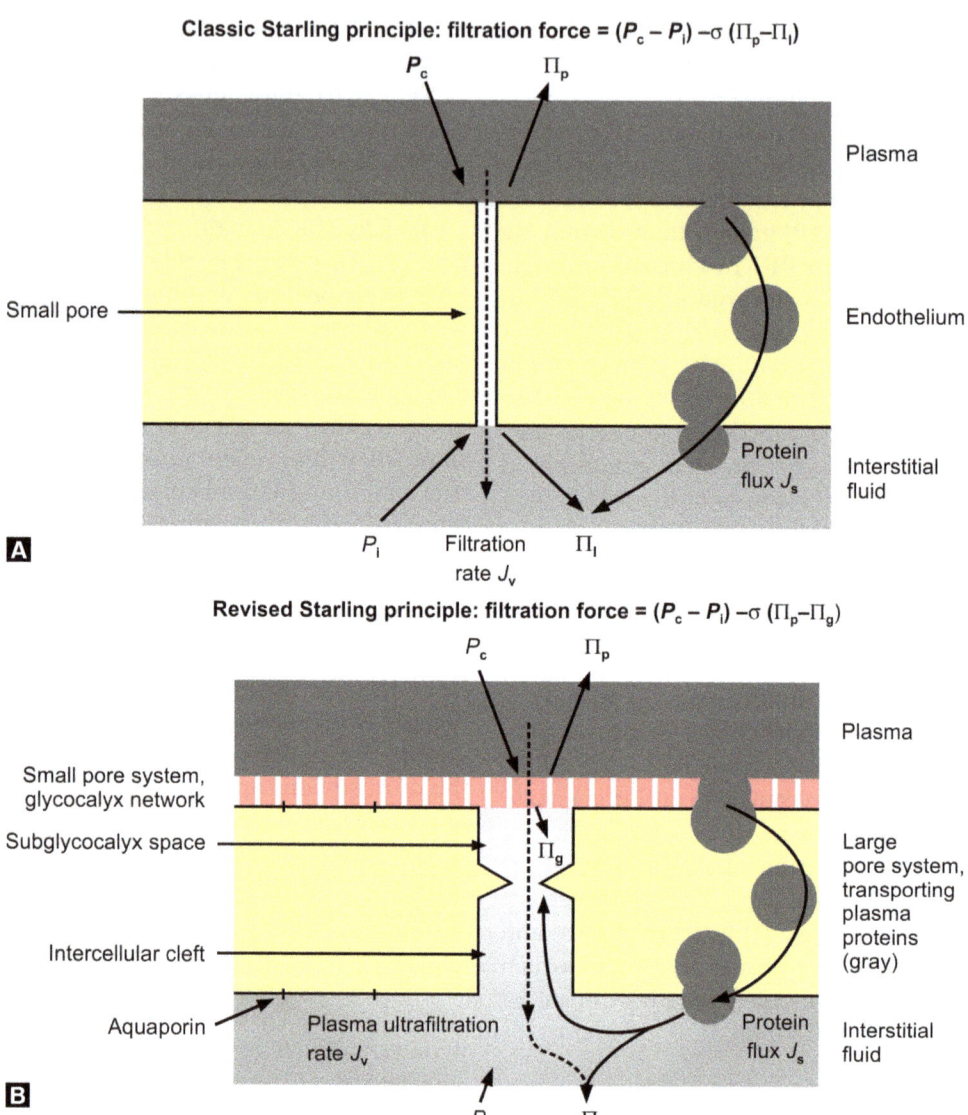

**Figs. 2A and B:** (A) In the classic Starling model, the endothelial layer is considered to be a continuous semi-permeable membrane; (B) The revised Starling model recognizes the glycocalyx-cleft model. *Gray shade indicates the colloid osmotic pressure (COP).* Note that the COP in the cleft is lower than the interstitial fluid (ISF).

output (CO).[14] To understand this, we have to understand the Frank–Starling curve. The response to fluids depends on the part of the curve the ventricle is operating. Also, the slope of the curve depends on the ventricular contractile function and differs between patients. When the ventricle is operating on the steep portion of the curve, there is a linear relationship between preload and cardiac output. After initial resuscitation, when the ventricle is operating on the flat portion of the curve, the increase in cardiac output in response to fluids is less. In other words, central venous pressure (CVP) or pulmonary capillary wedge pressure (PCWP) are static markers of volume, which do not give any information about which part of the Frank–Starling curve the ventricle is operating on. The volume responsiveness is a more clinically useful concept, which helps in identifying patients, whose ventricles are operating on the steep portion of the Frank–Starling curve. Dynamic markers of volume responsiveness like pulse pressure variation (PPV), stroke volume variation (SVV), inferior vena cava (IVC) collapsibility, and passive leg raise (PLR) test help in predicting fluid responsiveness.[15]

## ADVERSE EFFECTS OF FLUIDS

Intravenous fluid is a drug and needs careful consideration before administration. It is important to understand the adverse effects of giving fluids. Alsous et al. came to the conclusion that negative fluid balance achieved in any of the first 3 days of septic shock portends a good prognosis, based on their retrospective study.[16] The pan-European Sepsis Occurrence in Acutely Ill Patients (SOAP) study showed that positive fluid balance is a strong predictor of mortality among sepsis patient in the intensive care unit (ICU).[17] Boyd et al. reported that there was a correlation between positive fluid balance and 28-day mortality in septic shock patients in ICU.[18] The landmark Fluid And Catheter Treatment Trial (FACTT)[19] compared a liberal vs. conservative fluid management strategy, using fluid restriction and diuretics to maintain lower CVP and PCWP in the conservative arm in adults with acute respiratory distress syndrome (ARDS). The conservative fluid management arm had shorter duration of mechanical ventilation and ICU stay.

Fluids infused in large quantities at room temperature promote hypothermia by increasing the conductive heat loss.[20] Massive volume resuscitation with crystalloid can also dilute plasma proteins and affect coagulation. However, crystalloids actually strengthen the coagulation until the blood has been diluted by 40%, after which coagulopathy develops.[20]

In surgical patients, administering more than 2 liters of fluid results in a delay in the gastrointestinal recovery time of 2 days.[21] Normal saline, though an isotonic fluid, can cause hyperchloremic metabolic acidosis due to supraphysiologic levels of chloride.[22] Normal saline has been shown to increase extravascular fluid, and decrease renal BF velocity and renal cortical BF in human volunteers, which can contribute to acute kidney injury (AKI).[23] Excessive fluids can also damage the endothelial glycocalyx.[24] Chapell et al. showed that volume loading with 20 mL/kg of isotonic colloid solution to patients undergoing elective surgery causes a significant increase in serum glycocalyx components, hyaluronan, and syndecan. An intact glycocalyx is very important for the maintenance of vB function and fluid administration itself can affect endothelial permeability.

## CHOICES OF INTRAVENOUS FLUIDS

There has been a significant change in the type of IV fluids used in ICUs over the years. A study conducted in Australia and New Zealand between 2007 and 2013 demonstrated a significant increase in the use of crystalloids and decrease in use of colloids.[25] The introduction of balanced salt solutions like Hartmann's solution and Plasma-Lyte could be the reason behind the increased use of crystalloids. It is believed that solution with solutes and osmolarity like plasma should be preferred. In a murine model of septic shock, Hextend (a balanced colloid solution) infusion was associated with better short-term survival compared to normal saline. In this experimental study, Ringer's Lactate use did not improve survival but was associated with better plasma pH.[26] Other harmful effects of normal saline are detailed above including hyperchloremic metabolic acidosis and renal toxicity. But, in a large randomized clinical trial, normal saline use was not associated with increased risk of AKI compared to Plasma-Lyte.[27] In a nonblinded, cluster randomized, multiple crossover trial, 15,802 patients admitted to 5 ICUs were assigned to receive normal saline or balanced crystalloid solutions (lactated Ringer's solution or Plasma-Lyte-A) depending on the unit to which they were admitted. The investigators concluded that patients who received balanced salt solutions had lower incidence of major adverse kidney event (a composite outcome of death from any cause, renal replacement therapy, and persistent renal dysfunction).[28] The discussion about colloid use has been detailed in the section on "Septic Shock".

## INFUSION STRATEGIES—BOLUS VERSUS MAINTENANCE

Fluid bolus therapy (FBT) is commonly used in hospitalized patients with very little evidence of benefit. There is no standardized approach to what constitutes a fluid bolus leading to wide variation in practice. It is important to examine the clinically meaningful effects of a fluid bolus. There have been studies demonstrating that the effect is short-lasting and does not last beyond 60 minutes at best.[29] The rate of fluid infusion also varies based on physician or nurse discretion. There is some evidence that rapid infusion increases blood pressure without increase in cardiac index, unlike slow infusions.[30] When a convenience sample from the FACCT trial was studied for physiologic response to a fluid bolus, only small hemodynamic changes were noted. The urine output did not change, and there was minimal change in heart rate, MAP, and cardiac index. This immediate but nonsustained response often results in multiple fluid boluses and volume overload. The adverse effects of excess fluid administration have been described in a previous section of this chapter.

Maintenance fluid therapy (MFT) is rarely used in medical ICUs but is common in surgical ICUs and the perioperative setting. Often, it is used in patients who are unable to take oral fluids. The rate and type of fluid used is empiric and there is a paucity of evidence in this field. A recent study[31] concluded that hypotonic IV MFT (NaCl 0.32%) was associated with higher urine output, significantly less intravascular fluid retention compared with isotonic IV MFT (NaCl 0.9%). In line with a previous report by the same investigators, the authors argued that IV MFT should be hypotonic to avoid fluid overload. There is an ongoing prospective single-center double-blind randomized trial comparing isotonic versus hypotonic maintenance fluid strategy during and after surgery in patients undergoing different types of major thoracic surgery.[32]

## FLUID THERAPY IN SPECIFIC CIRCUMSTANCES

### Septic Shock

The landmark study by Rivers et al. changed the way physicians approached management of septic shock and brought early goal-directed therapy into focus.[33] It highlighted that early identification of sepsis and initiation of resuscitation within the first 6 hours of presentation improved outcomes. The patients in the early goal-directed therapy group received 1,500 mL more fluids than standard group in first 6 hours though the standard group received more fluids overall. Early goal-directed therapy resulted in decreased 28-day mortality due to sudden cardiovascular collapse as well as reduced requirement of vasopressors and mechanical ventilation. Subsequent meta-analysis also confirmed that early goal-directed therapy resulted in significant reductions in mortality.[34]

Septic shock is a distributive shock state, which results in impaired oxygen delivery and/or utilization. Hypovolemia resulting in reduced oxygen delivery to tissues is one of the mechanisms which is predominant in the initial stage. This could be due to true hypovolemia or relative hypovolemia because of vasodilation. Mitochondrial impairment of oxygen extraction caused by inflammation leads to impairments in utilization of delivered oxygen. Increase in lactate in septic shock were thought to result only from impaired BF and oxygen delivery. However, recent experiments have demonstrated that oxygen tension in skeletal muscle is increased during sepsis.[35] There is also evidence that increased stimulation of Na-K ATPase activity in skeletal muscle can cause increased lactate production.[36] Thus, IV fluids cannot completely reverse the defects in tissue oxygenation during sepsis (Flowchart 2).

A vitally important question is the end point of fluid resuscitation and determining when to stop therapy with IV fluids. There is no confirmation that higher CVP improves oxygen delivery and increases organ perfusion. MAP also remains a poor indicator of microcirculatory flow (see above). Venous oxygen saturation obtained from the superior vena cava or the pulmonary artery informs

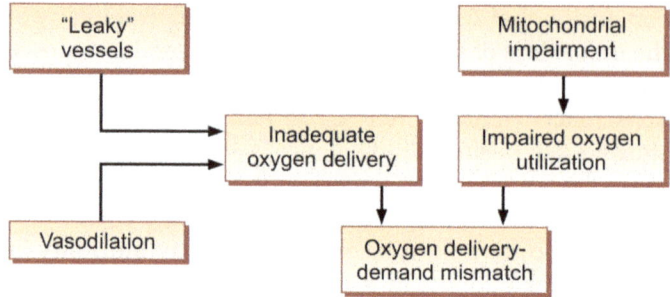

**Flowchart 2:** Pathophysiology of sepsis.

us about the relationship between oxygen delivery and oxygen demand. However, none of these markers reliably predicts response to fluid therapy. Ideally the goal of fluid resuscitation should be the achievement of a euvolemic state. This is difficult to discern in critically ill patients.[37-39]

A variety of techniques utilizing either changes in pleural pressure or increasing preload have been utilized to predict volume responsiveness. PPV and SVV use the concept of change in intrathoracic pressure to determine response to a fluid challenge in mechanically ventilated patients with peripheral arterial catheter.[40] Certain prerequisites, such as tidal volume of at least 8 mL/kg, complete patient-ventilator synchrony, constant R-R interval on ECG, absence of arrhythmia, absence of spontaneous efforts, and absence of right ventricular dysfunction are necessary for the validity of these tests using focused echocardiography; inspiratory increases in inferior vena cava diameter greater than 12% or 18% had greater than a 90% sensitivity and specificity for fluid responsiveness.[41,42] PLR is as good as 500 mL IV bolus and results in an increase aortic BF in fluid responsive patients.[43] The response to PLR requires monitoring of cardiac output or aortic flow, which can be assessed using intrapulmonary thermodilution methods, pulmonary artery catheters or noninvasive bioimpedance methods. It is also important to realize that presence of fluid responsiveness does not imply that a patient is hypovolemic or necessarily needs a fluid bolus.

The type of IV fluid (crystalloid versus colloid) is also surrounded by controversy. The Saline versus Albumin Fluid Evaluation (SAFE) trial in 2004 did not reveal differences in outcomes when albumin was compared to crystalloids in a large heterogeneous population.[44] However, albumin was associated with improvements in mortality in the subgroup with sepsis. The Colloid versus Crystalloid for the Resuscitation of the Critically Ill (CRISTAL) trial demonstrated no benefit between crystalloids and colloids in their primary outcome measure which was 28-day mortality. Mortality was however improved in the colloid arm at 90 days. Colloids were also associated with more days alive without ventilation and vasopressors at day 7 and 28.[45] Since these were secondary outcomes, they should be interpreted with caution and considered exploratory in nature. In the Albumin Italian Outcome Sepsis (ALBIOS) trial which studied albumin replacement in severe sepsis or septic shock, the investigators failed to demonstrate mortality differences at day 28 or day 90.[46] The Surviving Sepsis Campaign (SSC) guidelines suggest using albumin in sepsis and septic shock when patients require substantial amount of crystalloids, however, the evidence for this recommendation is weak.[4]

## Hypovolemic Shock

Hypovolemic shock occurs due to pathological decrease in total body fluid predominantly from the intravascular space. Extracellular fluid loss may also result in intracellular losses. Losses can occur at multiple sites including gastrointestinal (e.g. vomitus and diarrhea), renal (e.g. diuresis and salt-wasting nephropathies), and skin (e.g. burns and sweat) among others.

The general clinical principle is to replace the lost volume with a fluid of similar osmotic properties. Replacement with "balanced" or "buffered" crystalloid solutions (e.g. LR, Plasma-Lyte) is recommended. As mentioned earlier, there appears to be a trend in the literature toward worse renal outcomes with hyperchloremic, "nonbuffered" solutions such as normal saline.[47,48] Aggressive fluid resuscitation with bolus infusions, in small increments of 500 mL at a time of "balanced" crystalloid solutions should continue until clinical evidence of adequate perfusion and, ideally, resolution of the source of fluid losses is attained. As with other cases of shock, fluid resuscitation should be a closely-monitored, step-wise endeavor with the goal of achievement of euvolemia and adequate tissue perfusion. Further volume administration past this clinical endpoint has not been shown to be of benefit and may be deleterious to the microcirculatory environment. In the case of ongoing fluid losses, such as external drainage of the gastrointestinal (GI) tract or burns, maintenance IV fluid replacement should approximate ongoing volume and electrolyte losses and any insensible losses.

## Hemorrhagic Shock

Hemorrhagic shock occurs due to loss of whole blood with its main components of red blood cells and plasma. Fluid management in patients with hemorrhage is focused on replacing the loss with blood products as crystalloids alone do not adequately replace the oxygen-carrying capacity or the hemostatic properties of blood. In patients with massive blood loss and hemorrhagic shock, resuscitation with crystalloid alone without blood products can lead to hemodilution of clotting factors and platelets as well as hypothermia, all of which can interfere with hemostasis and lead to continued or even accelerated blood loss. Studies have shown that resuscitation with large-volume crystalloid (>1.5 L)[49] and high ratio of crystalloid to blood products (>1.5:1)[50] have been associated with worse outcomes.

However, because blood products are ideally typed and cross-matched to a specific patient or are not immediately available in the field during prehospital management or in the emergency department for patients with acute hemorrhage, crystalloid solutions are routinely used as the initial resuscitative fluid of choice until adequate quantities of blood products are available. IV fluid is ideally administered in small 500 mL boluses to prevent the end-organ damage of shock with swift transition to blood products as the main resuscitative fluid once available. Hypertonic fluids have been studied as ways to safely raise intravascular volume to maintain adequate perfusion using the smallest volume. But hypertonic crystalloid solutions have shown little benefit when compared to isotonic fluids.[51]

## Brain Injury/Cerebral Edema

Resuscitation targets in cerebral edema are no different than in general circumstances of fluid resuscitation. The target should always be euvolemia with avoidance of either hypovolemia or hypervolemia. As far as possible, isotonic crystalloids should be utilized. In the SAFE trial, the subset of patients with traumatic brain injury had worse neurological outcomes with 4% albumin administration, likely because of the relative hypotonic nature of this solution.[52] Administration of hypotonic solutions should be avoided as they are likely to exacerbate cerebral edema. 0.9% saline remains the most common resuscitation solution for patients with neurological injury. Hypertonic solutions (up to 23.4% saline) are used to raise serum sodium and decrease intracranial tension associated with cerebral edema. However, convincing data that these hypertonic solutions are better than conventional osmolar therapy such as mannitol are not available.[53] When hypertonic saline solutions are used as maintenance therapy in patients with brain injury and cerebral edema, they are frequently combined with equimolar amounts of sodium acetate to prevent hyperchloremic acidosis. Use of hypertonic saline solutions may also be required in the circumstance of cerebral salt-wasting syndrome that is sometimes seen with aneurysmal subarachnoid hemorrhage.[54]

## Acute Respiratory Distress Syndrome

The initial resuscitation phase of ARDS comprises of administering isotonic crystalloid to maintain euvolemia. There is no benefit to administration of albumin for resuscitation. A fluid conservative strategy in the FACCT trial was found to decrease the number of ventilator days in patients with ARDS.[19] Sepsis is the most common reason for ARDS and because of capillary leak syndrome many of these patients become hypervolemic during their ICU stay. Thus, consideration should be given to expeditiously removing fluid through diuretic administration or renal replacement therapy once they are hemodynamically stable. Major reasons for fluid overload in many of these patients is maintenance fluid therapy; this should be avoided. Instead serial assessments of volume status should be performed and bolus fluid therapy should be utilized when needed.

## Diabetic Ketoacidosis and Severe Hyperglycemic Syndromes

Initial fluid therapy consists of resuscitation with isotonic crystalloid to target euvolemia. Secondary to osmotic diuresis, there can be considerable volume deficits in these states. Administration of large amounts of saline can lead to hyperchloremic acidosis and consideration should be given to resuscitation with a balanced crystalloid such as lactated Ringer's solution. In many hyperglycemic states, a free water deficit may exist and very often, after achievement of euvolemia, ongoing administration of a hypotonic solution such as half normal saline is needed. As therapy with insulin infusions occurs, concomitantly dextrose is often added to solutions once the blood sugar falls below a certain value (most often 250 mg/dL).[55]

## Liver Failure/Chronic Liver Disease/Paracentesis

Liver failure is a hyperdynamic state resulting in increased cardiac output and decreased or near-normal blood pressure. The primary mechanism behind this hyperdynamic circulation is peripheral and splanchnic vasodilation.[56] As such, most patients are candidates for fluid resuscitation. Human serum albumin is synthesized in the liver and is the main plasma protein responsible for oncotic pressure. The rationale for its administration has traditionally rested on increasing intravascular volume, but albumin also has antioxidant, immunoregulatory, and endothelial regulatory functions.[57,58] In patients with liver failure, in addition to low circulating levels consequent to decreased production, albumin function may be impaired. As such, the rationale for albumin administration in patients with liver failure may be stronger than in other conditions. Administration of albumin in conjunction with high-volume paracentesis in patients with ascites has been shown by meta-analysis to prevent paracentesis-induced circulatory dysfunction and to decrease mortality.[59] This suggests that the benefit of albumin results at least in part from improved hemodynamics, but contributions from other effects remain possible. The administration of 20% albumin in patients with spontaneous bacterial peritonitis (SBP) and cirrhosis was found to prevent the development of hepatorenal syndrome and improve mortality.[60] However, the comparison was against placebo and not crystalloid. It is unclear whether the administration of crystalloids would have the same effect. In the absence of more robust data, it is reasonable to resuscitate patients with liver disease who have SBP or are undergoing large volume paracentesis with albumin. It is important to use a hyperoncotic solution of albumin (20–25%) in these circumstances.

## SALIENT POINTS

- The primary goal of fluid resuscitation is the achievement of euvolemia; hypervolemia should be avoided or corrected as soon as possible as it leads to organ failure.
- Hypotension is not always a trigger for fluid resuscitation; hypovolemia should be ascertained prior to initiating fluid resuscitation.
- Starling's equation of fluid flux has now been modified with expanded knowledge of the endothelial glycocalyx; it is no longer reasonable to give colloid solutions to pull fluid back from the interstitium.
- Intravenous fluids are drugs and are associated with many adverse reactions, the primary being fluid overload which deleteriously affects organ function.
- As far as possible, fluid should be used as boluses only; maintenance fluids are a leading cause of hypervolemia.
- Use of albumin should be avoided in patients with neurological injury.
- Hyperoncotic albumin solutions are a reasonable choice in patients with liver failure.
- Administration of normal saline, which is a hyperchloremic solution, is associated with metabolic acidosis and AKI. It is better to resuscitate with balanced crystalloid solutions.

## REFERENCES

1. Byrne L, Van Haren F. Fluid resuscitation in human sepsis: Time to rewrite history? Ann Intensive Care. 2017;7:4.
2. Legrand M, Mik EG, Balestra GM, et al. Fluid resuscitation does not improve renal oxygenation during hemorrhagic shock in rats. Anesthesiology. 2010;112(1):119-27.
3. Chawla LS, Ince C, Chappell D, et al. Vascular content, tone, integrity, and haemodynamics for guiding fluid therapy: a conceptual approach. Br J Anaesth. 2014;113(5):748-55.
4. Rhodes A, Evans LE, Alhazzani W, et al. Surviving Sepsis Campaign: International Guidelines for Management of Sepsis and Septic Shock: 2016. Crit Care Med. 2017;45(3): 486-552.
5. Asfar P, Meziani F, Hamel J-F, et al. High versus low blood-pressure target in patients with septic shock. N Engl J Med. 2014;370(17):1583-93.
6. Futier E, Lefrant JY, Guinot PG, et al. Effect of Individualized vs Standard Blood Pressure Management Strategies on Postoperative Organ Dysfunction Among High-Risk Patients Undergoing Major Surgery: A Randomized Clinical Trial. JAMA. 2017;318(14):1346-57.
7. Thooft A, Favory R, Salgado DR, et al. Effects of changes in arterial pressure on organ perfusion during septic shock. Crit Care. 2011;15(5):R222.
8. Taylor AE, Moore TM. Capillary fluid exchange. Am J Physiol. 1999;277(6 Pt 2):S203-10.
9. Starling EH. On the Absorption of Fluids from the Connective Tissue Spaces. J Physiol. 1896;19(4):312-26.
10. McDonald JN, Levick JR. Effect of extravascular plasma protein on pressure-flow relations across synovium in anaesthetized rabbits. J Physiol. 1993;465:539-59.
11. Levick JR, Michel CC. Microvascular fluid exchange and the revised Starling principle. Cardiovasc Res. 2010;87(2):198-210.
12. Rippe B, Haraldsson B. Fluid and protein fluxes across small and large pores in the microvasculature. Application of two-pore equations. Acta Physiol Scand. 1987;131(3):411-28.
13. Mortimer PS, Levick JR. Chronic peripheral oedema: the critical role of the lymphatic system. Clin Med. 2004;4(5): 448-53.
14. Cherpanath TG, Aarts LP, Groeneveld JA, et al. Defining Fluid Responsiveness: A Guide to Patient-Tailored Volume Titration. J Cardiothorac Vasc Anesth. 2014;28(3):745-54.
15. Guerin L, Monnet X, Teboul J. Monitoring volume and fluid responsiveness: from static to dynamic indicators. Best Pract Res Clin Anaesthesiol. 2013;27(2):177-85.
16. Alsous F, Khamiees M, Degirolamo A, et al. Negative fluid balance predicts survival in patients with septic shock: a retrospective pilot study. Chest. 2000;117(6):1749-54.
17. Ranieri VM, Reinhart K, Gerlach H, et al. Sepsis in European intensive care units: results of the SOAP study. Crit Care Med. 2006;34(2):344-53.
18. Boyd JH, Forbes J, Nakada TA, et al. Fluid resuscitation in septic shock: a positive fluid balance and elevated central venous pressure are associated with increased mortality. Crit Care Med. 2011;39(2):259-65.
19. National Heart, Lung, and Blood Institute Acute Respiratory Distress Syndrome (ARDS) Clinical Trials Network; Wiedemann HP, Wheeler AP, et al. Comparison of Two Fluid-Management Strategies in Acute Lung Injury. N Engl J Med. 2006;354:2564-75.
20. Hahn RG. Adverse effects of crystalloid and colloid fluids. Anaesthesiol Intensive Ther. 2017;49(4):303-8.
21. Li Y, He R, Ying X, et al. Ringer's lactate, but not hydroxyethyl starch, prolongs the food intolerance time after major abdominal surgery; an open-labelled clinical trial. BMC Anaesthesiol. 2015;15(1):72.
22. Wilkes NJ, Woolf R, Mutch M, et al. The effects of balanced versus saline-based hetastarch and crystalloid solutions on acid-base and electrolyte status and gastric mucosal perfusion in elderly surgical patients. Anesth Analg. 2001;93(4):811-6.
23. Chowdhury AH, Cox EF, Francis ST. A randomized, controlled, double-blind crossover study on the effects of 2-L infusions of 0.9% saline and plasma-lyte® 148 on renal blood flow velocity and renal cortical tissue perfusion in healthy volunteers. Ann Surg. 2012;256(1):18-24.
24. Chappell D, Bruegger D, Potzel J, et al. Hypervolemia increases release of atrial natriuretic peptide and shedding of the endothelial glycocalyx. Crit Care. 2014;18(5):538.
25. Hammond NE, Taylor C, Saxena M, et al. Resuscitation fluid use in Australian and New Zealand Intensive Care Units between 2007 and 2013. Intensive Care Med. 2015;41(9): 1611-9.
26. Kellum JA. Fluid resuscitation and hyperchloremic acidosis in experimental sepsis: improved short-term survival and acid-base balance with Hextend compared with saline. Crit Care Med. 2002;30(2):300-5.
27. Young P, Bailey M, Beasley R, et al. Effect of a Buffered Crystalloid Solution vs Saline on Acute Kidney Injury Among Patients in the Intensive Care Unit: The SPLIT Randomized Clinical Trial. JAMA. 2015;314(16):1701-10.
28. Semler MW, Self WH, Wanderer JP, et al. Balanced Crystalloids versus Saline in Critically Ill Adults. N Engl J Med. 2018;378(9):829-39.
29. Glassford NJ, Eastwood GM, Bellomo R. Physiological changes after fluid bolus therapy in sepsis: a systematic review of contemporary data. Crit Care. 2014;18(6):696.
30. Ho L, Lau L, Churilov L, et al. Comparative Evaluation of Crystalloid Resuscitation Rate in a Human Model of Compensated Haemorrhagic Shock. Shock. 2016;46(2): 149-57.
31. van Haren F. Personalised fluid resuscitation in the ICU: still a fluid concept? Crit Care. 2017;21(Suppl 3):313.
32. Hendrickx S, Van Vlimmeren K, Baar I, et al. Introducing TOPMAST, the first double-blind randomized clinical trial specifically dedicated to perioperative maintenance fluid therapy in adults. Anaesthesiol Intensive Ther. 2017;49(5):366-72.
33. Rivers E, Nguyen B, Havstad S, et al. Early goal-directed therapy in the treatment of severe sepsis and septic shock. N Engl J Med. 2001;345(19):1368-77.
34. Early Goal-Directed Therapy Collaborative Group of Zhejiang Province. [The effect of early goal-directed therapy on treatment of critical patients with severe sepsis/septic shock: a multi-center, prospective, randomized, controlled study]. Zhongguo Wei Zhong Bing Ji Jiu Yi Xue. 2010;22(6):331-4.

35. Boekstegers P, Weidenhöfer S, Kapsner T, et al. Skeletal muscle partial pressure of oxygen in patients with sepsis. Crit Care Med. 1994;22(4):640-50.
36. Levy B, Gibot S, Franck P, et al. Relation between muscle Na+K+ ATPase activity and raised lactate concentrations in septic shock: a prospective study. Lancet. 2005;365(9462):871-5.
37. Jones AE, Brown MD, Trzeciak S, et al. The effect of a quantitative resuscitation strategy on mortality in patients with sepsis: a meta-analysis. Crit Care Med. 2008;36(10):2734-9.
38. Nguyen HB, Kuan WS, Batech M, et al. Outcome effectiveness of the severe sepsis resuscitation bundle with addition of lactate clearance as a bundle item: a multi-national evaluation. Crit Care. 2011;15(5):R229.
39. Lee SW, Hong YS, Park DW, et al. Lactic acidosis not hyperlactatemia as a predictor of in hospital mortality in septic emergency patients. Emerg Med J. 2008;25(10):659-65.
40. Marik PE, Cavallazzi R, Vasu T, et al. Dynamic changes in arterial waveform derived variables and fluid responsiveness in mechanically ventilated patients: a systematic review of the literature. Crit Care Med. 2009;37(9):2642-7.
41. Feissel M, Michard F, Faller JP, et al. The respiratory variation in inferior vena cava diameter as a guide to fluid therapy. Intensive Care Med. 2004;30(9):1834-7.
42. Barbier C, Loubières Y, Schmit C, et al. Respiratory changes in inferior vena cava diameter are helpful in predicting fluid responsiveness in ventilated septic patients. Intensive Care Med. 2004;30(9):1740-6.
43. Monnet X, Rienzo M, Osman D, et al. Passive leg raising predicts fluid responsiveness in the critically ill. Crit Care Med. 2006;34(5):1402-7.
44. The SAFE Study Investigators. A Comparison of Albumin and Saline for Fluid Resuscitation in the Intensive Care Unit. N Engl J Med. 2004;350(22):2247-56.
45. Annane D, Siami S, Jaber S, et al. Effects of fluid resuscitation with colloids vs crystalloids on mortality in critically ill patients presenting with hypovolemic shock: the CRISTAL randomized trial. JAMA. 2013;310(17):1809-17.
46. Caironi P, Tognoni G, Masson S, et al. Albumin replacement in patients with severe sepsis or septic shock. N Engl J Med. 2014;370(15):1412-21.
47. Krajewski ML, Raghunathan K, Paluszkiewicz SM, et al. Meta-analysis of high- versus low-chloride content in perioperative and critical care fluid resuscitation. Br J Surg. 2015;102(1):24-36.
48. Yunos NM, Bellomo R, Hegarty C, et al. Association between a chloride-liberal vs chloride-restrictive intravenous fluid administration strategy and kidney injury in critically ill adults. JAMA. 2012;308(15):1566-72.
49. Ley EJ, Clond MA, Srour MK, et al. Emergency department crystalloid resuscitation of 1.5 L or more is associated with increased mortality in elderly and nonelderly trauma patients. J Trauma. 2011;70(2):398-400.
50. Neal MD, Hoffman MK, Cuschieri J, et al. Crystalloid to packed red blood cell transfusion ratio in the massively transfused patient: when a little goes a long way. J Trauma Acute Care Surg. 2012;72(4):892-8.
51. Wade CE, Grady JJ, Kramer GC. Efficacy of hypertonic saline dextran fluid resuscitation for patients with hypotension from penetrating trauma. J Trauma. 2003;54(Suppl 5):S144-8.
52. SAFE Study Investigators, Australian and New Zealand Intensive Care Society Clinical Trials Group, Australian Red Cross Blood Service, et al. Saline or albumin for fluid resuscitation in patients with traumatic brain injury. N Engl J Med. 2007;357(9):874-84.
53. Stocchetti N, Maas AI. Traumatic intracranial hypertension. N Engl J Med. 2014;370(22):2121-30.
54. Kirkman MA, Albert AF, Ibrahim A, et al. Hyponatremia and brain injury: historical and contemporary perspectives. Neurocrit Care. 2013;18(3):406-16.
55. Diabetes Canada Clinical Practice Guidelines Expert Committee, Goguen J, Gilbert J. Hyperglycemic Emergencies in Adults. Can J Diabetes. 2018;42 (Suppl 1):S109-14.
56. Sola E, Gines P. Renal and circulatory dysfunction in cirrhosis: current management and future perspectives. J Hepatol. 2010;53(6):1135-45.
57. Garcia-Martinez R, Caraceni P, Bernardi M, et al. Albumin: pathophysiologic basis of its role in the treatment of cirrhosis and its complications. Hepatology. 2013;58(5):1836-46.
58. Valerio C, Theocharidou E, Davenport A, et al. Human albumin solution for patients with cirrhosis and acute on chronic liver failure: Beyond simple volume expansion. World J Hepatol. 2016;8(7):345-54.
59. Bernardi M, Caraceni P, Navickis RJ, et al. Albumin infusion in patients undergoing large-volume paracentesis: a meta-analysis of randomized trials. Hepatology. 2012;55(4):1172-81.
60. Sort P, Navasa M, Arroyo V, et al. Effect of intravenous albumin on renal impairment and mortality in patients with cirrhosis and spontaneous bacterial peritonitis. N Engl J Med. 1999;341(6):403-9.

# CHAPTER 27

# Approach to the Patient with Hyponatremia and Hypernatremia

*Dharmendra Bhadauria, Harsh Vardhan*

## SODIUM HOMEOSTASIS

An abnormality in water homeostasis is the cause of disorders of serum sodium concentration, which leads to alteration in the relative ratio of sodium to body water. There are two main effectors in the defense of serum osmolality or osmoregulation: water intake and circulating arginine vasopressin (AVP); and defects in any one of them is responsible for most cases of hyponatremia and hypernatremia. In contrast, disorder of sodium homeostasis leads to a deficit or excess of whole body $Na^+$- $Cl^-$ content which a key determinant of the "volume regulations", henceforth effective circulatory fluid volume (ECFV).

### Regulation of Serum Sodium Concentration is Synonymous to Water Balance

Water is main constitution of body and it accounts for 50% and 60% of body weight in adult male and female, respectively. The quantity of water is mainly dependent upon the relative proportions of muscle and adipose tissue (fat) in the body. Fat does not require water to dissolve so it is stored without water while skeletal muscle being largest cellular organ, contains largest amount of body water. Adult male has more skeletal muscle and less fat than female, so has more water. Similarly, elderly people has relatively small proportion of muscle so having less total body water around 40–50% of body weight. On the other hand, new born has less fat so having more water around 70% of body weight. Obese persons have less water per kg body weight. The water in the body is distributed in two major compartments: (1) 55–75% is intracellular (ICF), and (2) 25–45% is extracellular (ECF), and in ECF water is distributed in 3:1 ratio as plasma water (intravascular) and interstitial (extravascular) spaces (Flowchart 1). In ECF and ICF, movement of water across the cell membranes lasts till the effective osmoles concentration becomes equal on both sides of these membranes. So, the number of effective osmoles decides the volume of each compartment. The chief ECF osmoles are cation $Na^+$ and its coexisting anions $Cl^-$ and $HCO_3^-$, whereas $K^+$ and organic compound like adenosine triphosphate (ATP), creatine phosphate, and phospholipids are the main ICF osmol.

Effective plasma osmolality is actually "tonicity" which is osmosis related activity of solutes that do not crosses cell membrane easily, hence responsible for distribution for water across the membrane. Extracellular $Na^+$ and extracellular $K^+$ are major determinant of effective plasma osmolality.

The volume of ECF compartment is mainly determined by *content* of $Na^+$ while the main factor deciding the ICF volume is the *concentration* of $Na^+$ in the ECF compartment. The $K^+$ retention, due to the presence of large macromolecular anions, is the main intracellular factor deciding the water accumulation in cells. The cells in the brain have ability to maintain near normal volume by changing the quantity of intracellular organic particles. Shift of water stops after the movement of an ultrafiltrate of plasma across capillary membranes, as there is no alteration in plasma $Na^+$. The two major factors or forces,

**Flowchart 1:** Distribution of water in a 70-kg person.

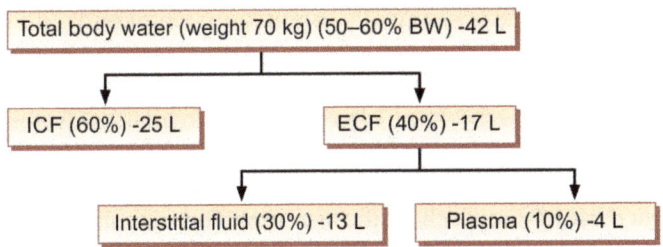

(BW: body weight; ECF: extracellular fluid; ICF: intracellular fluid)

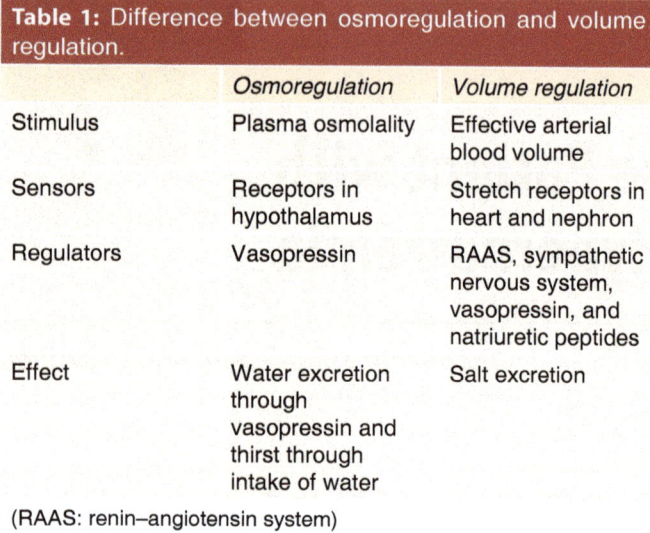

Table 1: Difference between osmoregulation and volume regulation.

|  | Osmoregulation | Volume regulation |
|---|---|---|
| Stimulus | Plasma osmolality | Effective arterial blood volume |
| Sensors | Receptors in hypothalamus | Stretch receptors in heart and nephron |
| Regulators | Vasopressin | RAAS, sympathetic nervous system, vasopressin, and natriuretic peptides |
| Effect | Water excretion through vasopressin and thirst through intake of water | Salt excretion |

(RAAS: renin–angiotensin system)

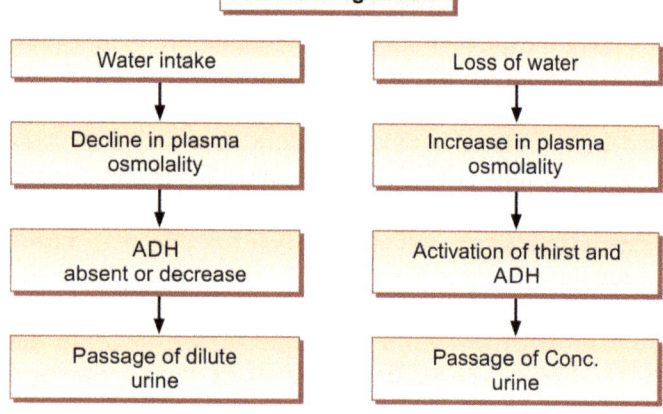

Flowchart 2: Water balance or osmotic regulation.

(ADH: antidiuretic hormone; Conc.: concentrated)

responsible for distribution of ECF volume between its intravascular and interstitial compartments, are the oncotic pressure across the capillary membrane and the hydrostatic pressure.

## WATER BALANCE

Water balance is essentially osmoregulation of body fluid hence different from volume regulation (Table 1). It is regulated by two regulators: (1) intake and (2) excretion of water (Flowchart 2). Thirst regulates the intake of water. Thirst stimulates water intake, which leads to fall of plasma Na (PNa) after ingesting adequate water followed by increase in size of cells of the osmostat. There is subsequent decline in thirst and inhibition of the secretion of vasopressin, followed by the excretion of dilute urine. Other regulator is excretion of water which is further regulated by two minor regulator: (1) the delivery of the volume of filtrate to the distal nephron and (2) lack of actions of vasopressin. Lack of action of vasopressin causes absence of aquaporin 2 (AQP2) channel from the apical membranes of the distal nephron, hence no reabsorption of water and excretion of dilute urine. But if there is lack of water in body causing a high PNa, it stimulates thirst and vasopressin release to enhance water reabsorption from distal nephron. This causes excretion of concentrated urine.

## HYPONATREMIA

### Case

A 27 year-old male known case of schizophrenia, in home for 12 weeks, presented to casualty with four episodes of generalized tonic-clonic seizures. Patient was on treatment with imipramine and chlorpropamide. Patient was evaluated and his investigations revealed: Serum Na$^+$ 116 mEq/L, serum K$^+$ 4 mEq/L, blood glucose 105 mg/dL, serum creatinine 1.0 mg/dL, blood urea nitrogen (BUN) 9 mg/dL, urine osmolality 79 mOsm/kg H$_2$O, and urine sodium 24 mEq/L. His diagnosis was severe hyponatremia with neurological manifestations in form of seizures. What is your approach to this man's hyponatremia?
- What emergency may arise during therapy, and how can they be avoided?
- What is the cause of hyponatremia in this patient?
- What is the emergency on admission?

### Definition

Hyponatremia is usually defined as a serum sodium concentration less than 135 mEq/L, chiefly caused by a water imbalance disorder.[1]

### Etiology/Mechanism

It is commonly due to dilutional decline in serum sodium concentration and associated with a proportional decline in the plasma osmolality, but not in all cases.

Hyponatremia is caused by the intravenous or oral intake of water and its subsequent retention in the body, associated with almost always due to an increase in circulating AVP and/or its enhanced sensitivity to the receptor in kidney, except in patients of hyponatremia caused by ingestion of fluids with low solute intake.[2,3] So in patients of hyponatremia, there is impairment in renal water excretion, mostly often due to an inability to suppress antidiuretic hormone (ADH) secretion or response. Patients may differ in underlying pathophysiology for the exaggerated or inappropriate AVP as a function of their ECFV.

It is required to understand the determinant of serum sodium concentration, to understand the development of hyponatremia and its therapy. It is of three types: (1) pseudohyponatremia, (2) translocational hyponatremia, and (3) true hyponatremia.

### Pseudohyponatremia

This condition is a laboratory artifact, in which value of the PNa is less than the PNa of the patient. Very high lipid or protein, nonaqueous content in plasma do decreases the water content of plasma. Although there is no effect on the sodium concentration in the water phase but, it leads to reduction in the Na concentration per unit of plasma. Hence, if measurements are in sodium concentration per volume of plasma by analyzer, then there will be reduction in serum Na. Sodium concentration is not affected, if measurement is directly done in the water phase. Serum osmolality remains normal and not affected by this artifact. It was seen more frequently with flame photometric measurement of Na, but now it is done with ion selective electrodes. Contrary to the belief, it still occurs because samples are diluted (indirect ion specific electrode). In undiluted sample, serum osmolality will be normal.

### Translocational Hyponatremia or Hypertonic Hyponatremia

Presence of an osmotically active exogenous substance in the plasma can cause movement of water into the plasma compartment causing hyponatremia like mannitol, glucose, and radiographic contrast agents. These are effective osmoles causing increases in tonicity, hence exit or translocation of water out of cell to exit cells and subsequent reduction in the serum sodium concentration.

### True Hyponatremia or Hyponatremia with a Low Serum Osmolality (Serum Osmolality Less than 275 mOsmol/kg)

Multiple classification system exists for this category of hyponatremia which are based on timing of onset of development of hyponatremia, biochemical severity of serum sodium concentration, and based on symptoms (Flowcharts 3A to C). Other systems of classification used for this type of hyponatremia are one which is based upon level of ADH levels either inappropriately elevated or appropriately suppressed (Flowchart 4),[2] and the other based upon volume status of patients (Flowchart 5) (hypovolemia, normovolemia, or hypervolemia).[4,5] In all cases for the development of hyponatremia, one requires inability to excrete ingested water.
- *Pathogenesis of hyponatremia with a low serum osmolality (Flowchart 6)*: Hyponatremia with a

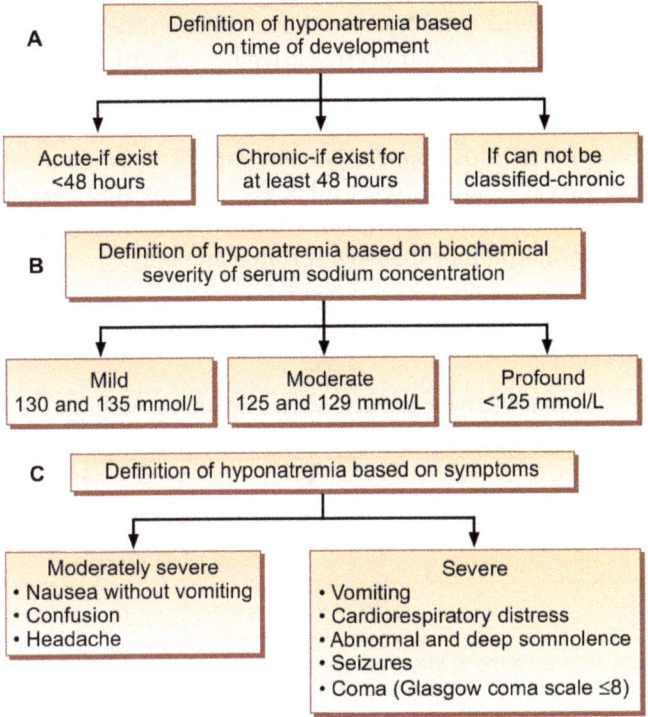

**Flowcharts 3A to C:** Different definitions of hyponatremia. (A) Based on time of development; (B) Based on sodium level; (C) Based on symptoms.

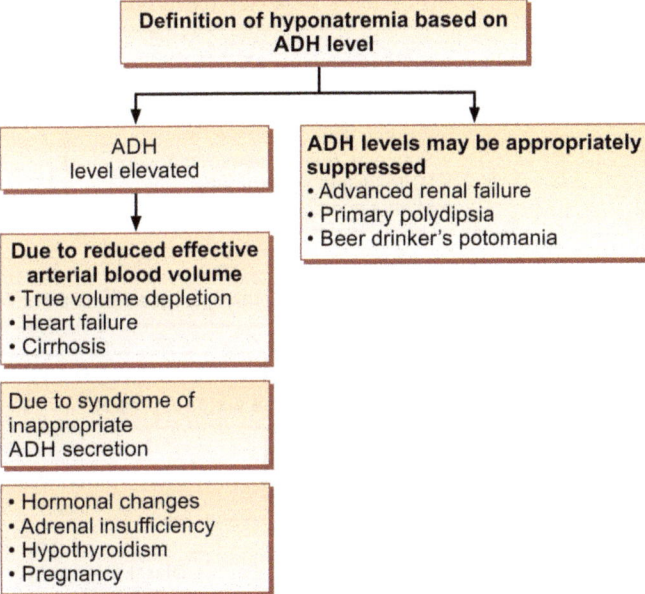

**Flowchart 4:** Definition of hyponatremia based on antidiuretic hormone (ADH) level.

low serum osmolality represents that there is an excess of water in relation to sodium in extracellular compartment and indicates more of total body water relative to total body sodium (Flowchart 6). These imbalances could occur either because of depletion of sodium more than water or by *dilution* of sodium because of more water in proportion of sodium. Although this concept is oversimplification, however it gives a simplified and logical understanding of pathogenesis, hence the diagnosis and management of hyponatremia with a low serum osmolality.

**Flowchart 5:** Definition of hyponatremia based on volume status.

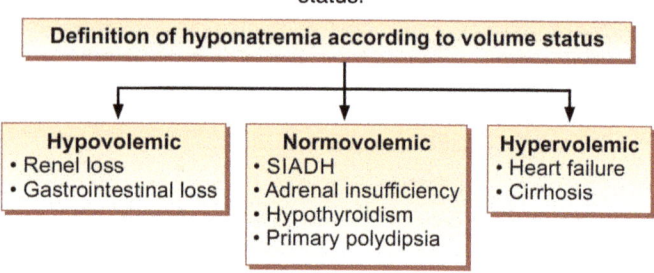

(SIADH: syndrome of inappropriate antidiuretic hormone)

## Clinical Effects

Hyponatremia is the most common electrolytes disorder, seen in 15–30% of acutely or chronically admitted patients in hospitals and responsible clinical symptom in around 20% of emergency admission. It can lead to a wide spectrum of clinical symptoms, from subtle to severe or even life-threatening.[6,7]

## Approach/Evaluation

Evaluation of hyponatremia should include attempt to identify for cause of hyponatremia such as a drug history in detail (Flowchart 7), history to search chest infection and malignancy causing activation of vasopressin, and an assessment of volume status. Severe hyponatremia is associated with multiple factors, so clinical assessment should include cause of high plasma AVP such as volume status, drugs, and stimulus like pain and nausea. One should use radiologic imaging to rule out pulmonary or central nervous system (CNS) etiologies for hyponatremia. A chest X-ray as screening tool may miss pulmonary neoplasm, hence, computed tomography (CT) thorax is better imaging in patients who have history of smoking.

**Flowchart 6:** Pathophysiology of hyponatremia.

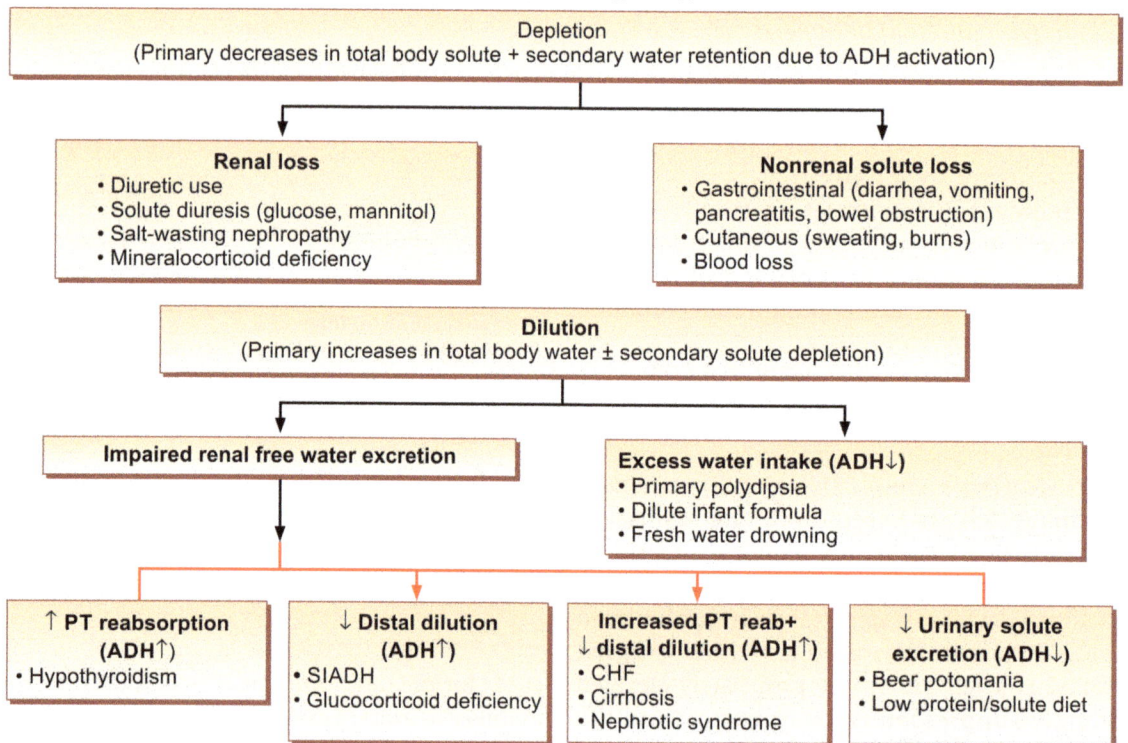

(ADH: antidiuretic hormone; CHF: congestive heart failure; PT: proximal tubule; Reab: reabsorption; SIADH: syndrome of inappropriate antidiuretic hormone)

- *Parameters and approach to be used to find out etiology of hypotonic hyponatremia (Flowchart 8)*

- *Serum sodium*: Ion specific electrode using direct potentiometry should be used to avoid laboratory artifact of pseudohyponatremia.
- *Serum osmolality*: Osmometer should be used, if unavailable then, random blood sugar, serum triglyceride, and serum protein helps in differentiating the causes. (Each 100 mg increase in blood glucose above 100 mg/dL decreases Na by 1.6 mEq/L.) When serum triglycerides are above 100 mg/dL, for every 500 mg/dL rise in serum triglycerides, fall in serum sodium will be about 1 mEq/L. When serum protein is above 8 g/L for every 1 g/dL rise in serum protein, fall in serum sodium will be about 4 mEq/L.
- *Urine osmolality*: It should be done in spot sample to assess vasopressin activity.

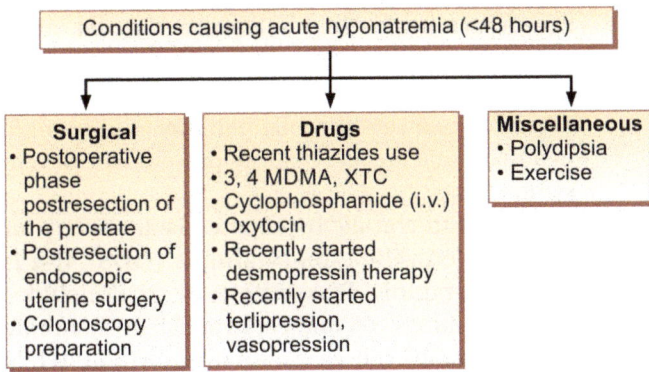

**Flowchart 7:** Causes of acute hyponatremia.

(MDMA: 3,4-methylenedioxymethamphetamine; XTC: Ecstacy)

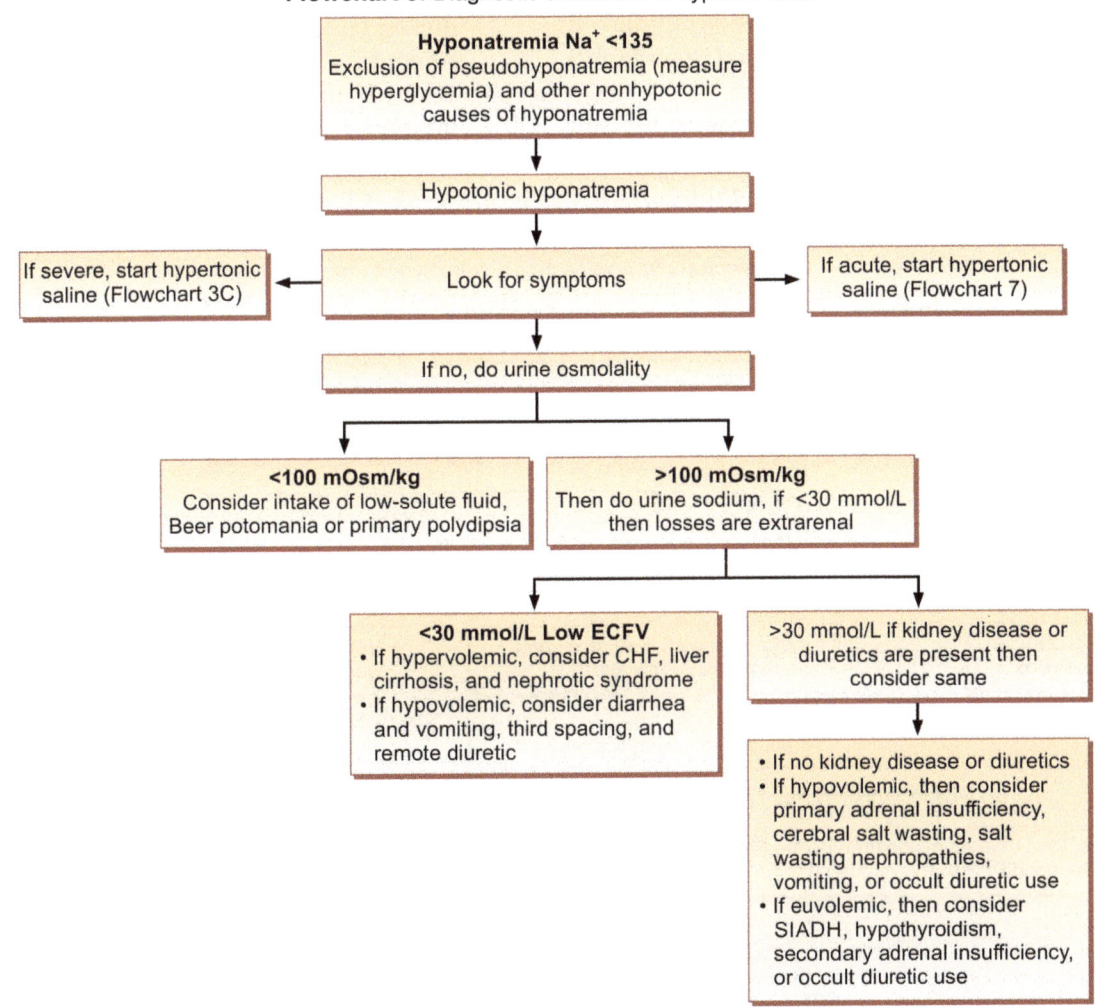

**Flowchart 8:** Diagnostic evaluation of hyponatremia.

(CHF: congestive heart failure; ECFV: effective circulatory fluid volume; SIADH: syndrome of inappropriate antidiuretic hormone)

- *Urine sodium concentration*: It should be done in spot sample for differentiating hypovolemia from euvolemia or hypervolemia.
- Other laboratory tests as serum urea concentration, serum uric acid concentration, fractional sodium excretion, and fractional uric acid excretion should also be sought (*see* Flowchart 8).

## Management

Objectives of management include determination of the duration of hyponatremia, the severity (degree) of hyponatremia, the severity of symptoms, and the need for hospitalization. Indications of hospitalization are acute hyponatremia, patients with severe hyponatremia (i.e. serum sodium less than 120 mEq/L), and patients with symptomatic hyponatremia. Goals of therapy are prevention of a further decline in serum sodium, prevention of brain herniation, to relieve symptoms of hyponatremia, and to avoid overcorrection (Flowcharts 9 to 11 and Boxes 1 to 3).

Therapy of hyponatremia includes hypertonic and isotonic saline, fluid restriction, vaptans [arginine vasopressin receptor 2 (AVPR2) antagonist], salt + furosemide and desmopressin, if cause of hyponatremia is rapidly reversible.

- *There are some important facts which need consideration to guide therapy for hyponatremia*:
  - Severe symptoms like headache, nausea, and/or vomiting to seizures, obtundation, and central herniation are usually seen in patients with acute hyponatremia, while patients with chronic hyponatremia are less likely to present with severe symptoms.
  - Patients with chronic hyponatremia are at risk for osmotic demyelination syndrome (ODS), if it is corrected rapidly. Risk factors for ODS includes serum sodium <105 mEq/L, hypokalemia, chronic alcoholism, liver disease, and malnutrition. While patients with acute hyponatremia are at risk for brain herniation.
  - Frequent monitoring of plasma Na plus concentration during corrective therapy is imperative because response to therapy is highly unpredictable.
  - Severe symptoms are used to improve on by a 4–6 mEq/L in serum sodium during the first 24 hours. There is no benefit rather potential harm on further faster increase, if symptoms persist thereafter.

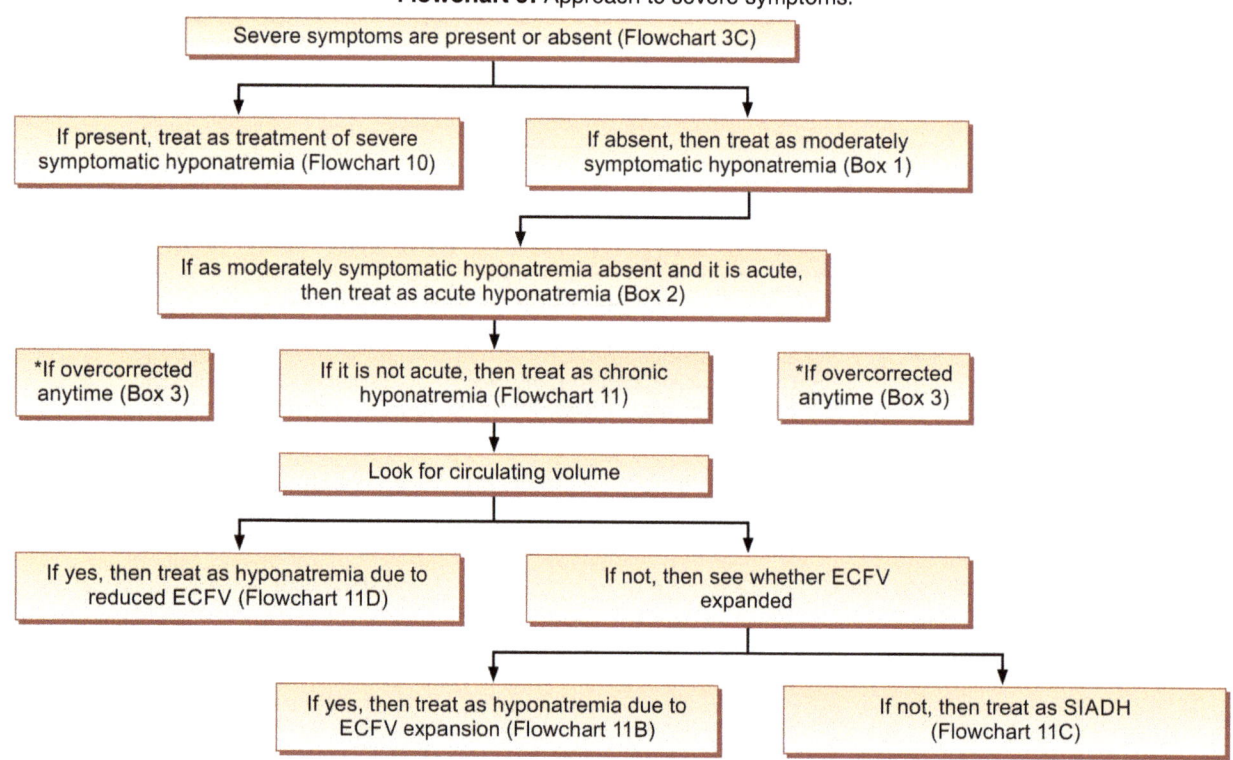

**Flowchart 9:** Approach to severe symptoms.

(ECFV: effective circulatory fluid volume; SIADH: syndrome of inappropriate antidiuretic hormone)

# Chapter 27
## Approach to the Patient with Hyponatremia and Hypernatremia

**Flowchart 10:** Hyponatremia with severe symptoms regardless of whether hyponatremia is acute or chronic.

**Hyponatremia with severe symptoms regardless of whether hyponatremia is acute or chronic**

**A. First-hour management**
- Admit the patient
- IV infusion of 150 mL 3% hypertonic over 20 minute
- Monitor the serum sodium concentration after 20 minute while repeating an infusion of 150 mL 3% hypertonic saline for the next 20 minute
- Repeat above if goal not achieved

**B. Follow-up management in case of improvement of symptoms after a 5 mmol/L increase in serum sodium concentration in the 1st hour**
- Stopping the infusion of hypertonic saline
- 0.9% saline until cause-specific treatment is started
- Limiting the increase in serum sodium concentration to a total of 10 mmol/L during the first 24 hours and an additional 8 mmol/L during every 24 hours thereafter until the serum sodium concentration reaches 130 mmol/L
- Checking the serum sodium concentration after 6 and 12 hours and daily afterward until the serum sodium concentration has stabilized under stable treatment

**C. Follow-up management in case of no improvement of symptoms after a 5 mmol/L increase in serum sodium concentration in the 1st hour**
- An IV infusion of 3% hypertonic saline or equivalent aiming for an additional 1 mmol/L per hour increase in serum sodium concentration
- Stopping the infusion of 3% hypertonic saline or equivalent when the symptoms improve, the serum sodium concentration increase 10 mmol/L in total or the serum sodium concentration reaches 130 mmol/L, whichever occurs first
- Additional diagnostic test
- Checking the serum sodium concentration every 4–6 hours as long as an IV infusion of 3% hypertonic saline or equivalent is continued.

(IV: intravenous)

**Flowchart 11:** Chronic hyponatremia without severe or moderately severe symptoms.

**Chronic hyponatremia without severe or moderately severe symptoms**

**A. General management**
- Stop unnecessary medication/fluid causing hyponatremia
- To start etiology-specific treatment
- Checking the serum sodium concentration 6 hourly in moderate or profound hyponatremia
- In mild hyponatremia, main aim is to increase serum sodium

**B. Patients with expanded extracellular fluid**
- Fluid restriction to prevent further fluid overload
- Cautious use of vasopressin receptor antagonists

**C. Patients with SIAD**
- Restricting fluid intake as first-line treatment in moderate or profound hyponatremia
- Consideration of equal second-line treatments like increasing solute intake with 0.25–0.50 g/kg/day of urea or a combination of low dose loop diuretics and oral sodium chloride if hyponatremia is moderate to profound
- Cautious use of vasopressin receptor antagonists

**D. Patients with reduced circulating volume**
- Restoration of extracellular volume with IV infusion of 0.9% saline or a balanced crystalloid solution at 0.5–1.0 mL/kg/hour
- Close monitoring of thermodynamically unstable patients

(SIAD: syndrome of appropriate deficiency; IV: intravenous)

**Box 1:** Hyponatremia with moderately severe symptoms.

- Diagnostic test for etiology
- Stop unnecessary medication causing hyponatremia
- To start etiology-specific treatment
- IV infusion of 150 mL 3% hypertonic over 20 minutes
- Aim is to increase 5 mmol/L per 24-hours serum sodium concentration
- In first 24 hours- the increase in serum sodium concentration to 10 mmol/L and a 8 mmol/L during every 24 hours thereafter, until a serum sodium concentration of 130 mmol/L is achieved
- Monitor sodium concentration after 1, 6 and 12 hours
- Additional diagnostic tests for other causes of the symptoms if no improvement of the symptoms
- If worsening of sodium occurs and became severe hyponatremia then manage as severely symptomatic hyponatremia

**Box 2:** Acute hyponatremia without severe or moderately severe symptoms.

- Use same method of sodium estimation
- Stop unnecessary medication/fluid causing hyponatremia
- Diagnostic assessment for etiology
- To start etiology-specific treatment
- If decline in serum sodium concentration >10 mmol/L, start a single IV infusion of 150 mL 3% hypertonic saline or equivalent over 20 minute
- The serum sodium concentration after 4 hours, using the same technique

(IV: intravenous)

**Box 3:** Rapidly reversible causes of hyponatremia.

*Rapidly reversible causes of hyponatremia*

- Hyponatremia due to volume depletion (after volume correction therapy)
- Hyponatremia due to adrenal insufficiency (after steroid therapy)
- Hyponatremia due to SIADH including post surgical or SIADH due to pain or drug

*Management of patients with rapidly corrected hyponatremia*

- Rapid intervention if it increases >10 mmol/L during the first 24 hours or >8 mmol/L in any 24 hours thereafter
- Discontinue the ongoing active treatment
- Start an infusion of 10 mL/kg body weight of electrolyte-free water (e.g. glucose solutions) over 1 hour under strict monitoring of urine output and fluid balance
- To add IV desmopressin 2 μg, should not be repeated more frequently than every 8 hours

(IV: intravenous; SIADH: syndrome of inappropriate antidiuretic hormone)

- *Things to be avoided during management of hyponatremia*:
  - Do not use isotonic saline in symptomatic or severe hyponatremia rather it should be used in true volume depletion.
  - Isotonic saline should not be used in edematous patients.
  - Isotonic saline should not be used in syndrome of inappropriate antidiuretic hormone (SIADH)
- *Formulas to calculate or to predict effect of infusate*:
  Sodium deficit = TBW × (desired SNa – actual SNa)
  Increase in serum sodium (SNa) = [Infusate (Na) – SNa] ÷ (TBW + 1)
  1 mL/kg body weight of 3% saline = 1 mEq/L increase in serum sodium

## Case Revisit

Patient presented to casualty with the severe symptoms, with four episodes of generalized tonic-clonic seizures. It is a case of acute hyponatremia due to self-induced acute water intoxication (Flowcharts 7 and 9). The goal of management is to prevent brain herniation. The emergency is both acute hyponatremia and severe symptoms in form of seizures. The initial 1st hour management is same in both situations. Patient was hospitalized and started with antiepileptic drug and with infusion of 3% hypertonic saline 150 mL, over 20–25 minutes. Serum sodium concentration should be measured after 20 minutes and repeating an infusion of 3% hypertonic saline 150 mL for the next 20–25 minutes (*see* Flowchart 9). The weight of patient is 70 kg, so 70 mL of 3% hypertonic saline will roughly increase 1 mEq/L. Seizure episodes were stopped and there was improvement in sensorium. Serum sodium improved to 120 mEq/L in first 5 hours. We should limit the increase in serum sodium concentration to a total of 10 mEq/L during the first 24 hours and an additional 8 mEq/L during every 24 hours thereafter until the serum sodium concentration reaches 130 mEq/L. After achieving improvement in symptoms, 0.9% saline infusion was started until cause-specific treatment is started (Flowchart 8). Pseudohyponatremia is ruled out as both blood sugars and triglyceride values were normal. It was a case of true hypotonic hyponatremia (plasma osmolality 245 mEq/L). Urine osmolality and urine sodium are 79 mOsm/kg $H_2O$ and 24 mEq/L, respectively, so it was a case of acute severe hyponatremia due to self-induced acute water intoxication, seen in patients of psychosis. Fluid restriction was started. Serum sodium was monitored 6 hourly after stabilization. After 4 days, his serum sodium was 131 mEq/L and patient was discharged from hospital after psychiatric consultation.

# HYPERNATREMIA

## Case

A 66-year-old lady presents with altered sensorium for 1 day with clinical features of dehydration, i.e. dry mucous membranes, decreased skin turgor. Her blood pressure is 136/70 mm Hg without postural drop. The serum sodium concentration is 177 mmol/L, and the body weight is 67 kg. What is your approach to this lady's hypernatremia?

## Definition

Hypernatremia is defined as plasma sodium (PNa) that is greater than 145 mmol/L. Severe hypernatremia is defined as a plasma sodium concentration above 150 mmol/L.[8] It can be primarily caused by a negative balance for water or a positive balance for sodium ions ($Na^+$). But the most common pattern is a negative balance of water and $Na^+$ ions, with a larger negative balance of water than that of $Na^+$.

## Etiology/Mechanism

The main mechanism for hypernatremia is either sodium gain or water loss. Some patients have both (Table 2).

Plasma sodium may rise in the setting of hypervolemia (positive balance of $Na^+$ ions) or normovolemia or hypovolemia (negative water balance, or a negative balance of both water and of $Na^+$ ions, but with a larger negative balance of water than that of $Na^+$ ions). The human body responds to rising PNa by either increasing thirst or reducing loss of water from urine.

Increased PNa stimulates osmoreceptors in hypothalamus, i.e. organum vasculosum laminae terminalis (OVLT) and stimulates thirst and also causes release of vasopressin from posterior pituitary gland which corrects PNa. For a patient to have significant degree of hypernatremia, either they cannot appreciate thirst or are unable to drink water. This commonly occurs in an unconscious state. Vasopressin secretion increases from posterior pituitary in response to increased PNa which in turn stimulates V2 receptors (V2R) in the basolateral membrane of principal cells in the cortical and medullary collecting ducts causing AQP2 water channels to shuttle from an intracellular store to the luminal membrane of principal cells. This results in conservation of water with the excretion of a small volume of urine with high concentration osmolality (Flowchart 12).

## Clinical Features

Clinical features depend on the rapidity of onset of hypernatremia. CNS signs and symptoms are prominent.

**Table 2:** Causes of hypernatremia.

**Primary Water Deficit**

*Increased water loss*

- *Renal loss:* Central DI, release of a vasopressinase form a necrotic tissue, nephrogenic DI, osmotic dieresis
- *Gastrointestinal loss:* Vomiting, osmotic diarrhea
- *Cutaneous loss:* Excessive sweating
- *Respiratory loss:* Hyperventilation

*Reduce water intake for many days*

- Lack of water
- Inability to gain access to, or to drink water
- Defective thirst caused by altered mental state, psychological disorder, or disease involving the osmoreceptor and/or the thirst center

*Shift of water into cell*

- Gain of effective osmoles, in the intracellular fluid compartment (e.g. because of seizures, rhabdomyolysis)

**Primary Gain of $Na^+$ Ions**

- Administration of intravenous fluid with a higher concentration of $NA^+ + K^+$ ions than their concentration in the urine during an osmotic or a water diuresis
- Infusion of hypertonic NaCl or $NaHCO_3$ in patient with oliguria
- Ingestion of sea water or replacing sugar by NaCl in feeding formula in infants

(DI: diabetes insipidus; NaCl: sodium chloride; $NaHCO_3$: sodium bicarbonate)

**Flowchart 12:** Response to increased plasma sodium.

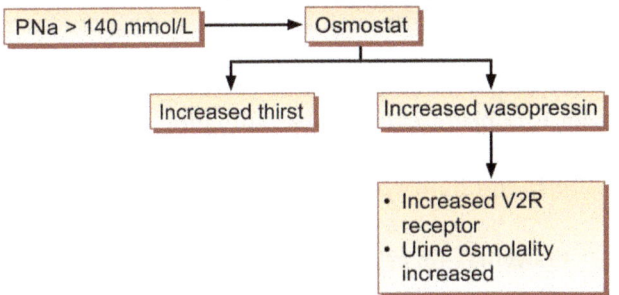

(PNa: plasma sodium; V2R: V2 receptors)

When the PNa raises acutely, the brain cell volume decreases, which causes blood vessels to stretch and possibly rupture. Over a 48-hour period, adaptive changes occur, which involves the gain of electrolytes and effective osmoles in brain cells and also an increase in the number of organic compounds in brain cells (e.g. taurine and myoinositol). As a result, water shifts from the ECF compartment into brain cells, which returns their volume toward normal. Most of the patients are in extremes of age. Elderly patients generally have few symptoms until the serum sodium concentration exceeds 160 mmol/L. The level of consciousness is correlated with the severity of the hypernatremia symptoms, which may include lethargy, weakness, irritability, seizures, and coma in acute hypernatremia. Convulsions are typically absent except in cases of inadvertent sodium loading or aggressive rehydration. In chronic hypernatremia (>48 hours), an osmotic adaptation is observed. Thus, patients may be relatively asymptomatic or with minimal symptoms.[9,10] Other features include symptoms and signs of volume expansion (e.g. peripheral and/or pulmonary edema) or volume depletion (e.g. postural hypotension, tachycardia, decreased skin turgor, dry mucous membrane, jugular venous pressure <5 cm H$_2$O). Common symptoms in infants include hyperpnea, muscle weakness, restlessness, a characteristic high-pitched cry, insomnia, lethargy, and even coma. Mortality rates in hypernatremic patients were reported to be dramatically increased as compared with normonatremic controls. This can be due to the severity of the underlying disease in intensive care unit (ICU) patients.[11]

## Approach/Evaluation

First step in the evaluation is to know whether it is acute (<48 hours) or chronic hypernatremia. And also to know, whether it is an emergency or not, because this decides the rapidity of correction. Most hypernatremia in clinical practice is chronic if not proved otherwise (Flowchart 13).

A detailed medical history including a detailed drug history is imperative to evaluate the cause of hypernatremia (Table 3).

Next step is the assessing extracellular volume status, on the basis of history, physical examination, and laboratory tests (Flowchart 14). Hypovolemic hypernatremia is by far the most common type of hypernatremia. The cause of hypovolemia, like decreased water intake, increased losses either extrarenal (such as gastrointestinal or insensible losses as in febrile illnesses) or renal (such as in diabetes insipidus or uncontrolled diabetes mellitus) should be carefully looked into. At the same time, examine for other signs of hypovolemia, such as decreased skin turgor, dry mucous membranes, orthostatic hypotension, postural tachycardia, prerenal acute renal failure, metabolic alkalosis, and/or hemoconcentration.[12]

Usually, patients with volume depletion exhibit low urinary excretion of sodium (<20 mEq/L). But in some circumstances like recent use of diuretics including osmotic, postobstructive nephropathy, or during recovery phase from acute tubular necrosis, an elevated urine sodium level (>20 mEq/L) might be observed. In these

**Table 3:** Drugs causing hypernatremia.

| Drug | Main mechanism(s) |
|---|---|
| Lithium | • Hypercalcemia leading to nephrogenic diabetes insipidus and causing water loss<br>• Central diabetes insipidus |
| Hypervitaminosis A and D | Hypercalcemia leading to nephrogenic diabetes insipidus |
| Cisplatin | Hypokalemia leading to nephrogenic diabetes insipidus |
| Aminoglycosides | Hypokalemia leading to nephrogenic diabetes insipidus |
| Demeclocycline | Nephrogenic diabetes insipidus |
| Amphotericin B | Nephrogenic diabetes insipidus |
| Phenytoin | Central diabetes insipidus |
| Ethanol | Central diabetes insipidus |
| Loop diuretics | Water loss |
| Manitol | Osmotic diuresis |
| Corticosteroids | Urea increase |
| Vasopressin receptor inhibitors (vaptans) | Water diuresis |
| Lactulose/sorbitol | Hypotonic gastrointestinal losses |
| Hypertonic NaHCO$_3$ or NaCl solution | Increased Na$^+$ administration |

(NaCl: sodium chloride; NaHCO$_3$: sodium bicarbonate)

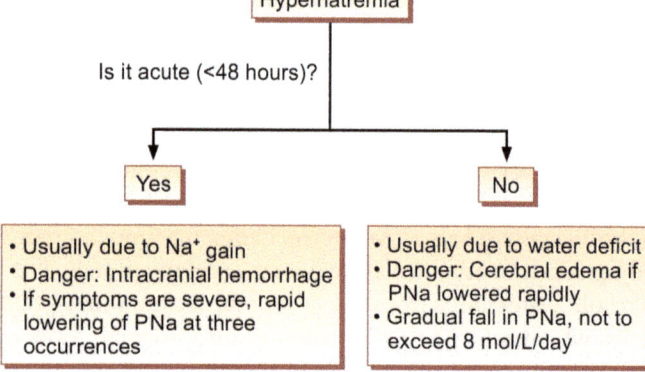

**Flowchart 13:** Initial assessment for hypernatremia.

(PNa: plasma sodium)

# Chapter 27
## Approach to the Patient with Hyponatremia and Hypernatremia

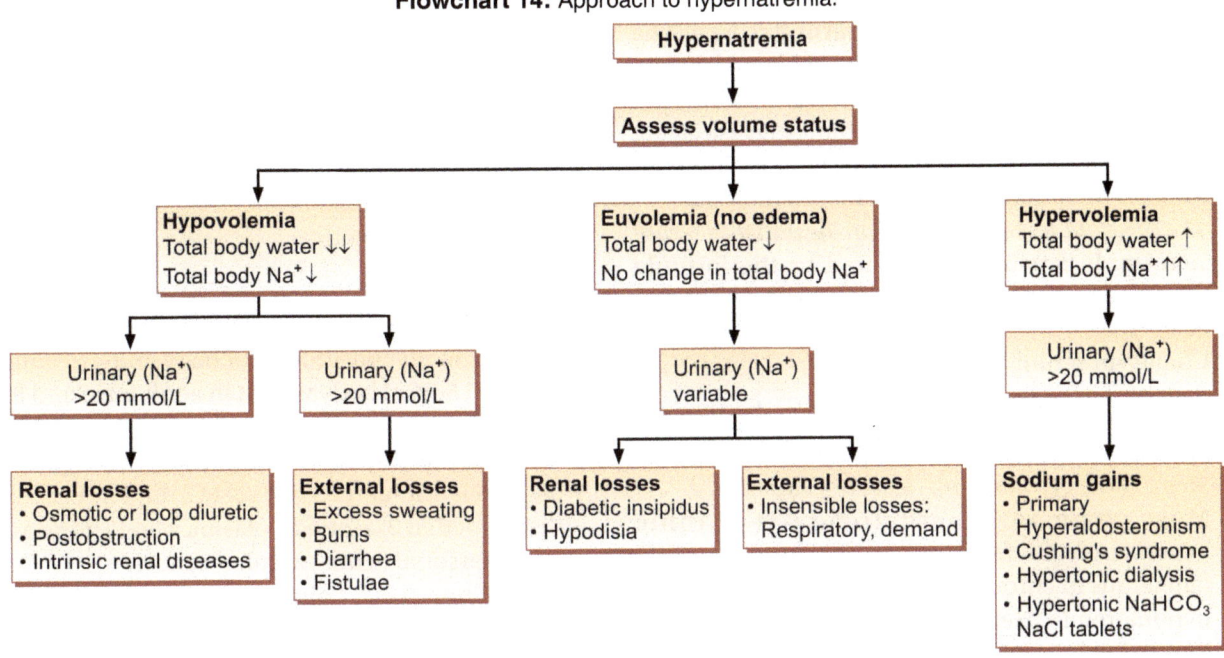

Flowchart 14: Approach to hypernatremia.

(Na: sodium; NaCl: sodium chloride; $NaHCO_3$: sodium bicarbonate)

cases, look for serum urea/creatinine ratio, >57 is a reliable index and suggestive of extracellular volume depletion.

The diagnosis of hypervolemic hypernatremia could be made from either physical examination and/or presence of history of administration of exogenous hypertonic sodium-containing solutions.

**Table 4:** Choice of fluid.

| | |
|---|---|
| Pure water loss (e.g. DI) | D5 |
| Hypotonic fluid loss | ½ Normal saline (NS) |
| Hypovolemic shock | NS till shock recovers |
| If patient is able to drink orally | Plain water |

(DI: diabetes insipidus; D5: 5% dextrose)

## Management

The steps to take in the clinical approach to patients with hypernatremia are similar to those with all other fluid, electrolyte, and acid-base disorders.
- First, recognize whether there are *emergencies* prior to therapy.
- Second, *anticipate and prevent dangers* that may arise during therapy; and
- Third, *proceed with therapy* and the diagnosis of the cause of hypernatremia. The correction of hypernatremia would include the following:
  - *Step 1: Calculate water deficit*
    Water deficit: TBW × (Sr. $Na^+$ − 140)/140
    [Total body water (TBW) = 0.45 × Body weight (in kg)]
    We also need to calculate the ongoing water loss. This will include insensible loss and electrolyte free water clearance (EFWC) from the urine.
    The estimated insensible water losses are usually 30–50 mL/hour or 10 mL/kg/day; in febrile patients, an additional 3.5 mL/kg/day per 1°C should be added. The renal water losses can be estimated by the EFWC as previously mentioned. This calculation is arbitrary. It can be in between 1 L/day and 1.5 L/day depending on the clinical situation.[13,14]
    EFWC = Urine × [1−(Na urine + K urine)/Na serum]
  - *Step 2: Choice of fluid*
    The correction is usually done with hypotonic fluids unless there is severe hypotension. The more hypotonic the infusate, the lower the rate of infusion. Because the risk of cerebral edema increases with the volume of the infusate, the volume should be restricted to that required to correct hypertonicity.[15] Available hypotonic fluids are shown in Table 4.
    There are practical issues with the available fluids. If we need to correct PNa by 10% in a 60-kg patient who has 25 L of total body water, we need to give around 2.5 L of fluids. Oral route would not be very effective as absorption from the gastrointestinal

tract will be slow. A large volume of 5% dextrose is also not advisable as some amount of glucose will be oxidized and there is a possibility of hyperglycemia which can cause osmotic diuresis and further worsening of hypernatremia. Some suggest giving distilled water through central vein as infusion through peripheral vein may cause hemolysis.

*The effect of 1 L of any infusate on the patient's serum sodium*: It is usually calculated by the formula proposed by Adrogue-Madias and verified by Liamis et al.[12]

Change in serum $Na^+$

$$= \frac{(Infusate\ Na^+ + Infusate\ K^+) - Serum\ Na^+}{Total\ body\ water + 1}$$

- *Step 3: Rate of correction: Acute or Chronic*
  Most common hypernatremia is chronic hypernatremia. Overly rapid correction is potentially dangerous in chronic hypernatremia, as in chronic hyponatremia. Hence, one should not permit the PNa to fall by more than 8–10 mmol/L per 24-hour period. In acute hypernatremia with significant symptoms (e.g. decreased level of consciousness, seizures), the PNa should be lowered rapidly, at least by 5% from its current level to prevent the devastating consequences of cellular dehydration including intracerebral or subarachnoid hemorrhages or even the demyelination syndrome. In asymptomatic acute hypernatremia, PNa should be lowered more slowly (e.g. by 1–2 mmol/L/hour). Hemodialysis may be the only option in some case to rapid fall in PNa.[16,17]

## Case Revisit

In this lady, most probable cause appears to be water loss. As the patient is altered, so she is not able to ingest the required amount of water.

- *Step 1: Calculate water deficit*
  Water deficit: TBW × (Sr. $Na^+$ – 140)/140
  [Total body water (TBW) = 0.45 × 67 kg = 30 L]
  Water deficit: 30 (150 – 140/140) = 2.1 L for target reduction of 10 mEq/L per day
  So, the total water which is to be replaced would be 2.1 L + 1.5 L = 3.6 L in next 24 hours @150 mL/hour.
- *Step 2: Choice of fluid*
  The fluid in this case can be 5% dextrose, ½ normal saline, and plain water through Ryle tube or orally when possible. The serum glucose concentration will be monitored, with insulin therapy started as required.

- *Step 3: Rate of correction: Acute or Chronic*
  As the patient is in altered sensorium, so initially the rate of correction should be rapid but not to permit the PNa to fall by more than 8–10 mmol/L per 24-hour period.
  So in the case presented above, total water which is to be replaced would be 2.1 L + 1.5 L = 3.6 L in next 24 hours @150 mL/hour.

## SALIENT POINTS

- Water is main constitution of body and it accounts for 50% and 60% of body weight in adult male and female, respectively.
- This water is distributed in two major compartments: 55–75% is ICF, and 25–45% is ECF and in ECF water is distributed in 3:1 ratio as plasma water (intravascular) and interstitial (extra vascular) spaces.
- The volume of ECF compartment is mainly determined by *content* of $Na^+$ while the major determinant of ICF volume is the *concentration* of $Na^+$ in the ECF compartment.
- Hyponatremia is usually defined as a serum sodium concentration less than 135 mEq/L.
- Hyponatremia is the most common electrolytes disorder, seen in 15–30% of acutely or chronically admitted patients in hospitals.
- Objectives of management include determination of the duration of hyponatremia, the severity (degree) of hyponatremia, the severity of symptoms, and the need for hospitalization.
- Hypernatremia is defined as plasma sodium (PNa) that is greater than 145 mmol/L.
- The most common clinical forms are chronic hypernatremia and hypernatremia due to volume loss.
- The objectives of management of hypernatremia are same as hyponatremia.

## REFERENCES

1. Spasovski G, Vanholder R, Allolio B, et al. Clinical practice guideline on diagnosis and treatment of hyponatraemia. Nephrol Dial Transplant. 2014;29(Suppl 2):i1-i39.
2. Rose BD, Post TW. Clinical Physiology of Acid-Base and Electrolyte Disorders, 5th edition. New York: McGraw-Hill; 2001. p. 699.
3. Sterns RH. Disorders of plasma sodium--causes, consequences, and correction. N Engl J Med. 2015;372:55.
4. Anderson RJ, Chung HM, Kluge R, et al. Hyponatremia: a prospective analysis of its epidemiology and the pathogenetic role of vasopressin. Ann Intern Med. 1985;102:164.

5. Chung HM, Kluge R, Schrier RW, et al. Clinical assessment of extracellular fluid volume in hyponatremia. Am J Med. 1987;83:905.
6. Beukhof CM, Hoorn EJ, Lindemans J, et al. Novel risk factors for hospital-acquired hyponatraemia: a matched case–control study. Clin Endocrinol. 2007;66:367-72.
7. Upadhyay A, Jaber BL, Madias NE. Epidemiology of hyponatremia. Semin Nephrol. 2009;29:227-38.
8. Adrogue HJ, Madias NE. Hypernatremia. N Engl J Med. 2000;342:1493-9.
9. Snyder NA, Feigal DW, Arieff AI. Hypernatremia in elderly patients: a heterogeneous, morbid, and iatrogenic entity. Ann Intern Med. 1987;107:309-19.
10. Arieff AI, Guisado R. Effects on the central nervous system of hypernatremic and hyponatremic states. Kidney Int. 1976;10:104-16.
11. Kraft MD, Btaiche IF, Sacks GS, et al. Treatment of electrolyte disorders in adult patients in the intensive care unit. Am J Health Syst Pharm. 2005;62:1663-82.
12. Liamis G, Tsimihodimos V, Doumas M, et al. Clinical and laboratory characteristics of hypernatraemia in an internal medicine clinic. Nephrol Dial Transplant. 2008;23:136-43.
13. Cox P. Insensible water loss and its assessment in adult patients: a review. Acta Anaesthesiol Scand. 1987;31:771-6.
14. Frost P. Intravenous fluid therapy in adult inpatients. BMJ. 2015;350:7620.
15. Kahn A, Brachet E, Blum D. Controlled fall in natremia and risk of seizures in hypertonic dehydration. Intensive Care Med. 1979;5:27-31.
16. Oh MS, Carroll HJ. Regulation of intracellular and extracellular volume. In: Arieff AI, De Fronzo RA (Eds). Fluid, Electrolyte, and Acid-Base Disorders, 2nd edition. New York: Churchill Livingstone; 1995. pp. 1-28.
17. Barsoum NR, Levine BS. Current prescriptions for the correction of hyponatraemia and hypernatraemia: are they too simple? Nephrol Dial Transplant. 2002;17:1176-80.

CHAPTER 28

# Approach to the Patient with Hypokalemia and Hyperkalemia

*Diego Luis Carrillo-Pérez, Gerardo Gamba*

## POTASSIUM HOMEOSTASIS

Potassium disorders are commonly encountered fluid and electrolyte abnormalities in critically ill patients, which are likely the result of comorbid disease, prolonged malnutrition, organ dysfunction, and polydrug therapy. Hyperkalemia and hypokalemia increase mortality in intensive care unit (ICU) patients; thus, early recognition and treatment are vital.[1]

Potassium ($K^+$) is the principal intracellular cation and is essential for regulation of a number of biological functions. The homeostasis of this cation relies on the balance between the intake (daily consumption is typically 50–100 mEq/day) versus renal excretion (that account to more than 95% of total excretion). Acutely, the internal balance, that is, the distribution of $K^+$ between extracellular and intracellular compartments, can momentarily affect serum $K^+$ concentration. External balance is mainly established by renal $K^+$ elimination, which depends on the glomerular filtration rate (GFR) and the distal nephron secretory capacity. On the other hand, internal balance of $K^+$ is modulated by hormonal mechanisms (involving insulin, beta-adrenergic agonist and aldosterone), which promote $K^+$ shift across the plasma membrane.

## HYPOKALEMIA

### Case

A 65-year-old man with chronic heart failure and type 2 diabetes mellitus was admitted to the ICU with a diagnosis of septic shock, secondary to community-acquired pneumonia. On physical examination, a temperature of 35.7°C, blood pressure of 98/56 mm Hg, pulse rate of 108/minute, and a respiration rate is 24/minute, jugular venous distention, pulmonary crackles and pedal edema were noted. The patient was treated with vasopressor support based on norepinephrine/dobutamine, insulin infusion, antibiotic therapy with penicillin, and furosemide infusion for overload management. On day 3, the patient developed hypokalemia of 2.8 mEq/L. Electrocardiogram (ECG) with ST-segment depression, decrease in T-wave amplitude and U-waves (Fig. 1). Which factors are involved in the development of hypokalemia in this patient?

### Definition

Hypokalemia is frequently encountered in clinical practice (21% of hospitalized patients), and it is defined as a $K^+$ concentration less than 3.5 mEq/L. A serum $K^+$ level of 2.5–3.0 mEq/L is classified as moderate hypokalemia and a level of less than 2.5 mEq/L as severe hypokalemia.[2]

### Etiology/Mechanism

Hypokalemia typically results from any one or combination of the following four causes: (1) pseudohypokalemia, (2) redistribution, (3) nonrenal potassium loss, and (4) renal potassium loss (Table 1). In critically ill patients, multiple causes frequently coexist. Redistribution usually causes transient hypokalemia, whereas disorders of external balance (inadequate intake or excessive potassium loss) cause sustained hypokalemia. Decreased intake rarely causes hypokalemia on its own because the kidney can significantly decreases potassium excretion in response to decreased intake. Nevertheless, it may contribute in hospitalized patients.[3]

### Pseudohypokalemia

Pseudohypokalemia presents secondary to a laboratory error. The most common cause is acute leukemia, in which the high leukocyte count takes up potassium when blood is stored at room temperature for prolonged periods. Rapid

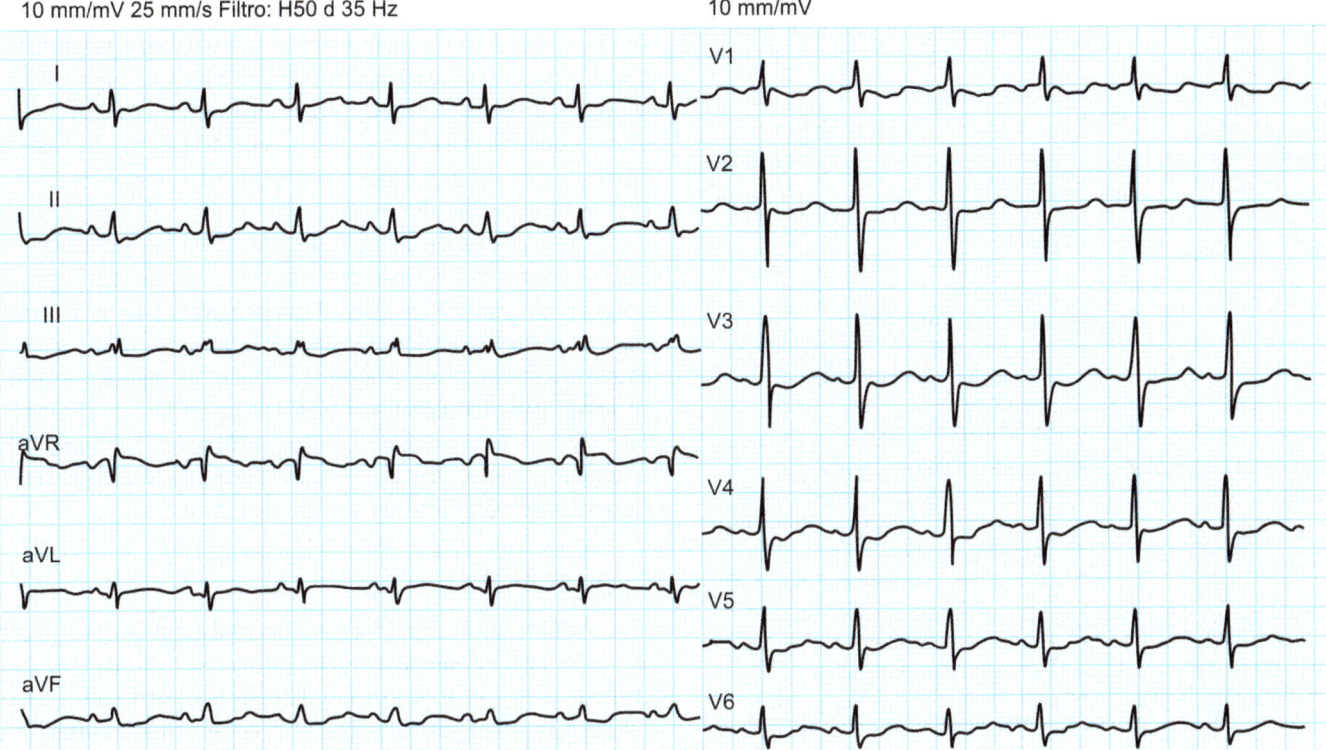

**Fig. 1:** Electrocardiogram of a hypokalemia patient, with ST-segment depression, decrease in T-wave amplitude and U-waves.

plasma separation and storage at 4°C corrects this artifact, which prevents inappropriate treatment.

### Redistribution (Cellular Shift)

Because less than 2% of total body potassium is extracellular, small potassium shifts from the extracellular to the intracellular compartment can results in hypokalemia. Multiple drugs and conditions can induce hypokalemia in critically ill patients due to transcellular shift of $K^+$ ($\beta_2$-adrenergic agonists, tocolytic agents, insulin, catecholamines, and xanthines all stimulate the intracellular uptake of $K^+$).

Drugs used to treat asthma (e.g. salbutamol), heart failure (e.g. dobutamine), chronic obstructive pulmonary disease (e.g. theophylline), or to prevent premature labor (e.g. terbutaline) can acutely decrease serum $K^+$ concentrations (>0.5–1 mEq/L) by increasing $Na^+$-$K^+$-ATPase activity secondary to $\beta$-adrenergic stimulation. Stressful events such as coronary ischemia, delirium tremens, and sepsis can also acutely induce a decreased of serum $K^+$ concentration, due to release of catecholamines and insulin, which both promote cellular $K^+$ uptake. This latter mechanism partly explains why patients with diabetes ketoacidosis treated with insulin develop hypokalemia. Moreover, insulin-induced cellular $K^+$ intake is also behind the hypokalemia in patients with refeeding syndrome.

Other causes of hypokalemia due to increased $K^+$ cellular uptake include: thyroxine administration, risperidone and quetiapine overdose, metabolic alkalosis, and hypothermia. Transfusion of previously frozen washed red blood cells also causes hypokalemia, presumably because of increase $K^+$ uptake by transfused cells. Barium poisoning from radiocontrast agents reduces the efflux of $K^+$ from muscle cells, causing hypokalemia.

### Nonrenal Potassium Loss

The skin and the gastrointestinal (GI) tract normally excrete small amounts of potassium. $K^+$ concentration in the stool is approximately 55–75 mEq/L, therefore, given the low stool volume daily losses of about 10 mEq/day are expected. With increased stool output seen with the use of laxatives, enemas, diarrhea, ileostomy, short bowel syndrome, $K^+$ losses can be significant. $K^+$ concentration in gastric secretions is about 5–10 mEq/L; thus, vomiting or excessive nasogastric suctioning induces chloride depletion and subsequent chloride-responsive metabolic alkalosis that indirectly stimulates renal $K^+$ excretion.

| Table 1: Differential diagnosis of hypokalemia. | |
|---|---|
| Mechanism | Differential diagnosis |
| Pseudohypokalemia | • Acute leukemia |
| Redistribution (cellular shift) | • B₂-adrenergic agonist (e.g. albuterol, terbutaline, epinephrine, dobutamine, etc.)<br>• Tocolytic agents (e.g. ritodrine)<br>• Insulin<br>• Theophylline<br>• Verapamil<br>• Metabolic alkalosis<br>• Hypothermia<br>• Risperidone and quetiapine overdose<br>• Barium poisoning |
| Nonrenal potassium loss | • Increased stool output (e.g. diarrhea, ileostomy, short bowel syndrome, laxatives, enemas, etc.)<br>• Vomiting<br>• Excessive nasogastric suction |
| Renal potassium loss ($K^+$ >20 mEq/day, spot urinary $K^+$ >15 mEq/L or PCR >1 mEq/mmol) | *High blood pressure with ↑ renin*<br>• Renin-secreting tumor<br>• Renovascular disease<br>• Malignant HTN<br>*High blood pressure with ↓ renin and ↑ aldosterone*<br>• Hyperaldosteronism<br>• Bilateral hyperplasia<br>*High blood pressure with ↓ renin and ↓ aldosterone*<br>• Cushing's syndrome<br>• Mineralocorticoid ingestion<br>• Adrenal hyperplasia<br>*Normal blood pressure with acidosis*<br>• Renal tubular acidosis<br>*Normal blood pressure with alkalosis and urinary chloride <10 mEq/day*<br>• Vomiting<br>*Normal blood pressure with alkalosis and urinary chloride >10 mEq/day*<br>• Diuretics<br>• Magnesium deficiency<br>• Bartter syndrome<br>• Gitelman syndrome |

($K^+$: potassium; PCR: potassium-creatinine ratio; HTN: hypertension)

### Renal Potassium Loss

This is the most common cause of hypokalemia. This mechanism is often iatrogenic, with diuretics reported to account for 36% of cases in hospitalized patients with severe hypokalemia. Loop diuretics that inhibit the Na-K-2Cl transporter in the thick ascending limb of the loop of Henle and thiazide diuretics that inhibit the Na-Cl cotransporter in the distal convoluted tubule indirectly stimulate $K^+$ secretion by increasing sodium and fluid delivery to the collecting duct. When used in the treatment of refractory congestive heart failure and metabolic alkalosis, acetazolamide increases sodium bicarbonate delivery in the collecting ducts and enhances potassium secretion. In cases of severe septic shock, the use of hydrocortisone can lead to excessive urinary $K^+$ wasting due to their mineralocorticoid effect.

Aminoglycosides, amphotericin B, cisplatin, tenofovir, and foscarnet all promote renal $K^+$ losses and can be caused of hypokalemia. Amphotericin B, cisplatin, and aminoglycosides also are associated with urinary magnesium wasting. Magnesium acts as a gate inhibitor of renal outer medullary potassium channel (ROMK), and its deficiency decreases this inhibition, increasing $K^+$ excretion. Penicillin and its synthetic derivatives act as nonreabsorbable anions, enhancing $K^+$ secretion.

## Clinical Effects

Hypokalemia has various detrimental effects in critically ill patients. The severity is dependent on the degree and duration of hypokalemia. Although hypokalemia can present as a myriad of signs and symptoms, cardiac and neuromuscular manifestations are the most clinically relevant. Both are related to alteration in the generation of the membrane action potential. In the heart, changes in the cardiomyocyte action potential translate into the following ECG manifestations: ST-segment depression, a decrease in T-wave amplitude, and an increase in U-wave amplitude, arrhythmias and conductions defects.

Neuromuscular manifestations include weakness, myalgias, muscle fatigue, and leg restlessness. Nevertheless, more severe hypokalemia (<2 mEq/L) can also present with paralysis that usually involves the extremities, but may progress to include the trunk and muscles of respiration, or frank rhabdomyolysis even in bed-bound patients.

## Approach/Evaluation

The cause of hypokalemia in most cases can be readily determined by clinical history, physical examination with assessment of volume status, and acid-base status. A focused history must include evaluation for possible GI losses, medications history, and assessment for underlying cardiac morbidities.

Assessment of urinary potassium excretion allows ones to determine whether hypokalemia is due to renal or extrarenal causes. The best method is a 24-hour urine collection, but it is cumbersome, so spot urinary $K^+$ concentration and potassium-creatinine ratio can also be used. A 24-hour urinary potassium excretion greater than 20 mEq, a spot urinary K+ concentration greater than 15 mEq/L or a potassium-creatinine ratio greater than 1 (mEq/mmol) suggests a renal cause of hypokalemia. In these patients, the following should be considered: high aldosterone levels or an acquired or inherited defect in distal nephron function (each of which affects distal nephron K+ secretion).

Plasma renin and aldosterone levels should be measured in hypertensive patients to exclude primary aldosteronism or adrenal hyperplasia, renovascular disease, exposure to glycyrrhizic acid in licorice or tobacco chewing. If the patient is normotensive, the differential diagnosis should include renal tubular acidosis, vomiting, diuretic abuse, Bartter or Gitelman syndrome and magnesium deficiency. These disorders can be better categorized according to plasma bicarbonate and urinary chloride. The approach to the patient with hypokalemia and renal losses is outlined in Table 1.

## Management

Management should be directed to the underlying cause and alleviate the primary disorder. It is essential to establish whether hypokalemia is caused by a cellular shift or by a K+ deficit. Hypokalemia should be treated to prevent the life-threatening complications like arrhythmias, paralysis, rhabdomyolysis, and diaphragmatic weakness. Older patients or those with heart conditions and taking digoxin are at a high risk of arrhythmias associated with hypokalemia.

Generally, serum K+ decreases by approximately 0.3 mEq/L for every 100-mEq reduction in total body K+, but it is highly dependent on body mass. The presence of ECG abnormalities or respiratory muscle paralysis mandates immediate treatment with intravenous K+. The maximum rate of K+ repletion should not exceed 20 mEq/hour in order to minimize the risk of iatrogenic hyperkalemia. Nevertheless, in the presence of unstable arrhythmias, infusions of up to 40 mEq/hour are indicated. In most cases, potassium chloride is preferred. Potassium phosphate administration is recommended in patients with concomitant hypophosphatemia (e.g. diabetic ketoacidosis and refeeding syndrome), and potassium bicarbonate is preferred in patients with concomitant metabolic acidosis. Hypomagnesemia promotes renal K+ wasting; therefore, adequate magnesium repletion is vital to allow for a more rapid correction of hypokalemia.

In the absence of a medical emergency and in cases of mild hypokalemia, oral repletion (60–80 mEq/day) is the preferred method as it minimizes the risk of rebound hyperkalemia.[4]

## Case Revisit

In this critically ill patient, multiple factors contributed to development of hypokalemia: (1) redistribution of K+ into the cells (insulin infusion, dobutamine, sepsis, hypothermia, and respiratory alkalosis) and (2) renal potassium loss (diuretics, and possibly by the use of penicillin that acts like a nonabsorbable anion which induces K+ secretion).

## HYPERKALEMIA

### Case

A 31-year-old woman with diabetes mellitus type 1 and chronic kidney disease KDIGO G4 A3 [serum creatinine 3.2 mg/dL, estimated GFR (eGFR) 18 mL/min/1.73m$^2$] is brought to the emergency room because of acute altered mental status. A few days earlier, she stopped her medications (including insulin, furosemide, and bicarbonate therapy). Leg edema was found on physical examination. ECG with sine wave appearance, absent P waves, broad QRS complex, with atypical right bundle branch block morphology, and peaked T waves (Fig. 2). Blood gases showed a metabolic acidosis (pH 7.2, $HCO_3^-$ of 12 mEq/L, $PaCO_2$ of 24 mm Hg), potassium of 7.3 mEq/L, and glucose of 513 mg/dL. Which factors are involved in this patient's hyperkalemia?

### Definition

Hyperkalemia is defined as a serum potassium concentration of K+ greater than 5.0 mEq/L, and occurs in up to 10% of hospitalized patients.[2,5]

### Etiology/Mechanism

Hyperkalemia is generally attributable to K+ cellular shifts or decreased renal potassium excretion (Table 2). As in hypokalemia, redistribution can also cause transient hyperkalemia, whereas disorders of external balance (decreased potassium excretion) cause sustained hyperkalemia. Excessive potassium intake is a rare cause of hyperkalemia by itself, but can exacerbate the severity of hyperkalemia in patients with renal insufficiency. Impaired renal potassium excretion can be caused by a decrease of the GFR with reduced distal salt delivery, a primary decrease in mineralocorticoid level or activity, or abnormal distal nephron function. Pseudohyperkalemia should be excluded before hyperkalemia can be attributed to cellular redistribution or decreased renal excretion.[6]

# Section 2
## Fluids and Electrolytes

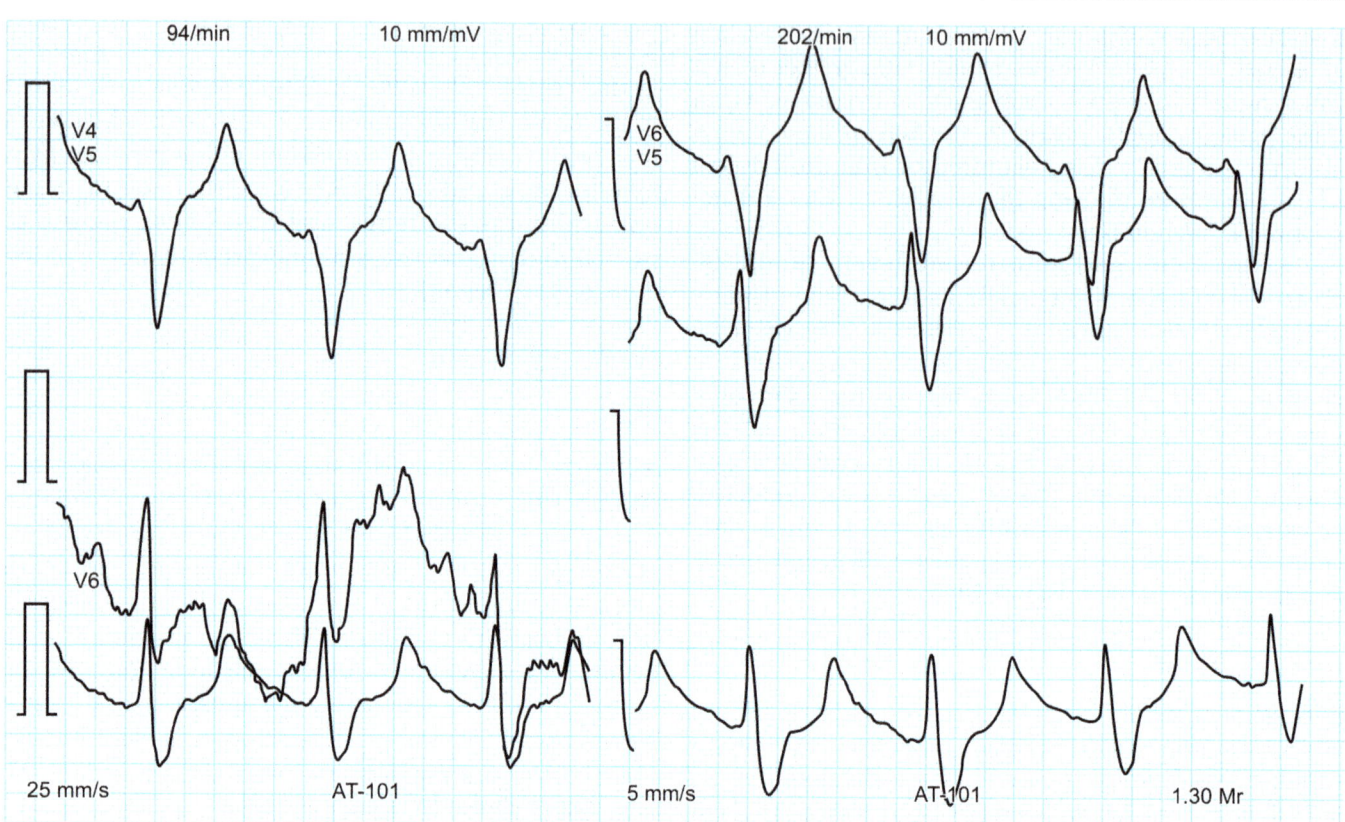

**Fig. 2:** Electrocardiogram of a hyperkalemia patient, with sine wave appearance, absent P waves, broad QRS complex, with atypical right bundle branch block morphology, and peaked T waves.

| Table 2: Differential diagnosis of hyperkalemia. | |
|---|---|
| Mechanism | Differential diagnosis |
| Pseudohyperkalemia | • Incorrect sample proceedings (e.g. small-bore needles, tourniquet application, etc.)<br>• Hematologic disorders (e.g. pronounced thrombocytosis and leukocytosis) |
| Redistribution (cellular shift) | • β2-adrenergic blockers (e.g. metoprolol, atenolol, propranolol, etc.)<br>• Succinylcholine<br>• Digoxin<br>• Insulin deficiency (e.g. diabetes)<br>• Hypertonicity (e.g. hyperglycemia)<br>• Metabolic acidosis<br>• Rhabdomyolysis<br>• Hemolysis |
| Exogenous potassium load | • Red blood cell transfusion<br>• Total parenteral nutrition<br>• Penicillin G potassium |
| Impaired renal excretion | • Decreased distal salt delivery (e.g. acute kidney injury, hypovolemia, Gordon syndrome, etc.)<br>• Decreased mineralocorticoid activity (e.g. RAAS inhibitors, NSAIDs, COX-2 inhibitors, calcineurin inhibitors, beta-adrenergic blockers, heparin, and diabetic nephropathy)<br>• Abnormalities of the cortical collecting tubule [e.g. potassium-sparing diuretics, ENaC blockers (e.g. amiloride), pentamidine, and trimethoprim] |

(RAAS: renin-angiotensin-aldosterone system; NSAIDs: nonsteroidal anti-inflammatory drugs; COX-2: cyclooxygenase-2; ENaC: epithelial $Na^+$ channel)

## Pseudohyperkalemia

Pseudohyperkalemia occurs by a mechanical release of K$^+$ from cells during the phlebotomy procedure inside blood collection tubes or by incorrect sample processing. Common reasons include tight and prolong fist clenching during the phlebotomy procedure, application of tourniquets, and use of small-bore needles. Other causes include hematologic disorders, such as thrombocytosis (platelets >1,000,000/cm$^3$) and pronounced leukocytosis (leukocytes >100,000/cm$^3$). Sometimes contamination with potassium ethylenediaminetetraacetic acid (EDTA) in certain sampling tubes can also cause a spurious increase in plasma K$^+$ concentration accompanied by a very low plasma calcium concentration.

## Cellular Shift

Cellular redistribution is more relevant as a cause of hyperkalemia than of hypokalemia. As little as a 2% shift in intracellular K$^+$ to the extracellular fluid can result in a serum K$^+$ level of 8 mEq/L. Insulin and catecholamines are the major physiologic regulators of potassium cellular shift, but other stimuli, including medications also affect transmembrane K$^+$ shifts. Beta-adrenergic blockers decrease K$^+$ cellular intake and can promote hyperkalemia in patients with decreased renal potassium excretion. Succinylcholine is commonly used as a muscle relaxant in ventilated patients in the ICU and promotes K$^+$ efflux from myocytes. In the setting of denervation, burns, trauma, or prolonged immobility, the hyperkalemic response can be severe. Digoxin is a cardiac glycoside that inhibits the cell membrane-bound Na$^+$-K$^+$-ATPase, which leads to a K$^+$ release into the extracellular space, mainly within toxic levels. Insulin resistance and/or insulin deficiency and hypertonicity can also favor K$^+$ shift and result in hyperkalemia.

## Disorders of Renal Potassium Excretion

Prolonged and severe hyperkalemia usually implies the presence of a concomitant decrease in renal potassium excretion. These conditions include a severely limit distal salt delivery, decrease mineralocorticoid levels or activity, or a distal nephron tubular defect. In many instances, one or more mechanisms can be present. By far the most common cause of hyperkalemia, seen first time in patient, is the decreased function of the kidneys. Patients with acute or chronic renal insufficiency often present with certain level of hyperkalemia. The K$^+$ levels, especially when associated with electrocardiographic evidences of arrhythmias, are one of the most common reasons to use hemodialysis to remove potassium from the body. Thus, serum K$^+$ levels are used to monitor the efficacy and requirement of dialysis therapy.

## Decreased Distal Salt Delivery

Clinical conditions where decreased renal perfusion occurs, aldosterone concentrations increase. As a result, the proximal absorption of sodium and water increases, which leads to decrease in distal delivery of sodium and water. Despite increased concentrations of aldosterone, the lack of availability of sodium can impair renal potassium secretion because the secretion of potassium in collecting duct is coupled with sodium reabsorption. Acute kidney injury may lead to a marked decrease in distal delivery of salt and water, which may secondarily decrease distal potassium secretion.

Decreased salt deliver in the content of normal GFR can be seen in a rare disordered known as pseudohypoaldosteronism type II or familial hyperkalemic hypertension. This is usually a dominant inherited disease due to mutations in genes that encode for regulatory proteins of the sodium chloride (NaCl) cotransporter of the distal convoluted tubule. The increase in the activity of this cotransporter leads to salt sensitive arterial hypertension, together with hyperkalemia and metabolic acidosis due to decreased delivery of salt to the collecting duct.

## Decreased Mineralocorticoid Activity

This mechanism of hyperkalemia can result from disturbances that originate at any point along the renin-angiotensin-aldosterone system (RAAS), which regulates the renal potassium excretion. Normally, aldosterone binds to a cytosolic receptor in the principal cell and stimulates sodium (Na$^+$) reabsorption across the luminal membrane through the epithelial Na$^+$ channel known as ENaC. This, in turn, drives potassium secretion by its electrochemical gradient through an apically located potassium channel. The permeability for the anion that accompanies sodium also influences potassium secretion, with less permeable anions having a greater stimulatory effect on potassium secretion.

Several conditions and drugs affect RAAS causing hypoaldosteronism by impairing renin release. Diabetic nephropathy is the most common cause of hyporeninemic hypoaldosteronism, accounting for about half of the cases. Drugs used in critically ill patients are also commonly known to cause hyporeninemic hypoaldosteronism. Nonsteroidal anti-inflammatory drugs (NSAIDs) and cyclo-oxygenase-2 (COX-2) inhibitors cause a reduction in renal prostaglandin synthesis which leads to a decrease in renin production, causing hyporeninemic hypoaldosteronism, leading to hyperkalemia and acidosis. Calcineurin inhibitors, such as cyclosporine and tacrolimus, suppress renin release, activate the salt reabsorption in the distal tubule, thus decreasing salt delivery to collecting duct, where in addition directly interfere with the secretion of $K^+$. Beta-adrenergic blockers inhibit the stimulatory effect of the sympathetic system on the release of renin. In addition, they interfere with the cellular uptake of potassium through decreased activity of the $Na^+$-$K^+$-ATPase.

Angiotensin-converting enzyme inhibitors (ACEIs) and angiotensin receptor blockers (ARBs) are associated with a greater risk of hyperkalemia due to decreased aldosterone activity. Heparin induces reversible hypoaldosteronism and hyperkalemia via a reduction in the number and affinity of angiotensin II receptors. This effect is independent of the route of heparin administration or the level of anticoagulation achieved. The azole antifungals (like ketoconazole) interfere with the biosynthesis of adrenal steroids and therefore can predispose to aldosterone deficiency.

### Abnormalities of the Cortical Collecting Tubule

The potassium-sparing diuretics (e.g. spironolactone, eplerenone) impair the ability of the cortical collecting tubule to secrete potassium by blocking the interaction of aldosterone with its receptor. Amiloride and triamterene block the ENaC in the collecting tubule. Blockade of sodium reabsorption through this channel abolishes the lumen's negative potential and drives secretion of potassium following its electrochemical gradient. A similar effect can be seen with pentamidine and trimethoprim. The structure of trimethoprim is similar to that of the potassium-sparing diuretic amiloride, and it may reduce urinary $K^+$ elimination by approximately 40%.

## Clinical Effects

Hyperkalemia is often asymptomatic, but severe hyperkalemia can present with generalized weakness, paralysis, and arrhythmias. The depolarizing effect of hyperkalemia on the heart is manifest by changes in the ECG, but ECG findings might not be sensitive in detecting mild and moderate hyperkalemia, therefore, any ECG change should be viewed as an emergency.

## Approach/Evaluation

The initial approach includes exclusion of pseudohyperkalemia, and identify if transcellular shift (redistribution) or renal defect in potassium excretion is present, through review the drugs and disorders (hypertonicity and insulin deficiency) that can move $K^+$ from the intracellular to extracellular space, and drugs and disorders (kidney disease or hypoaldosteronism) that can impair renal potassium excretion.

## Management

The most important goal of treating hyperkalemia is to prevent life-threatening cardiac arrhythmias. Patients with serum $K^+$ greater than or equal to 6.0 mEq/L or those with ECG abnormalities should be emergently treated. Therapeutic strategies are directed at antagonizing the effects of hyperkalemia at the cellular level (e.g. intravenous calcium), shifting $K^+$ from the extracellular to the intracellular space (e.g. insulin and dextrose, inhaled or intravenous β-adrenergic agonists, $NaHCO_3^-$), and removing $K^+$ from the body (e.g. diuretics and hemodialysis) (Table 3). A rapid correction of the primary cause should be addressed early and proactively, but emergent therapy, such as hemodialysis, should not be delayed if life-threatening manifestations are present.[7-9]

**Table 3:** Treatment options of hyperkalemia.

| Agent | Dose | Onset | Duration | Mechanism |
|---|---|---|---|---|
| Insulin plus glucose | 5–10 U IV with 50 mL IV D50W | 15 minutes | ≥2 hours | Redistribution (cellular shift) potassium into cells |
| B$_2$-agonists (albuterol) | 10–20 mg nebulized over 10 minutes | 30 minutes | ≥2 hours | |
| Sodium bicarbonate | 50–100 mEq IV over 2–5 minutes | 30 minutes | 2–6 hours | |
| Furosemide | 40 mg IV | 5–15 minutes | 4–6 hours | Potassium excretion |
| Sodium polystyrene sulfonate (Kayexalate) | Oral: 15 g, 1–4 times daily | 2–24 hours | 4–6 hours | |
| Hemodialysis | 2–4 hours | Immediate | Variable | Potassium removal |
| Calcium gluconate (10%) | 1 g IV over 5–10 minutes | Immediate | 30–60 minutes | Membrane potential stabilization |

(IV: intravenous; D50W: dextrose 50% in water)

## Case Revisit

Hyperkalemia on admission in the patient is most likely caused by the effects of hypertonicity and insulin deficiency on cellular K⁺ shifts, in addition to impaired K⁺ excretion secondary to a reduction in GFR, which decreases distal sodium delivery.

## SALIENT POINTS

- Hypokalemia can result from pseudohypokalemia, redistribution (cellular shift), nonrenal potassium loss (predominantly from GI tract) and renal potassium loss.
- The major causes of urinary potassium wasting include diuretics, hypomagnesemia and excretion of nonreabsorbable anions.
- In critically ill patients, multiple mechanisms contributed to the development of hypokalemia, and the treatment should be directed to the underlying causes.
- Hyperkalemia can result from pseudohyperkalemia, redistribution (cellular shift), or impaired renal potassium excretion (decreased distal salt delivery, decrease mineralocorticoid levels or activity, or a distal nephron tubular defect).
- The major cause of impaired renal potassium excretion is the decreased renal function (acute kidney injury and/or chronic kidney disease). Although one or more mechanisms can be present.
- The treatment of hyperkalemia includes redistribution of potassium into cells (insulin plus glucose, $B_2$-agonists, sodium bicarbonate), increase potassium excretion (furosemide and sodium polystyrene sulfonate), potassium removal (hemodialysis), and membrane potential stabilization (calcium gluconate).

## REFERENCES

1. Romito B, Dhillon A. Hyperkalemia and hypokalemia. In: Vincent JL, Moore F, Fink M (Eds). Textbook of Critical Care, 7th edition. Philadelphia: Elsevier; 2017. pp. 52-5.
2. Unwin RJ, Luft FC, Shirley DG. Pathophysiology and management of hypokalemia: a clinical perspective. Nat Rev Nephrol. 2011;7:75-84.
3. Palmer BF. A physiologic-based approach to the evaluation of a patient with hypokalemia. Am J Kidney Dis. 2010;56:1184-90.
4. Asmar A, Mohandas R, Wingo CS. A physiologic-based approach to the treatment of a patient with hypokalemia. Am J Kidney Dis. 2012;60:492-7.
5. Gumz ML, Rabinowitz L, Wingo CS. An integrated view of potassium homeostasis. N Engl J Med. 2015;373:60-72.
6. Palmer BF. A physiologic-based approach to the evaluation of a patient with hyperkalemia. Am J Kidney Dis. 2010;56:387-93.
7. Palmer BF. Managing hyperkalemia caused by inhibitors of the renin-angiotensin-aldosterone system. N Engl J Med. 2004;351:585-92.
8. Montford JR, Linas S. How dangerous is hyperkalemia? J Am Soc Nephrol. 2017;28:3155-65.
9. Pham AQ, Sexton J, Wimer D, et al. Managing hyperkalemia: stepping into a new frontier. J Pharm Pract. 2017;30:557-61.

# CHAPTER 29

# Approach to the Patient with Hypocalcemia and Hypercalcemia

*Bhuvana Krishna, Sriram Sampath*

## CALCIUM HOMEOSTASIS

Calcium is an abundant divalent cation found in the body, with important functions (Box 1).[1] Majority of the total body calcium (99%) is stored in the bone as hydroxyapatite and the remainder is found within the extracellular fluid (ECF). Calcium circulates in the ECF in three distinct forms—(1) 50% is ionized, (2) 40% is bound to plasma proteins, and the remaining 10% is chelated to anions like bicarbonate, lactates, ketones, phosphates, sulfates, and citrates.[2] Most of the protein bound calcium is bound to albumin (80%) and the remaining to globulins (20%). The normal total calcium concentration in the plasma varies between laboratories, but is generally in the range of 8.5–10.5 mg/dL (2.2–2.5 mmol/L). More than half of the plasma concentration exists as the biologically active ionized form of calcium, 4.5–5.0 mg/dL (1.1–1.3 mmol/L).

A change in the ionized form of calcium is mainly responsible for the clinical manifestations of hypocalcemia or hypercalcemia. There are conditions where the ionized form of calcium is low without a change in total plasma calcium concentration. This is commonly seen in conditions where anions like lactates, ketones, etc. increase, which chelate the ionized calcium resulting in hypocalcemia.

**Box 1:** Functions of calcium.

- For contraction of all muscles—especially duration and strength of cardiac muscle contraction
- Neurotransmitter release from neurons
- Cofactor for many enzymes
- Clotting of blood
- Proper bone formation
- Cardiac pacemaker activity
- Cell death and apoptosis
- Smooth muscle contraction in blood vessels
- Uterine contraction

## Hormonal Regulation

The plasma concentration of calcium is tightly regulated by a complex interplay between the (1) parathyroid hormone (PTH), (2) vitamin D, and (3) calcitonin; via the bone, kidney, and gastrointestinal tract (Fig. 1).

Parathyroid hormone is an 84-amino acid protein secreted by the chief cells of the parathyroid gland. The PTH hormone synthesis is affected by the concentration of ionized form of calcium, which binds to calcium sensing receptors (CaSRs) present on the parathyroid chief cells. The decrease in calcium levels causes a rapid increase in synthesis of PTH levels. The PTH increases the concentration of plasma calcium by:

- Acting directly on the kidneys to increase calcium reabsorption
- By increasing osteoclastic activity leading to bone resorption
- By stimulating the conversion of 25-hydroxyvitamin D to 1,25-hydroxyvitamin D or calcitriol in the kidneys, which in turn increases the calcium absorption from the small intestine.

The renal absorption of calcium occurs in the proximal tubule, loop of Henle, and the distal tubules. There are both passive and active mechanisms of calcium absorption from the distal tubules. The passive transport occurs due to an electropositive gradient created at the loop of Henle due to the reabsorption of sodium ($Na^+$) and potassium ($K^+$) anions. Drugs like diuretics which increase $Na^+$ excretion also increase calcium excretion. However, thiazide diuretics are an exception, where calcium reabsorption is increased in the distal tubules.

Parathyroid hormone secretion is also stimulated by hyperphosphatemia, which regulates the phosphate levels. The phosphate levels are increased by PTH through bone resorption and through vitamin D-mediated absorption

# Chapter 29
## Approach to the Patient with Hypocalcemia and Hypercalcemia

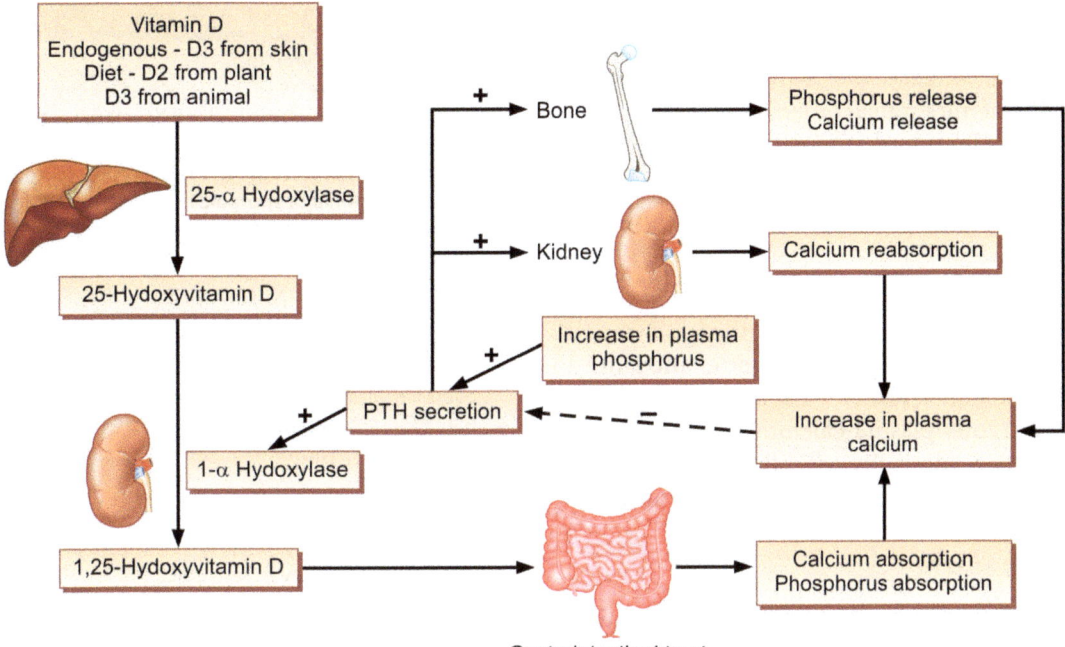

**Fig. 1:** Calcium metabolism.

from the gut. But these effects are negated by the direct effects of PTH on the kidneys by decreasing the renal absorption of phosphate.

A decrease in PTH levels results in hypocalcemia and hyperphosphatemia, and an increase in PTH production leads to hypercalcemia and hypophosphatemia.

Calcitonin is a 32-amino acid protein produced by the parafollicular cells of the thyroid gland in response to high levels of plasma calcium concentration. The action of calcitonin is opposite to that of PTH, it decreases plasma calcium levels by decreasing bone resorption.

## Metabolic Regulation

- Normally 1 g/dL (10 g/L) of albumin binds to 0.8 mg/dL (0.20 mmol/L) of calcium. Hence, changes in level of albumin significantly alter the total calcium concentration. An alkaline pH of plasma will increase the binding of ionized calcium to albumin without altering the total plasma concentration of calcium, leading to hypocalcemia.[3] An increase in pH by 0.1 results in decrease in ionized calcium by 0.1 mmol/L. Similarly, free fatty acids in plasma also increase the affinity of albumin to calcium.[4] Acidemia has an opposite effect.
- Increase in serum phosphate levels leads to binding of calcium to phosphate and deposition of calcium phosphate in tissues resulting in hypocalcemia with an increase in PTH levels.
- Magnesium is necessary for the synthesis of PTH by the parathyroid glands, thereby indirectly influencing the calcium levels.[5]
- Circulating cytokines suppress the synthesis of PTH leading to hypocalcemia.[6]
- Although a highly regulated system exists to maintain the ionized form of calcium in the narrow therapeutic range, changes in pH, albumin, lactates, phosphates, or magnesium, which are common in critically ill patients, may result in abnormalities in plasma calcium levels.[7]

## HYPOCALCEMIA

### Case

A 71-year-old lady presented to the emergency department with lethargy, decreased appetite disorientation, and speech disturbance for several days. Her clinical examination showed a heart rate of 64 beats/minute, a blood pressure of 108/70 mm Hg, and respiratory rate of 20/minute. She was drowsy and arousable but not oriented. Her laboratory investigations showed a serum creatinine of 3.2 mg/dL (282.8 μmol/L) and serum calcium was 4.8 mg/dL (1.20 mmol/L) with albumin values of 3.2 g/dL (32 g/L) and her phosphorus values were 2.5 mg/dL (0.81 mmol/L). Her ECG showed a prolonged QT interval (QTc-520 ms). Her PTH levels were sent which were high and vitamin D levels were very low.

Her past records showed that a month back she had a fall and had sustained a left fracture femur, for which she had undergone surgery. Her activities were severely restricted in spite of the surgical procedure.

How do you evaluate and manage this patient having hypocalcemia?

## Definition

Hypocalcemia is when the total plasma calcium level, corrected for albumin, is less than 8.5 mg/dL (2.13 mmol/L). Ionized calcium is a better measure to diagnose hypocalcemia (levels < 1.1 mmol/L) than the albumin adjusted total plasma calcium levels, which are prone for errors, especially in the critically ill patients, where hypoalbuminemia and pH abnormalities are common.

## Etiology/Mechanism

Hypocalcemia is more common than hypercalcemia in the critically ill, with an incidence of 65–88%.[6] There are many causes for hypocalcemia in the adults.[2,6,8] In general, there is a deficiency of PTH secretion by the parathyroid gland (hypoparathyroidism). Or hypocalcemia can result from vitamin D deficiency, where the PTH levels are elevated (secondary hyperparathyroidism). The etiological classification of hypocalcemia can be subdivided into hypocalcemia with hypoparathyroidism and hypocalcemia with hyperparathyroidism (Box 2).

*Hypocalcemia with hypoparathyroidism:*

- *Surgery or damage to parathyroid glands:* The most common cause for hypocalcemia in adults is due to surgical removal or damage to the parathyroid glands during thyroid surgeries or extensive head and neck surgeries for malignancies. Rarely, radiation to neck region can cause damage to the parathyroid glands. Hypoparathyroidism can also occur due to infiltrative diseases of the parathyroid glands as in, granulomatous diseases, Wilson's disease, iron overload, metastasis, and due to human immunodeficiency virus infection. In all these conditions, there is hypoparathyroidism leading to hypocalcemia with hyperphosphatemia.
- Hungry bone syndrome is a condition commonly seen after parathyroidectomy for hyperparathyroidism, thyroidectomy for thyrotoxicosis, and vitamin D supplementation for severe osteomalacia. These conditions already have a high bone turnover and the bone is undermineralized. With the correction of these disorders, the bone mineralization exceeds bone resorption resulting in hypocalcemia.[9]

**Box 2:** Etiology for hypocalcemia.

*Low PTH (hypoparathyroidism)*
- Genetic disorders
  - Abnormal parathyroid gland development
  - Abnormal PTH synthesis
  - Mutations of calcium-sensing receptor (autosomal dominant hypocalcemia or sporadic isolated hypoparathyroidism)
- Postsurgical (thyroidectomy, parathyroidectomy, and radical neck dissection)
- Autoimmune
  - Autoimmune polyglandular syndrome
  - Antibodies to calcium-sensing receptor
- Infiltration of the parathyroid gland (granulomatous, iron overload, and metastases)
- Radiation-induced destruction of parathyroid glands
- Hungry bone syndrome (postparathyroidectomy)
- HIV infection

*High PTH (secondary hyperparathyroidism in response to hypocalcemia)*
- Vitamin D deficiency or resistance
- Inadequate intake, malabsorption*, liver, or renal disease*
- PTH resistance
  - Missense mutation in PTH
  - Pseudohypoparathyroidism
    - Hypomagnesemia*
- Renal disease*
  - Loss of calcium from the circulation
  - Hyperphosphatemia*
    - Tumor lysis*
  - Acute pancreatitis*
    - Osteoblastic metastases
  - Acute respiratory alkalosis*
    - Sepsis or acute severe illness*

*Drugs*
- Inhibitors of bone resorption (bisphosphonates, calcitonin, and denosumab), especially in vitamin D deficiency
- Calcium chelators, citrate, massive blood transfusion*, or citrate dialysis*, EDTA- radiographic dyes, and phosphate
- Foscarnet (due to intravascular complexing with calcium)
- Phenytoin* (due to conversion of vitamin D to inactive metabolites)
- Fluoride poisoning
- Gadolinium—used for contrast study

*Disorders of magnesium metabolism**

Hypomagnesemia can reduce PTH secretion or cause PTH resistance and is therefore associated with normal, low, or high PTH levels

(EDTA: ethylenediaminetetraacetic acid; HIV: human immunodeficiency virus; PTH: parathyroid hormone)
*Common causes in the ICU

## Hypocalcemia with Hyperparathyroidism

- Vitamin D deficiency or resistance of target organs is associated with hypocalcemia and hypophosphatemia. Vitamin D deficiency can occur with poor dietary intake, malabsorption, or inadequate exposure to

sunlight. Renal failure or hepatic failure can also cause vitamin D deficiency due to poor conversion of vitamin D to the active form—calcitriol. Studies have associated vitamin D deficiency with cardiovascular disease and immune dysregulation, but the clinical relevance of this, in critically ill, is yet to be proven.
- Pseudohypoparathyroidism is a condition where there is a resistance of the target organ, i.e. bone, kidney, and gut to PTH, despite increased levels of circulating PTH. There is a genetic mutation in the receptors on the target organs, and the manifestation of hypocalcemia is seen in childhood.
- *Magnesium:* As mentioned earlier, is necessary for PTH production and its action on target organs. Hypomagnesemia at levels below 0.8 mEq/L (1 mg/dL or 4 mmol/L) causes hypocalcemia with normal, low or elevated PTH levels, and normal to low phosphate levels. Magnesium deficiency is commonly seen with malabsorption, chronic alcoholism, diuretic therapy, prolonged parenteral nutrition, and with use of drugs like aminoglycosides and cisplatin.
- Chronic kidney disease is a common cause for hypocalcemia where there is decreased renal production of 1,25-hydroxyvitamin D, or calcitriol. The other reason for hypocalcemia in renal failure is hyperphosphatemia. Hypocalcemia occurs only with end stage renal disease.
- *Loss of calcium from the circulation:* High phosphate levels bind with ionized calcium leading to deposition in bone and extraskeletal tissues, resulting in hypocalcemia. Hyperphosphatemia can occur in conditions that result in excessive tissue breakdown like, rhabdomyolysis or tumor lysis syndrome. In acute pancreatitis, there is deposition of calcium soap (saponification) in the abdominal cavity by an unknown mechanism, leading to hypocalcemia.
- *Osteoblastic metastasis:* Some tumors with osteoblastic metastasis as seen in breast and prostatic cancers have new bone formation resulting in hypocalcemia and elevation in alkaline phosphate levels.[10]
- Sepsis or acute severe illness can result in hypocalcemia due to multiple reasons.[6,8] The circulating inflammatory cytokines produced during an acute illness decrease the production of PTH, decrease the sensitivity of target organs to PTH, and impair production of calcitriol in the kidneys.
- *Drugs:* Calcium chelators like citrate, lactate, and ethylenediaminetetraacetic acid, chelate the ionized calcium in the blood causing hypocalcemia. Citrate is used as an anticoagulant in blood and blood products.

Citrate is rapidly metabolized in the liver. Citrate toxicity can occur only in cases of liver or kidney failure, with massive blood transfusions or during plasma exchange, leading to hypocalcemia.[11]

Severe lactic acidosis, as seen in critically ill, can also chelate the ionized calcium causing hypocalcemia. Other drugs like bisphosphonates, which inhibit bone resorption and chemotherapy drugs like cisplatin, can cause hypocalcemia. Phenobarbitone and phenytoin through vitamin D deficiency are some other drugs implicated in the causation of hypocalcemia.

## Clinical Effects

The presentation of hypocalcemia can be varied from asymptomatic, mild to severe hypocalcemia presenting with seizures, arrhythmias, heart failure, or laryngospasm (Table 1). The hallmark of presentation of hypocalcemia is tetany, which occurs due neuromuscular irritability secondary to abnormalities in conduction of action potential in the neuronal cells.
- Tetany can present as perioral numbness, paresthesia, muscle cramps, carpopedal spasm, and seizures. Tetany is generally seen in conditions, which cause acute severe hypocalcemia.

**Table 1:** Clinical presentation of hypocalcemia.

| Organ system | Manifestation |
|---|---|
| Nervous system | - Tetany<br>- Chvostek's and Trousseau's sign<br>- Carpopedal spasm and muscle cramps<br>- Paresthesia<br>- Seizures<br>- Weakness<br>- Lethargy |
| Respiratory system | - Apnea<br>- Bronchospasm<br>- Laryngeal spasm |
| Cardiovascular system | - Arrhythmias<br>- Heart failure<br>- Hypotension<br>- Insensitivity to digitalis<br>- ECG-QT and ST-interval prolongation, T wave inversion |
| Psychiatric | - Anxiety<br>- Dementia<br>- Depression<br>- Irritability<br>- Psychosis |

(ECG: electrocardiogram)

- Carpopedal spasm is flexion at the metacarpophalangeal joints and wrist, with extension at the interphalangeal joint and adduction of the digits.
- Trousseau's sign is manifestation of carpopedal spasm during inflation of the sphygmomanometer cuff on the arm.
- Chvostek's sign is twitching of perioral muscles when the facial nerve is tapped anterior to the earlobe.

Calcium is necessary for myocardial contractility. Hypocalcemia can cause hypotension, heart failure, and arrhythmias, and failure of response to drugs that act through the calcium-mediated mechanisms like digoxin, norepinephrine, and dopamine.[12,13]

Hypocalcemia should be considered in the critically ill patients when hypotension is refractory to fluids and vasopressor agents.[14] Calcium correction improves the myocardial contractility and restores vasomotor tone. Use of calcium channel blockers may exacerbate cardiovascular insufficiency in hypocalcemic patients. Acute hypocalcemia can also manifest as severe laryngospasm or bronchospasm in critically ill patients.[15]

### Approach/Evaluation

The systematic approach to a case of hypocalcemia is shown in Flowchart 1. The first step is to send a serum PTH levels.[16] The differential diagnosis for elevated PTH levels with hypocalcemia are many, the most common being vitamin D deficiency and renal failure. If PTH levels are low, the next test to be sent is serum magnesium levels, which if normal, a diagnosis of hypoparathyroidism is made, and if low, a diagnosis of functional hypoparathyroidism is made.

### Management

The rationale for treatment of hypocalcemia will depend on the severity, acuity of presentation, cause, and the presence of symptoms.

- Asymptomatic or mild hypocalcemia or chronic hypocalcemia (ionized calcium levels >0.8 mmol/L or corrected plasma calcium levels >7.5 g/dL)—oral supplementation of elemental calcium in the dosage of 1.5–2 g as calcium carbonate or calcium citrate in daily divided doses is sufficient. Calcium citrate has better bioavailability, but calcium carbonate is cheaper and preferred in patients with renal failure.
- Symptomatic hypocalcemia or severe hypocalcemia (ionized calcium levels <0.8 mmol/L or corrected plasma calcium levels <7.5 g/dL). These conditions warrant intravenous administration of calcium—a bolus of 100–200 mg of elemental calcium given over 10 minutes. Calcium given at a faster rate can cause arrhythmias. If hypocalcemic symptoms persist then an infusion is started in the dose of 15 mg/kg (3.75 mmol/kg) of elemental calcium given over 4–6 hours, which will raise the total serum calcium by 2–3 mg/dL (0.5–0.75 mmol/L).[2] Intravenous calcium is available in several forms; the most common are shown in Table 2.
- Definitive therapy for hypocalcemia is to treat the cause like, vitamin D supplementation in case of deficiency or stopping of offending drugs causing hypocalcemia like bisphosphonates, loop diuretics, calcitonin, or correction of hypomagnesemia and hyperphosphatemia.

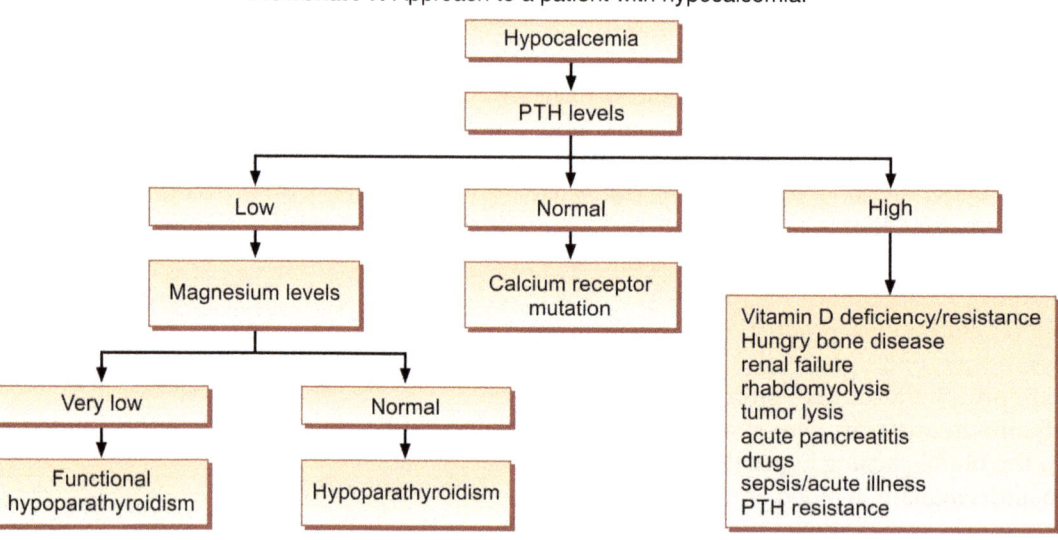

**Flowchart 1:** Approach to a patient with hypocalcemia.

(PTH: parathyroid hormone).

**Table 2:** Intravenous calcium preparations.

| Preparation | Ampoule | Elemental calcium mg (mmol) | Stat dose for acute hypocalcemia | Infusion preparation for acute hypocalcemia |
| --- | --- | --- | --- | --- |
| Calcium gluconate | 10 mL | 93 mg (2.3 mmol) | 1–2 ampoules | 10 ampoules in 900 mL of 5% Dextrose—930 mg/L infused over 4–6 hours or titrate to achieve calcium levels |
| Calcium chloride | 10 mL | 272 mg (6.8 mmol) | | Better bioavailable but more irritant to vein hence less desirable for a prolonged infusion |
| Calcium gluceptate | 5 mL | 90 mg | | Can be used when large volumes cannot be infused. 10 ampoules in 450 mL of 5% D–900 mg/500 mL |

- Vitamin D supplementation in the form of oral 1,25-hydroxyvitamin D or calcitriol in a dose of 0.5–1.0 µg daily is usually sufficient. But in some resistant cases larger doses may be required. Calcitriol is more expensive than vitamin $D_2$ (ergocalciferol) or vitamin $D_3$. Vitamin $D_2$ and vitamin $D_3$ are sufficient as nutritional supplementation in the doses of 400 units per day or in higher doses (50,000–100,000 units) in cases of malabsorption. But they need conversion to the biologically active form of 1,25-hydroxyvitamin D, hence of little use in patients with liver and renal dysfunction.

*Pearls in Managing Hypocalcemia*

There are some important points to remember, before treating hypocalcemia (Box 3).

*Hypocalcemia in critically ill patients*

Even in the absence of pre-existing diseases of calcium homeostasis, acute illness predisposes to hypocalcemia. In a recent review by Aberegg et al. incidence of hypocalcemia was reported up to 50% in intensive care unit (ICU) patients, when ionized calcium levels were measured.[17]

Sometimes, the reasons for hypocalcemia in the critically ill may be clearly evident, as listed in Box 2. Hypomagnesemia, acute renal failure, transfusion of citrated blood, plasma exchange, acute pancreatitis, tumor lysis, rhabdomyolysis and bicarbonate therapy, are some common etiologies for hypocalcemia in the ICU. In more than 50% of the cases of hypocalcemia, the cause may not be evident. Increased circulating cytokines,[18] relative hypoparathyroidism and acquired vitamin D deficiency are some proposed mechanisms for hypocalcemia in these patients.[18] The severity of hypocalcemia is associated with the severity of illness.

Hypocalcemia in critically ill patients may not manifest with the classical signs and symptoms of tetany.[19] The neuromuscular presentation may be masked by the coexisting disease state, or drugs like sedatives, paralytics, and anticonvulsants.

**Box 3:** Pearls in the treatment of hypocalcemia.

- Serum magnesium levels should be restored to normal levels for response to calcium supplementation
- Normalize phosphorus levels—administration of calcium in hyperphosphatemic patients will precipitate calcium phosphate in tissues
- Hypokalemia protects the patient form tetany. Correction of potassium without calcium correction can precipitate tetany
- Drugs that worsen hypocalcemia should be discontinued—like frusemide
- Calcium salts should not be administered with sodium bicarbonate—the mixture precipitates
- Intravenous calcium preparations are irritants to the vein–should be given as an infusion in dextrose solution, preferably through a central vein
- Calcium supplementation should be given cautiously in patients on digoxin—as hypercalcemia can precipitate digoxin toxicity.

As per Cochrane review, there is no clear evidence that parenteral supplementation of calcium impacts the outcome among ICU patients.[20] Calcium administration may actually increase the cytosolic calcium, which is an important second messenger, increasing reactive oxygen species, and may promote programmed cell death or apoptosis.[8]

Till date there are no clear-cut guidelines for routine measurement and correction of hypocalcemia in the critically ill. Critically ill patients probably experience a "sick eucalcemia syndrome",[17] as a defense mechanism, which may normalize with recovery from the illness.

## Case Revisit

Here is an elderly patient presenting with severe vitamin D deficiency leading to symptomatic severe hypocalcemia. Corrected calcium for albumin levels:

Total calcium concentration in serum (mg/dL) + [0.8 × 4.0 – serum albumin concentration (g/dL)] = 5.4 mg/dL (1.35 mmol/L).

In the presented case, severe hypocalcemia should be managed with intravenous 10% calcium gluconate, 1 ampoule given over 10 minutes, followed by an infusion of

10% calcium gluconate prepared with 10 ampoules in 900 mL of 5% D, infused over 6 hours. Serum ionized calcium to be monitored and continuation of intravenous infusion to be decided based on clinical response to therapy. The patient should be supplemented with oral calcium carbonate 500 mg three times a day and vitamin D in the form of calcitriol at a dose of 0.5 µg/day or vitamin $D_3$ at a dose of 400 units/day. The cause for vitamin D deficiency could be secondary to age, poor nutritional intake or malabsorption, and inadequate exposure to sunlight, as patient was bed bound after surgery.

## HYPERCALCEMIA

### Case

A 75-year-old man, with a longstanding history of hypertension and chronic kidney disease since 7 years, on maintenance hemodialysis twice weekly through an arteriovenous fistula, presents to the hospital with weakness of all four limbs and inability to walk for 15 days. Family members noticed that the patient has been excessively sleepy since last 3 days. Patient was brought to the emergency department with the above complaints. There were no other medication uses apart from antihypertensives. On performing his metabolic panel, creatinine was 9.4 mg/dL and corrected calcium was 14.8 mg/dL (ionized calcium was 1.6 mmol/L). The serum phosphorus levels were 2.2 mg/dL. Patient has had high PTH levels of 59.8 pmol/L (reference 1.4–6.8 pmol/L) 1 year back, but serum calcium levels were high normal at that time.

How do we evaluate a patient with hypercalcemia?

### Definition

Hypercalcemia is when calcium levels are more than 10.4 mg/dL (2.60 mmol/L) or ionized calcium levels more than 1.4 mmol/L. Mild-to-moderate hypercalcemia is when the plasma calcium levels are between 10.4 and 12.9 mg/dL (2.60–3.23 mmol/L) or severe hypercalcemia is when the calcium levels are more than 13 mg/dL (3.25 mmol/L). Different references give different values for classification of mild and severe hypercalcemia.

### Etiology/Mechanism

Hypercalcemia is not as common as hypocalcemia in the critically ill, and the incidence can vary from 3 to 32%, depending on the type of ICU population. Pseudohypercalcemia is noted when there is hemoconcentration during venipuncture[21] and in essential thrombocytosis. There are several etiologies for hypercalcemia and these are shown in Box 4.[22]

**Box 4:** Etiology for hypercalcemia.

*Primary hyperparathyroidism:*
- Malignancy:
  - Parathyroid hormone-related protein
  - Lytic bone metastasis
  - Ectopic production of 1,25-hydroxyvitamin D
- Nonparathyroid endocrine disorders:
  - Thyrotoxicosis
  - Pheochromocytoma
  - Adrenal insufficiency
  - Acromegaly
- Granulomatous diseases—producing excess of 1,25-hydroxyvitamin D:
  - Sarcoidosis
  - Tuberculosis
- Immobilization
- Drugs—thiazide diuretics, lithium toxicity
- Vitamin D toxicity
- Vitamin A toxicity
- Parenteral nutrition
- Milk-alkali syndrome
- Acute on chronic renal failure
- Treatment for hypocalcemia
- Hypovolemia
- Tertiary hyperparathyroidism seen in chronic renal failure

Primary hyperparathyroidism, due to increased production of PTH from a parathyroid adenoma, is one of the most common causes for hypercalcemia. It is incidentally detected during routine laboratory measurement of serum calcium levels. Patients generally have a mild hypercalcemia with an inappropriately elevated PTH levels, and rarely may present with renal stones secondary to hypercalciuria.

Severe symptomatic hypercalcemia requiring emergency treatment is generally associated with malignancy. Direct osteolytic lesions of the bone due to metastasis, or secretion of PTH-related protein (PTH-rP) by the malignant cells, are some reasons for hypercalcemia.[23] The PTH-rP, which acts through the PTH receptor is difficult to detect on routine PTH assays. Squamous cell lung cancers, breast cancers, multiple myeloma, T-cell tumors, and other squamous cell tumors are prone for hypercalcemia.

Drugs like thiazide diuretics increase calcium reabsorption from the kidneys causing hypercalcemia.

Granulomatous diseases like sarcoidosis and tuberculosis can cause hypercalcemia by conversion of 25 hydroxyvitamin D to 1,25-dihydroxyvitamin D in the granulomatous tissue.

Excessive consumption of vitamin D and vitamin A can cause hypercalcemia.

Immobilization, especially in young patients with renal insufficiency can cause rapid bone resorption and hypercalcemia.

Hypercalcemia can occur rarely in patients on dialysis who develop aluminum intoxication. Some renal failure patients with prolonged periods of secondary hyperparathyroidism can develop tertiary hyperparathyroidism; a state of autonomous excessive production of PTH resulting in hypercalcemia.

## Clinical Effects

Hypercalcemia can have varied clinical presentation (Table 3). Mild hypercalcemia is generally asymptomatic. Calcium levels more than 12 mg/dL (3.0 mmol/L) present with neurologic, renal, gastrointestinal, and cardiovascular manifestations. Patients present with neuropsychiatric manifestation, weakness, stupor, and coma. Renal manifestations are polyuria due to impaired salt and water absorption and nephrogenic diabetes insipidus. The polyuria results in dehydration and hypovolemia, compounded by poor oral intake due to anorexia, resulting in further impairment in renal excretion of calcium. Hypercalcemia also results in nephrocalcinosis secondary to hypercalciuria.

The clinical manifestations also depend on the age of the patient, the rapidity in increase in calcium levels, other comorbidities, and the duration of hypercalcemia.

## Approach/Evaluation

After rechecking the calcium levels including albumin corrected and ionized levels, check PTH level (Flowchart 2).[16] In case of high PTH level, look for 24-hour urine calcium excretion. While in case of normal or low PTH level, assess PTH-rP level, which further narrows down the differential diagnosis.

## Management[22]

There are four basic principles in the therapy of hypercalcemia:
1. Correct dehydration
2. Enhance renal excretion of calcium
3. Inhibit bone resorption
4. Treat the underlying cause.

### Mild Hypercalcemia

Asymptomatic or mild hypercalcemia that is seen with primary hyperparathyroidism, the treatment is controversial—should the patient be referred to a surgeon for removal of the parathyroid adenoma/gland? Or should the patient be managed medically? There are some generally accepted guidelines for surgical removal of parathyroid glands for hyperparathyroidism[24] as shown in Box 5. Frequent monitoring for symptoms, blood pressure, serum calcium levels, and creatinine levels at regular intervals is necessary in cases of mild hypercalcemia, managed conservatively.

### Severe Hypercalcemia

Management of severe hypercalcemia includes hydration, loop diuretics, and drugs to prevent bone resorption.
- Hydration with saline to restore the intravascular volume to normalcy is the first step in the management of severe hypercalcemia. The saline decreases the serum calcium levels by 1.6–2.4 mg/dL (0.40–0.60 mmol/L) per liter of hydration. Hydration also improves the glomerular filtration rate and thereby increases calcium excretion and decreases reabsorption from the tubules. Fluids should be adjusted based on patient's requirements and tolerance.
- Use of loop diuretics like furosemide helps in urinary excretion of calcium.[25] But the use of diuretics should be after adequate hydration with saline. Thiazide diuretics should be avoided as it increases serum calcium levels.

**Table 3:** Clinical presentation of hypercalcemia.

| Organ system | Manifestation |
|---|---|
| Neurologic | - Drowsiness<br>- Weakness<br>- Depression<br>- Lethargy<br>- Stupor<br>- Coma |
| Gastrointestinal | - Constipation<br>- Nausea<br>- Vomiting<br>- Anorexia<br>- Peptic ulcer disease<br>- Pancreatitis |
| Renal | - Polyuria<br>- Polydipsia<br>- Diabetes insipidus<br>- Nephrolithiasis<br>- Nephrocalcinosis<br>- Acute on chronic renal insufficiency |
| Musculoskeletal | - Bone pain<br>- Osteoporosis |
| Cardiovascular | - Shortening of QT interval<br>- Hypertension |

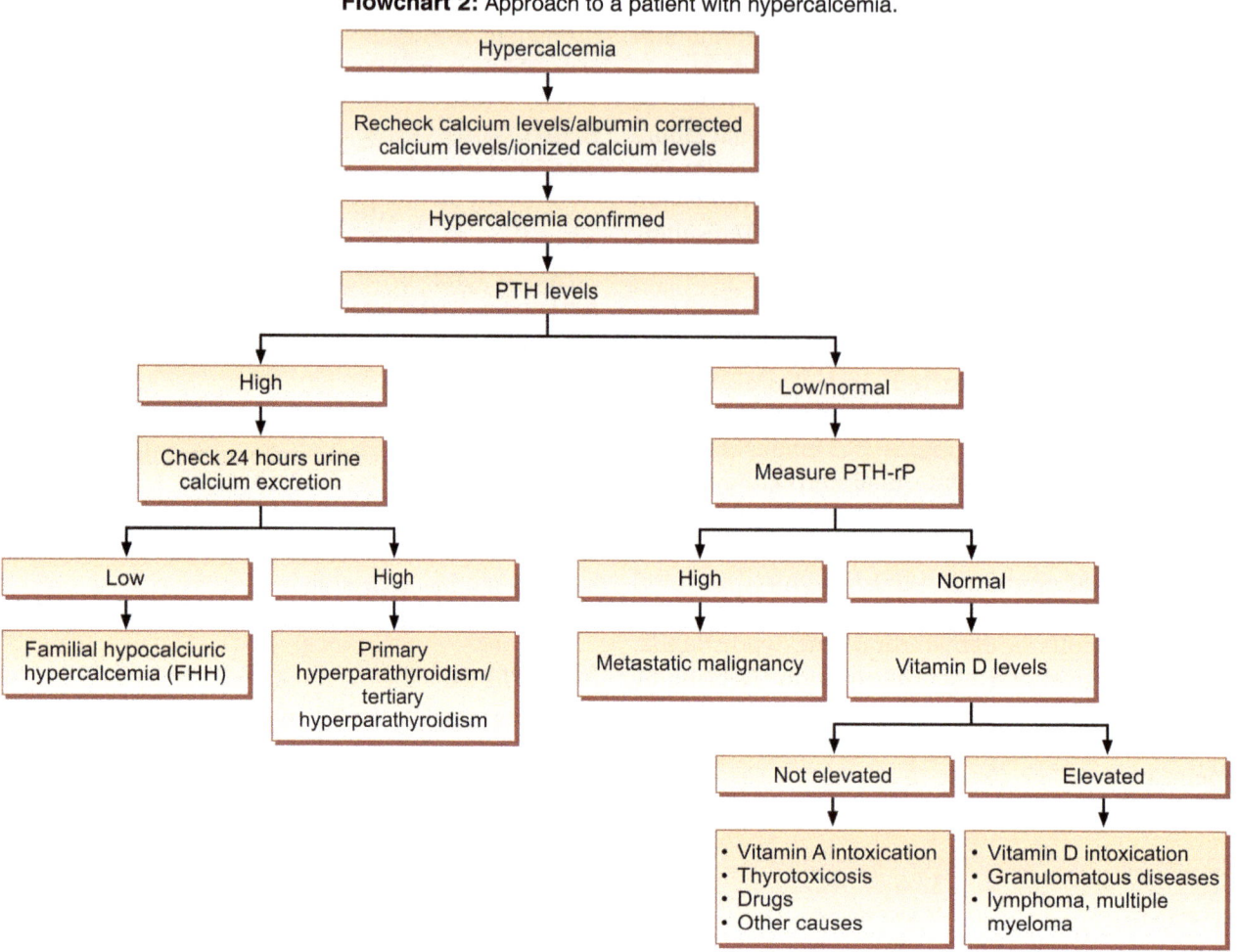

**Flowchart 2:** Approach to a patient with hypercalcemia.

(PTH: parathyroid hormone; rP: related protein).

> **Box 5:** Indications for surgical removal of parathyroid glands.
> - Serum calcium levels > 11.4 mg/dL
> - Previous episodes of life-threatening hypercalcemia
> - Renal insufficiency
> - Nephrocalcinosis
> - Substantial reduction in bone density of > 2 SD below mean for age, sex, and ethnic group
> - Increased 24 hours urinary calcium excretion of more than 400 mg
> - Age less than 50 years

- Drugs that prevent bone resorption:
  - Bisphosphonates (Table 4) are pyrophosphate compounds, which bind to hydroxyapatite in the bone and resist osteoclastic activity. Not only do they inhibit the osteoclastic bone resorption, they also decrease the viability of the osteoclasts.[22] Alendronate and risedronate are potent third generation oral bisphosphonates, not yet approved for treatment of malignancy-associated hypercalcemia. The bisphosphonates are nephrotoxic and need to be used cautiously in patients with impaired renal functions. Both dose reduction and increase in duration of infusion are necessary.
  - Calcitonin is a peptide hormone that inhibits bone resorption, inhibits intestinal absorption of calcium, and increases renal excretion of calcium. It is available as salmon calcitonin and is administered in the dose of 4 units/kg intramuscularly or subcutaneously every 12 hours. Calcitonin nasal spray—1 spray is 200 IU daily in alternating nostril. It has a rapid onset of action, and the effect is seen within hours, but it reaches a peak at 12–24 hours and wears out within 2–3 days. The reduction in calcium levels is very less, 2.0 mg/dL (0.5 mmol/L), hence it should be used with other medications, in case of severe hypercalcemia. But it is very useful for

## Chapter 29
### Approach to the Patient with Hypocalcemia and Hypercalcemia

**Table 4:** Bisphosphonates.

| Bisphosphonates | Dose | Onset/duration of action | Side effects |
|---|---|---|---|
| 1. Etidronate—first generation | 5–7 mg/kg body weight over 4 hours, 3–7 days | 1–2 days/ lasts 5–7 days | Transient increase in creatinine |
| 2. Pamidronate—second generation more potent | 60–90 mg 24 hour IV infusion every 4 weeks, 90 mg dose for severe hypercalcemia Oral 1,200 mg/day for 5 days | 1–2 days/lasts for 10–14 days | Well-tolerated transient leucopenia, a small reduction in phosphate levels, rarely osteonecrosis of the jaw |
| 3. Zoledronate | 4 mg IV over 15 minutes | 1–2 days/duration not known repeat every 3–4 weeks | Same as pamidronate rarely osteonecrosis of maxilla/mandible, renal impairment |
| 4. Ibandronate | 2–6 mg IV over 2 hours | 1–2 days/14 days | Same as pamidronate |

immediate reduction in calcium levels in patients with severe symptoms of hypercalcemia.[26] Calcitonin is generally well tolerated, rarely can cause transient nausea and abdominal cramps. Some patients may have hypersensitivity reactions to salmon calcitonin. Interestingly, it also has analgesic property and helps in reduction of bone pain in patients with skeletal disease.

- Other treatment modalities under investigation or less commonly used:
  - *Calcimimetics:* Calcimimetics are drugs, which mimic the action of calcium on tissues. Cinacalcet was the first calcimimetic drug to be approved. It mimics calcium at the parathyroid CaSRs, decreasing the production of PTH. It is useful for treating hypercalcemia due to primary and tertiary hyperparathyroidism. Dosage is oral tablets of 30 mg-90 mg every 6 hourly or 12 hourly. Common side effects are hypocalcemia, nausea, arthralgia, diarrhea, and paresthesia.
  - Plicamycin inhibits osteoclast formation by inhibiting ribonucleic acid (RNA) synthesis. It is given as an infusion in a dose of 25 µg/kg over 4–6 hours. A single dose is sufficient to normalize the calcium levels. The peak action is at 48–72 hours and the duration of action is for a few days to several weeks. Plicamycin has several side effects limiting its repeated usage. Nausea, local irritation, and extravasation can cause cellulitis, hepatotoxicity, nephrotoxicity, and thrombocytopenia are some side effects. The adverse effects can be reduced with use of recommended dosing and less frequent administration.
  - Glucocorticoids are useful in reduction of calcium levels in patients with hematological malignancies like lymphoma and multiple myeloma, by decreasing the activity of neoplastic tissue. It also counteracts the effects of vitamin D, hence useful in patients with hypercalcemia-associated vitamin D intoxication and granulomatous diseases. Recommended dose is 200-300 mg/day of hydrocortisone or 20–40 mg/day of prednisolone.
  - Gallium nitrate when given intravenously in a dose of 20 mg/sqm BSA in 1 liter of fluid daily for 5 days, adsorbs to hydroxyapatite and prevents bone resorption.[27] Main side effect is renal impairment, especially if given with other nephrotoxic drugs. Hydration can prevent the nephrotoxicity.
  - Intravenous sodium phosphate is to be considered only in severe life-threatening hypercalcemia, because it can precipitate as calcium phosphate in tissues. It causes a predictable reduction in calcium levels, but its use is superseded by other modalities of therapy. It is given as an infusion of 10-15 mmol of sodium phosphate.
- *Other modalities:* Dialysis with low calcium bath dialysate is a very effective means for reduction of calcium levels, especially in those with renal impairment and whom hydration and diuretics cannot be administered.

## Case Revisit

The patient with chronic renal failure on regular hemodialysis with pre-existing secondary hyperparathyroidism (previously elevated PTH levels), developing hypercalcemia, makes us suspect tertiary hyperparathyroidism. The PTH level was repeated and was found to be 192 pmol/L. Since the patient has symptoms of severe hypercalcemia, he should be treated with calcitonin injections 4 U/kg intramuscularly or subcutaneously every 12 hours or a single nasal spray of calcitonin (200 IU)/day. Urgent hemodialysis with a low calcium bath could be used to decrease the calcium levels. Bisphosphonates are not routinely recommended in chronic renal failure. Cinacalcet should be started for decreasing the PTH production, which will decrease the calcium levels. Evaluate for a parathyroid adenoma.

## SALIENT POINTS

- Calcium is an abundant ion found in the ECF that is tightly regulated by hormones, with important biological functions.
- More than half of the plasma concentration of calcium that is unbound to protein, exists in the ionized form.
- The ionized form of calcium is more important than serum calcium, as it is responsible for the symptoms of hypo- and hypercalcemia.
- Acute illness predisposes to hypocalcemia, but routine measurement and correction of hypocalcemia in critically ill patients has not found to be beneficial.
- A systematic approach must be followed for the evaluation and management of hypo- and hypercalcemia.

## REFERENCES

1. Ariyan CE, Sosa JA. Assessment and management of patients with abnormal calcium. Crit Care Med. 2004;32(Suppl 4):S146-54.
2. Bushinsky DA, Monk RD. Electrolyte quintet: Calcium. Lancet. 1998;352(9124):306-11.
3. Watchko J, Bifano EM, Bergstrom WH. Effect of hyperventilation on total calcium, ionized calcium, and serum phosphorus in neonates. Crit Care Med. 1984;12(12):1055-6.
4. Zaloga GP, Willey S, Tomasic P, et al. Free fatty acids alter calcium binding: a cause for misinterpretation of serum calcium values and hypocalcemia in critical illness. J Clin Endocrinol Metab. 1987;64(5):1010-4.
5. Rude RK, Oldham SB, Singer FR. Functional hypoparathyroidism and parathyroid hormone end-organ resistance in human magnesium deficiency. Clin Endocrinol. 1976;5(3):209-24.
6. Zaloga GP. Hypocalcemia in critically ill patients. Crit Care Med. 1992;20(2):251-62.
7. Slomp J, van der Voort PH, Gerritsen RT, et al. Albumin-adjusted calcium is not suitable for diagnosis of hyper- and hypocalcemia in the critically ill. Crit Care Med. 2003;31(5):1389-93.
8. Kelly A, Levine MA. Hypocalcemia in the critically ill patient. J Intensive Care Med. 2013;28(3):166-77.
9. Brasier AR, Nussbaum SR. Hungry bone syndrome: clinical and biochemical predictors of its occurrence after parathyroid surgery. Am J Med. 1988;84(4):654-60.
10. Riancho JA, Arjona R, Valle R, et al. The clinical spectrum of hypocalcaemia associated with bone metastases. J Intern Med. 1989;226(6):449-52.
11. Kahn RC, Jascott D, Carlon GC, et al. Massive blood replacement: Correlation of ionized calcium, citrate, and hydrogen ion concentration. Anesth Analg. 1979;58:274-8.
12. Ginsburg R, Esserman LJ, Bristow MR. Myocardial performance and extracellular ionized calcium in a severely failing human heart. Ann Intern Med. 1983;98(5 Part 1):603-6.
13. Connor TB, Rosen BL, Bleaustein MP, et al. Hypocalcemia precipitating congestive heart failure. N Engl J Med. 1982;307:869-72.
14. Bristow MR, Ginsburg R, Minobe W, et al. Decreased catecholamine sensitivity and beta adrenergic receptor density in failing human hearts. N Engl J Med. 1982;307:205-11.
15. Chernow BA, Zaloga GA, McFadden EL, et al. Hypocalcemia in critically ill patients. Crit Care Med. 1982;10(12):848-51.
16. Body JJ, Bouillon R. Emergencies of calcium homeostasis. Rev Endocr Metab Disord. 2003;4(2):167-75.
17. Aberegg SK. Ionized Calcium in the ICU: Should it Be Measured and Corrected? Chest. 2016;149(3):846-55.
18. Canaff L, Hendy GN. Calcium-sensing receptor gene transcription is up-regulated by the proinflammatory cytokine, interleukin-1β role of the NF-κB pathway and κB elements. J Biol Chem. 2005;280(14):14177-88.
19. Zaloga GP, Chernow B. The multifactorial basis for hypocalcemia during sepsis: studies of the parathyroid hormone-vitamin D axis. Ann Intern Med. 1987;107(1):36-41.
20. Forsythe RM, Wessel CB, Billiar TR, et al. Parenteral calcium for intensive care unit patients. Cochrane Database Syst Rev. 2008;(4):CD006163.
21. McMullan AD, Burns J, Paterson CR. Venepuncture for calcium assays: should we still avoid the tourniquet? Postgrad Med J. 1990;66:547-8.
22. Bilezikian JP. Management of acute hypercalcemia. N Engl J Med. 1992;326(18):1196-203.
23. Mundy GR, Guise TA. Hypercalcemia of malignancy. Am J Med. 1997;103:134-45.
24. Complete Proceedings of the Consensus Development Conference. Diagnosis and management of asymptomatic primary hyperparathyroidism. J Bone Miner Res. 1991;6(Suppl 2):S1-165.
25. Suki WN, Yium JJ, Von Minden M, et al. Acute treatment of hypercalcemia with furosemide. N Engl J Med. 1970;283(16):836-40.
26. Silva OL, Becker KL. Salmon calcitonin in the treatment of hypercalcemia. Arch Intern Med. 1973;132:337-9.
27. Leyland-Jones B. Treatment of cancer-related hypercalcemia: the role of gallium nitrate. Semin Oncol. 2003;30(2 Suppl 5):13-19.

# CHAPTER 30
# Approach to the Patient with Hypophosphatemia and Hyperphosphatemia

*Nasirul J Ekbal, Andrew Davenport, Banwari Agarwal*

## PHOSPHATE HOMEOSTASIS

Phosphate is the most abundant intracellular anion. It contains four oxygen atoms and a central phosphorus atom. 85% of the body's phosphate stores exist as hydroxyapatite, the main mineral component of bone.[1] However, phosphate also forms an integral part of various cell structures, present in both intra- and extra-cellular fluids and participates in most biological processes. Only 0.1% of total body phosphate is present in extracellular fluid and the serum concentration ranges from 0.80 to 1.40 mmol/L (2.5–4.3 mg/dL). Normal dietary intake (dairy products, meat, and eggs) is usually about 700–1400 mg per day.[2] Phosphate absorption is highly efficient (~70%) and occurs predominantly via the active type IIb sodium phosphate cotransporters (Npt2b) on the apical brush border of the small intestine (duodenum and jejunum). The kidneys play a key role in phosphate homeostasis, the majority of phosphate is recovered by reabsorption (85%) by three renal sodium phosphate cotransporters—Npt2a, Npt2c, and PiT-2; all located in the apical border in the proximal convoluted tubule.[3] Parathyroid hormone and fibroblast growth factor 23 (FGF23) decrease tubular phosphate reabsorption, whereas 1,25-dihydroxycholecalciferol (calcitriol) increases reabsorption and enhances absorption from the gastrointestinal tract.[4]

## HYPOPHOSPHATEMIA

### Case

A 45-year-old man with a history of chronic pancreatitis (secondary to alcohol abuse) is admitted to intensive care unit and diagnosed with severe community pneumonia. He is currently being mechanically ventilated and requiring 0.30 µg/kg/min of noradrenaline to maintain a mean arterial pressure of 65 mm Hg. He has a body weight of 45 kg and a body mass index (BMI) of 18 kg/m². He is due to commence enteral feeding. Five days after initiation of feeding he has the following blood tests (Table 1).

### Definition

Approximately 5% of hospitalized patients have hypophosphatemia, which is defined as mild, moderate, and severe for serum phosphate levels of 0.65–0.81 mmol/L (2–2.5 mg/dL), 0.32–0.65 mmol/L (1–2 mg/dL), and 0.32 mmol/L (<1 mg/dL), respectively.

### Etiology/Mechanism

Hypophosphatemia is particularly more frequent in certain patient groups, such as diabetic ketoacidosis, sepsis, and postoperative patients thus, has a high prevalence in the critically ill patients.[5] Hypophosphatemia can occur by several different mechanisms:

### Inadequate Intake

All living organisms rely on energy rich phosphate moieties; adenosine triphosphate (ATP), adenosine diphosphate (ADP), and adenine monophosphate (AMP) to drive cellular metabolism. As such it would be very unusual for patients to

**Table 1:** Laboratory values of a case presented with hypophosphatemia.

| | |
|---|---|
| Na⁺ | 138 mmol/L (mEq/L) |
| K⁺ | 2.8 mmol/L (mEq/L) |
| HCO₃⁻ | 24 mmol/L (mEq/L) |
| PO₄⁻ | 0.53 mmol/L (mEq/L) |
| Mg²⁺ | 0.85 mmol/L (mEq/L) |
| Urea | 6.0 mmol/L (mEq/L) |
| Creatinine | 70 µmol/L (0.2 mg/L) |

have insufficient dietary phosphate intake, unless they had a severe sicca syndrome, anorexia, or starvation, or bulimia.

### Internal Redistribution of Phosphate

Internal distribution is the most common cause of hypophosphatemia in critically ill patients. Increased production of glycolytic phosphorylated compounds during stress uses up extracellular stores of phosphate. Low phosphate levels occur after major surgery particularly after major hepatic surgery, where almost all patients develop hypophosphatemia in the first week.[6] In addition, use of insulin either during treatment of diabetic ketoacidosis or to control hyperglycemia decreases serum phosphate due to intracellular movement with glucose.[7] Commonly used drugs, such as epinephrine and norepinephrine, potentiate this effect. In patients with hyperglycemia, the subsequent osmotic diuresis exacerbates hypophosphatemia and requires careful monitoring. Influx of phosphate into cells is a primary manifestation of the refeeding syndrome during the anabolic stage. Another cause of redistribution is respiratory alkalosis in which the increase in intracellular pH stimulates glycolysis and causes phosphate to enter cells.[8]

### Decreased Intestinal Absorption

Decreased intestinal absorption of phosphate is unlikely to cause hypophosphatemia as a low-phosphate diet results in upregulation of both intestinal uptake and renal absorption.[9] However, this should still be considered in patients with intestinal malabsorption, either due to primary intestinal disorders, chronic diarrhea, vomiting, or use of aluminum or magnesium-containing antacids. Phosphate is absorbed in the small intestine by a series of sodium-phosphate cotransporters (NaPi-IIb) predominantly in the duodenum compared to jejunum and ileum. Phosphate may also be absorbed to a lesser extent by sodium-independent mechanisms in the ileum and the colon. 1,25-dihydroxyvitamin D3 is an important physiological regulator of intestinal phosphate absorption increasing phosphate transport in both the duodenum and jejunum. Specific regions of the small intestine adapt differently to acute or chronic changes in dietary phosphate load and phosphatonins, FGF23 and secreted frizzled-related protein 4 (SFRP4), inhibit both renal and intestinal phosphate transport. It had been thought that increased intestinal phosphate absorption stimulated the kidneys to rapidly excrete phosphate, mediated by a gut-derived phosphaturic factor. However, no phosphaturic factor has yet been identified, and it is now thought that hyperphosphatemia and increased parathyroid hormone concentrations are most likely the drivers for phosphaturia following supraphysiological intestinal phosphate absorption, by downregulation of renal sodium-phosphate cotransporters (NaPi-IIa).

### Increase Urinary Phosphate Excretion

Renal loss of phosphate is commonly due to the use of diuretic therapy but may also be seen with other drugs (Table 2). Primary hyperparathyroidism and vitamin D deficiency are causes of acquired phosphate wasting whereas X-linked hypophosphatemia (XLH) of which 39 mutations in the PHEX gene have been identified so far, and autosomal recessive vitamin D-resistant rickets are genetic causes.[7] Hypophosphatemia is also seen in Fanconi's syndrome due to a global defect in proximal tubular function and has numerous etiologies.[4] Fanconi's syndrome may be inherited as with cystinosis, Dent's disease; Dent 1 [a defect of chloride voltage-gated channel 5 (CLCN5 transporter)] and Dent 2 and Lowe's syndrome [variants of inositol polyphosphate 5-phosphatase (OCRL-1)], tyrosinemia, Wilson's disease, galactosemia, glycogen storage diseases, hereditary fructose intolerance, and more recently mutations of the bifunctional peroxisomal protein with the N terminal having enoyl-CoA hydratase activity while the C-terminal region contains 3-hydroxyacyl-CoA dehydrogenase activity (EHHADH). Acquired forms of the Fanconi syndrome include drugs (Table 2), lead poisoning, multiple myeloma, or monoclonal gammopathy of undetermined significance, autoimmune forms of interstitial nephritis, including Sjögren's syndrome.

**Table 2:** Drug-induced hypophosphatemia.

| Drug class | Example | Mechanism |
| --- | --- | --- |
| Tyrosine kinase inhibitor | Sorafenib Regorafenib Tipifarnib | Renal tubular injury |
| Reverse transcriptase inhibitors | Adefovir Tenofovir Ledipasvir Didanosine Sofosbuvir | Fanconi syndrome |
| Cytotoxic drugs | Ifosfamide Cisplatin | Renal tubular injury |
| Anticonvulsants | Valproic acid | Fanconi syndrome |
| Antibiotics | Gentamicin Amikacin | Renal tubular injury |
| | Out of date tetracycline | Fanconi syndrome |
| Iron preparations | Deferasirox Ferric carboxymaltose | Fanconi syndrome |

Mesenchymal tumors may also cause hypophosphatemia, sometimes referred to as oncogenic osteomalacia. These tumors can produce FGF23 and to a lesser extent SFRP4. FGF23, in particular inhibits the production of 1,25 dihydroxylated vitamin D3, and also causes internalization of NaPi cotransporters leading to reduced renal proximal tubular reabsorption and urinary phosphate wasting. These mesenchymal tumors include oat cell and small cell cancers, ovarian and renal cell cancers, neurofibromatosis type II, and anaplastic thyroid cancers. The bone lesions in acromegalic patients with the McCune-Albright syndrome can also produce FGF23 and leading to urinary phosphate wasting. Both primary hyperparathyroidism and parathyroid hormone (PTH) secreted by tumors can also lead to renal tubular phosphate wasting.

### Renal Replacement Therapies

Finally, phosphate has a molecular weight of only 95 Daltons and is therefore easily cleared, with potential rapid changes in serum concentrations, in the effluent fluid during hemodialysis and hemofiltration with renal replacement therapy in critical care patients, particularly with continuous forms of renal replacement therapy (CRRT), as the longer treatment times allow greater phosphate transfer, compared to the shorter session times of intermittent hemodialysis treatments, from intracellular stores into the plasma and then clearance into the dialysate or filtrate.[9]

### Clinical Effects

Hypophosphatemia most often remains asymptomatic, however, physiological disturbances usually occur with severe hypophosphatemia (serum phosphate <0.4 mmol/L (1.2 mg/dL)) and fatal complications have been described. Hypophosphatemia impairs intracellular energy production causing cellular dysfunction. Weakness of skeletal or smooth muscle, ranging from ophthalmoplegia to proximal myopathy, is the most common clinical consequence of phosphate deficiency.[10] More importantly, phosphate depletion results in impaired myocardial contractility and a relationship between hypophosphatemia and acute heart failure exists.[11] Indeed, increased inotropic support is associated with hypophosphatemia following cardiac surgery[12] and correction of phosphate may improve cardiac output in patients with concomitant heart failure.[13] A reduced threshold for both supraventricular and ventricular arrhythmias in the hypophosphatemic myocardium is also reported, and these arrhythmias may prove refractory until phosphate concentrations are restored.[14]

Respiratory insufficiency with diaphragmatic dysfunction is impaired in severe hypophosphatemia presenting with acute respiratory failure or failure to wean from ventilation.[15] Phosphate deficiency also reduces tissue oxygen delivery due to depletion of 2,3-diphosphoglycerate (2,3-DPG) and shift of the oxygen dissociation curve to the left and this effect may be more marked in those with chronic lung disease.[9] Hematologic dysfunction, such as impaired phagocytosis is also seen, and may explain the association with gram-negative bacteremia developing in hypophosphatemic patients. Multiple studies show an association between hypophosphatemia and increased mortality; however, it remains unclear whether a low serum phosphate is directly causal in itself, or merely a marker of illness severity.[5]

### Approach/Evaluation

In addition to serum phosphate studies, a bone profile (including serum calcium, albumin parathyroid hormone, vitamin D levels, both 25-hydroxylated vitamin D3 and 1,25 dihydroxylated vitamin D3, FGF23, and tumor secreted PTH fragments) can be helpful. High calcium with low PTH indicates primary hyperparathyroidism. High PTH levels with low calcium and phosphate suggest intestinal malabsorption or vitamin D deficiency. Low levels of other serum electrolytes, e.g. magnesium and potassium is seen in poor nutritional states.[7] An arterial blood gas may also be helpful if a respiratory alkalosis is suspected. If the diagnosis of hypophosphatemia is not apparent, a 24-hour urine collection can be measured or a fractional excretion of filtered phosphate ($FEPO_4$) calculated. Less than 100 mg of phosphate in 24 hours or an $FEPO_4$ less than 5% indicates appropriate low tubular phosphate excretion suggesting internal redistribution or decreased intestinal absorption. Phosphate excretion of over 100 mg or a $FEPO_4$ greater than 5% indicates renal phosphate wasting.[16]

### Management

Depending on the severity of hypophosphatemia, replacement may be enteral or parenteral. However, though hypophosphatemia is associated with increased mortality in patient subgroups, e.g. sepsis,[17] no randomized controlled evidence exists to whether correction, or the speed of correction of hypophosphatemia in asymptomatic patients improves outcomes. Therefore, currently no widely agreed guidelines exist for the monitoring of serum levels and treatment of hypophosphatemia in critically ill patients.[5] Indeed, mild hypophosphatemia may not necessarily require specific treatment. A reasonable approach would be enteral replacement is asymptomatic patients with a serum phosphate below 0.64 mmol/L (2.0 mg/dL), who are absorbing feed. Oral forms include Phosphate-Sandoz® which contains 16.1 mmol (mEq) of $PO_4^{2-}$. Recognized regimes include up to six tablets daily, in divided doses, which must be dissolved in water and care must be taken to avoid combination with calcium or magnesium salts due to the risk of both aggregation and blocking of fine bore nasogastric tubes, and also binding in the gut and reduced phosphate absorption.[18]

Intravenous correction of hypophosphatemia is in the form of a phosphate Polyfuser® [containing $PO_4^{2-}$ 100 mmol/L (mEq/L), $K^+$ 19 mmol/L (mEq/L), and $Na^+$ 162 mmol/L (mEq/L)] and should be given via a central venous catheter due to the risk venous thrombophlebitis. Intravenous correction should be reserved for patients who are symptomatic or phosphate levels of below 0.32 mmol/L (12.4 mg/dL). Replacement is usually 9 mmol (mEq) every 12 hours, however, in critically ill patients the dose may be increased to 30–50 mmol (mEq) according to severity over 6–12 hours. This is because although multiple studies have confirmed the safety of phosphate regimens,[5] intravenous administration is not without complications. Large intravenous phosphate doses may exacerbate hypocalcemia (due to precipitation) and calcium should be corrected before phosphate replacement. In addition, hypomagnesemia and hypotension may result.[5] In theory rapid infusion of phosphate also risks precipitation of small crystals of calcium and phosphate. Rare cases of calcification in the lungs resulting in a stiff lung syndrome and difficulty in ventilation and also in the kidney leading to acute or chronic kidney injury have been reported. In patients with renal impairment, the risk of hyperphosphatemia is high and caution should be taken in this particular group. Caution should also be taken as intravenous phosphate has a volume of at least 500 mL and a relatively high sodium load and therefore may be unsuitable for patients at risk of volume overload. Alternative replacement regimes include nonproprietary potassium phosphates, which reduce the need for high-sodium content fluid with lower volume solutions (usually containing 1 mmol/mL (mEq/mL) phosphate and 1 mmol/mL (mEq/mL) potassium). These solutions can be added to both intravenous fluid and total parenteral nutrition.[9] Traditionally dialysis fluids have been phosphate free, but recently commercial dialysates and replacement solutions designed for CRRT containing 1.2 mmol/L (3.7 mg/dL) concentration of phosphate have become available to prevent hypophosphatemia developing during CRRT.

## Case Revisit

The results of the index case show hypokalemia, hypophosphatemia and hypomagnesemia, and are consistent with refeeding syndrome. This patient is particularly at risk, as he appears to be severely malnourished with a history of alcoholism. Refeeding syndrome is defined as clinical complications that occur due to the derangement in fluids and electrolytes after rapid nutritional rehabilitation (enteral or parental) to malnourished patients.[19] Starvation results in a shift to fat and protein metabolism, however, the change from catabolic to anabolic metabolism with reinstitution of a carbohydrate load, triggers a surge of insulin release that shifts electrolytes into intracellular compartments.[20] The hallmark biochemical feature is *hypophosphatemia*. Alterations in potassium and/or magnesium, as well as water, sodium and thiamine balance also feature.[21] Life-threatening clinical features include neuromuscular dysfunction, respiratory insufficiency, cardiac arrhythmias, heart failure, and death.[22] Prevention of refeeding syndrome involves lower rates of nutritional support, e.g. 10 kcal/kg/day, ensuring careful monitoring of fluids and electrolytes with appropriate early replacement in addition to providing multivitamin supplementation (specifically thiamine).[23]

## HYPERPHOSPHATEMIA

### Case

A 35-year-old man undertook a 20-mile marathon. After 6 hours, toward the end of the finish line, he collapsed due to severe leg weakness and cramps. He was taken to the nearest emergency department with his partner, who revealed that he had no past medical or family history of illness and did not take any regular medication. This was also his first attempt at long distance running.

The patient had the following blood and arterial blood gas results (Table 3).

### Definition

Hyperphosphatemia is defined as levels above 1.45 mmol/L (4.5 mg/L).

### Etiology/Mechanism

Hyperphosphatemia can result from four different mechanisms:

#### Increase Phosphate Load

Exogenous phosphate intake alone is an uncommon cause of hyperphosphatemia, particularly in the presence

# Chapter 30
## Approach to the Patient with Hypophosphatemia and Hyperphosphatemia

**Table 3:** Laboratory and arterial blood gas values of a case of hyperphosphatemia.

| Blood test results | | Arterial blood gas results on air | |
|---|---|---|---|
| Na+ | 145 mmol/L (mEq/L) | pH | 7.20 |
| K+ | 6.5 mmol/L (mEq/L) | pO2 | 11.0 kPa (82.5 mm Hg) |
| Urea | 22.0 mmol/L (mEq/L) | pCO2 | 3.3 kPa (24.7 mm Hg) |
| Creatinine | 300 µmol/L 3.39 mg/dL | HCO3− | 16.3 mmol/L (mEq/L) |
| Albumin | 38 g/L | Cl− | 92 mmol/L (mEq/L) |
| Bilirubin | 12 µmol/L | Lactate | 5.0 mmol/L (mEq/L) |
| AST | 260 IU/L | BE | −6.8 mmol/L (mEq/L) |
| ALP | 60 IU/L | | |
| Corrected Ca2+ | 1.95 mmol/L (6.0 g/dL) | | |
| PO4− | 2.5 mmol/L (7.7 g/dL) | | |
| CK | 40,000 IU/L | | |

of normal renal function; however, a number of reports exist of hyperphosphatemia after excessive use of sodium phosphate laxatives leading to acute phosphate nephropathy.[24] However, volume contraction, due to diarrhea caused by the laxatives and preexisting chronic kidney disease (CKD) may contribute in this setting. Excessive phosphate loads from the intracellular compartment due to tissue breakdown and release into the extracellular space is more likely to be encountered in critical care practice. Clinical conditions include tumor lysis syndrome, caused by cytotoxic chemotherapy in patients with large tumor burdens can lead to hyperphosphatemia, as can extensive crush injury and rhabdomyolysis. In addition, malignant hyperthermia, burns, and acute severe organ damage including acute red blood cell lysis (glucose-6-phosphate dehydrogenase deficiency), fulminant hepatitis, and acute kidney injury.

### Acute Intracellular to Extracellular Shift

Intracellular shifts of phosphate from intact cells are uncommon but may be seen in conditions with severe lactic acidosis and hyperglycemia. Metabolic acidosis reduces the glycolytic pathway and in diabetic ketoacidosis, with insulin deficiency, results in diminished cellular phosphate utilization with subsequent hyperphosphatemia.[9]

### Decreased Phosphate Excretion/Increase in Tubular Phosphate Reabsorption

However, the most common cause of hyperphosphatemia is acute or CKD. Once GFR falls below 20–25 mL/min, free serum calcium levels fall and phosphate rises. Stimulation of the parathyroid glands produce PTH which leads to maximal suppression of reabsorption of phosphate and increased phosphaturia however as GFR continues to fall, these compensatory mechanisms fail and tubular excretion is overwhelmed by ongoing intestinal absorption.[3] Conversely, an increase in proximal tubular phosphate reabsorption in patients with otherwise normal renal function is seen in conditions such as hypoparathyroidism which may be due to developmental abnormalities, autoimmune diseases, postneck surgery, or irradiation, and activating mutations of the calcium-sensing receptor. The genetic forms are very rare and relate to defects in G-coupled proteins; type 1a Albright's hereditary osteodystrophy (gene *GNAS1*), type 1b associated with a methylation defect (gene *GNAS1/STX16*), and type 2 which has a normal response to cyclic AMP. In addition, hyperphosphatemia may be due to a lack of PTH effects, as with bisphosphonate use, and secondary to hypercalcemia seen with vitamin D toxicity, milk-alkali syndrome, sarcoidosis, hyper- and hypomagnesemia, immobilization, osteolytic metastases, and tumoral calcinosis. Other causes include vitamin A toxicity and acromegaly.

### Pseudohyperphosphatemia

Delay in analyzing samples and excessive pressure applied during venepuncture increase phosphate leakage from red blood cells causing pseudohyperphosphatemia. Interference with biochemical analysis may produce falsely raised serum phosphate. This has been described in conditions with excess immunoglobulins (e.g. multiple myeloma), hyperlipidemia and hyperbilirubinemia. Amphotericin B and heparin are also noted to cause spurious hyperphosphatemia.[25]

## Clinical Effects

Even severe hyperphosphatemia is for the most part asymptomatic, however, rapid increases may cause acute hypocalcemic symptoms and present with tetany. In prolonged hyperphosphatemia, calcium and phosphate are at the limits of solubility in plasma therefore a raised calcium × phosphate product (Ca × P) is associated with increased risk precipitation and ectopic soft tissue calcifications.[26] Hyperparathyroidism is an independent risk factor contributing to calciphylaxis, a severe form of vascular thrombotic occlusion with endoluminal calcification inducing painful skin and subcutaneous fat infarction, affecting up to 4% of patients with end-stage renal disease.[27] In response to elevated phosphate concentrations, genes such as *CBFA1* are activated and trigger vascular smooth muscle cells to differentiate and undergo osteogenic transformation, which promotes vascular calcification of blood vessel walls and arteriosclerosis. This increase in vascular stiffness predisposes to systolic hypertension and left ventricular hypertrophy.[28]

### Approach/Evaluation

In addition to the investigations described above for hypophosphatemia, elevated creatinine values help to determine whether kidney disease is the cause of hyperphosphatemia. Serum calcium and magnesium levels are typically low. Additional tests include serum creatine kinase (CK) and urine myoglobin (rhabdomyolysis) and exclusion of tumor lysis syndrome with serum urate and lactate dehydrogenase if clinically indicated.[7] Rarely, if the cause of hyerphosphatemia remains unclear, a 24-hour measurement of urinary phosphate can be performed; $FEPO_4$ exceeding 15% confirms massive phosphate ingestion (e.g. laxative abuse) or tissue lysis whereas a $FEPO_4$ less than 15% suggests either renal impairment or hypoparathyroidism.[29]

### Management

No treatment is usually required in the acute setting and hyperphosphatemia may be corrected by treating the underlying cause; however, severe hyperphosphatemia can be life-threatening if associated with sudden hyperkalemia or symptomatic hypocalcemia. In patients with normal kidney function, a phosphate diuresis can be induced with volume resuscitation using normal saline. Renal replacement therapy may be required, particularly if renal function is severely impaired in cases of rapid cell turnover or breakdown. In chronic hyperphosphatemia, unnecessary dietary phosphate (e.g. cola, preprepared sauces) should be restricted, in favor of adequate protein intake (e.g. eggs). However, oral phosphate binders, both calcium- (Calcichew/OsvaRen) and noncalcium (Sevelamer/Lanthanum) containing preparations reduce absorption from the small bowel, are usually required to control serum phosphate for patients with CKD stages 4 and 5 (estimated glomerular filtration rate <30 mL/min, <15 mL/min).[26] All agents lower serum phosphate by binding phosphate in the GI tract thereby reducing intestinal absorption. Hence, these medication need to be taken with food to bind any phosphate present.

### Case Revisit

The history and classical biochemical picture of hyperkalemia, hyperphosphatemia, hypocalcemia, high aspartate aminotransferase (AST) and an acute kidney injury, is suggestive of exercise-induced rhabdomyolysis. Rhabdomyolysis is the "dissolution" skeletal muscle and is a clinical syndrome characterized by the leakage of extravasation of muscle cell contents including electrolytes and sarcoplasmic proteins, e.g. myoglobin into the circulation.[30] Although myoglobinuria is pathognomonic for rhabdomyolysis, the significantly raised serum CK is a more useful marker for the diagnosis and assessment of severity because of its delayed clearance from plasma.[31] The underlying precipitant may be traumatic or nontraumatic as in the case above, and causes the energy-dependent Na-K-ATPase pump on myocyte membranes to fail. This causes impairment of sarcoplasmic calcium efflux from the cell and activation of cytolytic enzymes leading to subsequent myocyte disintegration.[32] Regardless of cause, acute kidney injury is one of the most severe complications of rhabdomyolysis and develops in up to a third of patients. The mechanism of injury is believed to be triggered by conversion of $Fe^{3+}$ to the highly reactive $Fe^{4+}$ species, which causes free radical production and oxidative cellular damage, and myoglobin precipitation in the renal tubules.[33] Goals in the treatment of rhabdomyolysis includes avoidance of further renal injury by ensuring adequate hydration and possible urinary alkalization with bicarbonate to keep pH more than 6.5,[34] although evidence is limited.[35] Further management includes management of electrolyte disturbances (e.g. hyperkalemia) and consideration of renal replacement therapy.

## SALIENT POINTS

- Phosphate homeostasis is under tight physiological control.
- Hypophosphatemia is common in critically ill patients, and may cause a multitude of systemic effects.
- No widely agreed guidelines exist for the thresholds of treatment of hypophosphatemia in critically ill patients.
- Hyperphosphatemia is unusual in critically ill patients. However, in the context of acute cellular destruction or breakdown, prompt recognition of the underlying cause and institution of treatment is required.

## REFERENCES

1. Waldmann C, Soni N, Rhodes A (Eds). Oxford Desk Reference: Critical Care. London: Oxford University Press; 2008.
2. Kalantar-Zadeh K, Gutekunst L, Mehrotra R, et al. Understanding sources of dietary phosphorus in the treatment of patients with chronic kidney disease. Clin J Am Soc Nephrol. 2010;5(3):519-30.
3. Blaine J, Chonchol M, Levi M. Renal control of calcium, phosphate, and magnesium homeostasis. Clin J Am Soc Nephrol. 2015;10(7):1257-72.
4. Johnson RJ, Feehally J, Floege J. Comprehensive Clinical Nephrology, 5th edition. Philadelphia, PA: Saunders; 2014. pp. 1-1320.
5. Geerse DA, Bindels AJ, Kuiper MA, et al. Treatment of hypophosphatemia in the intensive care unit: a review. Crit Care. 2010;14(4):R147.
6. Salem RR, Tray K. Hepatic resection-related hypophosphatemia is of renal origin as manifested by isolated hyperphosphaturia. Ann Surg. 2005;241(2):343-8.
7. Barratt J, Harris K, Topham P. Oxford Desk Reference: Nephrology. Oxford: Oxford University Press; 2008.
8. Paleologos M, Stone E, Braude S. Persistent, progressive hypophosphataemia after voluntary hyperventilation. Clin Sci (Lond). 2000;98(5):619-25.
9. Wadsworth RL, Siddiqui S. Phosphate homeostasis in critical care. BJA Education. 2016;16(9):305-9.
10. Knochel JP. The pathophysiology and clinical characteristics of severe hypophosphatemia. Arch Intern Med. 1977;137(2):203-20.
11. Keşkek ŞÖ, Sağlıker Y, Kırım S, et al. Low serum phosphorus level in Massry's phosphate depletion syndrome may be one of the causes of acute heart failure. J Nutr Sci Vitaminol (Tokyo). 2015;61(6):460-4.
12. Cohen J, Kogan A, Sahar G, et al. Hypophosphatemia following open heart surgery: incidence and consequences. Eur J Cardiothorac Surg. 2004;26(2):306-10.
13. Davis SV, Olichwier KK, Chakko SC. Reversible depression of myocardial performance in hypophosphatemia. Am J Med Sci. 1988;295:183-7.
14. Ognibene A, Ciniglio R, Greifenstein A, et al. Ventricular tachycardia in acute myocardial infarction: the role of hypophosphatemia. South Med J. 1994;87(1):65-9.
15. Alsumrain MH, Jawad SA, Imran NB, et al. Association of hypophosphatemia with failure-to-wean from mechanical ventilation. Ann Clin Lab Sci. 2010;40(2):144-8.
16. Yu ASL, Stubbs JR. (2017). Evaluation and Treatment of Hypophosphatemia. [online] Available from http://www.uptodate.com [Last accessed January, 2019].
17. Shor R, Halabe A, Rishver S, et al. Severe hypophosphatemia in sepsis as a mortality predictor. Ann Clin Lab Sci. 2006;36(1):67-72.
18. White R, Bradnam V. Handbook of Drug Administration Via Enteral Feeding Tubes, 1st edition. UK: Pharmaceutical Press; 2007.
19. Mehanna HM, Moledina J, Travis J. Refeeding syndrome: what it is, and how to prevent and treat it. BMJ. 2008;336(7659):1495-8.
20. Crook MA. Refeeding syndrome: problems with definition and management. Nutrition. 2014;30(11-12):1448-55.
21. Scott R, Bowling TE. Enteral tube feeding in adults. J R Coll Physicians Edinb. 2015;45(1):49-54.
22. Ziegler TR. Parenteral nutrition in the critically ill patient. N Engl J Med. 2009;361(11):1088-97.
23. National Collaborating Centre for Acute Care. (2006). NICE Guidelines [CG32]. Nutritional Support for Adults: Oral Nutrition Support, Enteral Tube Feeding and Parental Nutrition. [online] Available from https://www.nice.org.uk/guidance/gc32 [Last accessed January, 2019].
24. Markowitz GS, Stokes MB, Radhakrishnan J, et al. Acute phosphate nephropathy following oral sodium phosphate bowel purgative: an underrecognized cause of chronic renal failure. J Am Soc Nephrol. 2005;16(11):3389-96.
25. Stubbs JR, Yu AS, Chir B. (2017). Overview of the Causes and Treatment of Hyperphosphatemia. [online] Available from http://www.uptodate.com [Last accessed January, 2019].
26. Steddon S, Chesser A, Cunningham J, et al. Oxford Handbook of Nephrology and Hypertension, 2nd edition. London: Oxford University Press; 2014.
27. Magro CM, Simman R, Jackson S. Calciphylaxis: a review. J Am Col Certif Wound Spec. 2010;2(4):66-72.
28. Alesutan I, Voelkl J, Feger M, et al. Involvement of vascular aldosterone synthase in phosphate-induced osteogenic transformation of vascular smooth muscle cells. Sci Rep. 2017;7(1):2059.
29. Lederer H. (2018). Hyperphosphatemia Treatment & Management. [online] Available from https://emedicine.medscape.com [Last accessed January, 2019].
30. Bosch X, Poch E, Grau JM. Rhabdomyolysis and acute kidney injury. N Engl J Med. 2009;361(1):62-72.
31. Keltz E, Khan FY, Mann G. Rhabdomyolysis. The role of diagnostic and prognostic factors. Muscles Ligaments Tendons J. 2013;3(4):303-12.
32. Petejova N, Martinek A. Acute kidney injury due to rhabdomyolysis and renal replacement therapy: a critical review. Crit Care. 2014;18(3):224.
33. Torres PA, Helmstetter JA, Kaye AM, et al. Rhabdomyolysis: pathogenesis, diagnosis, and treatment. Ochsner J. 2015;15(1):58-69.
34. Slater MS, Mullins RJ. Rhabdomyolysis and myoglobinuric renal failure in trauma and surgical patients: a review. J Am Coll Surg. 1998;186(6):693-716.
35. Scharman EJ, Troutman WG. Prevention of kidney injury following rhabdomyolysis: a systematic review. Ann Pharmacother. 2013;47(1):90-105.

# CHAPTER 31

# Approach to the Patient with Hypomagnesemia and Hypermagnesemia

Dharshan Rangaswamy

## MAGNESIUM HOMEOSTASIS

Magnesium ($Mg^{++}$), a divalent cation is the most abundant intracellular cation after potassium. Majority of the intracellular $Mg^{++}$ in the body (99%) is mainly present in the bone (50-60%, hydroxyappetite crystals), muscles (20%), and soft tissues including liver. In bone, $Mg^{++}$ stores are dynamic, with increased turnover and osteopenia in low serum $Mg^{++}$ states.[1] Only 1% of the body $Mg^{++}$ is found in extracellular space. The normal serum $Mg^{++}$ concentration ranges between 1.7 and 2.6 mg/dL (0.7-1.1 mmol/L or 1.4-2.2 mEq/L).[2] Approximately 70% of serum $Mg^{++}$ is in the free form and 30% is albumin bound. The nonbound form is ultrafiltrable in the kidney and majority is present as free, ionized, and physiologically active $Mg^{++}$ with only a small portion bound to other serum anions.[3-6]

$Mg^{++}$ serves as a co-factor for many biological processes that utilize ATP. It is essential for intracellular signaling, protein, and DNA synthesis, oxidative phosphorylation, mineralization of bone, maintaining cardiovascular tone, and for neuromuscular excitability and relaxation. Release of parathyroid hormone (PTH) and its target organ sensitivity is regulated by $Mg^{++}$.[1,7] It also plays an important role in maintaining calcium and potassium homeostasis.[2-6]

$Mg^{++}$ homeostasis is mainly regulated by the interplay of kidney, gastrointestinal tract and the bone. A regular diet contains about 300 mg/day of $Mg^{++}$ and is mainly absorbed in the small intestine (jejunum and ileum) and to a lesser extent from the sigmoid colon. The absorption ranges from 25% (during $Mg^{++}$ rich diet) to 75% (during $Mg^{++}$ depleted diet) depending on dietary $Mg^{++}$ content and a small amount of $Mg^{++}$, approximately 25-30 mg/day gets secreted in the gastrointestinal tract.[1,8] Absorption occurs majorly by a nonsaturable paracellular passive pathway (70%) and by saturable transcellular pathway (30%). The percentage of absorption by transcellular pathway increases when diet is deficient for $Mg^{++}$.[9,10] It occurs mainly by the transient receptor potential melastatin (TRPM) cationic channels, TRPM6, and TRPM7. Absorption by paracellular pathway is regulated by proteins which comprise the tight junction, such as claudins, occludin, and zona-occludens-1. By altering the phosphorylation of these tight junctional proteins, ionic permeability of the paracellular pathway can be increased or decreased. Also, paracellular absorptive transport depends on the positive luminal transepithelial electrical voltage and concentration gradient.[2,11]

## Renal Regulation of $Mg^{++}$

Normally, up to 96% of filtered $Mg^{++}$ is reabsorbed by the renal tubules. Proximal tubule accounts for 10-20% of the reabsorbed $Mg^{++}$, mainly by paracellular pathway. The main segment for renal reabsorption of $Mg^{++}$ occurs at the thick ascending limb of the loop of Henle (TALLOH) accounting for up to 70% of reabsorbed $Mg^{++}$ and a minor fine tuning occurs at the distal convoluted tubule (DCT).[12] At the TALLOH, absorption is mainly by paracellular pathway driven by a lumen positive transepithelial voltage, generated by recycling of potassium through the apical renal outer medullary potassium (ROMK) channel. The tight junction proteins belonging to the claudin family (claudin-16/claudin-19/paracellin-1) mediates the paracellular transport. They are negatively charged proteins with cationic selectivity responsible for paracellular reabsorption of $Ca^{2+}$ and $Mg^{++}$.[13] Also regulating the paracellular reuptake at the TALLOH are the PTH and the calcium sensing receptor (CaSR). PTH stimulates $Ca^{++}$ and $Mg^{++}$ reabsorption while stimulation of CaSR inhibits paracellular reabsorption of $Mg^{++}$.[1,2] At the DCT (5-10%), reabsorption is mainly by active transcellular transport mediated by TRPM6. Epidermal growth factor (EGF) enhances $Mg^{++}$ transport through TRPM6. Other transport proteins involved in $Mg^{++}$ regulation at the DCT are apical K channel Kv1.1, basolateral K channel Kir4.1,

# Chapter 31
## Approach to the Patient with Hypomagnesemia and Hypermagnesemia

Mg$^{++}$/sodium exchanger (SLC41A1 family), γ-subunit of Na/K-ATPase and cyclin M2.[2]

## HYPOMAGNESEMIA

### Case

A 74-year-old male, occasional alcoholic was admitted in an intensive care unit for supraventricular tachycardia and altered sensorium. He was recently diagnosed to have carcinoma of the colon, during evaluation for chronic diarrhea, weight loss, and easy fatigability. His previous medication included a proton pump inhibitor (PPI) and hydrochlorothiazide (12.5 mg) for hypertension. Since last three months patient is on treatment with cetuximab (an epidermal growth factor receptor blocker) for his colonic malignancy. His laboratory parameters at admission were as shown in Table 1.

The etiological agent for hypomagnesemia in the above case is likely due to:
a. Proton pump inhibitor
b. Alcohol
c. Chronic diarrhea
d. Thiazide diuretic
e. Cetuximab.

### Definition

A serum Mg$^{++}$ concentration of <1.7 mg/dL or <0.7 mmol/L (<1.4 mEq/L) is defined as hypomagnesemia. Its prevalence ranges from 10% in hospitalized patients to 60% in intensive care unit patients.[14]

### Etiology/Mechanism

It occurs due to decreased intake, redistribution, gastrointestinal losses, or renal losses. Isolated hypomagnesemia is rare and if present one may have to evaluate for rare genetic causes of isolated Mg$^{++}$ wasting such as isolated dominant hypomagnesemia with hypocalciuria (FXYD2 mutation). Often it is associated with abnormalities of other ions and acid base disturbance.[2] Common causes for hypomagnesemia are summarized in Box 1.

**Box 1:** Causes of hypomagnesemia.

- *Gastrointestinal causes*:
  - Diet deficient in Mg$^{2+}$
  - Malabsorption/chronic diarrhea
  - Laxative abuse
  - Continuous nasogastric drainage
  - Intestinal fistula
  - Proton pump inhibitors
- *Renal loss*:
  - *Hereditary/congenital cause*:
    - FHHNC (mutations in claudin-16 and claudin-19)
    - HSH (mutations in *TRPM6*)
    - Bartter's syndrome [mutations in NKCC2 (type 1), ROMK (type II), ClC-Kb (type III), or CaSR (type V)]
    - Gitelman's syndrome (mutations of NCC)
    - EAST/SeSAME syndrome (mutations in Kir4.1)
    - Other: Mutations of the *FXYD2* gene, HNF1B, CNNM2, Kv1.1 or pro-EGF
  - *Postobstructive diuresis*: Diuretic phase of ATN
  - *Drugs*:
    - Loop and thiazide diuretics
    - Cisplatin
    - Aminoglycosides
    - Pentamidine
    - Foscarnet
    - Immunosuppressants (tacrolimus, cyclosporine, rapamycin)
    - EGF receptor antagonists (panitumumab, cetuximab)
  - *Endocrine*:
    - Hyperaldosteronism
    - Diabetes and diabetic ketoacidosis
    - Hypoparathyroidism
    - Hyperthyroidism
  - *Redistribution*:
    - Hungry bone syndrome
    - Acute pancreatitis
    - Blood transfusions
    - Insulin treatment
  - *Miscellaneous*:
    - Chronic alcoholism
    - Preeclampsia

ATN: acute tubular necrosis; CaSR: calcium sensing receptor; ClC-Kb: Cl channel Kb; CNNM2: cyclin M2; EAST (epilepsy, ataxia, sensorineural deafness, and tubulopathy)/SeSAME (seizures, sensorineural deafness, ataxia, mental retardation, and electrolyte imbalance); EGF: epidermal growth factor; FHHNC: familial hypomagnesemia with hypercalciuria and nephrocalcinosis; FXYD2: sodium/potassium-transporting ATPase gamma chain (a protein that in humans is encoded by the *FXYD2* gene); HFN1B: hepatocyte nuclear factor 1 beta; HSH: hypomagnesemia with secondary hypocalcemia; NCC: thiazide-sensitive NaCl cotransporter; NKCC2: Na1-K1-2Cl2 cotransporter; ROMK: renal outer medullary potassium; TRPM6: transient receptor potential melastatin 6

**Table 1:** Biochemical values at admission for presented case of hypomagnesemia.

| Biochemical variable | Value |
| --- | --- |
| Serum creatinine | 0.9 mg/dL |
| Serum sodium | 140 mEq/L |
| Serum potassium | 2.8 mEq/L |
| Serum chloride | 98 mEq/L |
| Serum magnesium | 0.8 mEq/L |
| Serum calcium (corrected) | 7.1 mEq/L |
| Serum bicarbonate | 22 mEq/L |
| Urine sodium | 38 mEq/L |
| Fractional excretion of magnesium | 8% |

## Clinical Effects

Because of its predominant intracellular distribution, deficiency of $Mg^{++}$ is underrecognized. Symptoms of hypomagnesemia depend on the severity of $Mg^{++}$ deficiency and the presence of associated electrolyte abnormalities (like serum calcium and serum potassium). Majority of patients have only mild $Mg^{++}$ deficiency and are often asymptomatic. Symptoms appear in severe hypomagnesemia when serum $Mg^{++}$ falls below 1.2 mg/dL (<0.5 mmol/L; <1 mEq/L) and include, neuromuscular irritability symptoms such as an extensor plantar reflexes, positive Trousseau's and Chvostek's signs, fatigability, and tetany.[15,16] As these symptoms are also seen in hypocalcemia, when present one should suspect hypoparathyroidism. Other central nervous system symptoms include vertigo, ataxia, depression, and seizure activity. Patients with severe hypomagnesemia are at an increased risk for tachycardia, ventricular, and supraventricular arrhythmia. Electrocardiogram (ECG) often demonstrates widening of the QRS complex, prolonged QT interval, peaked or diminished T waves, and prolonged PR interval. Sinus tachycardia, ventricular extrasystolic beats, and/or torsades de pointes are other ECG abnormalities observed in hypomagnesemia.[17]

## Approach/Evaluation

When evaluating a case of hypomagnesemia, estimation of corrected serum calcium, serum potassium, acid base abnormality, and urine calcium excretion should be an integral part. At the TALLOH, calcium competes with $Mg^{++}$ for uptake. In conditions, where the filtered load of calcium increases, it competes and impairs $Mg^{++}$ reabsorption. Hypomagnesemia, in turn, leads to PTH resistance and decrease in PTH secretion.[18] This would result in decreased mobilization of calcium and $Mg^{++}$ from bone, impaired proximal tubule active reabsorption of calcium, and renal $Mg^{++}$ wasting, further intensifying $Mg^{++}$ deficiency (Flowchart 1).

More than 50% of clinically significant hypokalemia have concomitant $Mg^{++}$ deficiency. At the distal renal tubule a decrease in intracellular $Mg^{++}$, secondary to $Mg^{++}$ deficiency, releases the $Mg^{++}$ mediated inhibition on the inward rectifying ROMK channels resulting in increased distal potassium secretion. However, this gets self-limited as the intracellular potassium concentration falls in $Mg^{++}$ deficient states due to decreased activity of basolateral $Na^+/K^+$ ATPase, limiting its ability to cause hypokalemia. But in conditions when $Mg^{++}$ deficiency is accompanied by an increased distal sodium delivery (e.g. diuretics) or when aldosterone levels are elevated, it would exacerbate the hypokalemia by aggravating renal potassium wasting.[19]

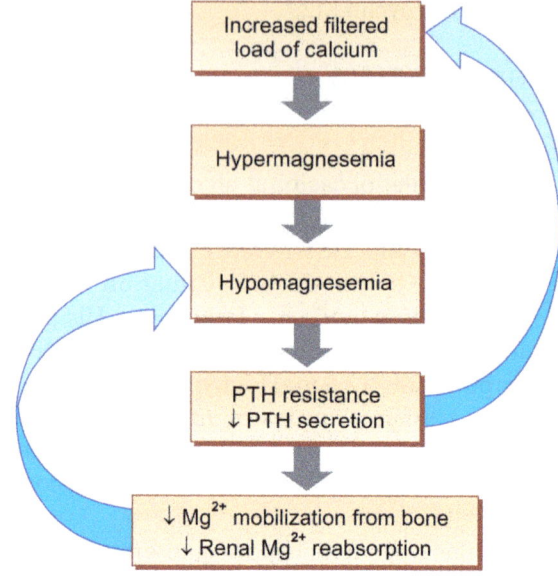

**Flowchart 1:** Amplification loop of hypomagnesemia.

(PTH: parathyroid hormone).

Proton pump inhibitors cause hypomagnesemia after prolonged use in up to 1% of patients, by preventing both transcellular and paracellular absorption in the small intestine. One should carefully monitor for serum $Mg^{++}$ in patients taking a PPI in conjunction with antiarrhythmic drugs.[20,21] Gastrointestinal causes for $Mg^{++}$ deficiency have fractional excretion of $Mg^{++}$ ($FeMg^{++}$) <2%, due to an intact renal compensatory absorptive capacity. Renal losses of $Mg^{++}$ are either primarily due to a defect in $Mg^{++}$ absorption or secondary to defects in tubular sodium reabsorption. When hypomagnesemia is secondary to renal losses, $FeMg^{++}$ is >2%. The formula to calculate the $FeMg^{++}$ is:

$FeMg^{++}$ = (urine $Mg^{++}$ × serum creatinine)/[0.7 (serum $Mg^{++}$ × urine creatinine)] × 100

The serum $Mg^{++}$ level is multiplied by 0.7, as only 70% of serum $Mg^{++}$ is ionized and freely filterable by glomerulus.[22] Since $Mg^{++}$ is a necessary co-factor for ATP synthesis, hypomagnesemia is associated with decreased ATP synthesis. This in turn affects the function of high energy consuming nephron segments like TALLOH, resulting in associated electrolyte abnormalities.[23] Drugs (like, loop diuretics) and genetic causes (like, FHHNC, Bartters' syndrome) which mainly affect the TALLOH, often also causes metabolic alkalosis, hypokalemia, hypercalciuria, and nephrocalcinosis. While hypocalciuria, metabolic alkalosis, and hypokalemia are often associated with hypomagnesemia due to drugs (like, thiazide diuretics, cetuximab) and genetic causes (e.g. Gitelmans' syndrome) affecting the DCT. Ethanol has a direct inhibitory effect on $Mg^{++}$ reabsorption in the kidney causing a mild reversible hypomagnesemia. However, it can be severe when patients have associated complications of chronic ethanol consumption like pancreatitis, alcohol-induced osmotic diuresis, or malnutrition secondary to poor dietary intake.[24]

## Management

Incidentally detected and asymptomatic hypomagnesemia (serum $Mg^{++}$ > 1.2 mg/dL), does not merit aggressive management.[25] Patients should be encouraged to consume foods which are rich source of $Mg^{++}$ such as green vegetables especially spinach, whole, unrefined grains, legumes such as beans and peas, nuts and seeds, dairy products, and meat and sea food. Various oral formulations commercially available for maintenance supplementation include $Mg^{++}$ oxide (400 mg), $Mg^{++}$ hydroxide (200 mg), $Mg^{++}$ orotate (500 mg), $Mg^{++}$ chloride, and $Mg^{++}$ lactate. Each 400 mg of $Mg^{++}$ oxide tablet contains 242 mg of elemental $Mg^{++}$. Its absorption is less efficacious with only one-third being bio-available. In India, $Mg^{++}$ hydroxide is commercially available as 200 mg tablet (Meyer vitabiotics, ultra $Mg^{++}$). Two tablets (2 × 200 mg) of ultra-$Mg^{++}$ contains 375 mg of elemental $Mg^{++}$, providing 100% recommended daily allowance of $Mg^{++}$.

In more severe cases of hypomagnesemia (serum $Mg^{++}$ < 1.2 mg/dL) with symptoms such as neuromuscular irritability or ventricular arrhythmias, patients should be managed as a medical emergency requiring intravenous replacement of $Mg^{++}$.[1,26] Commercially available preparation contains 50% $Mg^{++}$ sulfate as 0.5 gm/mL injection (2 mL single dose vial). $Mg^{++}$ replenishment should be achieved by 1–4 g of $Mg^{++}$ sulfate diluted in 100 mL of D5W as a slow intravenous infusion over 8–24 hours on day 1. The dose should be repeated if serum $Mg^{++}$ continues to be less than 1.0 mg/dL. Serum $Mg^{++}$ should not be measured immediately following an infusion as it is subject to slow equilibration between serum and the intracellular spaces and tissues and is subject to falsely high serum values when measured immediately following an infusion.[26] With an abrupt rise in serum $Mg^{++}$ level following an infusion, the stimulus for reabsorption of $Mg^{++}$ at the TALLOH is lost resulting in approximately 50% of the infused dose getting eliminated from the kidney. In patients with impaired renal function the dose of replacement should be reduced to 25–50% of patients with normal renal function. Further, patients should receive 2–4 g of daily intravenous $Mg^{++}$ infusions for next 3–5 days to replenish the $Mg^{++}$ stores. All associated electrolyte abnormalities should be addressed simultaneously especially calcium and potassium supplementation in presence of hypocalcemia and hypokalemia. Following $Mg^{++}$ sulfate infusion, the sulfate ions complexes with calcium and gets excreted in urine. This would reduce the ionized calcium concentration further worsening hypocalcemia. Sulfate ions also cause kaliuresis, necessitating careful monitoring and replacement of these electrolytes.[27] Also, all patients should be monitored for symptoms of hypermagnesemia during $Mg^{++}$ infusion, such as areflexia or respiratory depression.

## Case Revisit

In the above patient, the fractional excretion of $Mg^{++}$ is more than 2%, indicating a renal loss as the cause of hypomagnesemia. Options (a) and (c) are ruled out as they lead to gastrointestinal loss of $Mg^{++}$. As the patient was an occasional alcoholic with no complications related to alcoholism, it is unlikely to be the etiological agent (option b) for his hypomagnesemia. Hydrochlorothiazide (option d) can cause hypomagnesemia, hyponatremia, and hypokalemia. Patient was on a very low dose of the thiazide diuretic and is unlikely to cause such severe hypokalemia and hypomagnesemia as indicated by the absence of hyponatremia. The most likely etiology in the above patient is cetuximab (option e) (Flowchart 2).

Cetuximab is a monoclonal antibody against epidermal growth factor (EGF) receptor, used for the treatment of colorectal cancer, nonsmall cell cancer of the lung, and head and neck cancer. Hypomagnesemia is seen in approximately one-third of patients who receive cetuximab and the incidence increases with prolonged duration of exposure to the drug and is an indirect marker of the efficacy of the drug.[28] EGF on binding to its receptor on the basolateral surface of the DCT, stimulates $Mg^{++}$ reabsorption by activation of TRPM6 on the apical surface. Cetuximab by its blocking effect, prevents the interaction of normally secreted EGF with its receptor causing impaired renal reabsorption and urinary losses of $Mg^{++}$, leading to hypomagnesemia.[29,30] Hypomagnesemia in turn causes hypokalemia and hypocalcemia as previously explained and correction of hypomagnesemia is central to the correction of these electrolyte abnormalities.

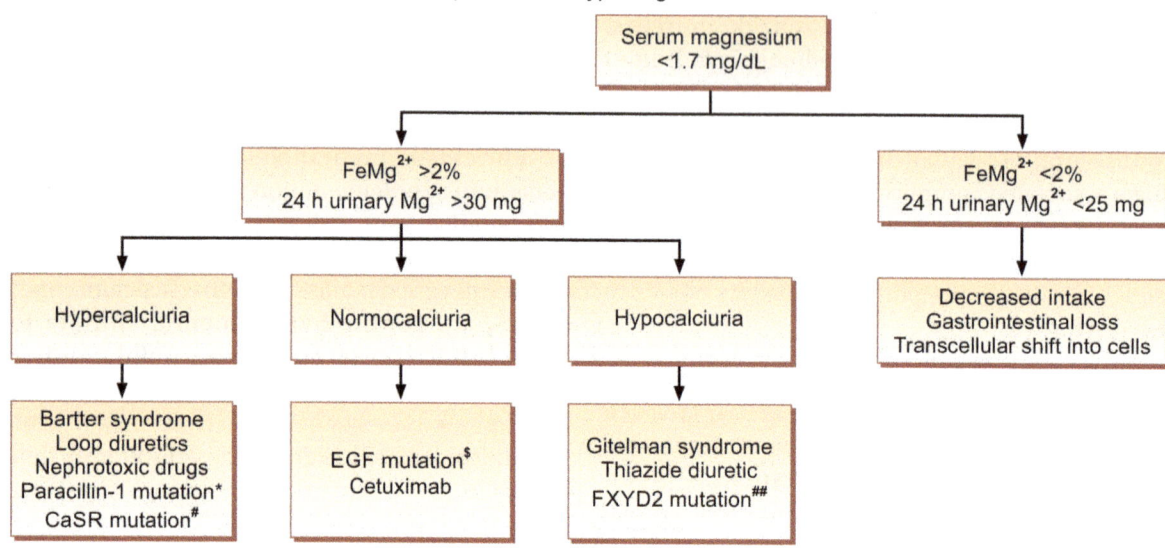

**Flowchart 2:** Approach to a patient with hypomagnesemia and normal renal function.

(CaSR: calcium-sensing receptor; FeMg$^{2+}$: fractional excretion of magnesium)
*Familial hypomagnesemia with hypercalciuria and nephrocalcinosis.
#Autosomal dominant hypocalcemia with hypercalciuria.
$Isolated recessive hypomagnesemia with normocalciuria.
##Isolated dominant hypomagnesemia with hypocalciuria.

## HYPERMAGNESEMIA

### Case

A 26-year-old pregnant female was brought to the emergency with history of seizures and altered sensorium. She had no preceding illness and had a single antenatal visit at fourth month of gestation. She was currently in her 30th week of gestation. On examination patient was arousable on deep stimulus and had no focal neurological deficit. Her pulse rate was 110 beats/min and her blood pressure was 190/110 mm Hg. She was provisionally diagnosed to have eclampsia with a postictal phase and was started on 6 g of Mg$^{++}$ sulfate infusion as bolus followed by a maintenance dose of 2 g/h over next 6 hours. She was also started on antiepileptic drugs and calcium channel blockers for her hypertension management. Over the next 4 hours, patient developed severe respiratory depression, hypotension and her ECG showed a prolonged PR and QT interval and an increased QRS duration. Her urine output in last 4 hours was less than 100 mL and laboratory investigations showed an elevated serum creatinine (4.5 mg/dL), low normal serum calcium (8.5 mg/dL), a normal phosphorus (3.5 mg/dL) and a high normal serum potassium (5.2 mEq/L). On physical examination she had an absent patellar deep tendon reflex. She was intubated and put on mechanical ventilation. A fresh venous sample drawn 4 hours after admission demonstrated a serum Mg$^{++}$ level of 10.4 mEq/L.

1. What is the mostly likely cause of her hypermagnesemia?
   a. Unmonitored Mg$^{++}$ sulfate administration
   b. Renal failure
   c. Rhabdomyolysis secondary to prolonged seizures
   d. All of the above
   e. Both (a) and (b)
2. What is the best therapeutic approach for acute reduction of her serum Mg$^{++}$ levels?
   a. Stop Mg$^{++}$ infusion and repeat serum Mg$^{++}$ levels after 2 hours
   b. Intravenous bolus furosemide every fourth hourly
   c. Hemodialysis
   d. Peritoneal dialysis
   e. Intravenous calcium gluconate infusion.

### Definition

Serum Mg$^{++}$ levels of more than 2.6 mg/dL (1.1 mmol/L or 2.2 mEq/L) amounts to hypermagnesemia.

### Etiology/Mechanism

Not commonly encountered, it can occur under three clinical settings[31]
1. In presence of renal failure:—As kidneys are the main route for excretion of Mg$^{++}$. In patients with end-stage renal disease on dialysis, serum levels of Mg$^{++}$ correlate principally with dietary Mg$^{++}$ intake.[32]

2. Exogenous Mg$^{++}$ supplementation:—Either intravenous, oral, or as an enema. Intravenous Mg$^{++}$ infusion used as an emergency among pregnant women, to reduce neuromuscular irritability in eclampsia/preeclampsia requires careful and frequent monitoring of deep tendon reflexes and respiratory rate to determine hypermagnesemia.[33] Intravenous infusion is also used as a smooth muscle relaxant and bronchodilator in children with status asthmaticus.[34] Massive oral ingestion of Mg$^{++}$ based antacids, accidental intake of gypsum salts (Mg$^{++}$ sulfate) or use of Mg$^{++}$ based cathartics (Mg$^{++}$ citrate) can result in hypermagnesemia especially when accompanied by renal failure[35,36] Also, large bowel can absorb a substantiate quantity of Mg++ from retention enemas resulting in hypermagnesemia.[37]
3. Increased absorption secondary to impaired gut motility (mechanical bowel obstruction, secondary to anticholinergics, etc.) or in presence of gastrointestinal disorders (colitis, active ulcer disease, etc.).[31] Rarely hypermagnesemia can occur in patients with lithium toxicity, tumor-lysis syndrome, adrenal insufficiency, and familial hypocalciuric hypercalcemia.[38]

## Clinical Effects

Clinical presentation in hypermagnesemia primarily depends on the serum Mg$^{++}$ level and in general involves neuromuscular and cardiovascular system and from those occurring secondarily to hypocalcemia (Table 2). Neuromuscular symptoms occur secondarily to an impaired impulse transmission across neuromuscular junction in presence of hypermagnesemia, producing a curare like effect.[39] In mild cases patient presents with lethargy, drowsiness, nausea, and an absent deep tendon reflexes on examination. In more severe cases, it can result in muscle paralysis, flaccid quadriplegia, respiratory muscle weakness, and apnea. Cardiovascular manifestation ranges from conduction abnormalities, bradycardia, hypotension, ECG changes such as prolonged PR interval, increased QRS duration, tall "T" waves, prolonged QT interval to complete heart block, and cardiac arrest in more severe cases. ECG changes are like those seen in hyperkalemia and it is common to miss hypermagnesemia in the absence of a good clinical history. Cardiovascular manifestations of hypermagnesemia are primarily due to the intracellular and extracellular calcium channel blocking and from intracellular cardiac potassium channel blocking effect of Mg$^{++}$.[40] Hypermagnesemia impairs the PTH secretion resulting in mild hypocalcemia.[41]

## Approach/Evaluation

Hypermagnesemia is seen rarely in clinical practice and symptoms closely mimic to those from hypocalcemia. Along with serum magnesium levels, corrected serum calcium, and renal function test should be part of initial investigation. A careful history to elicit the clinical situation which led to hypermagnesemia holds the key for management. As previously mentioned, the three clinical scenarios which are the likely etiologies for clinical hypermagnesemia should be carefully ruled out.

## Management

Management of hypermagnesemia primarily depends on the renal function. In patients with normal renal function, careful monitoring (clinical and biochemical, especially during Mg$^{++}$ infusion) and stopping Mg$^{++}$ supplementation after the desired correction is vital.[42] If hypermagnesemia persists even after stopping supplementation, patient should receive hydration with normal saline followed by loop diuretic (furosemide). Majority of the patients with normal renal function and preserved urine output respond to the above measures. In presence of renal failure, oliguria and other metabolic or acid-base derangements, it is acceptable to start patients on dialysis.[43] Presence of neurological and cardiovascular features of hypermagnesemia should be treated as an emergency and hemodialysis is preferred over peritoneal dialysis for rapid correction.[44] Expecting a logistic delay of 1–2 hours for the preparation of hemodialysis, patients should be immediately started on intravenous calcium infusion as an antagonist to Mg$^{++}$. The dose of 100–200 mg of calcium gluconate should be administered over 5–10 minutes under an ECG monitor.[31,43]

**Table 2:** Serum magnesium levels and manifestations in patients with hypermagnesemia.[5,32,44]

| Serum magnesium level (mg/dL) | Clinical effects |
| --- | --- |
| <3.6 | Asymptomatic |
| 5–8 | Nausea, headache, light headedness, cutaneous flushing, diminished deep tendon reflexes |
| 9–12 | Absent deep tendon reflexes, somnolence, hypotension, ECG changes |
| 12–15 | Sinoatrial and atrioventricular block, muscle paralysis, hypoventilation |
| >15 | Cardiac asystole, respiratory arrest, coma |

## Case Revisit

In the above case the most likely cause for hypermagnesemia is a combination of unmonitored $Mg^{++}$ sulfate infusion and the presence of renal failure (option e). Absence of hyperphosphatemia and significant hyperkalemia makes option c less likely. The low normal serum calcium level is most likely to decrease PTH release secondary to hypermagnesemia. The rapid therapy to antagonize the action of $Mg^{++}$ especially when associated with ECG changes is to start patient of calcium infusion. However, hemodialysis is required for elimination of excess $Mg^{++}$ in presence of renal failure and oliguria. In the above patient option (e) would only antagonize the effect of hypermagnesemia but patient would require to be stated on urgent hemodialysis for acute reduction of serum $Mg^{++}$ levels (option c). Hemodialysis, with its higher flow rates, works more acutely than peritoneal dialysis in poisonings and lowers $Mg^{++}$ levels to a nontoxic range within hours.

## SALIENT POINTS

- Magnesium is the second most abundant intracellular cation and only 1% of the body $Mg^{++}$ found in extracellular space. The normal serum $Mg^{++}$ concentration ranges between 1.7 and 2.6 mg/dL (0.7–1.1 mmol/L or 1.4–2.2 mEq/L).
- $Mg^{++}$ serves as a co-factor for many biological processes that utilize ATP. It is essential for intracellular signaling, protein and DNA synthesis, oxidative phosphorylation, mineralization of bone, neuromuscular excitability, calcium, and potassium homeostasis.
- Up to 96% of filtered $Mg^{++}$ is reabsorbed by the renal tubules. The TALLOH accounts for up to 70% of reabsorbed $Mg^{++}$ and is mainly by paracellular pathway. Tight junction proteins belonging to claudin family mediates paracellular transport.
- Symptoms appear in severe hypomagnesemia when serum $Mg^{++}$ falls below 1.2 mg/dL and include neuromuscular irritability symptoms such as an extensor plantar reflexes, positive Trousseau's and Chvostek's signs, tetany, seizures, and risk for tachycardia, ventricular, and supraventricular arrhythmia.
- When evaluating hypomagnesemia, estimation of corrected serum calcium, serum potassium, acid base abnormality, and urine calcium excretion should be an integral part. $Mg^{++}$ replenishment should be achieved by 1–4 g of $Mg^{++}$ sulfate diluted in 100 mL of D5W as a slow intravenous infusion over 8–24 hours.
- Serum $Mg^{++}$ levels of >2.6 mg/dL amounts to hypermagnesemia. Not commonly encountered, it can occur in presence of renal failure, exogenous $Mg^{++}$ supplementation and increased absorption, secondary to impaired gut motility, or in presence of gastrointestinal disorders.
- Clinical presentation in hypermagnesemia involves neuromuscular, cardiovascular, and those occurring secondarily to hypocalcemia. Neuromuscular symptoms produce a curare like effect. Cardiovascular manifestation ranges from conduction abnormalities, bradycardia, and hypotension.
- Management of hypermagnesemia primarily depends on the renal function. In presence of renal failure, oliguria, and other metabolic or acid-base derangements, hemodialysis should be initiated. In case of delay, 100–200 mg of calcium gluconate should be administered over 5–10 minutes under an ECG monitor.

## REFERENCES

1. Martin KJ, González EA, Slatopolsky E. Clinical consequences and management of hypomagnesemia. J Am Soc Nephrol. 2009;20(11):2291-5.
2. Blaine J, Chonchol M, Levi M. Renal control of calcium, phosphate, and magnesium homeostasis. Clin J Am Soc Nephrol. 2015;10(7):1257-72.
3. Whang R, Hampton EM, Whang DD. Magnesium homeostasis and clinical disorders of magnesium deficiency. Ann Pharmacother. 1994;28(2):220-6.
4. Konrad M, Schlingmann KP, Gudermann T. Insights into the molecular nature of magnesium homeostasis. Am J Physiol Renal Physiol. 2004;286(4):F599-605.
5. Topf JM, Murray PT. Hypomagnesemia and hypermagnesemia. Rev Endocr Metab Disord. 2003;4(2):195-206.
6. Ayuk J, Gittoes NJ. How should hypomagnesaemia be investigated and treated? Clin Endocrinol (Oxf). 2011;75(6):743-6.
7. Freitag JJ, Martin KJ, Conrades MB, et al. Evidence for skeletal resistance to parathyroid hormone in magnesium deficiency. Studies in isolated perfused bone. J Clin Invest. 1979;64(5):1238-44.
8. Brannan PG, Vergne-Marini P, Pak CY, et al. Magnesium absorption in the human small intestine. Results in normal subjects, patients with chronic renal disease, and patients with absorptive hypercalciuria. J Clin Invest. 1976;57(6):1412-8.
9. Quamme GA. Recent developments in intestinal magnesium absorption. Curr Opin Gastroenterol. 2008;24(2):230-5.
10. Fine KD, Santa Ana CA, Porter JL, et al. Intestinal absorption of magnesium from food and supplements. J Clin Invest. 1991;88(2):396-402.

11. Anderson JM, Van Itallie CM. Physiology and function of the tight junction. Cold Spring Harb Perspect Biol. 2009;1(2):a002584.
12. Ferre S, Hoenderop JG, Bindels RJ. Insight into renal Mg2+ transporters. Curr Opin Nephrol Hypertens. 2011;20(2):169-76.
13. Haisch L, Almeida JR, Abreu da Silva PR, et al. The role of tight junctions in paracellular ion transport in the renal tubule: lessons learned from a rare inherited tubular disorder. Am J Kidney Dis. 2011;57(2):320-30.
14. Reinhart RA, Desbiens NA. Hypomagnesemia in patients entering the ICU. Crit Care Med. 1985;13(6):506-7.
15. Dyckner T. Serum magnesium in acute myocardial infarction. Relation to arrhythmias. Acta Med Scand. 1980;207(1-2):59-66.
16. Vallee BL, Wacker WE, Ulmer DD. The magnesium-deficiency tetany syndrome in man. N Engl J Med. 1960;262:155-61.
17. Fox C, Ramsoomair D, Carter C. Magnesium: its proven and potential clinical significance. South Med J. 2001;94(12):1195-201.
18. Chase LR, Slatopolsky E. Secretion and metabolic efficacy of parathyroid hormone in patients with severe hypomagnesemia. J Clin Endocrinol Metab. 1974;38(3):363-71.
19. Huang CL, Kuo E. Mechanism of hypokalemia in magnesium deficiency. J Am Soc Nephrol. 2007;18(10):2649-52.
20. Lameris AL, Hess MW, van Kruijsbergen I, et al. Omeprazole enhances the colonic expression of the Mg(2+) transporter TRPM6. Pflugers Arch. 2013;465(11):1613-20.
21. Hess MW, Hoenderop JG, Bindels RJ, et al. Systematic review: Hypomagnesaemia induced by proton pump inhibition. Aliment Pharmacol Ther. 2012;36(5):405-13.
22. Elisaf M, Panteli K, Theodorou J, et al. Fractional excretion of magnesium in normal subjects and in patients with hypomagnesemia. Magnes Res. 1997;10(4):315-20.
23. Skou JC. The influence of some cations on an adenosine triphosphatase from peripheral nerves. J Am Soc Nephrol. 1998;9(11):2170-7.
24. De Marchi S, Cecchin E, Basile A, et al. Renal tubular dysfunction in chronic alcohol abuse—effects of abstinence. N Engl J Med. 1993;329(26):1927-34.
25. Augus ZS. Hypomagnesemia. J Am Soc Nephrol. 1999;10(7):1616-22.
26. Kraft MD, Btaiche IF, Sacks GS, et al. Treatment of electrolyte disorders in adult patients in the intensive care unit. Am J Health Syst Pharm. 2005;62(16):1663-82.
27. Navarro J, Oster JR, Gkonos PJ, et al. Tetany induced on separate occasions by administration of potassium and magnesium in a patient with hungry-bone syndrome. Miner Electrolyte Metab. 1991;17(5):340-4.
28. Palmer BF, Glassock RJ, Bleyer AJ, et al. Nephrology quiz and questionnaire: electrolytes. Clin J Am Soc Nephrol. 2012;7(6):1047-52.
29. Cao Y, Liao C, Tan A, et al. Meta-analysis of incidence and risk of hypomagnesemia with cetuximab for advanced cancer. Chemotherapy. 2010;56(6):459-65.
30. Saif MW. Management of hypomagnesemia in cancer patients receiving chemotherapy. J Support Oncol. 2008;6(5):243-8.
31. Khairi T, Amer S, Spitalewitz S, et al. Severe symptomatic hypermagnesemia associated with over-the-counter laxatives in a patient with renal failure and sigmoid volvulus. Case Rep Nephrol. 2014;2014:560746.
32. Wyskida K, Witkowicz J, Chudek J, et al. Daily magnesium intake and hypermagnesemia in hemodialysis patients with chronic kidney disease. J Ren Nutr. 2012;22(1):19-26.
33. Lu JF, Nightingale CH. Magnesium sulfate in eclampsia and preeclampsia: pharmacokinetic principles. Clin Pharmacokinet. 2000;38(4):305-14.
34. Kokotajlo S, Degnan L, Meyers R, et al. Use of intravenous magnesium sulfate for the treatment of an acute asthma exacerbation in pediatric patients. J Pediatr Pharmacol Ther. 2014;19(2):91-7.
35. Birrer RB, Shallash AJ, Totten V. Hypermagnesemia-induced fatality following epsom salt gargles(1). J Emerg Med. 2002;22(2):185-8.
36. Woodard JA, Shannon M, Lacouture PG, et al. Serum magnesium concentrations after repetitive magnesium cathartic administration. Am J Emerg Med. 1990;8(4):297-300.
37. Schelling JR. Fatal hypermagnesemia. Clin Nephrol. 2000;53(1):61-5.
38. Shinall MC Jr, Dahir KM, Broome JT. Differentiating familial hypocalciuric hypercalcemia from primary hyperparathyroidism. Endocr Pract. 2013;19(4):697-702.
39. Krendel DA. Hypermagnesemia and neuromuscular transmission. Semin Neurol. 1990;10(1):42-5.
40. Agus ZS, Morad M. Modulation of cardiac ion channels by magnesium. Annu Rev Physiol. 1991;53:299-307.
41. Cholst IN, Steinberg SF, Tropper PJ, et al. The influence of hypermagnesemia on serum calcium and parathyroid hormone levels in human subjects. N Engl J Med. 1984;310(19):1221-5.
42. Vissers RJ, Purssell R. Iatrogenic magnesium overdose: two case reports. J Emerg Med. 1996;14(2):187-91.
43. Mordes JP, Wacker WE. Excess magnesium. Pharmacol Rev. 1977;29(4):273-300.
44. Jhang WK, Lee YJ, Kim YA, et al. Severe hypermagnesemia presenting with abnormal electrocardiographic findings similar to those of hyperkalemia in a child undergoing peritoneal dialysis. Korean J Pediatr. 2013;56(7):308-11.

**SECTION 3**

# Blood Gases

32. Acid-base Homeostasis
33. Approach to the Patient with Metabolic Acidosis and Alkalosis
34. Approach to the Patient with Respiratory Acidosis and Alkalosis
35. Basics of Arterial Blood Gas Interpretation
36. Arterial Blood Gas Interpretation in Clinical Practice

# Acid-base Homeostasis

*Saurabh Saigal*

## INTRODUCTION

Acid is defined as any substance that is capable of releasing H⁺ into solution whereas the base is defined as any substance capable of combining with/accepting H⁺ in solution.[1] In body, there are two types of acids which are produced—volatile acid i.e. $CO_2$ which is produced as a result of all metabolic processes and around 13,000 mEq/day is produced. Other acid is fixed acid which is produced by protein catabolism predominantly and is buffered immediately (Table 1). Base is defined as the substance capable of accepting H⁺ ion. The most common base in our body is $HCO_3^-$ which accepts H⁺ ion to form $H_2CO_3$ and then ultimately dissociates to form $CO_2 + H_2O$.

## ACID-BASE HOMEOSTASIS

The acid-base homeostasis has to be maintained if we want to maintain our pH. The free hydrogen ion concentration or [H⁺] needs to be maintained in a narrow range. The normal value of H⁺ ion concentration is 0.00000004 Eq/L. pH is the negative (–) log of this value.[2]

- pH and [H⁺] have inverse relationship
- Large changes in [H⁺] lead to small changes in pH.

According to Henderson–Hasselbalch equation:[2]

$$pH = pKc + \log [HCO_3]/[H_2CO_3]$$
$$[H_2CO_3] = PaCO_2 \times 0.03 \sim PaCO_2$$

pKc is a constant

$$pH \alpha [HCO_3]/[PaCO_2]$$

Hence, to maintain a normal pH, the ratio $[HCO_3]/[PaCO_2]$ must be maintained. The human body responds to the change in pH by basically three mechanisms in a stepwise manner (Fig. 1):

1. *First defense:* Buffering
2. *Second defense:* Respiratory alteration, i.e. alteration in $PaCO_2$
3. *Third defense:* Renal, i.e. alteration in $HCO_3$ excretion.

## Buffering

It is the body's first defense against the change in pH and is a fast physiochemical phenomenon. The body has a large buffer capacity. The bicarbonate is used for buffering of fixed acids; hence in numerator the amount of bicarbonate decreases and this is reflected as fall in pH as $pH \alpha HCO_3/CO_2$. Four common buffers in the body are:[3]

1. Bicarbonate buffers [in extracellular fluid (ECF)]
2. Hemoglobin (in intracellular fluid)
3. Plasma protein (in intracellular fluid)
4. Phosphates (in intracellular fluid).

**Table 1:** Production of various fixed acids in the body.

| Metabolism | Acid production |
| --- | --- |
| Protein catabolism | Sulfuric and phosphoric acids |
| Incomplete lipid metabolism | Acetoacetate and β-hydroxy butyric acid |
| Anaerobic metabolism of carbohydrate | Lactic acid |

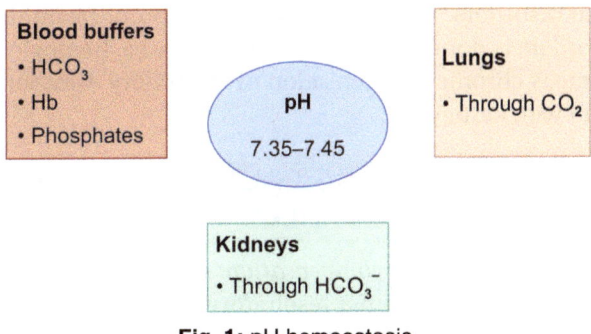

**Fig. 1:** pH homeostasis.

The bicarbonate buffers in the ECF are a part of $CO_2$-bicarbonate buffer system. It is responsible for major extracellular buffering (up to 80%). The bicarbonate buffer is the most common buffer for neutralizing metabolic acids but it cannot buffer respiratory acid-base disorders. These are ineffective in buffering changes in $H^+$ ions produced by it.

The hemoglobin is the only intracellular effective buffer because of its high concentration and histidine residues; it buffers most of the respiratory acid-base disorders i.e. 99% for respiratory acidosis and 97% for respiratory alkalosis. Deoxygenated hemoglobin is a better buffer than oxyhemoglobin.

In short, respiratory disorders are predominantly buffered in the intracellular compartment. Metabolic disorders have a larger buffering contribution from ECF (ECF buffering of 40% for metabolic acidosis and 70% metabolic alkalosis).

### Respiratory Response

It is affected by alteration of ventilation; the respiratory centers are located in medulla. These centers are stimulated by central and peripheral chemoreceptors.[3] The central chemoreceptors located in carotid and aortic bodies are stimulated by acidity of cerebrospinal fluid (CSF); the peripheral chemoreceptors are stimulated by hypoxia.[3] These receptors in turn stimulate the inspiratory muscles and hence respiratory rate is altered. The power and strength of respiratory muscles decide the respiratory rate and tidal volume, hence $PaCO_2$ levels. The respiratory compensation takes approximately 12–24 hours.

### Renal Response

The kidney is responsible for compensation of chronic respiratory disorders. The kidney takes usually longer response time, i.e. in days which involve the adjustment of bicarbonate excretion by kidney. The renal response is responsible for excretion of fixed acids and compensatory changes in plasma $HCO_3$ in the presence of respiratory acid-base disorders.[3] The acute compensation of respiratory disorders is done by intracellular buffers, i.e. hemoglobin whereas chronic compensation of respiratory disorders is dealt with kidneys.

### NORMAL PHYSIOLOGICAL RESPONSE FOR RESPIRATORY DISORDERS

*Respiratory disorders compensation:* Respiratory disorders can be classified as either respiratory acidosis or alkalosis. These can be further classified as acute or chronic. Acute

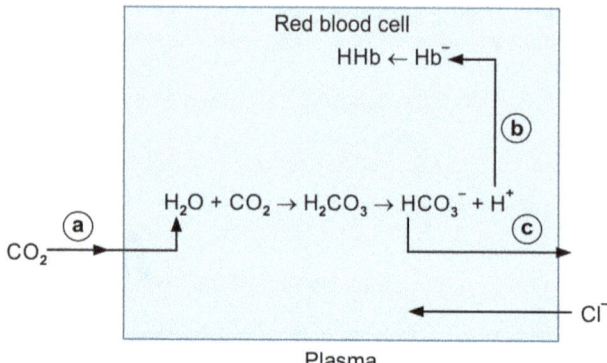

**Fig. 2:** Acute respiratory acidosis compensation. (a) $CO_2$ combines with $H_2O \rightarrow H_2CO_3$ is formed; (b) $H_2CO_3$ dissociates into $HCO_3^- + H^+$. $H^+$ ion combines with $Hb^-$; (c) $HCO_3^-$ is effluxed into plasma in exchange of $Cl^-$ ion.

disorders are buffered by intracellular buffers whereas as chronic disorders are buffered by kidney.

### Normal Response for Respiratory Acidosis

#### Acute Respiratory Acidosis

The compensatory response to acute respiratory disorder is limited to buffering. About 99% of this buffering occurs intracellularly. Proteins are the most important intravascular buffers for $CO_2$ but their concentration is low in respect to $CO_2$ required for buffering.

The bicarbonate system is most important extracellular buffer but is not responsible for any buffering of a respiratory acid-base disorder.[3] The reason is that for bicarbonate system to buffer $H^+$ produced by dissociation of $H_2CO_3$ would just result in production of equal amount of $CO_2$.

The chloride shift at the tissue level leads to intracellular buffering which is described in Figure 2.

The $CO_2$ from plasma diffuses into the RBC, where in presence of $H_2O$ and enzyme carbonic anhydrase it is converted to $H_2CO_3$. This $H_2CO_3$ is broken down to $H^+$ and $HCO_3^-$; the $H^+$ ions combine with Hb to form deoxy Hb and $HCO_3^-$ diffuses out of the RBC into the plasma in exchange of $Cl^-$ i.e. chloride shift.

#### Chronic Respiratory Acidosis

The kidneys respond by retaining bicarbonate. The response to a chronic respiratory acidosis is slower and takes around 72–96 hours. The response occurs because intracellular carbon dioxide rises in the tubular cell and combines with $H_2O$ to form $H_2CO_3$. The $H_2CO_3$ dissociates to form $H^+$ and $HCO_3^-$. This leads to increased $H^+$ ions secretion from proximal convoluted tubule (PCT) cells

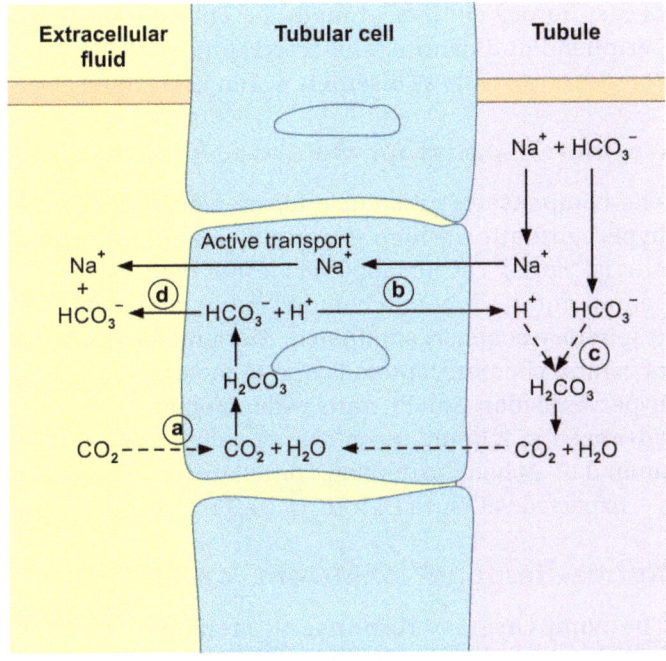

Fig. 3: Chronic respiratory acidosis compensation. (a) $CO_2$ level in the tubular cell rises and combines with $H_2O$ to form $H_2CO_3$. $H_2CO_3$ dissociates itself to $HCO_3^- + H^+$; (b) $H^+$ ions are secreted from tubular cell into tubule in exchange of $Na^+$; (c) $HCO_3^-$ itself cannot cross the apical membrane, it combines with $H^+$ ions which are secreted from tubular cell and form $H_2CO_3$ which dissociates to $CO_2 + H_2O$ and $CO_2$ diffuses into tubular cell; (d) As a result, more $HCO_3^-$ is generated and it is reabsorbed along with $Na^+$.

into tubular lumen in exchange of $Na^+$ ions. The $HCO_3^-$ itself cannot cross the apical membrane; the $HCO_3^-$ in the tubule combines with $H^+$ ions and forms $H_2CO_3$ which ultimately dissociates to $H_2O + CO_2$; where $CO_2$ diffuses into the tubular cell. As a result more and more of $HCO_3^-$ is generated and reabsorbed along with $Na^+$ (Fig. 3).

The $H^+$ ions, which are secreted in the tubular fluid, are to be neutralized. There is renal ammoniagenesis in which ammonia is released from glutamine. This $NH_3$ which is generated, diffuses across the proximal tubular cell into tubular luminal fluid and this in turn combines with $H^+$ ions and $NH_4^+$ ions are formed; these are combined with $Cl^-$ ion in order to maintain electroneutrality (Fig. 4). The final result is:

- There is increased bicarbonate production which finally crosses the basolateral membrane and enters the circulation
- Increased $Na^+$ reabsorption in exchange for $H^+$
- Increased $NH_3$ production to buffer the $H^+$ ion in the tubular lumen (as a result urinary $NH_4Cl$ increases).

## Normal Response for Respiratory Alkalosis

The compensatory response is fall in $HCO_3^-$. Initially there is a physiochemical response which lowers the bicarbonate dramatically. The effector organ for compensation is kidney. The renal response is slow and it takes 2–3 days for a maximal response.

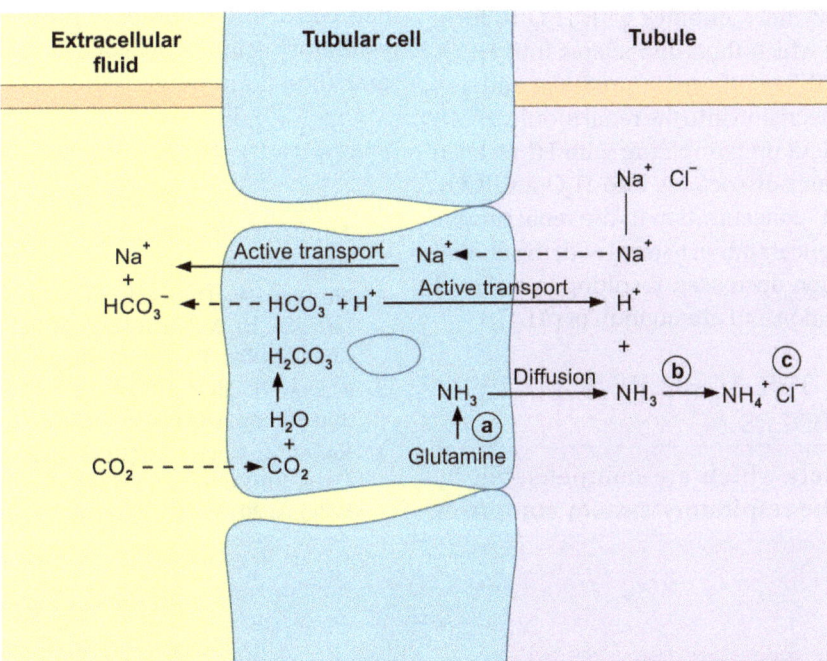

Fig. 4: Renal ammoniagenesis. (a) $H^+$ ions secreted in tubular fluid combine with $NH_3$ which is formed from Glutamine; (b) They ultimately form $NH_4^+$ ion; (c) They combine with $Cl^-$ and excreted as $NH_4Cl$ in urine.

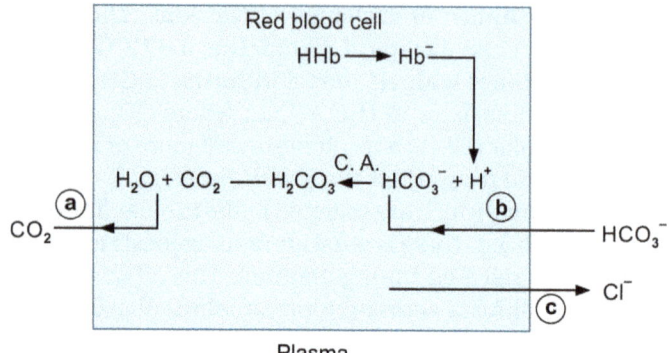

**Fig. 5:** Compensation in acute respiratory alkalosis. (a) Low levels of PaCO₂ in plasma lead to diffusion of CO₂ from RBC into plasma; (b) To compensate for it, HCO₃⁻ enters the RBC where it combines with H⁺ to form H₂CO₃. H⁺ ion dissociates from HHb; (c) To compensate for HCO₃⁻ entry, the Cl⁻ moves out into the plasma (C.A.: carbonic anhydrase).

### Acute Respiratory Alkalosis

Low levels of $CO_2$ in plasma lead to less diffusion of $CO_2$ into the plasma. To compensate for it, $HCO_3^-$ enters the RBC where it combines with H⁺ and forms $H_2CO_3$, and to compensate for it, chloride moves from RBC into the plasma (Fig. 5).

### Chronic Respiratory Alkalosis

Within the renal tubular cells, $CO_2$, under the influence of carbonic anhydrase enzyme, combines with $H_2O$ to form carbonic acid ($H_2CO_3$), which then dissociates into $HCO_3^-$ and H⁺. Alkalemia inhibits carbonic anhydrase activity, resulting in reduced H⁺ secretion into the renal tubule. $HCO_3^-$ reabsorption is dependent on combining with H⁺ to form carbonic acid, which later dissociates into $H_2O$ and $CO_2$. Owing to the reduced H⁺ concentration in the renal tubule, there is inadequate H⁺ concentration to react with the filtered $HCO_3^-$. $HCO_3^-$ reabsorption decreases, resulting in reduced plasma $HCO_3^-$ concentration and attenuation of pH.

## NORMAL PHYSIOLOGICAL RESPONSE FOR METABOLIC DISORDERS

These are the disorders which are compensated by respiratory system. The respiratory system comprises of respiratory centers in medulla, chemoreceptors—peripheral and central, and respiratory muscles. Lung compensates for these disorders within 12–24 hours.

### Normal Response for Metabolic Acidosis

The compensatory response for metabolic acidosis is hyperventilation which eventually leads to decrease arterial PaCO₂. The metabolic acidosis is detected by both central and peripheral chemoreceptors and eventually respiratory center is stimulated. The initial stimulation of central chemoreceptors is due to increase in H⁺. The hyperventilation usually starts within minutes and is well advanced at 2 hours but maximal compensation takes around 12–24 hours to develop. Formula for compensation:[4]

Expected $PaCO_2 = (1.5 \times HCO_3^-) + 8 \pm 2$

### Normal Response for Metabolic Alkalosis

The compensatory response to metabolic alkalosis is hypoventilation. The hypoventilation leads to compensatory rise in arterial PaCO₂. The central and peripheral chemoreceptors which respond to CSF acidity are not stimulated due to relative alkalinity of CSF. Thus it leads to hypoventilation. Formula for compensation:[4]

Expected $CO_2 = (0.7 \times HCO_3^-) + 21 \pm 1.5$

The compensatory process tries to bring pH toward normal but never near normal. If pH is near normal then coexisting disorder is present whether it is primary respiratory acidosis or alkalosis; $HCO_3^-$ changes with $CO_2$ in same direction; similar is the case in metabolic disorders.

### REFERENCES

1. Fencel V, Leith DE. Stewarts quantitative acid base chemistry. Applications in biology and medicine. Respir Physiol. 1993;91:1-16.
2. Neligan PJ, Deutschman CS. Perioperative acid-base balance. In: Miller R (Ed). Miller's Anesthesia, 7th edition. Philadelphia, PA: Churchill Livingstone/Elsevier; 2010.
3. Malley WJ. Clinical Blood Gases: Assessment and Intervention, 2nd edition. US: Elsevier; 2005.
4. Kollef M, Isakow W (Eds). Washington Manual of Critical Care, 2nd edition. Philadelphia: Lippincott Williams & Wilkins; 2013.

# CHAPTER 33

# Approach to the Patient with Metabolic Acidosis and Alkalosis

*Jeroen Tahon, Niels Van Regenmortel*

## INTRODUCTION

Metabolic acidosis and alkalosis are extremely common in the hospital and the intensive care unit. Although some disorders are mild and self-limiting, others are life-threatening. The assessment of metabolic acid-base disorders can assist clinicians in making a correct and timely diagnosis of the underlying disease, act as a measure of severity of illness, unmask on current problems and physiological reserves, and guide treatment. Therefore, a thorough knowledge of their mechanisms and differential diagnosis is of paramount importance to any critical care physician. In this chapter, we will describe how to approach metabolic acidosis and alkalosis and illustrate the stepwise analysis using different cases. The two main methods, (1) the traditional bicarbonate-centered approach (including the base excess methodology) and (2) the physicochemical Stewart approach will be discussed.

## APPROACH TO THE PATIENT WITH METABOLIC ACID-BASE DISORDERS

### The Traditional, Bicarbonate-centered Approach

The bicarbonate-centered approach focuses on the carbonic acid and bicarbonate buffering system to maintain acid-base homeostasis. The metabolic component is assessed by measuring or calculating bicarbonate level ($HCO_3^-$). The serum bicarbonate level is not a pure metabolic marker, as it is influenced by the partial pressure of carbon dioxide ($pCO_2$). Even in the absence of metabolic compensation, an increase in bicarbonate level can be observed in respiratory acidosis and a decrease in case of respiratory alkalosis. To deal with this problem, the *base excess* concept was introduced in 1960 as an index of the metabolic component of acid-base balance.[1] Base excess is defined as the amount of acid that must be added to a liter of blood to return its pH to 7.40 at a temperature of 37°C and a $pCO_2$ of 40 mm Hg (5.3 kPa). The *standard* or *in vivo* base excess (SBE) improves the accuracy of the base excess by considering the whole extracellular fluid compartment. It is calculated using a standard value for the hemoglobin concentration (5 g/dL or 3 mmol/L). It must be acknowledged that the metabolic compensation of a chronic respiratory problem will influence SBE, thereby mitigating SBE as a purely metabolic factor. This critique formed the basis of the so-called "Great Transatlantic Acid-base Debate", eventually leading to the development of a set of rules of thumb relating $pCO_2$ and bicarbonate level to each other.[2,3] The so-called Boston or Winters' rules remain the most popular way of assessing acid-base disorder in North America, while the base excess approach is prominent in Europe. Whatever the chosen approach, a systematical analysis is of paramount importance. We think, from a bicarbonate-centered point of view, the "Rules of Five" methodology, as described by Whittier et al. is an efficient and complete tool to assess a metabolic acid-base problem.[4]

*First step: Assessment of the net deviation of pH from its normal range*

If an acidemia (pH < 7.35) is present, an acidosis always must be present. In case of alkalemia (pH > 7.45), there must always be an alkalosis. A normal pH does not rule out an acid-base problem—a mixed disorder can be present. A compensatory process rarely pushes pH back into its normal range.

*Second step: Assessment of the primary acid-base disorder*

- Respiratory alkalosis: $pCO_2$ below 35 mm Hg
- Respiratory acidosis: $pCO_2$ over 45 mm Hg

- Metabolic alkalosis: $(HCO_3^-)$ over 26 mmol/L or a SBE more than 2 mmol/L
- Metabolic acidosis: $(HCO_3^-)$ below 22 mmol/L or a SBE less than 2 mmol/L[5]

If a complex acid-base disorder is suspected, the most likely cause of the disturbance (the one that matches with the direction of the pH) will be taken as primary disorder. The other components of the complex disorder will be unmasked in later steps.

*Third step: Calculation of the anion gap*

Serum anion gap = $[(Na^+) + (K^+)] - [(Cl^-) + (HCO_3^-)]$ (normal value: 7–15 mmol/L)

The anion gap concept is based on the principle of electroneutrality—by subtracting the commonly measured anions, chloride, and bicarbonate from the cumulative concentration of sodium and potassium, a virtual difference or gap can be found.[5,6] Depending on the laboratory method, the normal range is between 7 mmol/L and 15 mmol/L. This gap is "filled" with negative charges—albumin, phosphate, and a large number of unmeasured anions, originating from metabolism. It is important to calculate the anion gap in case of metabolic acidosis or mixed disorders as it can distinguish between two important, but totally different clinical problems. In normal anion gap metabolic acidosis (NAGMA), the main problem lies in the electrolyte balance (most frequently due to a net chloride gain—the concomitant decrease in $(HCO_3^-)$ in the presence of increased chloride results in an unchanged anion gap), where high anion gap metabolic acidosis (HAGMA) is characterized by the presence of unmeasured anions. Even if the pH is normal, it is important to calculate the anion gap. It can unmask a mixed acid-base disorder (e.g. a high anion gap metabolic acidosis and metabolic alkalosis) rather than a compensated primary disorder. The anion gap concept is demonstrated by the gamblegrams in Figure 1.

The interpretation of the anion gap assumes a normal concentration of albumin. To avoid false negative results, a correction should be applied if the serum albumin concentration is abnormally low.[7] Therefore, we need to increase the actual anion gap with the charged fraction of the decrease in albumin from its normal value. Approximately 25% of the albumin in human plasma is present in its charged state, therefore we increase the anion gap with 0.25 times the difference between the actual level (in g/L) and the normal level (40 g/L). Sometimes an abnormally low anion gap is encountered. This can be the result of hyponatremia without concomitant hypochloremia (rare) or the presence of unmeasured cations [heavy chains produced in multiple myeloma (especially IgG), hypermagnesemia, hypercalcemia, and lithium amongst others].

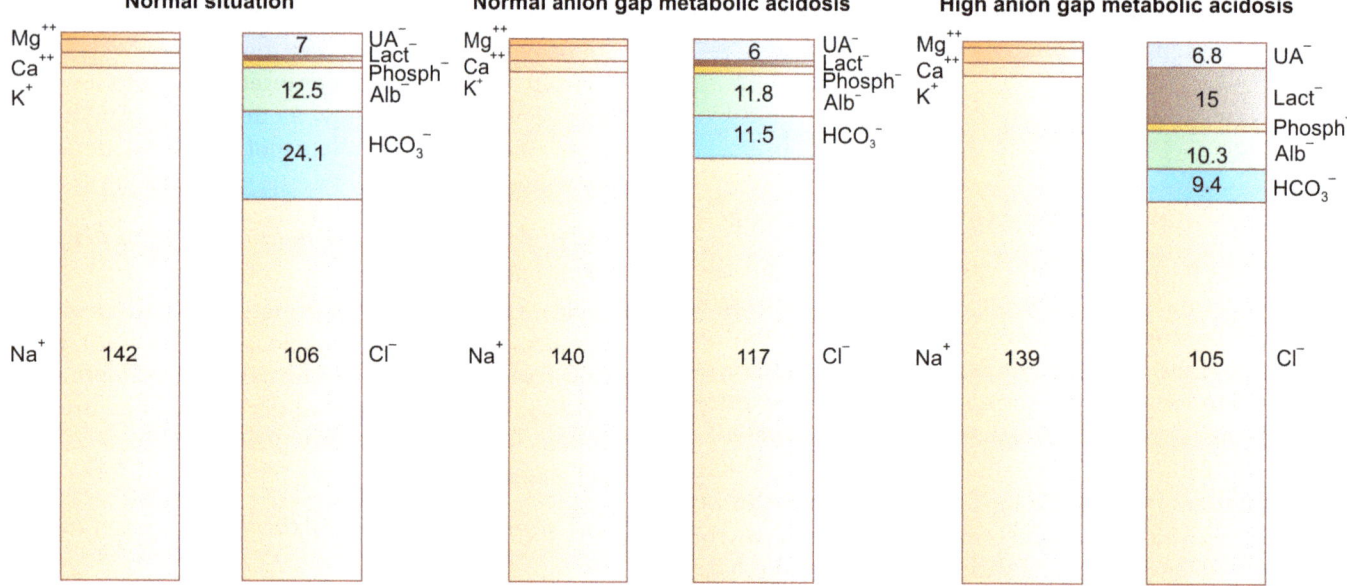

**Fig. 1:** Gamblegrams illustrating the normal situation (left), normal anion gap metabolic acidosis (middle) and high anion gap metabolic acidosis due to lactate (middle). UA⁻: unmeasured anions.

*Fourth step: Assessment of compensatory response*

Compensatory mechanisms will try to minimize fluctuations of pH. Metabolic disturbances will be compensated by the respiratory system and *vice versa*. As a compensatory process will rarely return pH within its normal range, abnormal values of $pCO_2$, bicarbonate or SBE in the presence of a normal pH usually indicate a mixed acid-base disorder. Different rules are used to calculate the relationship between the degree of change in one component of acid-base (metabolic or respiratory) and the compensatory change in the other. We summarize these rules of thumbs below:

- *Metabolic acidosis*: Respiratory compensation by hyperventilation

  $\Delta pCO_2 = 1 - 1.3\, \Delta(HCO_3^-) \rightarrow$ a decrease in $pCO_2$ that equals 1–1.3 times the decrease in bicarbonate from its normal value of 25 mmol/L is regarded as complete respiratory compensation.

  *Alternative formula*:
  Predicted $pCO_2 = 1.5 \times (HCO_3^-) + 8$

- *Metabolic alkalosis*: Respiratory compensation by hypoventilation

  $\Delta pCO_2 = 0.6\, \Delta[HCO_3^-] \rightarrow$ an increase in $pCO_2$ that equals 0.6 times the increase in bicarbonate from its normal value of 25 mmol/L is regarded as complete respiratory compensation. Since, on a physiological level, alkalosis is preferred above potentially deleterious hypoventilation, which would be necessary for complete respiratory compensation, the latter formula is less reliable. It is also the reason that the degree of compensation is lower—$pCO_2$ will increase only 0.6 times the increase in bicarbonate from its normal value.

  *Alternative formula:*
  Predicted $pCO_2 = 0.7 \times (HCO_3^-) + 21$ [in case is $(HCO_3^-) <$ 40 mmol/L]

  Predicted $pCO_2 = 0.75 \times [HCO_3^-] + 19$ [in case is $(HCO_3^-) >$ 40 mmol/L]

- *Respiratory acidosis*: Renal metabolic compensation
  - *Acute respiratory acidosis (minutes to hours)*—every 10 mm Hg increase in $pCO_2$ (from 40 mm Hg), is accompanied by a 1-mmol/L-increase in $(HCO_3^-)$. This increase is not due to compensation, but a mere consequence of the Henderson equilibrium. It should not lead to a rise in SBE.
  - *Chronic respiratory acidosis (over 12 hours)*—every 10 mm Hg increase in $pCO_2$ (from 40 mm Hg), should be compensated by a 4-mmol/L—increase in $(HCO_3^-)$.

- *Respiratory alkalosis:* Renal metabolic compensation
  - *Acute respiratory alkalosis (minutes to hours)*—every 10 mm Hg decrease in $pCO_2$ (from 40 mm Hg), is accompanied by a 2-mmol/L-decrease in $(HCO_3^-)$. Again, this is no real compensation and SBE should not be decreased.
  - *Chronic respiratory alkalosis*—every 10 mm Hg decrease in $pCO_2$ (from 40 mm Hg), is accompanied by a 5-mmol/L-decrease in $(HCO_3^-)$.

*Fifth step: Determination of the delta gap*

The delta gap, in the same way as the anion gap, relies on the concept of serum electroneutrality. It is based on the assumption that for every mmol/L increase in anion gap, there should be an equal drop in bicarbonate level. If bicarbonate level is lower than expected from the increased anion gap, a concomitant normal anion gap metabolic acidosis is present. If, on the other hand, bicarbonate level is higher, there is an additional metabolic alkalosis. We therefore calculate the delta gap in situations where there is an increased anion gap. To calculate the delta gap, the change in anion gap will be compared with the change in bicarbonate. It should be applied especially when there is no metabolic alkalosis diagnosed up to now or when a combination of high and normal anion gap is suspected. Sometimes delta gap is denoted by a ratio (1:1 being normal), rather than in the absolute values of their two components. We find the latter more intuitive.

## Introduction to the Physicochemical or "Stewart" Approach

While the above-mentioned set of rules enables a detailed assessment of an acid-base problem, their use requires repeated training and can be time-consuming even for experienced users. Important aspects of metabolic disorders or compensation, electrolyte and albumin levels, only come into view after extensive calculations. In 1981, Peter Stewart introduced a different view, the physicochemical approach to acid-base disorders.[8,9] The main advantage of this approach is its more complete picture, by drawing electrolytes and albumin in the picture early in the assessment, thereby making complex rules to calculate compensation redundant. It also makes a detailed quantitative analysis possible. A full exploration of Stewart's approach is beyond the scope of this chapter, but for daily practice, it should be sufficient to understand some of its basic principles. Stewart's equations predict that only changes in three independent variables will result in changes in the dissociation of water, thereby influencing the concentration of (H⁺) and thus pH. There are not more than three independent variables:

*pCO₂, the partial pressure of CO₂*
It follows from the Stewart equations that if pCO₂ increases, [H⁺] will increase as well. This is not different from other approaches to acid-base physiology.

*SID, the strong ion difference*
Strong ions are essentially completely dissociated, they exist in charged form only. In human plasma, the strong ions include $Na^+$, $K^+$, $Ca^{2+}$, $Mg^{2+}$, $Cl^-$, and lactate⁻. SID is the sum of strong cations minus the sum of strong anions. In plasma, it is mainly determined by $Na^+$ and $Cl^-$ and its normal value is about 40 mEq/L. It follows from the Stewart equations, that if SID decreases, H⁺ must increase and *vice versa*. Any pathological process that disturbs the balance between strong cations and strong anions will directly affect pH. This includes lactic acidosis, renal acidosis, vomiting-induced alkalosis, contraction alkalosis, and most importantly iatrogenic fluid administration due to an increase in chloride that is larger than the increase in sodium.

*$A_{TOT}$, the total amount of weak acids*
Weak acids are molecules that exist both in their charged and uncharged forms. They are grouped as $A_{TOT}$, the total amount of weak acids and consist mainly of plasma proteins. From an acid-base perspective, albumin and to a lesser extent phosphate, are the most important contributors. It follows from the Stewart equations that if $A_{TOT}$ increases, (H⁺) must also increase. This implies that hypoalbuminemia causes to alkalosis. Similarly, hyperphosphatemia, as seen in renal failure, causes acidosis.

The effect of these different variables on acidity is summarized in Figure 2. It is easily appreciated that a decrease in (SID) exerts the strongest effect. Stewart considers ($HCO_3^-$) and (H⁺)-dependent variables, of which changes in concentration are induced by changes in SID, pCO₂, and $A_{TOT}$.

In analogy with the anion gap in the traditional approach, it is also possible to assess unmeasured anions using the Stewart approach. Therefore, we need to know the value of the SID by measuring the known strong anions (the apparent SID or $SID_A$) and the value of SID by assessing the electric charge attributable to the weak anions (the effective SID or $SID_E$). Both values can be calculated using the following formulas:

Apparent SID or $SID_A$ = [($Na^+$) + ($K^+$) + ($Mg^{2+}$) + ($Ca^{2+}$)] − [($Cl^-$) − (lactate⁻)] (by convention in mEq/L)

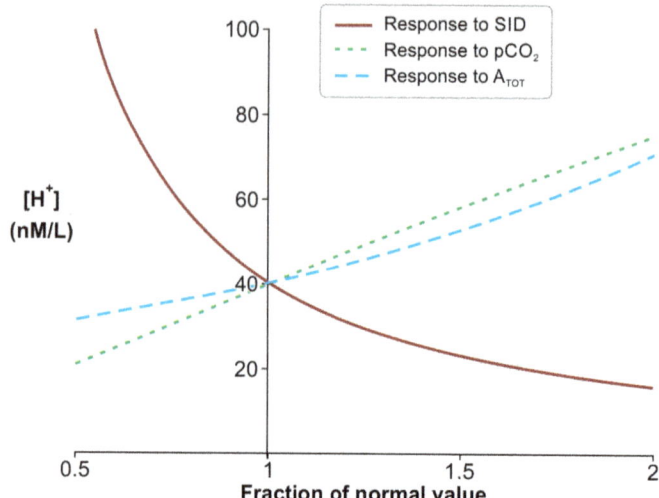

**Fig. 2:** Spider plot showing the dependence of plasma pH on changes in the three independent variables strong ion difference (SID) (normal value = 40 mEq/L), pCO₂ (normal value = 40 mm Hg) and total concentration of nonvolatile weak acids ($A_{TOT}$) (normal value = 17.2 mmol/L).

Effective SID or $SID_E$ = ($HCO_3^-$) + (albumin) in g/L × (pH × 0.123 − 0.631) + (phosphate) in mmol/L × (pH × 0.309 − 0.469)[10,11]

The difference ($SID_E$ − $SID_A$) is called the strong ion gap or SIG and is an estimate of unmeasured anions. The assessment of unmeasured anions could be viewed as an improvement over the classic anion gap, as it excludes disturbances due to albumin, phosphate, and lactate.

In daily practice, the physicochemical approach can be used on two levels of complexity. First, mostly for complex cases, the different elements of an acid-base problem (pH, pCO₂, electrolytes, lactate, phosphate, and albumin) can be introduced in a dedicated calculator (e.g. www.acidbase.org), leading to a very precise prediction of the impact of every factor (pCO₂, $A_{TOT}$, SID, and SIG) on plasma pH. The acid-base status can be visualized by plotting a gamblegram, illustrating every aspect of a patient's acid-base profile at a glance. The second way of applying the Stewart approach is more easily applicable at the bedside. After having determined the primary process according to the traditional approach, the clinician has a "quick-look" at the most important elements of the physicochemical approach to unmask the disease states responsible for metabolic acidosis and alkalosis and assess their impact on standard base excess.[12] An easy surrogate for $SID_A$ is the calculation of the difference between sodium and chloride. Normally this value lies around 35–38 mmol/L. Whenever the sodium-chloride difference is smaller, low-SID acidosis can be expected (e.g. after resuscitation with NaCl 0.9%), while the opposite is also true (high-SID alkalosis) due to an increased sodium-chloride difference. Also, the impact of hypoalbuminemia (or, less frequent, hyperalbuminemia) could be assessed by estimating the charged portion of the difference from the normal albumin level, analogy with the corrected anion gap, sees above). The part of the standard base excess that is not explained by the SID-effect and the albumin-effect must be caused by unmeasured anions.

This approach can be illustrated by the following case study. A 45-year-old male with a medical history of hypertension and chronic kidney failure is admitted in the emergency room presenting with fever, chills, and hypotension with mottled skin. An urgent blood gas analysis shows the following values: pH 7.18, pCO$_2$ 20 mm Hg, bicarbonate 8 mmol/L, standard base excess 20 mmol/L, sodium 130 mmol/L, potassium 3 mmol/L, chloride 105 mmol/L and lactate 5 mmol/L. Using the rules of five, it would take the full five steps to unmask the underlying normal anion gap metabolic acidosis, since the increased anion gap (normal 15 mmol/L, here 20 mmol/L) does not match with the severely decreased bicarbonate (normal 25 mmol/L, here 8 mmol/L), leading to delta gap of 12 mmol/L. A bedside calculation of the sodium-chloride difference, here decreased from 35 mmol/L to 25 mmol/L and therefore approximately responsible for 10 mmol of the negative standard base excess, quickly unmasks the main factor of the problem: low SID acidosis, due to relative hyperchloremia in relation to a low sodium level. The importance is stressed by the fact that if point-of-care lactate measurement had not been available, the situation could have been misinterpreted as a dramatic lactic acidosis and might have led to an unnecessary aggressive clinical approach.

## METABOLIC ACIDOSIS

### Case

A 67-year-old Caucasian female is admitted to the emergency department with pain in the right ankle and dyspnea. Her medical history includes type 2 diabetes mellitus, arterial hypertension, chronic kidney disease (CKD-EPI of 17.6 mL/min/1.73 m$^2$), atrial fibrillation, heart failure with preserved ejection fraction (HFpEF) with moderate mitral regurgitation and a right hemicolectomy for adenocarcinoma. Her regular medications include bumetanide, amlodipine, warfarin, tramadol hydrochloride, atenolol, and sitagliptin. Osteomyelitis complicated with acute congestive heart failure is suspected. After initiating treatment with intravenous loop diuretics and antibiotics [ciprofloxacin (250 mg twice daily)] and flucloxacillin [2 g (six times daily)] in the emergency department, she is hospitalized. Despite all efforts during the course of her stay, she develops oliguria with acute on chronic renal failure due to cardiorenal syndrome and—4 weeks after her initial admission—she is referred to the nephrologist.

Clinical examination shows signs of congestion (bilateral crackles and pitting edema of the lower limbs up to the knees) without much respiratory distress. Further physical examination is unremarkable. Chest X-ray looks largely decongested. The arterial blood gas analysis shows the following values: pH 7.29, pCO$_2$ 22 mm Hg, bicarbonate 11 mmol/L, standard base excess 14 mmol/L, sodium 145 mmol/L, potassium 3 mmol/L, chloride 108 mmol/L, lactate 1 mmol/L. Her renal function has worsened (CKD-EPI 8.9 mL/min/1.73 m$^2$). Further electrolyte analysis shows hyperphosphatemia (2.65 mmol/L), hypocalcemia (2.03 mmol/L), and a normal magnesium level (0.81 mmol/L). Her blood glycemia equals 4 mmol/L. There is profound hypoalbuminemia (22 g/L). No ketones are demonstrated in the urine.

## Different Causes of Metabolic Acidosis

### High Anion Gap Metabolic Acidosis

The most important distinction that must be made after the diagnosis of metabolic acidosis is whether unmeasured anions are present. Using the traditional approach, this is assessed by distinguishing high from normal anion gap metabolic acidosis (after having corrected the anion gap for abnormalities in albumin level). Using the Stewart approach, we assess SIG. Table 1 summarizes common and less common causes of unmeasured anions. Although many mnemonic acronyms are available (such as KUSMALE and MUDPILES), the newer "GOLDMARK" resembles the most complete list of causes.[13,14]

L-lactate is the most frequent cause of unmeasured anions in acutely ill patients.[15] Before advancing to the

**Table 1:** Frequent causes of metabolic acidosis due to unmeasured anions ("GOLDMARK").

| | |
|---|---|
| G | Glycols (e.g. ethylene and propylene) |
| O | 5-Oxoproline |
| L | L-lactate |
| D | D-lactate |
| M | Methanol |
| A | Aspirin |
| R | Renal failure |
| K | Ketoacidosis |

causes of this important marker of a wide array of clinical problems, we would like to stress the fact that there is no such thing as "lactic acidosis"![16] On a physiological level, glycolysis is the catabolic reaction that converts glucose to pyruvate. This process takes place in the cytosol of virtually all cells, after which—in aerobic conditions—pyruvate will be further metabolized and enter the Krebs cycle to produce a large amount of ATP. In anaerobic conditions or when mitochondrial respiration is saturated, there will be a need for greater reliance on ATP regeneration from nonmitochondrial sources such as glycolysis, a process causing cellular acidosis.[16] As for each molecule of pyruvate that is metabolized into lactate, one proton is captured—the production of lactate thus counteracts and delays acidosis. As such, lactate is a marker, rather than the cause of intracellular acidosis, making the terminology "lactic acidosis" an incorrect denominator that should not be used in clinical practice.

Anaerobic breakdown of glucose due to local (mesenteric ischemia, burns, seizures, or excessive muscle activity, etc.) or generalized hypoperfusion (shock, carbon monoxide intoxication, etc.) are well-known causes of lactate elevation. However, clinicians should be aware of many other conditions causing a rise in serum lactate. Beta-mimetics, excessive adrenergic stimulation (e.g. severe sepsis, acute lung injury, or asthma) and thiamine deficiency can cause elevated lactate levels, even in aerobic conditions due to an increased energy demand. In case of shock, a persistent high lactate level after 24 hours is associated with poor clinical outcomes. This also applies for septic patients with very high lactate levels at time of admission. Lactate can be helpful to diagnose mesenteric ischemia but be aware that lactate develops late in the course of mesenteric ischemia. Shortly after an epileptic insult, a steep rise in lactate level can be noticed. However, the peak is temporary and will decline within a few hours after seizures are resolved. An impaired clearance of lactate, as seen in acute liver failure, can also cause hyperlactatemia. It is in these situations that lactate used as a buffer in balanced solutions (see below) cannot be metabolized adequately, will continue to act as a strong anion and cause metabolic acidosis. Finally, L-lactate can also appear due to medication (biguanides, propofol, and nucleoside reverse transcriptase inhibitors), ethanol, leukemia or lymphoma and rarely in case of inborn errors of metabolism.

D-lactate is a different stereoisomeric form of lactate.[17] The production of D-lactate is strongly associated with short bowel syndrome. Carbohydrate malabsorption in the small intestine delivers a high carbohydrate load in the colon, where it can be fermented by bacteria to D-lactate. It is not possible to measure D-lactate with the current lactate tests, although it can be confirmed by specific laboratory analysis.

When unmeasured anions are detected, it is important to assess the osmolal gap, the difference between the osmolality that is calculated using the classic formula $[2 \times (Na^+) + glucose + urea]$ (all values in mmol/L) and the "true" measured osmolality. A normal osmolal gap is lower than 10 mmol/L. An increased osmolal gap (>20 mOsm/L) is an indication for the presence of osmotically active substances. Frequently, it concerns alcohols (ethanol, methanol, ethylene glycol, propylene glycol—components of antifreeze, windshield wiper fluid, and cleaners), but sugars (mannitol, sorbitol), proteins, and lipids (hypertriglyceridemia) are also possible causatives. Ketoacidosis, lactic acidosis, and renal failure only induce a mild osmolal gap (15–20 mOsm/L).

The presence of toxic alcohols should always be in the differential diagnosis when a high osmolal gap coexists with a high anion gap metabolic acidosis is found (also called "double gap acidosis"). Early after the ingestion of a toxic alcohol, the osmolal gap reaches its peak due to the serum concentration of the alcohol itself. The anion gap, on the other hand, will rise after a few hours when the un-ionized alcohols are metabolized into their toxic metabolites.[18] The osmolal gap due to methanol intoxication is frequently higher than with glycols because it has the lowest molecular weight of alcohols. The toxicity of methanol is mainly attributed to its metabolites (formaldehyde and then formic acid) formed by alcohol dehydrogenase. These metabolites are neurotoxic and may result in blindness due to retinal injury. Glycols (e.g. ethylene, propylene, and diethylene glycol) will be metabolized to toxic glycolic acid, glyoxylic acid, and oxalate. First, they cause neurologic complications, followed by specific end-organ damage (cardiopulmonary and renal). Often, lactate will be found false positive, as metabolites of ethylene glycol cross-react with L-lactate oxidase used in blood gas analyzers. Urinary calcium oxalate crystals, found in half of the cases at presentation, appear 4–8 hours after intake and are helpful in making the diagnosis.[19,20] It should be acknowledged that even in serious intoxications, the serum osmolal gap can be normal, especially in late presentations.[21] Concomitant intake of ethanol can also mitigate signs of profound toxicity because it inhibits the hepatic metabolism of the parent alcohol.[22]

5-Oxoprolineor pyroglutamic acid are toxic metabolites of the γ-glutamyl cycle after exposure to acetaminophen (glutathione depletion), high doses of flucloxacillin (inhibitor of 5-oxoprolinase) or both. Depletion of hepatic glutathione stores has a central role in the pathophysiology of 5-oxoproline-induced acidosis. Predisposing risk factors for acquired 5-oxoproline acidosis include age, female gender, cachexia or malnutrition, liver or renal disease and chronic alcohol abuse. It can be diagnosed by measuring serum and/or urinary 5-oxoproline levels. Inherited enzyme defects as a cause of 5-oxoproline accumulation are extremely rare.[23,24]

Salicylate overdose is a rare cause of high anion gap metabolic acidosis. It is often accompanied by a respiratory alkalosis due to stimulation of the respiratory system. Due to analytic issues, high salicylate levels can cause false negative normal anion gap acidosis.[25,26] Renal failure is a common cause of metabolic acidosis. Only advanced renal failure will lead to substantially increased unmeasured anions, where early stage renal failure will provoke normal anion gap acidosis (see below).[27] Renal failure leads to impaired excretion of acid anions (urea, phosphoric acid, and sulfate). Due to skeletal buffering of hydrogen ($H^+$), the serum bicarbonate level usually never drops below 10 mmol/L. If this occurs, it is necessary to screen for other causes of unmeasured anions.[28]

Ketones are responsible for the high anion gap in ketoacidosis, an acute complication of diabetes mellitus type 1, and sometimes the first presentation of undiagnosed diabetes. Because of a depletion of insulin and thus glucose as the main energy source, free fatty acids, metabolized to ketones will be used to maintain the body's energy needs. Acetoacetic acid, beta-hydroxybutyric acid, and acetone are the most important ketoacids. Note that a urinary dipstick (nitroprusside test) will especially react with acetoacetic acid, less with acetone, but not with β-hydroxybutyric acid (the predominant ketone).[29] Often, a precipitating event can be identified in patients admitted with ketoacidosis (infection, acute coronary syndrome, cerebral attack, pancreatitis, etc.). Euglycemic ketoacidosis is known in patients treated with SGLT2-inhibitors.[30] Severe alcoholism, severe starvation, or both may contribute to nondiabetic ketoacidosis.[31,32]

Other causes of unmeasured anions include toluene (a solvent of some types of paint thinners and glue), the tuberculostatic isoniazid, paraldehyde intake, and citrate toxicity. Citrate accumulation can be seen after massive transfusion or after administering of citrate as regional anticoagulant (renal replacement therapy). Toxicity of citrate is usually seen in patients with concomitant liver failure because of the inadequate conversion of citrate to bicarbonate. It is characterized by low systemic ionized calcium ($iCa^{2+}$) and a high total serum calcium ($tCa^{2+}$). The diagnosis of citrate intoxication is likely if the $tCa^{2+}/iCa^{2+}$ ratio is more than 2.5.[33]

### Normal Anion Gap or Low Strong Ion Difference Metabolic Acidosis

Normal anion gap metabolic acidosis is most frequently caused by an increase in chloride in the absence of a concomitant rise in sodium concentration, causing a decrease in SID. Therefore, it is usually called hyperchloremic metabolic acidosis, although low SID acidosis would be an even more appropriate term. The causes are summarized in Box 1.

The most frequent cause is the administration of intravenous fluids with zero SID.[34] When resuscitating a patient with large amounts of fluids, plasma SID will be forced in the direction of the SID of the fluid. The clinical importance of this disturbance is currently unclear.[35] Fluid-induced disorders of the acid-base equilibrium can

**Box 1:** Causes of normal anion gap metabolic acidosis.

- *Fluid resuscitation:*
  - Unbalanced crystalloids (the administration of zero-SID solutions, e.g. NaCl 0.9%, decreasing plasma strong ion difference)
- *Gastrointestinal:*[37]
  - *Diarrhea:* Large-volume losses of sodium, potassium, and bicarbonate
  - *Biliary and pancreatic drainage:* Mostly postoperative depletion of bicarbonate-rich (chloride-poor) fluids
  - *Laxative abuse:* Typically characterized by severe hypokalemia and metabolic alkalosis. Metabolic acidosis will arise only when laxative abuse is accompanied with diarrhea.[39]
  - Ureterosigmoidostomy, less frequent with Bricker deviation (ileal conduit), due to enteral resorption of urinary chloride[40]
  - Small intestinal fistulas or villous adenomas (rare tumors)
- *Renal:*
  - Early stage of renal failure: Decline of the ability to excrete ammonium due to the loss of functional nephrons
  - Carbonic anhydrase inhibitor, resulting in hyperchloremia[41]
  - Renal tubular acidosis (RTA):[42]
    - Type I RTA: Impaired acidification in the distal tubule: urinary pH should be > 5.5 despite of metabolic acidosis.
    - Type II RTA: Impaired $HCO_3^-$-reabsorption in proximal tubule, but distal acidification is intact so urinary pH can be reduced to < 5.3.
    - Type IV RTA: Due to aldosterone deficiency or resistance and characterized by patients with serum hyperkalemia without an obvious cause (e.g. renal failure or drug induced).
- *Others*:
  - Hyperalimentation
  - Hippuric acid

(SID: strong ion difference)

be avoided by using solutions that do not alter plasma SID. We call these solutions "balanced" and their common characteristic lies in the fact that they contain more strong cations (mostly sodium) than strong anions (mostly chloride) and the electrical "gap" hereby created is filled by agents, like lactate, acetate or gluconate that will quickly be metabolized by the liver or muscles.

Normal anion gap or low SID acidosis can also be caused by gastrointestinal or renal problems.[36,37] Assessing the urinary anion gap can help to differentiate between these two causes. In analogy with serum anion gap, urinary anion gap is the difference between the urinary cations sodium and potassium and the anion chloride (the amount of urinary bicarbonate is negligible).[38] A negative urinary anion gap hints at the presence of the unmeasured cation ammonium ($NH_4^+$). Ammonium is used by the kidney to excrete chloride without the concomitant excretion of sodium. A normal anion gap or low SID acidosis in the presence of a negative urinary anion gap indicates an adequate renal response to acidosis, pointing out a gastrointestinal cause (neGUTive). Normal anion gap acidosis with a positive urinary anion gap indicates impaired ammonium excretion as seen in renal causes, such as the different forms of renal tubular acidosis.

## Case Revisit

Using the traditional approach, we apply the "Rules of Five". First step: Acidosis or alkalosis. Acidemia, and thus acidosis is present as the pH has decreased below 7.35. Second step: Metabolic or respiratory. The primary cause seems to be metabolic, as bicarbonate and SBE are below normal values. Third step: Anion gap. The anion gap is 29 mmol/L, so there is a high anion gap metabolic acidosis. The anion gap needs to be corrected for the underlying hypoalbuminemia. As albumin has decreased from its normal value of 40 g/L to 22 g/L and around 25% of albumin in human plasma is present in its charged state, the anion gap should be increased with 4.5 mmol/L. The corrected anion gap thus amounts to ±34 mmol/L or around 20 mmol/L of unmeasured anions. Fourth step: Compensatory response. Respiratory compensation is clearly present, as $pCO_2$ decreased to 22 mmol/L. The Boston rules can predict whether this compensation is adequate. As bicarbonate has decreased with 14 mmol/L (25 mmol/L to 11 mmol/L), a complete respiratory compensation would lead to a decrease in $pCO_2$ of 1–1.3 times this amount (a decrease of 14–18 mm Hg from a normal value of 40 mmol/L, or a $pCO_2$ of 22–26 mm Hg). This corresponds to the measured $pCO_2$ (22 mm Hg). Fifth and final step: Delta gap. The increase in (actual, not corrected!) anion gap (15–29 = 14 mmol/L) is accompanied by an equal decrease in serum bicarbonate of 14 mmol/L, so no concomitant normal anion gap metabolic acidosis nor metabolic alkalosis is present.

When applying the bedside principles of the physicochemical approach according to Stewart, it can be easily appreciated that the sodium-chloride difference (37 mmol/L) is more or less normal, so there are no relevant disturbances due to an altered strong ion. On the other hand, hypoalbuminemia is responsible for a decreased $A_{TOT}$ (4.5 mmol/L). The SBE of –14 mmol/L consists of a negligible SID-effect, so taking again 4.5 mmol/L of hypoalbuminemic metabolic alkalosis into account, around 20 mmol/L of unmeasured anions is once more unmasked. A complete Stewart analysis can precisely quantify the acid-base effects of all components of the acid-base disorder (Fig. 3A), further visualized by a gamblegram (Fig. 3B).

Whatever the approach used, it is clear that the primary disorder is a metabolic acidosis due to unmeasured anions. Potential causes are evaluated based on the GOLDMARK mnemonic. The patient has a medical history of type 2 diabetes mellitus, but dipstick for urinary ketones is negative. (Apart from this case, it should be noted that treatment with the oral antidiabetic SGLT-2 inhibitors can induce ketoacidosis in the absence of hyperglycemia). On arterial blood gas analysis, no elevation of L-lactate (1 mmol/L) is detected. Although her medical history reveals a right hemicolectomy, this is not a common cause of short bowel syndrome. Also, the absence of diarrhea renders D-lactate as the cause of metabolic acidosis extremely unlikely. An unremarkable osmolal gap and the absence of ingestion of alcohols virtually rules out an intoxication with methanol or ethylene glycol. There is no record of salicylate intake. Renal failure is the most obvious cause of the high anion gap acidosis. On the other hand, even in end-stage renal disease (ESRD), the plasma bicarbonate level is maintained between 12 mmol/L and 20 mmol/L by buffer systems other than bicarbonate. A bicarbonate level below 12 mmol/L is very unusual, which should be taken into consideration when a high anion gap acidosis is assigned to renal failure. A second cause of high anion gap is thus suspected. Given she was treated with high doses flucloxacillin for 6 weeks, the patient is screened for the accumulation of 5-oxoproline. The serum level of 5-oxoproline is clearly elevated (6.74 mmol/L), with a urinary oxoproline concentration of 5.4 mg/mg creatinine. We conclude the combination of renal failure and the presence of 5-oxoproline are responsible for the metabolic acidosis, counteracted by respiratory compensation and

# Chapter 33
## Approach to the Patient with Metabolic Acidosis and Alkalosis

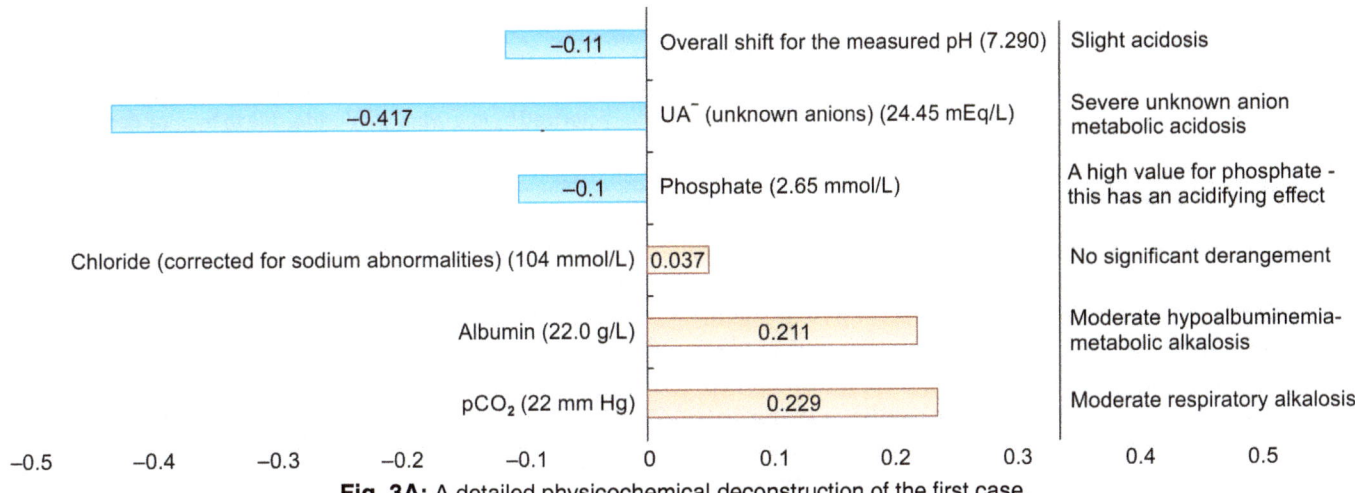

**Fig. 3A:** A detailed physicochemical deconstruction of the first case.
*Source:* www.acidbase.org.

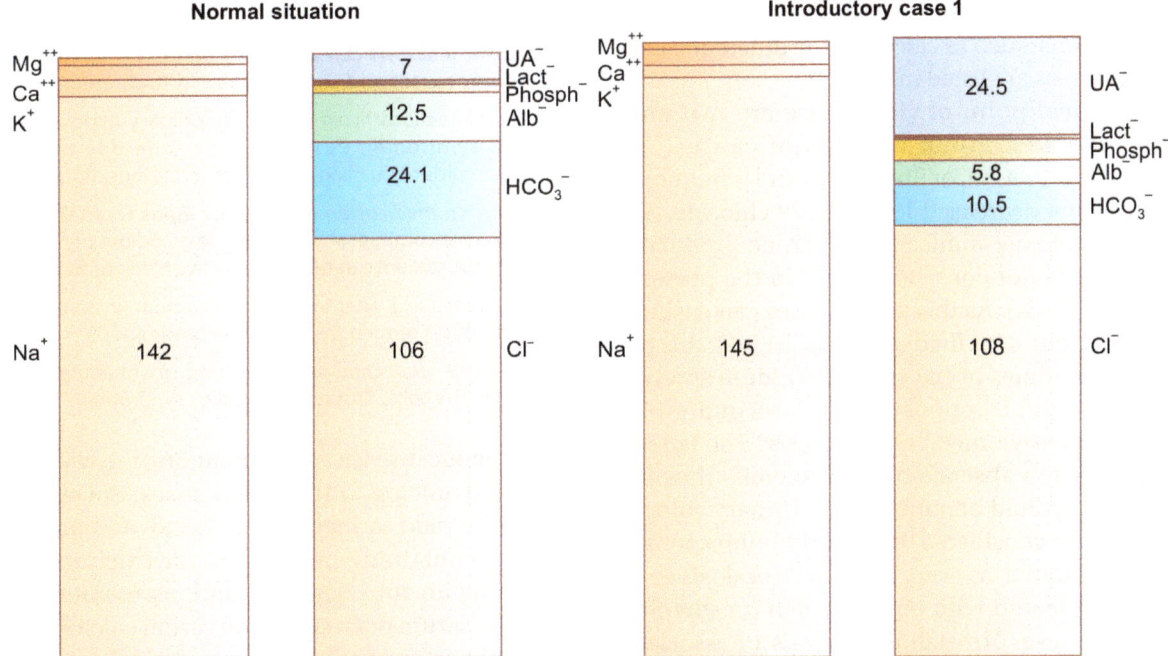

**Fig. 3B:** Precise visualization of the first case using a gamblegram. Left: normal situation, Right: data from the first case.
*Source:* www.acidbase.org.

hypoalbuminemia. Flucloxacillin was immediately stopped and intravenous acetylcysteine was started. Continuous venovenous hemofiltration (CVVH) was initiated on the intensive care unit.

## METABOLIC ALKALOSIS

### Case

In the late afternoon, the hospital's emergency team is called to the surgical ward, where a patient was found unconscious by the attending nurse. Two days earlier, the patient had been admitted for acute alcoholic pancreatitis and had been unable to ingest food or fluids since admission. Postpyloric feeding had not been initiated yet. In the meantime, he had been treated with Plasmalyte A (Na 140 mmol/L, potassium 5 mmol/L, chloride 98 mmol/L) at a rate of 166 mL per hour. On arrival of the emergency team, the following parameters are noted: blood pressure 110/60 mm Hg, a regular pulse 94 beats/minute, respiratory rate 10 breaths/minute, Glasgow Coma Scale 8/15 (E1M5V2). The patient has a nasogastric tube in place, that has produced 1 L of gastric fluid over the last

12 hours. An arterial blood gas analysis is quickly drawn and shows the following values: pH 7.55, $pCO_2$ 52 mm Hg, bicarbonate 45 mmol/L, standard base excess 21 mmol/L, sodium 135 mmol/L, potassium 3 mmol/L and chloride 85 mmol/L.

## Causes of Metabolic Alkalosis

According to the bicarbonate-centered approach, primary metabolic alkalosis is characterized by an elevated pH and an increased [$HCO_3^-$] and SBE due to a loss of [$H^+$] or a gain in [$HCO_3^-$]. From a physicochemical perspective, there are two different types of metabolic alkalosis: an increased SID or a decreased $A_{TOT}$. Hypoalbuminemia is by far the most frequent cause of a decreased $A_{TOT}$. An increased SID is characterized by an increase in the difference between strong cations and anions. In clinical practice, this is mostly frequently caused by a decrease in chloride, sometimes due to an increase in sodium and very rarely to an increment in strong other cations, such as calcium. The different causes of high SID alkalosis are listed in Box 2.

From a clinical point of view, there are two main categories—the first group consists of causes, e.g. hypovolemia, dehydration, or fluid losses and is frequently characterized by a decreased low urinary chloride, as a marker of hypovolemia-induced aldosterone-production (urinary sodium is not consistently low in the presence of metabolic alkalosis). As this set of causes can easily be treated with chloride-rich fluids (e.g. NaCl 0.9%), this first category has sometimes been called "chloride-responsive metabolic alkalosis", as opposed to the second group, "chloride-unresponsive metabolic alkalosis". The latter is characterized by the absence of hypovolemia, thus less easily corrected by fluid administration. Urinary chloride is high. It should be considered that chloride-unresponsive alkalosis is a misnomer, as every metabolic alkalosis could be successfully treated with chloride-rich (or low-SID) solutions. Many causes of metabolic alkalosis are associated with hypokalemia. Hypokalemia itself maintains metabolic alkalosis by different mechanisms, e.g. it results in an intracellular shift of ($H^+$), impairs chloride reabsorption in the distal tubule and stimulates renal ammonium production, leading to the loss of chloride without the concomitant loss of sodium. Metabolic alkalosis can also be seen when chronic hypercapnia is suddenly corrected (e.g. mechanical ventilation of a patient with long-term chronic obstructive pulmonary disease).[45,46] Long-term hypoalbuminemic metabolic alkalosis is frequently compensated by hyperchloremic metabolic acidosis.

In clinical practice, a useful approach to the patient with metabolic alkalosis is to screen first for chloride- or

**Box 2:** Causes of metabolic alkalosis.

**Metabolic alkalosis caused by chloride loss or hypovolemia-induced aldosterone-production with sodium retention. Characterized by low urinary chloride, due to hyperaldosteronism (exception: diuretic-induced alkalosis)**

*Gastrointestinal:*
- Loss or removal of chloride-rich gastric secretions, due to vomiting or losses through nasogastric tube (including self-induced vomiting)
- Chloride-losing diarrhea (including laxative abuse)

*Renal:*
- Loop or thiazide diuretics (urinary chloride can be high)
- Rare genetic renal tubulopathies with a loop diuretic-type defect (Bartter's syndrome) or a thiazide-type defect in the distal tubule (Gitelman's syndrome)

*Skin:*
- Chloride-containing sweat losses in cystic fibrosis

*Contraction or chloride depletion alkalosis:[43]*

**Metabolic alkalosis caused by a gain in strong cations. Mostly euvolemic causes and characterized by high urinary chloride.**

*Primary mineralocorticoid excess,* e.g. primary hyperaldosteronism (Conn's syndrome), Cushing's syndrome due to exogenous corticosteroids or Cushing's disease, licorice ingestion

*Sodium-rich medication or high-SID fluids* (containing sodium without a concomitant strong anion), e.g. sodium penicillin, sodium bicarbonate, sodium citrate due to massive blood product transfusion.

*Hypercalcemia,* e.g. after ingestion of calcium (in combination with antacids, this is termed the milk-alkali syndrome)[44]

*Rare, genetic renal conditions,* resulting in enhanced retention of sodium in the collecting tubule (Liddle's syndrome).

hypovolemic disease states, including the use of diuretics, before advancing to the rarer causes. Specific attention should be paid to ingestion of laxatives, corticosteroids, sodium-containing medication, or calcium-rich fluids. If nothing obvious can be found, assessment of urinary chloride, serum potassium, and serum calcium will enable the clinician to exclude other prominent causes. In the case of high urinary chloride, specific inherited renal and endocrinological disease should be ruled out by specialized professionals.

## Case Revisit

Alkalemia (step 1) in combination with high bicarbonate and SBE quickly leads to the diagnosis of metabolic alkalosis (step 2). Calculation of the anion gap (step 3) could in this case be interesting to check—although unlikely—whether an underlying high anion gap metabolic acidosis could be present. This is not the case as the anion gap is within the normal range (8 mmol/L). To determine the level of

# Chapter 33
## Approach to the Patient with Metabolic Acidosis and Alkalosis

compensation (step 4), we check whether the change in pCO₂ is around 0.6 times the change in bicarbonate from its normal value of 25. In this case, bicarbonate has increased with 20 mmol/L, thus the increase in pCO₂ of 12 mm Hg means there is an adequate compensatory effort. The calculation of the delta gap is unnecessary, as metabolic alkalosis has already been diagnosed and high anion gap metabolic alkalosis has already been excluded. From a physicochemical point of view, there is an obvious increase in sodium-chloride difference (50 mmol/L), acting as a quick assessment of high SID. No values of albumin or phosphate are available. Although, the diagnosis is clear without the need for a detailed analysis, for the sake of completeness, we provide a full physicochemical analysis in Figure 4A and the according gamblegrams in Figure 4B.

The clinical picture can thus be explained by convulsions due to metabolic alkalosis, possibly enhanced by alcohol withdrawal. The origin of the metabolic alkalosis

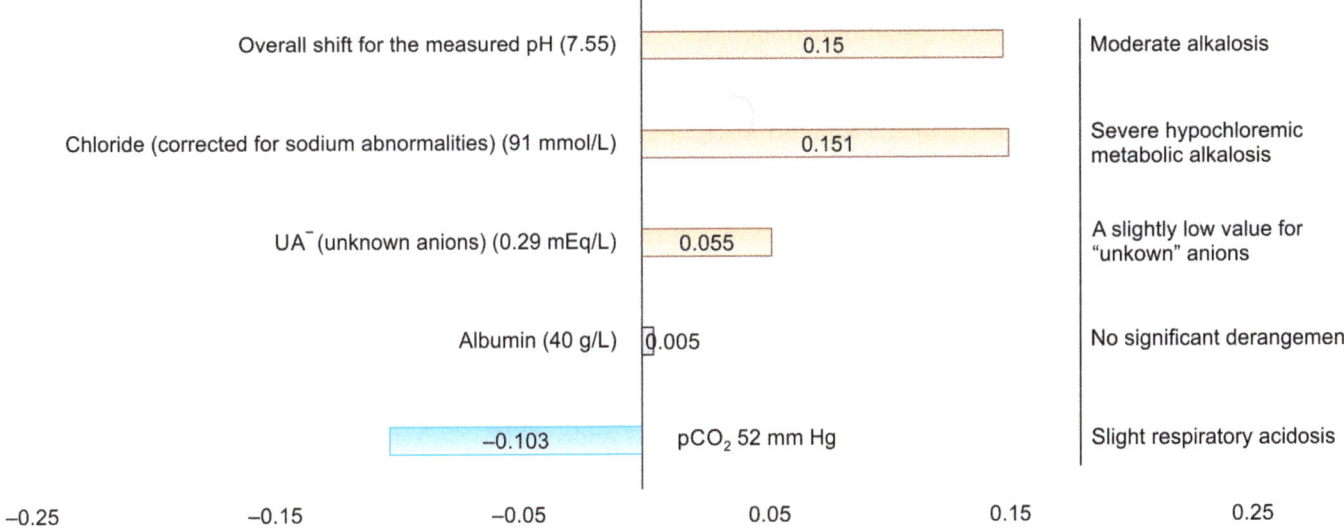

**Fig. 4A:** A detailed physicochemical deconstruction of the second case.
*Source:* www.acidbase.org.

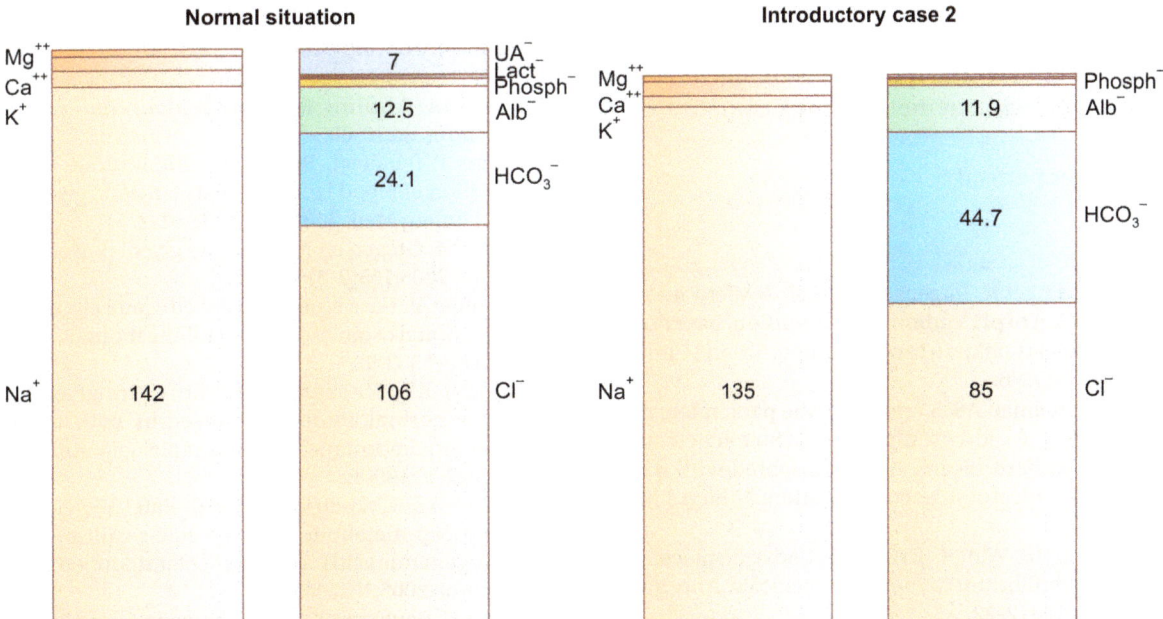

**Fig. 4B:** Precise visualization of the second case using a gamblegram. Left: normal situation, Right: data from the second case.
*Source:* www.acidbase.org.

is threefold. Loss of gastric fluid, induced by pancreatitis-associated paralytic ileus, is the most important cause, as illustrated by the important hypochloremia. The treatment with a high SID solution such as Plasmalyte is not the best choice in this particular situation. With its *in vivo* SID of 50 mEq/L, it is likely that this solution has aggravated the metabolic alkalosis. Zero-SID solutions, e.g. NaCl 0.9% remain the option of choice in patients that loose chloride-rich gastric fluid. Finally, hypokalemia certainly contributes to the metabolic alkalosis as described earlier. In summary, this is a typical case of chloride-responsive metabolic alkalosis. In a hypovolemic or euvolemic patient, the administration of NaCl 0.9% will sufficiently correct the disturbances rapidly. In the unlikely case of hypervolemia, it would be possible to administer a concentrated negative SID solution, such as ammonium chloride.

## SALIENT POINTS

- Both metabolic acidosis with a high and normal anion gap and metabolic alkalosis can coexist and therefore need to be approached stepwise and methodically.
- The "traditional", bicarbonate-centered approach includes a set of rules of thumb to find mixed disorders and to evaluate the degree of a compensatory process.
- The physicochemical or "Stewart" approach offers the most complete tools to break down an acid-base disorder to its individual components and draws electrolytes and weak acids such as albumin in the picture.
- A little insight in these physicochemical principles is extremely helpful in the quick bedside diagnosis of mixed disorders without the need for a complex set of rules.
- Practice makes perfect!

## REFERENCES

1. Andersen OS, Engel K, Jorgensen K, et al. A Micro method for determination of pH, carbon dioxide tension, base excess and standard bicarbonate in capillary blood. Scand J Clin Lab Invest. 1960;12:172-6.
2. Schwartz WB, Relman AS. A critique of the parameters used in the evaluation of acid-base disorders. "Whole-blood buffer base" and "standard bicarbonate" compared with blood pH and plasma bicarbonate concentration. N Engl J Med. 1963;268:1382-8.
3. Albert MS, Dell RB, Winters RW. Quantitative displacement of acid-base equilibrium in metabolic acidosis. Ann Intern Med. 1967;66(2):312-22.
4. Whittier WL, Rutecki GW. Primer on clinical acid-base problem solving. Dis Mon. 2004;50(3):122-62.
5. Reddy P, Mooradian AD. Clinical utility of anion gap in deciphering acid-base disorders. Int J Clin Pract. 2009;63(10):1516-25.
6. Kraut JA, Madias NE. Serum anion gap: its uses and limitations in clinical medicine. Clin J Am Soc Nephrol. 2007;2(1):162-74.
7. Chawla LS, Shih S, Davison D, et al. Anion gap, anion gap corrected for albumin, base deficit and unmeasured anions in critically ill patients: implications on the assessment of metabolic acidosis and the diagnosis of hyperlactatemia. BMC Emerg Med. 2008;8:18.
8. Gattinoni L. Foreword. In: Kellum JA, Elbers PW (Eds). Stewart's Textbook of Acid-Base, 2nd edition. Amsterdem: PW Elbers and Acidbase.org; 2009. pp. 21-3.
9. Stewart PA. Modern quantitative acid-base chemistry. Can J Physiol Pharmacol. 1983;61(12):1444-61.
10. Figge J, Rossing TH, Fencl V. The role of serum proteins in acid-base equilibria. J Lab Clin Med. 1991;117(6):453-67.
11. Fencl V, Jabor A, Kazda A, et al. Diagnosis of metabolic acid-base disturbances in critically ill patients. Am J Respir Crit Care Med. 2000;162(6):2246-51.
12. Story DA. Stewart acid-base: a simplified bedside approach. Anesth Analg. 2016;123(2):511-5.
13. Berend K, de Vries AP, Gans RO. Physiological approach to assessment of acid-base disturbances. N Engl J Med. 2014;371(15):1434-45.
14. Mehta AN, Emmett JB, Emmett M. GOLD MARK: an anion gap mnemonic for the 21st century. Lancet. 2008;372(9642):892.
15. Andersen LW, Mackenhauer J, Roberts JC, et al. Etiology and therapeutic approach to elevated lactate levels. Mayo Clin Proc. 2013;88(10):1127-40.
16. Robergs RA, Ghiasvand F, Parker D. Biochemistry of exercise-induced metabolic acidosis. Am J Physiol Regul Integr Comp Physiol. 2004;287(3):R502-16.
17. Uribarri J, Oh MS, Carroll HJ. D-lactic acidosis. A review of clinical presentation, biochemical features, and pathophysiologic mechanisms. Medicine (Baltimore). 1998;77(2):73-82.
18. Kraut JA, Mullins ME. Toxic alcohols. N Engl J Med. 2018;378(3):270-80.
19. Pernet P, Bénéteau-Burnat B, Vaubourdolle M, et al. False elevation of blood lactate reveals ethylene glycol poisoning. Am J Emerg Med. 2009;27(1):132.e1-2.
20. Leth PM, Gregersen M. Ethylene glycol poisoning. Forensic Sci Int. 2005;155(2-3):179-84.
21. Steinhart B. Case report: severe ethylene glycol intoxication with normal osmolal gap—"a chilling thought". J Emerg Med. 1990;8(5):583-5.
22. Ammar KA, Heckerling PS. Ethylene glycol poisoning with a normal anion gap caused by concurrent ethanol ingestion: importance of the osmolal gap. Am J Kidney Dis. 1996;27(1):130-3.
23. Fenves AZ, Kirkpatrick HM 3rd, Patel VV, et al. Increased anion gap metabolic acidosis as a result of 5-oxoproline (pyroglutamic acid): a role for acetaminophen. Clin J Am Soc Nephrol. 2006;1(3):441-7.
24. Lanoy C, Bouckaert Y. Metabolic acidosis and 5-oxoprolinuria induced by flucloxacillin and acetaminophen: a case report. J Med Case Rep. 2016;10(1):184.

25. Gabow PA, Anderson RJ, Potts DE, et al. Acid-base disturbances in the salicylate-intoxicated adult. Arch Intern Med. 1978;138(10):1481-4.
26. Jacob J, Lavonas EJ. Falsely normal anion gap in severe salicylate poisoning caused by laboratory interference. Ann Emerg Med. 2011;58(3):280-1.
27. Warnock DG. Uremic acidosis. Kidney Int. 1988;34(2):278-87.
28. Taboulet P, Haas L, Porcher R, et al. Urinary acetoacetate or capillary beta-hydroxybutyrate for the diagnosis of ketoacidosis in the emergency department setting. Eur J Emerg Med. 2004;11(5):251-8.
29. Adrogue HJ, Wilson H, Boyd AE 3rd, et al. Plasma acid-base patterns in diabetic ketoacidosis. N Engl J Med. 1982;307(26):1603-10.
30. Peters AL, Buschur EO, Buse JB, et al. Euglycemic diabetic ketoacidosis: A potential complication of treatment with sodium-glucose cotransporter 2 inhibition. Diabetes Care. 2015;38(9):1687-93.
31. Levy LJ, Duga J, Girgis M, et al. Ketoacidosis associated with alcoholism in nondiabetic subjects. Ann Intern Med. 1973;78(2):213-9.
32. Toth HL, Greenbaum LA. Severe acidosis caused by starvation and stress. Am J Kidney Dis. 2003;42(5):E16-9.
33. Kramer L, Bauer E, Joukhadar C, et al. Citrate pharmacokinetics and metabolism in cirrhotic and noncirrhotic critically ill patients. Crit Care Med. 2003;31(10):2450-5.
34. Kellum JA. Saline-induced hyperchloremic metabolic acidosis. Crit Care Med. 2002;30(1):259-61.
35. Van Regenmortel N, Verbrugghe W, Van den Wyngaert T, et al. Impact of chloride and strong ion difference on ICU and hospital mortality in a mixed intensive care population. Ann Intensive Care. 2016;6(1):91.
36. Kraut JA, Madias NE. Differential diagnosis of nongap metabolic acidosis: value of a systematic approach. Clin J Am Soc Nephrol. 2012;7(4):671-9.
37. Gennari FJ, Weise WJ. Acid-base disturbances in gastrointestinal disease. Clin J Am Soc Nephrol. 2008;3(6):1861-8.
38. Goldstein MB, Bear R, Richardson RM, et al. The urine anion gap: a clinically useful index of ammonium excretion. Am J Med Sci. 1986;292(4):198-202.
39. Oster JR, Materson BJ, Rogers AI. Laxative abuse syndrome. Am J Gastroenterol. 1980;74(5):451-8.
40. McDougal WS. Metabolic complications of urinary intestinal diversion. J Urol. 1992;147(5):1199-208.
41. Moviat M, Pickkers P, van der Voort PH, et al. Acetazolamide-mediated decrease in strong ion difference accounts for the correction of metabolic alkalosis in critically ill patients. Crit Care. 2006;10(1):R14.
42. Rodríguez Soriano J. Renal tubular acidosis: the clinical entity. J Am Soc Nephrol. 2002;13(8):2160-70.
43. Luke RG, Galla JH. It is chloride depletion alkalosis, not contraction alkalosis. J Am Soc Nephrol. 2012;23(2):204-7.
44. Medarov BI. Milk-alkali syndrome. Mayo Clin Proc. 2009;84(3):261-7.
45. Polak A, Haynie GD, Hays RM, et al. Effects of chronic hypercapnia on electrolyte and acid-base equilibrium. I. Adaptation. J Clin Invest. 1961;40:1223-37.
46. Schwartz WB, Hays RM, Polak A, et al. Effects of chronic hypercapnia on electrolyte and acid-base equilibrium. II. Recovery, with special reference to the influence of chloride intake. J Clin Invest. 1961;40:1238-49.

# CHAPTER 34

# Approach to the Patient with Respiratory Acidosis and Alkalosis

*John Botha, Ravindranath Tiruvoipati*

## RESPIRATORY ACIDOSIS

### Case

A 45-year-old male presented to his family physician with acute shortness of breath. He had a past medical history of asthma. His asthma was well controlled in the past and he had not previously been admitted to hospital for his asthma. He was a current smoker and was experiencing flu-like symptoms few days prior to presentation to his family physician. His physician suspected an acute exacerbation of asthma with clinical features suggestive of a pneumothorax. He was transferred to the emergency department of a large hospital and shortly after presentation suffered a respiratory arrest. He was intubated, resuscitated and a confirmed left pneumothorax was decompressed after placement of an intercostal catheter. He was subsequently admitted to the intensive care unit (ICU) and was difficult to ventilate with uncontrollable hypercapnia and respiratory acidosis. Partial pressure of carbon dioxide ($PaCO_2$) was 73 mm Hg with a pH of 7.22 and worsening surgical emphysema.

### Definition

Respiratory acidosis arises from acute or chronic hypercapnia defined as an elevation in the arterial $CO_2$ tension ($PaCO_2$) associated with acidosis (arterial pH <7.35).

### Etiology/Mechanism

The arterial $CO_2$ level is directly proportional to the rate of production of $CO_2$ and inversely proportional to $CO_2$ elimination by the lung (alveolar ventilation). As illustrated in Table 1, there are many causes of hypercapnic respiratory failure. Conditions that depress the respiratory center include therapeutic or recreational drug administration, traumatic brain injury, a cerebrovascular

**Table 1:** Causes of respiratory acidosis.

| | |
|---|---|
| Inadequate alveolar ventilation | *Central respiratory depression*:<br>• Hypoventilation of obesity<br>• Drug-induced depression of the respiratory center<br>• CNS trauma, infarct or hemorrhage<br>• High central neural blockade<br>• Cervical cord trauma or lesions<br>• Poliomyelitis<br>• Tetanus<br>*Nerve or muscle disorders*:<br>• Muscle relaxant drugs<br>• Myasthenia gravis<br>• Guillain-Barré syndrome<br>• Myopathies<br>• Toxins<br>*Lung or chest wall pathology*:<br>• Adult respiratory distress syndrome<br>• Pneumonia<br>• Pulmonary edema<br>• Restrictive lung disease<br>• Chronic obstructive pulmonary disease (COPD)<br>• Chest trauma<br>• Pneumothorax<br>• Diaphragmatic paralysis or splinting<br>*Airway disorders*:<br>• Bronchospasm/asthma<br>• Upper airway obstruction<br>• Laryngospasm |
| Overproduction of $CO_2$ | • Malignant hyperthermia<br>• Neuroleptic malignant syndrome<br>• Hypercatabolic disorders |
| Increased intake of $CO_2$ | • Insufflation of $CO_2$ into a body cavity<br>• Addition of $CO_2$ to inspired gas<br>• Rebreathing of $CO_2$-containing expired gas |

event or meningoencephalitis. More caudal neurological conditions are cervical cord trauma, infections, tumors or demyelinating pathologies. Pathology of the anterior horn cells such as motor neuron disease would need to be considered particularly if the clinical examination provided features suggestive of this diagnosis such as skeletal muscle atrophy and fasciculation. Peripheral neuropathy remains a rare but potentially life-threatening cause of hypoventilation and the clinician needs to remain vigilant when considering rapidly progressive neuropathy such as the Guillain-Barré syndrome. Dysfunction of the neuromuscular junction may be more problematic to diagnose particularly if there is no history of recent anesthetic administration. A history of muscle fatigability may be the only clue to unrecognized myasthenia gravis. A family history of muscular weakness is important if muscular dystrophy is considered and the cutaneous manifestations of an immune-mediated myopathy should be sought. The clinical examination remains invaluable in eliciting the signs of muscular weakness and muscle enzymes, autoantibodies and nerve conduction studies are usually confirmatory. The respiratory examination and chest radiograph are required to make a diagnosis of chest wall, pleural, airway or a lung parenchymal disease process that may impede ventilation and cause respiratory acidosis. Occasionally elevated levels of $CO_2$ may be due to increased production in conditions such as malignant hyperthermia, shivering, hyperpyrexia, and neuroleptic malignant syndrome.

## Clinical Effects

The physiological consequences of hypercapnia and hypercapnic acidosis are that various organ systems may be affected including the respiratory, cardiovascular,[1,2] central nervous, neuromuscular and renal systems. Hypercapnia has many effects on the cardiovascular system by influencing preload, afterload and myocardial contractility. Hypercapnic acidosis increases heart rate but decreases myocardial contractility and systemic vascular resistance. The net effect of these changes is an increase in cardiac output. The respiratory effect of acute hypercapnia is one of induced air hunger and an increased respiratory drive. Contrary to the vasodilatory effects of hypercapnia on the systemic circulation, hypercapnic acidosis induces hypoxic pulmonary vasoconstriction with a reduction in the shunt induced decrease in $PaO_2$. The exact consequences of hypercapnia on oxygen carriage and oxygen dissociation are complex and not clearly understood. Hypercapnia and acidosis shifts the hemoglobin-oxygen dissociation curve toward right reducing the affinity of hemoglobin to oxygen. This has two important implications. It augments the tissue release of oxygen as well as reduces the oxygen uptake from pulmonary alveoli to pulmonary capillary blood. The overall effect of hypercapnia is an unchanged or improved tissue oxygenation due to increase in cardiac output. The implication of reduction in oxygen affinity with the right shift of the dissociation curve remains unknown in clinical practice. The central nervous system effects of hypercapnia include an increase in intracranial pressure due to cerebral vasodilation.[3] Acute hypercapnia may also cause $CO_2$ narcosis and this is particularly relevant in patients with $CO_2$ retention who are administered narcotics. Hypercapnic acidosis has also been shown to reduce renal blood flow but the clinical consequences of this effect are unclear.[4]

In the early stages of many disease processes, physiological compensation may occur at the expense of an increased work of breathing. With time and appropriate renal compensation, acute respiratory acidosis may progress to chronic respiratory acidosis as bicarbonate is retained. This presentation is usually a manifestation of long-standing chronic obstructive airways disease. What remains a more life-threatening complication of ventilatory failure is the onset of muscle and diaphragmatic fatigue, particularly if associated with an altered level of consciousness as a consequence of hypercarbia.

## Approach/Evaluation

Respiratory acidosis is usually the physiological manifestation of decreased alveolar ventilation and a useful approach to diagnosis is to consider the anatomical sites where pathology may compromise ventilation. If there is depression of the respiratory center, there is usually an altered level of consciousness and the history, clinical examination and sometimes neuroimaging is required to confirm the diagnosis. Table 1 provides a useful mechanistic guide to conditions that may cause respiratory acidosis.

As respiratory acidosis may be acute or chronic in presentation, a detailed history and clinical examination is invaluable in elucidating the pathophysiology. It may also be helpful to revert to radiological imaging and arterial blood gas interpretation to further understand the disease process. Arterial blood gasses are useful in distinguishing acute from chronic respiratory acidosis. As the kidneys take time to compensate for acidosis, acute hypercapnic failure is associated with acidemia as opposed to chronic respiratory acidosis where renal compensation has occurred.[5,6] It has been established that unless there are confounders in the setting of acute respiratory acidosis, the serum $HCO_3$ increases by 0.8 mmol/L up to 30 mmol/L for each 7.5 mm Hg increase in $PaCO_2$. In chronic respiratory acidosis, the serum $HCO_3$ increases by 3 mmol/L up to 36 mmol/L for each 7.5 mm Hg increase in $PaCO_2$. The clinical application of these findings may be hampered in patients with disordered renal function or where loop diuretics have been administered.

## Management

The management of respiratory acidosis will be determined by the physiological and clinical consequences of the acidosis and whether the process is acute or chronic.[7] Chronic respiratory acidosis is unlikely to be life-threatening unless acute decompensation has occurred. Furthermore, chronic respiratory acidosis is usually associated with long-standing pathophysiology with a variable response to therapy. Typical examples are obstructive sleep apnea and chronic obstructive pulmonary disease. Progressive neuromuscular disease may also present as chronic hyperbaric respiratory failure and therapy will be guided by treating reversible factors and establishing the appropriateness of permanent ventilator support.

Acute respiratory acidosis usually requires urgent intervention particularly if the hypercarbia is profound, resulting in an altered level of consciousness and/or organ dysfunction. Under these circumstances reversible causes should be identified and treated. Supportive treatments including mechanical ventilation may be required. The past decade has witnessed a marked increase in the use of noninvasive ventilation with evidence indicating it is particularly advantageous in respiratory failure attributed to chronic obstructive pulmonary disease. Should invasive mechanical ventilation be required, careful consideration should be given to the consequences of mechanical ventilation in patients with acute airflow obstruction from asthma. In these patients, the focus of therapy should be to maintain the airway plateau pressure below 25 cm $H_2O$, provide adequate time for expiration to prevent dynamic hyperinflation and to focus on changes in pulmonary mechanics rather than arbitrary $CO_2$ measurements. Where ventilator support is required in patients with extensive parenchymal disease, decreased lung compliance and increased physiological dead space due to ventilation perfusion mismatch, ventilator settings should be judicious. Elimination of $CO_2$ is mostly dependent on alveolar ventilation and the determinants of alveolar ventilation are expressed as follows:

Alveolar ventilation = Respiratory rate × (Tidal volume – Dead space)

In the ventilated patient, increasing the respiratory rate is a less efficient method of increasing alveolar ventilation as dead space ventilation is also increased. However, an excessive increase in tidal volume that results in overdistention of alveoli and compression and stretching of alveolar capillaries will reduce perfusion to these alveoli and increase dead space ventilation. Despite the potential adverse consequences of increasing tidal volume in ventilated patients, this is the preferred strategy to increase alveolar ventilation in ventilated patients. Unless the patient has limited pulmonary reserve, increased production of $CO_2$ rarely results in clinically significant hypercapnia.

When ventilating patients with respiratory failure, surrogate markers of arterial $CO_2$ tension ($PaCO_2$) may be used. End-tidal $CO_2$ measurements are commonly used to evaluate alveolar ventilation and end-tidal $CO_2$ pressure monitors ($PETCO_2$) are used routinely to ensure endotracheal tube placement. Usually the $PETCO_2$ is several mm Hg less than the $PaCO_2$. The two important factors that alter this gradient are lung disease and changes in cardiac output. Increases in physiological dead space are likely to cause a widened $PETCO_2$ to $PaCO_2$ gradient with the potential complication of hypercarbia and respiratory acidosis.

The available data from clinical studies on mechanically ventilated patients with severe respiratory failure are conflicting. Hickling KG et al. reported improved survival in patients with acute respiratory distress syndrome (ARDS) where lung-protective ventilation was used with permissive hypercapnia, in their noncomparative observational study.[8] Further studies investigating restrictive tidal volumes to prevent ventilator associated lung injury suggested detrimental effects of hypercapnic acidosis associated with low volume/pressure-limited ventilation. In the landmark ARDS net study,[9] the investigators actively managed hypercapnic acidosis, aiming to maintain pH greater than 7.30 for all patients, and allowed for protocol violations in tidal volume and airway pressure limits if the pH dropped below 7.15. In summary, while the effect of low-volume/low-pressure ventilation was found to be beneficial, the effects of hypercapnia and resultant acidosis remain unclear and potentially harmful. With current evidence, it appears that mild to moderate hypercapnia ($PCO_2$ 50–60 mm Hg), especially when the pH is greater than or equal to 7.3, is usually tolerated.

A recent multicenter, binational, retrospective study assessed the impact of compensated hypercapnia and resultant acidosis in patients receiving mechanical ventilation.[10] These data confirmed that hypercapnic acidosis during the first 24 hours of intensive care admission is more strongly associated with increased hospital mortality than compensated hypercapnia or normocapnia. This large observational study of 252,812 ventilated ICU patients suggests that hypercapnic acidosis is deleterious in the critically ill. Similar results were reported in other studies and the concept of permissive hypercapnia is not supported by the recent data.[11,12]

Hypercapnic acidosis that is severe and life threatening is most commonly managed using ventilator support. In recent years, extracorporeal techniques are sometimes used to manage patients with respiratory failure where mechanical ventilation is difficult. If oxygenation can be maintained and the most profound physiological derangement is hypercapnic acidosis, extracorporeal $CO_2$ ($ECCO_2$) removal may be indicated.[13] With these devices, it is possible to remove all metabolically produced $CO_2$ using blood flow rates between 1 L/min and 2 L/min of venous blood flow through the artificial membrane lung. The potential advantages of these devices are that lung-protective ventilation may be delivered and the consequences of hypercapnic acidosis mitigated.

## Case Revisit

His medical management was optimized with bronchodilators and eventually muscle relaxants to facilitate ventilation. The patient was ventilated using volume-controlled mode of ventilation and his positive end-expiratory pressure (PEEP) was frequently measured with attempts to maintain the pressure below 10 cm $H_2O$, thus avoiding dynamic hyperinflation. Despite adhering to the recommended guidelines for ventilation of patients with severe airflow obstruction, there was ongoing barotrauma with worsening subcutaneous emphysema and the development of a further pneumothorax. A decision was reached to initiate $ECCO_2$ removal. Over the subsequent 24 hours, the patient showed clinical signs of improvement and after a prolonged admission he was discharged from the ICU.

# RESPIRATORY ALKALOSIS

## Case

A 35-year-old female presents to the emergency department in the early morning with shortness of breath, pleuritic chest pain and a productive cough for 5 days. Clinically she has central cyanosis, a fever of 38.2°C, tachycardia of 120/min and a blood pressure of 110/76 mm Hg. Auscultation of the lungs reveals scattered crackles and the breath sounds are diminished in both lung bases. The chest radiograph indicates bilateral pneumonia and blood gasses are as follows—pH 7.44, $PaCO_2$ 28 mm Hg, $HCO_3$ 24 mm Hg and the $PaO_2$ 50 mm Hg on room air. She is fluid resuscitated and commenced on broad-spectrum antibiotics.

## Definition

Respiratory alkalosis is a condition characterized by a primary reduction in arterial $PaCO_2$ (<35 mm Hg) causing an elevation of blood pH beyond the normal range (>7.45).

## Etiology/Mechanism

Respiratory alkalosis is caused by a reduction in $CO_2$ which often accompanies increased alveolar ventilation. There are many causes for this condition[14] (Table 2).

## Clinical Effects

Respiratory alkalosis may be a manifestation of a life-threatening condition but hypocarbia *per se* has less life-threatening physiological consequences as opposed to hypercarbia. There are numerous potential physiological consequences of respiratory alkalosis. Respiratory alkalosis alters electrolyte homeostasis, separate from its renal compensatory mechanisms. In the early stages of respiratory alkalosis, hyperkalemia may occur as a consequence of hyperventilation-induced augmentation of alpha-adrenergic activity. Subsequently, hypokalemia develops from transcellular shift, reduced renal reabsorption, and the renal excretion of bicarbonate.[15] The consequence of bicarbonaturia is increased renal potassium excretion. Hypokalemia is usually mild, but may be severe in pregnant women due to high circulating progesterone levels causing hyperventilation and respiratory alkalosis. There have been case reports of respiratory alkalosis-induced hypokalemia leading to flaccid paralysis. Acute respiratory

**Table 2:** Causes of respiratory alkalosis.

| | |
|---|---|
| Central causes | - Head injury<br>- Stroke<br>- Anxiety-hyperventilation syndrome<br>- Pain<br>- Drugs<br>- Endogenous compounds<br>- Raised intracranial pressure<br>- Encephalopathy |
| Pulmonary causes | - Hypoxemia<br>- Pulmonary embolism<br>- Pneumonia<br>- Asthma<br>- Pulmonary edema |
| Other causes | - Sepsis<br>- Pregnancy<br>- Thyrotoxicosis |

alkalosis may cause hypophosphatemia as a consequence of increased cellular uptake. With chronic respiratory alkalosis, hyperphosphatemia and hypocalcemia may develop from parathyroid hormone resistance. Respiratory alkalosis may induce bronchoconstriction and can induce pulmonary arterial vasodilation. Tachycardia may develop as a consequence of increased sympathetic activity and chest pain may occur through coronary vasospasm. Atrial and ventricular arrhythmias have also been reported both in acute and chronic respiratory alkalosis. Gastrointestinal (GI) and hepatic symptoms have been described in acute respiratory alkalosis. These symptoms may include nausea, vomiting, and increased GI motility. Hypocapnia (when $PaCO_2$ <20 mm Hg) can affect central and peripheral nervous systems. Diverse signs and symptoms have been described and these include vertigo, dizziness, anxiety, hallucinations and seizures. Somatic symptoms have also been reported that includes migraines, stroke-like symptoms or partial seizures. These changes have been attributed to reduced cerebral blood flow, causing cerebral ischemia. Peripheral manifestations may occur as tetany and paresthesias. These neurological manifestations are thought to be mediated by hyperventilation-induced increased neuronal excitability caused by hypocalcemia and possibly by hypophosphatemia.

## Approach/Evaluation

A useful approach in establishing the cause of respiratory alkalosis is to consider the anatomical location of the pathology. Table 2 provides a diagnostic approach to respiratory alkalosis. Some common central causes are a head injury or stroke, anxiety-hyperventilation syndrome and various drugs such as salicylate intoxication. Central hyperventilation may also be a consequence of an encephalopathy such as hepatic and septic encephalopathy. Hypoxemia from any cause may lead to hyperventilation via the peripheral chemoreceptors. Pulmonary conditions such as pulmonary emboli, pneumonia, asthma and pulmonary edema may activate pulmonary receptors and cause hyperventilation. The physiological and metabolic consequences of pregnancy and thyrotoxicosis are also well described causes of respiratory alkalosis.

## Management

The management of respiratory alkalosis is to treat the underlying cause of the hyperventilation. Hyperventilation due to anxiety may require reassurance and sometimes anxiolytics. Central neurological causes need to be identified and managed with appropriate neurological or neurosurgical interventions. Pulmonary causes of hyperventilation and respiratory alkalosis are usually a physiological response to hypoxia or decreased pulmonary compliance and improve as the underlying condition responds to therapy. Diverse causes of respiratory alkalosis such as pregnancy, endocrine and metabolic causes are usually not of clinical significance and the alkalosis resolves with disappearance of the underlying stimulus. In situations when management requires intubation and mechanical ventilation, sedation and muscle relaxants may effectively control hyperventilation if clinically indicated.

## Case Revisit

The patient is likely to meet criteria for the ARDS complicating community-acquired pneumonia. The alkalosis need not be treated directly and her hyperventilation is a consequence of decreased lung compliance and hypoxia. The consequences of this altered physiology are hyperventilation and resultant respiratory alkalosis as she compensates for the hypoxia. Appropriate antibiotics should be administered and oxygen delivery optimized. Both high-flow nasal cannula and noninvasive ventilation will improve oxygenation and provide PEEP but intubation and mechanical ventilation is indicated if she progresses to severe ARDS. Her hemodynamic and volume status should be optimized with judicious attention to fluid management. Should hyperventilation lead to ventilator asynchrony, she should be sedated and consideration given to muscle relaxants. The ventilation strategy should include protective lung ventilation with restrictive tidal volumes and limitation of plateau airway pressures. After satisfactory clinical and radiological improvement of her ARDS, she should be changed to a mode that delivers spontaneous ventilation. Should hyperventilation persist after resolution of her pulmonary pathology, consideration should be given to an encephalopathy or an alternate cause for ICU delirium.

## SALIENT POINTS

- Respiratory acidosis may be acute or chronic in presentation. A detailed history, clinical examination, arterial blood gases and radiological imaging are important in elucidating the pathophysiology and understanding the disease process. The serum bicarbonate is a useful indicator in differentiating acute from chronic respiratory acidosis.
- Acute and acute-on-chronic respiratory acidosis usually requires urgent intervention particularly if the

hypercarbia is profound, resulting in an altered level of consciousness and/or organ dysfunction.
- Respiratory alkalosis may be a manifestation of a life-threatening condition but hypocarbia *per se* has less life-threatening physiological consequences as opposed to hypercarbia.
- Respiratory alkalosis is usually a consequence of neurological or respiratory pathology and is managed by treating the underling disorder.

## REFERENCES

1. Price HL. Effects of carbon dioxide on the cardiovascular system. Anesthesiology. 1960;21:652-63.
2. Juan G, Calverley P, Talamo C, et al. Effect of carbon dioxide on diaphragmatic function in human beings. N Engl J Med. 1984;310:874-9.
3. Zhou Q, Cao B, Niu L, et al. Effects of permissive hypercapnia on transient global cerebral ischemia-reperfusion injury in rats. Anesthesiology. 2010;112(2):288-97.
4. Bersentes TJ, Simmons DH. Effects of acute acidosis on renal hemodynamics. Am J Physiol. 1967;212(3):633-40.
5. Williams MH Jr, Shim CS. Ventilatory failure: etiology and clinical forms. Am J Med. 1970;48:477-83.
6. West JB. Causes of carbon dioxide retention in lung disease. N Engl J Med. 1971;284:1232-6.
7. Davidson AC, Banham S, Elliott M, et al. BTS/ICS guideline for the ventilatory management of acute hypercapnic respiratory failure in adults. Thorax. 2016;71 Suppl 2:ii1-35.
8. Hickling KG. Lung-protective ventilation in acute respiratory distress syndrome. Am J Respir Crit Care Med. 2000;162(6):2021-2.
9. Acute Respiratory Distress Syndrome Network, Brower RG, Matthay MA, et al. Ventilation with lower tidal volumes as compared with traditional tidal volumes for acute lung injury and the acute respiratory distress syndrome. N Engl J Med. 2000;342:1301-8.
10. Tiruvoipati R, Pilcher D, Buscher H, et al. Effects of hypercapnia and hypercapnic acidosis on hospital mortality in mechanically ventilated patients. Crit Care Med. 2017;45(7):e649-56.
11. Nin N, Muriel A, Peñuelas O, et al. Severe hypercapnia and outcome of mechanically ventilated patients with moderate or severe acute respiratory distress syndrome. Intensive Care Med. 2017;43:200-8.
12. Barnes T, Zochios V, Parhar K. Re-examining permissive hypercapnia in ARDS: a narrative review. Chest. 2018;154:185-95.
13. Tiruvoipati R, Buscher H, Winearls J, et al. Early experience of a new extracorporeal carbon dioxide removal device for acute hypercapnic respiratory failure. Crit Care Resusc. 2016;18(4):261-9.
14. Gardner WN. The pathophysiology of hyperventilation disorders. Chest. 1996;109:516-34.
15. Krapf R, Beeler I, Hertner D, et al. Chronic respiratory alkalosis. The effect of sustained hyperventilation on renal regulation of acid-base equilibrium. N Engl J Med. 1991;324:1394-401.

# CHAPTER 35

# Basics of Arterial Blood Gas Interpretation

*Roop Kishen*

## INTRODUCTION

Arterial blood gases (ABGs) are one of the most common investigations performed in the critically ill, both in emergency departments (ED) and on those admitted to intensive care unit (ICU) routinely; possible these days with the availability of easy-to-use point-of-care equipment. However, as many clinicians are either not familiar with ABG interpretation, or have inadequate understanding of the subject,[1] it is easy to get distracted by abnormal ABG results and spend a lot of time and effort in trying to "correct the abnormality". There are also many books and articles detailing many formulae, graphs, and tables as "causes" of acidosis and alkalosis; this only adds to the general confusion.[2] It should be emphasized that any abnormality in ABG should only be interpreted with reference to the clinical condition of that patient. A fundamental knowledge of cardiovascular, respiratory, and fluid/electrolyte physiology is essential for proper understanding and interpretation of ABG abnormalities. There are several "approaches" for interpreting acid-base abnormalities, all have their followers; however, none of these approaches are without flaws. This chapter will briefly deal with these approaches and discuss basics of ABG interpretation. It is also the purpose of this chapter to make ABG interpretation easy and interesting without relying on too many formulae and equations but by using simple mental arithmetic.

## WHY MEASURE ABG?

Critically ill patients presenting to ED or admitted to ICU suffer from acute and often multi-system physiological disturbances and pathology. Multiple physiologic parameters (e.g. blood pressure, heart rate, etc.) are employed to monitor and evaluate these patients as well as to gauge the effects of therapy; ABGs being one such, albeit, an invasive parameter. ABGs not only provide data about oxygenation and respiratory status as well as important metabolic derangements (e.g. acidosis, etc.) in the critically ill but may also provide meaningful information about prognosis (e.g. clearance of lactate in patients with sepsis). However, ABGs are not a substitute for a thorough clinical evaluation of the patient but only form an adjunct in their management. ABGs should only be ordered when and if their interpretation will result in change/escalation in patient management and the clinician is confident in interpreting their results *vis a vis* the patient's clinical presentation and findings.

## GENERAL PRINCIPLES AND TECHNICAL ASPECTS

### Appropriate Sampling, Care and Transport of Arterial Blood

Arterial blood samples for ABG analysis are either obtained from a direct arterial puncture or from an indwelling arterial line. The most common site for direct arterial puncture is the radial artery of nondominant hand; second most common site being the femoral artery and the least common site, the brachial artery. Radial artery is superficial and easily palpable as is the femoral artery. The procedure is painful in conscious patents, thus ABG estimation should not be undertaken lightly. Thorough asepsis is essential as are the tests for distal circulation integrity (Allen test), especially when performing radial artery punctures; however, Allen test is not mandatory, and many do not perform it.

Arterial blood samples are more often drawn from indwelling arterial cannulae, especially in ICU patients. The sample is collected from the three-way tap a few centimeters proximal to the cannula. The saline (often heparinized) is withdrawn in a 5 mL syringe and discarded. The actual sample is then drawn in a heparinized syringe and sent for ABG analysis. Detailed description of ways to perform arterial punctures is outside the scope of this chapter.

Sampling errors can lead to erroneous results and therefore wrong clinical conclusions. Care must be taken in sampling and transporting arterial blood samples drawn. Following Do's and Don'ts help in reducing sampling errors and improve accuracy:

- Do not draw a blood sample for ABGs immediately after an intervention, e.g. applying an oxygen mask, changing fractional inspired oxygen concentration ($FiO_2$), and/or changing critically ill patient's position. Wait for a steady state which may take a while especially in patients with pulmonary pathology.
- Ensure that the sampling syringe does not have excess heparin in it. As it is an acid, too much heparin may cause faulty results. Usually a small volume of heparin (0.25 mL of 1,000 U/mL) is drawn into the syringe, the plunger withdrawn to allow heparin to coat the syringe barrel and then heparin expelled completely; this leaves adequate amount necessary to keep blood anticoagulated for the test. Alternatively, commercially available syringes for the purpose may be used but they may drive up the cost of each ABG test.
- Make sure laboratory knows that you are sending a sample for ABG estimation or ensure the point-of-care machine is available, ready to use, and you or another person present know how to use it. Point-of-care equipment should be calibrated daily and be regularly subjected to quality control.
- Samples should be kept in ice if the transport/test time is expected to exceed 5–6 minutes. Cooling the sample slows the metabolic activity of blood component cells which might otherwise affect the results.
- Hazardous samples should be clearly marked as such. $FiO_2$ should be mentioned on the request slip as this not only helps to put the results in context but also helps the laboratory staff to check the validity of their equipment.
- Expel any air bubbles from the syringe as gases from blood can diffuse into the bubbles and vice versa—producing erroneous results.
- Ensure that arterial blood has been drawn and not venous; it is not always possible to tell arterial blood from venous blood by just looking at its color.
- And last but not the least; if arterial puncture has failed a couple of times, do not persist as arterial punctures are painful and may cause vessel damage, including creation of false aneurysms.

## Gas Partial Pressure (Tension)

Pressure of gas is defined as the pressure exerted by the number of its molecules that collide with the wall of the container. The total pressure of a mixture of gases (e.g. air) is the sum of individual pressures (called partial pressure and denoted by the letter "P") exerted by its components. Partial pressure of a gas in a mixture is directly related to the proportion of that gas in the mixture. Thus:

Total pressure of air (simplified): 593.5 + 159.0 + 0.5 + 7.0 = 760 (mm Hg) at sea level. (Representing partial pressures, P, of $N_2$, $O_2$, $CO_2$ and inert gases, respectively).

P for a component gas can be determined from the total pressure of the mixture, if the proportion of the component gas is known. Thus P for $O_2$ in dry air at sea level is:

$PO_2$ (Air) = 760 × (20.98/100) = 159 mm Hg, where 20.98 is the percentage of $O_2$ in dry air.

P can be expressed as mm Hg or kPa (kilo Pascal, in SI units; *Le System International d'Unités*). Whereas kPa is commonly used in Europe and Australasia, mm Hg is in common use in the US and Indian subcontinent (to convert mm Hg into kPa divide pressure in mm Hg by 7.5). To avoid confusion and mistakes, when denoting a gas partial pressure P, it is customary to mention the medium in which it has been measured. Thus, we can denote P in various media, e.g. $PO_2$ (partial pressure of oxygen in atmosphere), $PAO_2$ (in alveolus), $PaO_2$ (in arterial blood), $PvO_2$ (in venous blood) and so on and so forth.

Saturation usually refers to $O_2$ saturation in blood and is denoted as $SaO_2$ (when measured in arterial blood), as $SpO_2$ (when measured peripherally with a pulse oximeter) or $SvO_2$ (in venous blood). Readers must note that saturation is different from P and for $O_2$, the relationship between the two is not linear.

## INTERPRETING ABG (WITH EMPHASIS ON INTERPRETING ACID-BASE DISTURBANCES)

Previous chapter has dealt with the basic acid-base physiology, so this will not be repeated here. However, for the sake of recall, and to understand Stewart or modern approach, a short discussion of acids, bases and other terminology follows.

Clinicians have adopted the so-called modern definition of acids and bases after Brönsted and Lowry[3] where acids are defined as "proton ($H^+$) donors" and bases defined as "proton acceptors". Stewart, a Canadian physiologist, argues that this definition of acids and bases is a source of great confusion among clinicians concerning acid-base physiology and prefers an earlier definition (according to Arrhenius)[4] of acids as "those substances which, when dissolved in water, produce an increased concentration of $H^+$". Stewart further argues that this, earlier (Arrhenius's) definitions, allows us to call $CO_2$ an acid, which the Brönsted-Lowry definition does not.

Strong ions are those ions which are completely dissociated at body temperature and pH. Thus $Na^+$, $Cl^-$, $K^+$, $Ca^{++}$, $SO_4^-$ etc. are strong ions, whereas ions like $HCO_3^-$ do not dissociate completely and are therefore called weak ions. Weak acids (e.g. albumin) are also incompletely dissociated and their dissociation is pH and temperature dependent.

## Approaches to Interpreting Acid-base Abnormalities

Over the last 60 years or so, several approaches have been proposed to interpret acid-base abnormalities; all approaches have their merits and demerits. Earlier approaches were based solely on the famous Henderson–Hasselbalch equation, familiar to almost all clinicians, having been taught to generations of medical students. Henderson[4] applied the law of mass action to the equilibrium reaction for carbonic acid to derive $H^+$. This equation was subsequently modified by Hasselbalch[5] to calculate pH.

$$pH = pK + \log \frac{[HCO_3^-]}{S_{CO_2} \times PaCO_2}$$

(where $S_{CO_2}$ is the solubility coefficient of $CO_2$ and pK is the negative logarithm of a constant).

Earlier (pre 1950) approach to acid-base interpretation was based entirely on the above traditional theory. During 1952 polio epidemic in Denmark, physicians caring for these patients were intrigued by "a strange metabolic alkalosis" killing their patients who were suffering from paralysis (and thus hypoventilating). $CO_2$ could only be measured at that time in blood as dissolved $CO_2$ (higher dissolved $CO_2$ increasing plasma $HCO_3^-$).[6] With high levels of $HCO_3^-$ in their patients, these physicians sought to "correct this fatal metabolic alkalosis"! It was soon pointed out by a young anesthetist, Bjørn Ibsen, that high dissolved $CO_2$ (and therefore "alkalosis") was, in fact reflection of $CO_2$ retention due to inadequate ventilation. (That intensive care was born with this astute observation is another story).[7] Soon pH measurements were instituted and $PaCO_2$ was shown to be high in these patients, along with a low pH and modern respiratory acid-base physiology was born.[6] Work was already underway to refine this "purely bicarbonate based" approach with the concept of Buffer Base in 1948[8] proposed by Singer and Hastings, Standard Bicarbonate proposed by Astrup in 1960[9] and that of Base Excess in the same year by Siggaard-Andersen and Engle.[10]

Acid-base abnormalities are common and frequent in critically ill. Although analysis of ABG results tells us about the state of oxygenation, respiratory adequacy, and if a state of acidosis or alkalosis (i.e. a metabolic abnormality) exists, these are only the effects and not the actual nature of pathology. Patient's history and a thorough clinical examination cannot be overemphasized. There are four approaches for interpreting acid-base disorders. Of these the first three are qualitative in that they tell us that acidemia and alkalemia (the physiological abnormality) exists. Although traditionalists disagree,[11,12] the fourth approach (after Stewart) is quantitative and sheds more light on the nature of pathology. These approaches are described as follows:

### The $CO_2/HCO_3^-$ (Boston) Approach

Based entirely on Henderson–Hasselbalch equation and ignoring the noncarbonate buffers (e.g. hemoglobin, albumin), this approach uses mathematical relationship between $PaCO_2$ and plasma $HCO_3^-$ (or total $CO_2$) to assess the nature of acid-base disorders. It was developed at Tufts University, Boston, USA (hence, its name) by Swartz and Relman[13] after studying several hundreds of patients with known and chronic *but* stable (compensated!) acid-base disorders. The degree of "compensation" from the normal was measured in a number of diseased states, using linear equations, to describe a variety of abnormal acid-base states.[14] This approach relates $H^+$ to $CO_2$ in respiratory disorders and $H^+$ to $CO_2/HCO_3^-$ in metabolic acid-base disturbances. These authors argue that, despite existence of other buffers like hemoglobin, these are the only parameters that "an expert clinician needs to know, besides clinical history" to analyze simple and complex acid-base abnormalities.[13] They called this approach physiological and discounted *whole-blood buffer base, standard bicarbonate,* and *base excess* as "superfluous and misleading"! However, this approach requires various corrections (see below) as well as "knowledge of expected response" etc. to interpret acid-base disturbances. Besides, $HCO_3^-$ varies with $PaCO_2$, which also influence $H^+$, therefore, this approach cannot be used to analyze metabolic disturbances on its own. This approach is easy to use in simple and uncomplicated, especially chronic disorders, e.g. chronic respiratory failure. Its usefulness in critical care is somewhat limited.

### Base Excess/Deficit (Danish or Copenhagen) Approach

To better qualify and recognize nonrespiratory components of acid-base disturbance, Danish workers added refinements to acid-base physiology.[6,8,9,10] These refinements [whole-blood buffer base, standard bicarbonate, and base excess (BE)] moved us away from Henderson–Hasselbalch equation in order to identify acid-base changes independent of prevailing $PaCO_2$. Of these, BE still survives and is extensively used in ED, ICU, and acute medicine. However, the concept was not accepted by all, the "Boston" school laboratories still refusing to report BE![15] This Transatlantic debate continues still and many clinicians either refuse to use BE or classify it as a "nonphysiologic" variable with no place in acid-base physiology.[16]

Simple rules of thumb can be applied in interpreting acid-base abnormalities using BE approach. Thus, in acute respiratory acidosis and alkalosis, BE does not change. Metabolic acidosis reduces BE, i.e. it becomes negative (e.g. –4.0; –6.3 etc.; also called base deficit) and in metabolic alkalosis it becomes positive (e.g. +2.8, +7.3 etc.). Changes in BE represent the sum-total of all acidifying or alkalinizing effects which are independent of $CO_2$ changes. Having said that, it is an *in vitro* calculated value and changes slightly *in vivo* with changes in $PaCO_2$ due to equilibration across whole extracellular space. BE equation has been modified to take account of this fact and thus improve its accuracy *in vivo*. This is termed as *standard base excess* (SBE). Despite the corrections applied, *in vivo* BE can still drift with $PaCO_2$.[5]

### Anion Gap Approach

Emmett and Nairns[17] developed Anion Gap (AG) approach to address the limitations of above two approaches. Derived from principles of electroneutrality, AG is calculated as:

$$AG = \{[Na^+] + [K^+]\} - \{[Cl^-] + [HCO_3^-]\}$$

(where, [ ] represent molar concentrations of various ions)

The sum of differences in concentrations of these commonly measured extracellular ions reveals a "gap" of about 14 ± 2 mmol/L, its value usually being positive. The gap accounts for unmeasured anions (e.g. lactate, phosphate, sulfate, and proteins) not accounted for in the above equation. In metabolic acidosis, a widened AG (>16) is due to unmeasured anions like lactate or ketones; conversely, if AG does not widen, then most likely cause of acidosis is heperchloremia. AG is suggested as a useful approach in diagnosis hyperlactatemia and various poisonings. Unfortunately, most critically ill are hypoproteinemic as well as hypophosphatemic. Under these conditions, deciding what is a normal AG in critically ill can be problematic. With modern point-of-care blood gas analyzers capable of measuring lactate directly as well as AG having been shown to be poor at diagnosis hyperlactatemia in critically ill, utility of this approach is highly questionable in ICU patients. Hypoproteinemia affects AG as well and, despite correction for low albumin, AG still does not perform very well in the critically ill.[5]

### Stewart–Fencl Approach

The "Modern" approach, Stewart approach (later modified by Fencl), is based on the principle of electroneutrality (not to be confused with AG). This approach, thought to be complex and, therefore, not known to many clinicians, provides a more accurate reflection of acid-base status and is especially useful in complex disorders. The original multinomial equations solved by Stewart to arrive at his conclusions required a computer and so the approach did not become popular and remained unknown, indeed it still is not known to many clinicians. This approach discards $HCO_3^-$ in analysis of acid-base abnormalities and original approach by Stewart did not take BE into account either. The idea of discounting $HCO_3^-$ and BE in any discussion of acid-base physiology seemed so preposterous to many so much so that Stewart approach was labeled as "absurd and anachronistic".[18] Subsequent modifications by Fencl, Gilfix and Story have made this one of the easiest and useful approaches to use by bedside.[19]

Detailed description of Stewart approach is outside the scope of this chapter; therefore, only a few basic principles will be described here. Stewart rejected the Brönsted and Lowry[3] definition of acids and bases and went back to an earlier definition proposed by Arrhenius in 1887, which states that acids are substances that when dissolved in water increase $H^+$ and bases ionize in water to increase $OH^-$. This allowed Stewart to call $CO_2$ an acid, which earlier definition did not. Stewart based his approach on principles of physical chemistry as applied to body fluids and applied the *Law of conservation of mass, Law of mass action,* and *Law of electroneutrality* to arrive at his approach. Thus, Stewart rejected Henderson–Hasselbalch equation and suggested that pH of body fluids does not change because of addition or loss of acid or base (as proposed by traditional approaches) but because of a change in $CO_2$, strong ions [actually strong ion difference (SID)] and total weak acid; he called these three variables the *independent variables* (variables that cannot be influenced by other factors). He therefore proposed that $H^+$ and $HCO_3^-$ are dependent variables and are changed/influenced by a change in above three independent variables. This sounds very confusing to traditionalists as generations of clinicians have been taught that addition of $H^+$ and loss of $HCO_3^-$ are the reasons for metabolic acidosis and vice versa.[20]

- In Stewart approach, $CO_2$ affects pH in the familiar way, increase in $CO_2$ reduces pH (causing respiratory acidosis) and a reduction in $CO_2$ causes respiratory alkalosis.
- Strong ions are those ions which dissociate completely in body fluids; thus, cations like $Na^+$, $K^+$, $Ca^{++}$, $Mg^{++}$, and anions like $Cl^-$, lactate are strong ions whereas $HCO_3^-$ is not. SID can be calculated as:

    SID = $[Na^+ + K^+ + Ca^{++} + Mg^{++}] - [Cl^- + Lactate]$

    If SID decreases due to an increase in anions while cations stay more or less stable (e.g. increase in plasma $Cl^-$ after 0.9% saline infusion), electroneutrality is upset and water, an abundant source of $H^+$, dissociates to produce $H^+$ to restore the balance, thus increasing $H^+$ and causing acidosis. Decrease in cations relative to anions has the same effect. Conversely, a widened SID (e.g. due to reduced anions, e.g. $Cl^-$ loss by diuretic therapy) relative to cations causes alkalosis as $H^+$ (taken up by $OH^-$) reduces to restore electroneutrality. Increase in cations relative to anions also causes alkalosis—e.g. the mechanism behind sodium bicarbonate infusion in metabolic acidosis ($Na^+$ is added to the system which widens SID).
- Weak acids in Stewart's description are acids that dissociate incompletely at body pH and temperature. They are plasma proteins, phosphate, etc., the effect of plasma proteins being almost entirely due to albumin. These are represented as $A_{TOT}$ in Stewart equations. Increase in albumin causes a metabolic acidosis and a decrease causes metabolic alkalosis. Most critically ill are hypoalbuminemic, thus exhibit small but significant metabolic alkalosis due to lowered albumin.

    It has already been mentioned that many clinicians shun Stewart approach, believing it to be complex. Nothing could be further from the truth. A few points need to be kept in mind while using this approach to analyze acid-base disturbances.

- Clinicians need to "park" $HCO_3^-$ while trying to understand Stewart approach as it has no place in this approach.
- Acidosis/alkalosis is not a disease in itself; it is a signal that a pathology exists. The best clue to that pathology is history and clinical examination of the patient concerned.
- Although clinicians try and see if the state of acidosis (or alkalosis) is "compensated or not", there seems to be little merit in trying to do so as it does not help in solving the clinical problem.
- Stewart approach does not lay emphasis on "compensation" that is supposed to have taken place. Some clinicians view these changes in response to an acid-base disturbance not as "compensation" but physiological response to altered pH. It may or may not actually have happened.
- Acidosis is apparent when there are anions (like lactate, ketones, and other unmeasured anions) present in blood.
- As changes in electrolyte composition of plasma (via SID) and of weak acid (via $A_{TOT}$) affect pH and therefore acid-base status, these must be accounted for when analyzing ABGs with Stewart approach.

A simplified Stewart–Fencl approach as suggested by Gifix[21] and others[22] is the preferred method for ABG analysis for most clinicians who use this approach. This approach combines classical Stewart approach with BE excess (Danish) approach. To analyze ABGs by this approach, we need ABG results, including BE [usually reported as standard base excess (SBE)] from the blood gas machine as well as plasma $Na^+$ and $Cl^-$ and plasma albumin (almost all point-of-care machines now report plasma $Na^+$ and $Cl^-$ and some, but not all, report plasma albumin as well). A couple of simple calculations will evaluate the effect of SID and $A_{TOT}$ on acid-base status of the blood sample. As seen above, SID is calculated as:

SID = $[Na^+ + K^+ + Ca^{++} + Mg^{++}] - [Cl^- + Lactate]$

However, for bedside calculations, only $Na^+$ and $Cl^-$ are used (and lactate, if abnormal) as changes in other cations will only minimally affect the result and can be easily ignored for purposes of bedside calculation. Thus, SID = $[Na^+] - [Cl^-]$ for bedside use. Following calculations are used:

Effect of SID on BE (or $BE_{SID}$):    $([Na^+] - [Cl^-]) - 38$
(where 38 is average SID in the critically ill)

Albumin or $A_{TOT}$ effect (or $BE_{ATOT}$)   $(42 - [Albumin]) \times .25$
(where 42 g/L or 4.2 g/dL is normal albumin)

Actual BE (True BE)    Measured BE − $[BE_{SID} + BE_{ATOT}]$

It sounds very complex but in practice it is very easy. A simple example will illustrate the point:

## Case

A female patient, 38 years old, in respiratory failure and sepsis is admitted to ICU from surgical ward after a bout of fever and hypotension. She was given oxygen and

2,000 mL of 0.9% saline as initial resuscitation measures. Hypotension did not improve and $SpO_2$ stayed less than 85%, hence admission to ICU. With $O_2$ saturations less than 88% on high flow oxygen, she is commenced on noninvasive respiratory support. Arterial line is inserted and after an hour or so, ABG results are as follows:

- pH = 7.28
- $PCO_2$ = 32.5 mm Hg
- $PO_2$ = 75.7 mm Hg (on continuous positive airway pressure; $FiO_2$ 0.6)
- $HCO_3^-$ = 14.5
- BE = –11.1
- Na = 142 mEq
- Cl = 112 mEq
- Albumin = 2.3 g/dL (23 g/L).
- Serum Creatinine = 2.4 mg/dL

Calculating by Stewart–Fencl approach:

NaCl effect or $BE_{SID}$ on measured BE = [142 – 112] – 38
= –8

$A_{TOT}$ effect or $BE_{ATOT}$ on measured BE = [42 – 23] × 0.25
= 4.75

Total effect on measured BE = –8 + 4.75 = –3.25

Actual BE = –11.1 – [–3.25] = –7.85

This patient clearly has a metabolic acidosis. Her SID is narrowed and that contributes to acidosis (–8 mEq/L). However, her weak acid (albumin) is decreased which makes her moderately alkalotic (+4.75 mEq/L) thus offsetting some of the acidosis. The rest of the metabolic acidosis (–7.85 mEq/L) is contributed by unmeasured anions due to deranged renal function (elevated creatinine) as well as sepsis. These results fit the clinical picture as clearly there is a moderate to severe metabolic acidosis, some of which was iatrogenic—due to fluid resuscitation with 0.9% saline on the ward which has increased $Cl^-$ (decreased SID) and diluted albumin (reduced weak acid—$A_{TOT}$). In Stewart approach, "compensatory" mechanisms are not catered for. In any case, trying to find "compensatory" changes adds little to clinical management of the patient.

## CORRECTIONS AND CONCORDANCE: DO WE REALLY NEED THEM?

There are clinicians who still believe that ABG results that we get from blood gas machines must be "tested" for accuracy. This was true a few decades ago as the machines were not reliable. However, with modern day laboratory and point-of-care machines that are regularly calibrated and checked according to well-established laboratory quality control criteria, this is not necessary. Besides, these accuracy checks (referred to as concordance) follow fixed formulae, as if blood that has been tested, is in an isolated compartment. The reality is vastly different; blood is an "open" system, constantly in contact with other fluid compartments in the body. Beside this, critically ill do not follow one single formula during their acid-base disturbances. Thus, a test for concordance may or may not be accurate in these situations and insisting on such tests may only lead to mistakes.

There has been interest in correcting ABG results to patient's temperature. Most clinicians do not temperature correct them as the validity of ABG results at different temperatures has not been established. However, with application of therapeutic hypothermia in some patients, this debate is about to raise its head again.

For Boston approach, various formulae (e.g. Winter's formula)[23] are given to "calculate" the "expected $PaCO_2$ and/or $HCO_3^-$. Again, as Boston approach was initially developed after analysis of chronic stable patients, these formulae worked. In the critically ill, these formulae do not work and with applying BE or Stewart approach to analyze ABG, are not required in any case.

The example quoted earlier illustrates some of these points. Calculating the expected $PaCO_2$ by Winter's formula tells us that expected $PaCO_2$ should be about 29.5 mm Hg; it is 32.5! So accordingly, she has some respiratory acidosis but that hardly matters as she is already on NIV! Also, does it mean that we should now reduce her $PaCO_2$ by increasing ventilatory support? Similarly, anion gap calculation tells us that she has a high anion-gap acidosis, but we already know that from Stewart approach. Thus, these corrections and additional calculations are neither warranted nor add any further insight into the clinical problem.

## CONCLUSION

Acid-base disturbances are common in the critically ill. In themselves, such disturbances are not a disease but a mark of disease. Interpreting acid-base abnormalities requires proper training and understanding. Various systems are available for interpreting acid-base abnormalities; all of these systems or approaches have their dedicated followers. Boston approach is simple and works well with simpler situations. Siggaard-Andersen brought order to chaos within acid-base physiology, with his pioneering work on BE approach. However, Stewart gave us a newer way of looking at acid-base physiology by applying laws of physical chemistry to body fluids. It is not a perfect system; no experimental evidence exists about water dissociation to form $H^+$! However, it is an approach that works well clinically and even outperforms other approaches especially in complex disorders. It must be re-emphasized, that no matter what approach or system a clinician follows, ABG results cannot and should not be interpreted without reference to the patient and the clinical condition at hand.

## SALIENT POINTS

- Acid-base abnormality in a patient is not the disease per se but a pointer to existence of severe pathology.
- The exact "amount" of acid-base abnormality is of less significance than the fact that an abnormality exists.
- There are various approaches to interpreting acid-base disturbances; none of them are perfect.
- Boston and AG approaches are inadequate in the critically ill. BE approach is currently the most popular among critical care physicians, anesthetists, and acute physicians. Stewart approach, as modified by Fencl is becoming increasingly popular, despite many criticisms. It is the only quantitative approach available at present.
- Acid-base abnormalities should never be interpreted without reference to the patient in whom the investigation has been performed.
- The best way to treat any acid-base abnormality is to treat the patient.
- Finally, it cannot be overemphasized that clinicians should always treat the patient *and not* the number.

## REFERENCES

1. Gattinoni L. Foreword. In: Kellum JA, Elber PWG (Eds). Stewart's Textbook of Acid-Base, 2nd edition. Amsterdam, The Netherlands: Paul WG Elbers; 2009. pp. 21-3.
2. Introduction. In: Driscoll P, Brown T, Gwinnutt C, Wardle T, (Eds). A Simple Guide to Blood Gas Analysis. London, UK: BMJ Publishing Group. BMA House; 2000. p. vii.
3. Story DA. Bench-to-bedside review: a brief history of clinical acid-base. Crit Care. 2004;8(4):253-8.
4. Astrup P, Severinghaus JW. The History of Blood Gases, Acids and Bases. Munksgaard: Copenhagen; 1986. pp. 1-318.
5. Kishen R. Acid-base disorders in critical care and emergency medicine. In: David S (Ed). Textbook of Emergency Medicine. New Delhi, India: Wolters Kluwar; 2012. pp. 66-78.
6. West JB. The physiological challenges of the 1952 Copenhagen poliomyelitis epidemic and a renaissance in clinical respiratory physiology. J Appl Physiol (1985). 2005;99(2):424-32.
7. Kishen R. Perceptions, perspectives and progress: Intensive care 50 years on. In: Nayyar V, Peter JV, Kishen R, Srinivas S (Eds). Critical Care Update 2010. New Delhi, India: Jaypee Brothers; 2010. pp. 5-17.
8. Singer RB, Hastings AB. An improved clinical method for the estimation of disturbances of acid-base balance of human blood. Medicine (Baltimore). 1948;27(2):223-42.
9. Astrup P, Jorgensen K, Andersen OS, et al. The acid-base metabolism: A new approach. Lancet. 1960;1(7133):1035-9.
10. Andersen OS, Engle K, Jorgensen K, et al. A micro method of determination of pH, carbon dioxide tension, base excess and standard bicarbonate in capillary blood. Scand J Clin Lab Invest. 1960;12:172-6.
11. Rastegar A. Clinical utility of Stewart's method in diagnosis and management of acid-base disorders. Clin J Am Soc Nephrol. 2009;4(7):1267-74.
12. Doberer D, Funk GC, Kirchner K, et al. A critique of Stewart's approach: the chemical mechanism of dilutional acidosis. Intensive Care Med. 2009;35(12):2173-80.
13. Schwartz WB, Relman AS. A critique of the parameters used in the evaluation of acid-base disorders. "Whole-blood buffer base" and "standard bicarbonate" compared with blood pH and plasma bicarbonate concentration. N Eng J Med. 1963;268:1382-8.
14. Neligan PJ, Deutschman CS. (2005). Acid-base balance in critical care medicine. Department of Anesthesia, University of Pennsylvania. [online] Available from: http://www.areac54.it/public/acid%20base%20balance%20in%20critical%20care%20medicine.pdf [Last Accessed January 2019].
15. Severinghaus JW. Siggaard-Andersen and the "Great Trans-Atlantic Acid-Base Debate". Scand J Clin Lab Invest Suppl. 1993;214:99-104.
16. Martin L (Ed). All You Really Need to Know to Interpret Arterial Blood Gasses, 2nd edition. Baltimore, USA: Lippincott Williams & Wilkins; 1999. pp. 125-7.
17. Emmett M, Nairns RG. Clinical use of anion gap. Medicine (Baltimore). 1977;56(1):38-54.
18. Siggaard-Andersen O, Fogh-Andersen N. Base excess or buffer base (strong ion difference) as measure of a nonrespiratory acid-base disturbance. Acta Anaesthesiol Scand Suppl. 1995;107:123-8.
19. Kishen R, Honoré PM, Jcobs R, et al. Facing acid-base disorders in the third millennium—the Stewart approach revisited. Int J Nephrol Renovasc Dis. 2014;7:209-17.
20. Kishen R. (2010). Trouble with bicarbonate. A brief review of Stewart approach for interpreting acid-base disorders. Indian Anaesthetists Forum 2010. [online] Available from: https://www.researchgate.net/publication/230595051 [Last Accessed January 2019].
21. Gilfix BM, Bique MN, Magder S. A physical chemical approach to the analysis of acid-base balance in the clinical setting. J Crit Care. 1993;8(4):187-97.
22. Story DA, Morimatsu H, Bellomo R. Strong ions, weak acids and base excess: a simplified Fencle-Stewart approach to clinical acid-base disorders. Br J Anaesth. 2004;92(1):54-60.
23. Albert MS, Dell RB, Winter RW. Quantitative displacement of acid-base equilibrium in metabolic acidosis. Ann Intern Med. 1967;66(2):312-22.

# CHAPTER 36

# Arterial Blood Gas Interpretation in Clinical Practice

*Roop Kishen*

## INTRODUCTION

Acid–base disturbances are not diseases *per se*, rather they are "symptoms" of disturbance and a set of blood gas results [arterial blood gases (ABGs)] is only an aid to clinical diagnosis and nothing more. Not all acid–base disturbances are pathologic, e.g. lactic acidosis seen after a severe and prolonged asthmatic attack. Many acid–base disturbances are also self-limiting, e.g. "hyperchloremic" acidosis seen after infusion of large volumes of "0.9% saline". However, moderate to severe acid–base disturbances in the critically ill are pointers to underlying pathology and need careful assessment of the patient. It must be emphasized that ABGs should never be interpreted in isolation but with the reference to the patient they have been taken from and correlated with the clinical condition.

## ARTERIAL BLOOD GAS INTERPRETATION IN CLINICAL PRACTICE

After reading chapter on "Basics of arterial blood gas interpretation", readers should be familiar with various ways (approaches) for interpreting ABG results. In the following sections a few case scenarios are presented. Each case scenario will begin with a short history, followed by ABG results. These will be interpreted according to three approaches that have already been discussed in previous chapter; e.g. (a) Boston approach along with anion gap (AG) approach (also called physiological approach); (b) base excess (BE) approach (also called Danish approach); and (c) Stewart-Fencl approach which combines Stewart and BE approach (also called Modern approach). It should be noted that this is not a comparative analysis between these approaches, rather the intention is to illustrate the utility of these approaches in interpreting complex ABG results in the critically ill. (*These are genuine patients managed by the author and not made up scenarios*).

### Important Note about Methodology Used in Interpreting Arterial Blood Gas Results in this Chapter

The author is of the view that ABG interpretation is unnecessarily made complex by looking at the "expected" changes in $HCO_3$ and $pCO_2$. Clinicians should understand that these "expected" changes were worked out in stable patients with background of chronic respiratory failure. These "expected" changes rarely hold good in acutely ill patients in our intensive care units (ICUs), even if they have a background of chronic respiratory disease. Similarly, looking for "compensations" of various types (e.g. a respiratory alkalosis in "primary" metabolic acidosis) in acute acid–base disturbances is futile as well, as these only confuse the issue at hand and do not help clinical management. The author takes the view that ABG interpretation should be kept simple and to the point without causing confusion. Hence, ABG interpretation is made very simple here so that there is clear understanding of the clinical problem without distractions. This view may be at variance with commonly accepted teaching!

## STEPS IN INTERPRETING ARTERIAL BLOOD GAS RESULTS

A busy clinician in a busy ICU (especially out-of-hours), looking after several critically ill patients should take care in interpreting ABG results as with many distractions present (e.g. demands made by clinical condition of more than one patient in ICU), mistakes are easily made. A stepwise analysis of ABG results for quick bedside interpretation should follow a set pattern in order not to miss important acid–base disturbances.

- Ensure you are looking at the intended/correct patient's ABG results—mix-ups in patients are not unknown!
- Look at $pO_2$ first—is the oxygenation adequate and that life threatening hypoxemia is not evident ($pO_2$ should be > 75 mm Hg or 10 kPa)? This is because quick remedies (e.g. administration of high flow oxygen) are easy first step, should the patient be seriously hypoxemic!
- Look at pH—is there an acidosis (i.e. pH <7.35) or alkalosis (i.e. pH >7.45)?
- Decide what type of disturbance is present—respiratory or nonrespiratory (metabolic) by looking at $pCO_2$.
- A respiratory acidosis is present if $pCO_2$ is high (>44 mm Hg or 5.8 kPa); conversely, a respiratory alkalosis is present if it is low (<35 mm Hg or 4.5 kPa).
- Look at the BE—is it <2.5 (metabolic acidosis) or >2.5 (metabolic alkalosis)?
- Having dealt with any life-threatening clinical situation (e.g. severe hypoxemia with appropriate measures like high flow oxygen mask) further note can be made of electrolytes ($HCO_3$, $Na^+$, $K^+$, $Cl^-$, etc.) as well as albumin (useful in Stewart approach[1]).
- Only now can one arrive at full interpretation of ABG disturbance and formulate a detailed plan as to the proper clinical interpretation (e.g. metabolic acidosis related to renal failure) and clinical management plan (e.g. dialysis).

*It must be emphasized that the best way to treat acid-base disturbance is to treat the patient and NOT THE NUMBER.*

## Case 1: Treat the Patient and not the Number!

After an unexpectedly long operation for open total cystectomy and ileal conduit formation, a postoperative patient (62-year-old-female) was referred to ICU for further monitoring. The anesthetists and the surgeons were concerned about the patient's progressive metabolic acidosis (BE increasing from –2.9 to –12.0) over the course of surgery which had lasted nearly 8 hours. Upon admission to ICU the patient was awake, pain free (analgesia being provided with epidural infusion), hemodynamically stable and warm to touch. Urinary output from the newly formed ileal conduit was satisfactory. She was receiving 40% oxygen by a face mask and her ABGs results soon after ICU admission were as follows (Table 1A).

Following the "steps" mentioned above, she is not hypoxemic and does not need immediate intervention (she is already receiving oxygen). Looking at her pH, she clearly has an acidosis (as her pH is <7.35). Boston approach suggests that she has a mixed disorder. Her bicarbonate is low, so she has a metabolic acidosis.

**Table 1A:** Arterial blood gas (ABG) parameters and values of case 1.

| Parameter | Value |
|---|---|
| pH | 7.17 |
| $pCO_2$ | 43 mm Hg |
| $pO_2$ | 110 mm Hg |
| Bicarbonate | 13.8 mEq/L |
| BE | –12.5 mEq/L |
| Lactate | 21.6 mg/dL |
| Na | 144 mEq/L |
| Cl | 115 mEq/L |
| Albumin | 3.2 g/dL (32 g/L) |

However, her "expected $pCO_2$" should be 26.7–30.7 and therefore she also has a respiratory acidosis! Her AG is 15.2 (144 – [115 + 13.8]); so she has a "normal anion gap" metabolic acidosis. Danish approach suggests that although her $pCO_2$ is slightly elevated at 43 mm Hg, she has a metabolic acidosis as her BE is less than 2.5 mEq/L. Both approaches are correct in diagnosing metabolic acidosis; however, neither approaches point out to an etiology for her metabolic acidosis. Boston approach also labels her having a "respiratory acidosis". A clinician can only guess that "hyperchloremia" may be responsible for her acidosis by noting high serum $Cl^-$. Neither of these approaches suggest interventions to correct her metabolic acidosis.

Modern (Stewart-Fencl) approach also suggests that she has a metabolic acidosis and points out the reason for her acidosis being low strong ion difference (SID) caused by increased $Cl^-$ ion. Her SID is 29 (144–115) and causes a narrow SID acidosis of the order of –9 ([144 – 115] –38). This is off-set by a mild metabolic alkalosis because of somewhat low albumin (effect on BE is +2.5; ([42 – 32]/4 = +2.5). Therefore, her actual BE is –6 (–12.5 – [–9 + 2.5]), i.e. she only has a moderate metabolic acidosis. This is in keeping with her clinical condition, a stable postoperative patient who underwent a rather prolonged operation.

On examining her anesthetic records, it was noted that she had received 3 L of 0.9% saline and 3 L of high chloride containing colloid perioperatively. Thus, her metabolic acidosis was almost entirely due to low SID (commonly called hyperchloremic metabolic acidosis due to infusion of fluids containing more than physiological levels of $Cl^-$). Her maintenance fluids were changed to Hartmann's (with no other intervention) and her metabolic acidosis resolved overnight. Next morning her ABG results were as follows (Table 1B).

Her albumin has dropped which will cause small metabolic "alkalosis". She is also exhibiting slightly more

## Chapter 36
### Arterial Blood Gas Interpretation in Clinical Practice

**Table 1B:** Arterial blood gases (ABG) parameters and values (16 hours apart) of case 1.

| Parameter | Initial values | Later in ICU |
|---|---|---|
| pH | 7.17 | 7.38 |
| pCO$_2$ | 43 mm Hg | 41 mm Hg |
| pO$_2$ | 110 mm Hg | 132 mm Hg |
| Bicarbonate | 13.8 mEq/L | 22.3 mEq/L |
| BE | −12.5 mEq/L | +1.4 mEq/L |
| Lactate | 21.6 mg/dL | 34.2 mg/dL |
| Na | 144 mEq/L | 141 mEq/L |
| Cl | 115 mEq/L | 108 mEq/L |
| Albumin | 3.2 g/dL (32 g/L) | 2.6 g/dL (26 g/L) |

(ICU: intensive care unit).

**Table 2:** Arterial blood gas (ABG) parameters and values of case 2.

| Parameter | Value |
|---|---|
| pH | 6.94 |
| pCO$_2$ | 22.7 mm Hg |
| pO$_2$ | 105 mm Hg |
| Bicarbonate | 4.6 mEq/L |
| BE | −26.0 mEq/L |
| Na | 141 mEq/L |
| Cl | 110 mEq/L |
| Albumin | 2.8 g/dL (28 g/L) |
| Lactate | 45.9 mg/dL (5.1 mmol/L)* |

(*To convert lactate mg/dL to mmol/L, divide by 9).

hyperlactatemia which might worry a lot of clinicians; however, this hyperlactatemia is temporary, does not indicate there is anything amiss clinically as the patient is stable, and is entirely due to infusion of Hartmann's overnight. The patient recovered completely and was discharged to the ward the following day and eventually discharged home.

### Case 2: Sepsis and Acute Kidney Injury Produce Anions that We Do not Normally Measure

A young female patient (32 years) with pneumonia and possible developing sepsis was referred to ICU for further clinical management. The patient was tachypneic (RR- 32 breaths/min), tachycardic (HR 127 beats/min) but normotensive (BP 118/84 mm Hg). Her urine output over the last 12 hours had been only 250 mL. High-flow oxygen mask had been applied. ABG results were as follows (Table 2).

Although clearly unwell and in respiratory distress, she is not hypoxemic; however, she does need resuscitation and ventilatory support.

From the ABG results, she has severe acidosis. Boston approach suggests a mixed metabolic acidosis; a severe metabolic acidosis (bicarbonate 4.6) and a mild respiratory acidosis (expected pCO$_2$ should be 13–17 mm Hg). Calculating AG, we see there is a high AG acidosis which is partly accounted for by increased lactate ([141] − [110 + 4.6 + 5.1] = 21.3). Danish approach suggests a severe metabolic acidosis (BE −26.0) and a moderate respiratory alkalosis (pCO$_2$ of 22.7 mm Hg)—many clinicians would interpret this low pCO$_2$ as "respiratory compensation" (although pH has not moved much toward normal!). Both approaches also suggest that there is a moderate lactic acidosis.

Modern approach also suggests a severe metabolic acidosis. SID and low albumin affect her BE. Her SID is narrow and SID effect on BE is −12.1 ({[141] − [110 + 5.1] − 38 = −12.1}, lactate is included here as it is high). Her albumin is also low at 2.8 g/dL affecting her pH by +3.5 ([42 − 28]/4 = 3.5). Therefore, her actual BE = −17.4 (−26 − [−12.1 + 3.5] or −17.4). Having accounted for narrow SID and low albumin effect, a large quantity of unmeasured anions [found in sepsis and/or acute kidney injury (AKI)], besides lactate, are the cause of her severe metabolic acidosis.

This severe metabolic acidosis fits her clinical picture. She was almost anuric and further laboratory results showed that her serum urea was 42 mg/dL (normal range: 8–20 mg/dL) and serum creatinine was 4.07 mg/dL (normal up to 1.3 mg/dL). Her severe acidosis was, therefore, due to AKI with sepsis contributing to it. She required fluids, vasopressors and renal replacement therapy. Hyperlactatemia in her case can be due to either sepsis or increased work of breathing (as she had been tachypneic for several hours) or the combination of the two. Patient eventually recovered and after a couple of weeks was transferred to a lower level of care (surgical HDU) and was finally discharged home.

### Case 3: Electrolyte and Fluid Disturbances can Cause Acid-Base Perturbations[2]

A young (34 years old) woman was admitted to surgical HDU (a lower level of care than ICU) of our institution from another hospital. She was a known patient of our specialist surgical unit (Intestinal Failure Unit). Previously, she had had abdominal sepsis (couple of years before the current admission), had been operated upon and was left with an upper gastro-intestinal fistula (from her jejunum) with high output, controlled with codeine phosphate and loperamide.

She was on home parenteral nutrition but could eat and drink freely. Recently, the patient had experienced "flu" like symptoms, was admitted to another hospital where she was kept for a couple of days. As she did not recover from her "flu" she was transferred to our surgical unit because she was thought to have abdominal sepsis. Her codeine and loperamide had been stopped at the first hospital for some "unknown" reason (increasing her fistula output). On presentation at our institution, she was breathless but did not look in respiratory distress. She still had a generalized body ache and low-grade pyrexia (37.5–38.0°C). Clinically, there was nothing else abnormal. Along with routine investigations, ABGs were ordered, which showed "severe metabolic acidosis" (Table 3). Sepsis (because of fever and acidosis) and/or pulmonary embolism (because she was tachypneic) were suspected. Despite a normal white cell count, platelet count and coagulation profile, she underwent an abdominal computerized tomography (CT) scan as well as a pulmonary CT-angiogram; both were normal. Various specialists (pulmonologists, nephrologists, etc.) including ICU senior resident were consulted; however, none could find anything abnormal except tachypnea and severe acidosis and recent low urine output. Infusion of 1.4% $NaHCO_3$ did not help the situation. The ABG results that caused a lot of anxiety amongst her attending clinicians are given in Table 3.

It is clear that although she is tachypneic, she is not in immediate danger as she is not hypoxemic (receiving oxygen by face mask). All approaches recognize that the patient has moderate to severe acidosis. Boston approach suggests this as her bicarbonate is low; it also suggests that, as her actual $pCO_2$ is higher than that "expected" (expected $pCO_2$ should be 12–16 mm Hg), she also has a "respiratory acidosis"! Her AG is normal as is her lactate; thus, no cause of metabolic acidosis is apparent. Danish approach also suggests a metabolic acidosis (BE of –22.2) and a "respiratory compensation" (low $pCO_2$ of 21.8 mm Hg). However, the cause of metabolic acidosis is not apparent.

Modern approach also suggests that a metabolic acidosis is present. It suggests that, because of low Na, her SID has narrowed. Calculating the SID effect, its contribution to BE is –20 mEq/L [(127 – 109) – 38 = –20]. Her albumin is nearly normal and contributes +1.5 mEq/L to her acid–base disturbance [(42 – 36/4) = 1.5]. Thus, the combined SID and albumin contribution to her BE is –18.5 mEq/L (–20 + 1.5); therefore her actual BE is –3.7 mEq/L [–22.2 – (–18.5) = –3.7]. Thus, after accounting for SID and albumin effect, she has a mild metabolic acidosis; her $pCO_2$ is low because of the effect of low pH on respiratory center, stimulating it. So, the modern approach suggests low SID as the main cause of her low BE (and therefore pH) thus pointing the clinician to, first, resolve this issue.

Why should this lady have a low SID? On further examination and inquiry, it was noted that her fistula output had increased to about 6 L a day. On analysis, fistula fluid contained 106 mEq/L of Na and 88 mEq/L of Cl. Her codeine phosphate and loperamide were reinstituted and fistula losses were replaced by Hartmann's in equal amounts. Her "severe" acidosis resolved in a couple of days without any other intervention, leaving her with mild metabolic acidosis (BE –4 to –5) because of her chronically narrower than normal SID due to residual fistula fluid loss ("normally" about 1 L/day on codeine and loperamide). She did have flu which resolved in another 3 days without causing any further problems. She was discharged home after a few days without requiring ICU admission. A year later she was admitted for closure of her jejunal fistula successfully and discharged home after her surgery.

## Case 4: A High $CO_2$ but does She Require Ventilatory Support?

A female patient (58 years old) was referred to ICU for ventilatory support as ABG showed a very high $pCO_2$. This patient had suffered a subarachnoid hemorrhage (grade II) the previous night and been taken to a local hospital. She was admitted to a medical ward there, pending transfer to our institution (being the regional neurosciences center) for definitive care. Next morning she was transferred to our Neurosciences High Dependency unit (NHDU—lower level of care from ICU). She was a bit confused but had a Glasgow Coma Scale (GCS) of 14 (E = 4, M = 6, and V = 4). She had a urinary catheter *in situ*, with a large quantity of very dilute urine in her collecting bag. Clinically there was little else to find. An arterial line was sited in preparation for a cerebral

**Table 3:** Arterial blood gas (ABG) parameters and values of case 3.

| Parameter | Value |
| --- | --- |
| pH | 7.11 |
| $pCO_2$ | 21.8 mm Hg |
| $pO_2$ | 142.0 mm Hg |
| Bicarbonate | 4.4 mEq/L |
| BE | –22.2 mEq/L |
| Na | 127 mEq/L |
| Cl | 109 mEq/L |
| Albumin | 3.6 g/dL (36 g/L) |
| Lactate | 10.8 mg/dL |

# Chapter 36
## Arterial Blood Gas Interpretation in Clinical Practice

| Table 4A: Arterial blood gas (ABG) parameters and values of case 4. | |
|---|---|
| Parameter | Value |
| pH | 7.52 |
| pCO$_2$ | 102.0 mm Hg |
| pO$_2$ | 66.7 mm Hg* |
| Bicarbonate | 46.0 mEq/L |
| BE | +14.7 mEq/L |
| Na | 132 mEq/L |
| Cl | 78 mEq/L |
| Albumin | 3.7 g/dL (37 g/L) |
| Lactate | 10.8 mg/dL |

(*On air as her O$_2$ mask had been removed as it was (erroneously) thought that she was retaining CO$_2$ because of O$_2$ therapy!)

| Table 4B: Arterial blood gas (ABG) parameters and values of case 4 after intervention. | |
|---|---|
| Parameter | Value |
| pH | 7.48 |
| pCO$_2$ | 62.5 mm Hg |
| pO$_2$ | 118.5 mm Hg |
| Bicarbonate | 29.8 mEq/L |
| BE | +5.3 mEq/L |
| Na | 141 mEq/L |
| Cl | 91 mEq/L |

angiogram and aneurysmal coiling later that evening. ABGs were taken and the results were as follows (Table 4A).

One look at the ABGs shows that this patient is hypoxemic and requires an intervention—supplemental O$_2$ despite her elevated CO$_2$. This was promptly instituted by the senior ICU clinician who saw her later. Boston approach suggests a "mixed" disorder! A metabolic alkalosis is present (high HCO$_3$ of 46.0 mEq/L) and a respiratory acidosis as her expected pCO$_2$ should be about 77 mm Hg but actual pCO$_2$ is higher at 102 mm Hg. Her AG is normal at 8 [132 − (78 + 46)] and does not add to our understanding of her problem. Danish approach suggests a "primary" metabolic alkalosis (high pH) and "compensatory" respiratory acidosis (again, pH is not actually "compensated" very well!). However, this again does not explain what is happening? Both approaches also do not suggest what next to do, except perhaps institute some form of respiratory support.

Modern approach also suggests a severe metabolic alkalosis. It immediately points out to a wide SID of 54 mEq/L (132 − 78) affecting her BE by a quantum of +16 [(132 − 78) − 38]. The albumin effect is +1.25 [(42 − 37)/4]. Accounting for both SID and albumin effect, her actual BE is −2.55 mEq/L [14.7 − (16 + 1.25)].

When the referral to ICU was made, a senior clinician (author) clinically evaluated her in the NHDU. First, despite her high pCO$_2$ an oxygen mask delivering 28% O$_2$ was applied as she was hypoxemic. As noted above, she was conscious (GCS 14) and hemodynamically stable. She had just finished her breakfast! The history revealed that she had received a large dose of furosemide in the referring hospital (the reason for which was not immediately apparent) and serum electrolytes revealed a significant hypochloremia, almost certainly as consequence of unnecessary diuretic administration. After careful evaluation and making sure there were no physical signs of pathological rise in intracranial pressure (ICP—which would be the reason for invasive ventilation) she was prescribed 0.9% saline to correct both the electrolyte abnormality (correction of widened SID and volume deficit due to unwarranted diuretic therapy). Two liters intravenous fluid and 4 hours later, her ABG were as follows (Table 4B).

Although not completely resolved, her BE, pCO$_2$, SID, etc. are moving towards normal with 0.9% saline. Thus, the etiology of her severe metabolic alkalosis (and the CO$_2$ response) was the result of widened SID which could be corrected with saline infusion.

This was a complex case in that a high pCO$_2$ was present on the background of an unresolved intracranial pathology. However, a decision not to ventilate but correct her biochemistry was taken in her best interest. She was kept under very close observation lest her high pCO$_2$ should adversely affect her ICP in which case she would have been transferred to ICU for invasive ventilation. She continued to improve with further 2 L of saline and underwent a successful cerebral angiography and coiling of her aneurysm later that evening. She was discharged home in due course. The reason for her unwarranted diuretic therapy in the referring hospital could not be ascertained!

## Case 5: Where have All the Acidoses Gone?

An elderly man (69 years age) was being treated on medical wards for his exacerbation of his chronic obstructive airways disease (COPD, now called chronic air flow limitation) with steroids, bronchodilators, and antibiotics. He was also receiving diuretics as he was also thought to be suffering from left ventricular failure. After about 4 days on the ward he developed abdominal distention with generalized tenderness. He became tachycardic and hypotensive with a decreased conscious level (GCS − 11; E = 3, V = 3, M = 5). Surgical consultation was sought. He was diagnosed with abdominal sepsis, probably due to a perforated intestinal diverticulum. He was taken to operating room; an arterial and a central line were sited and he was appropriately resuscitated with fluids and vasopressors. At laparotomy, surgeons found that there was a perforated diverticulum and generalized fecal peritonitis as expected. He had bowel resection, a thorough abdominal washout and ileostomy. He was admitted to ICU for further care. On the ward, his ABGs were as follows (this made some clinicians think that he did not have a pathology in his abdomen as he did not have metabolic acidosis!) (Table 5).

All clinicians involved in this patient's care were puzzled by a lack of any indication of metabolic acidosis (except a raised lactate) in this patient preoperatively which would be in keeping with his clinical condition! In fact, ABGs had consistently shown a positive (+) BE with high $HCO_3$.

His $pO_2$ was suboptimal, so the first step is to increase the inspired oxygen to about 40% (this had been done immediately after he was assessed by the anesthetist on the ward). Boston approach suggests a metabolic alkalosis (as $HCO_3$ and pH, both are high). The expected $pCO_2$ should be 75–79 mm Hg as against actual $pCO_2$ of only 60.2 mm Hg, so accordingly, Boston approach would suggest that part of high pH is in part due to a "respiratory alkalosis". AG is normal at 14 mEq/dL ([132 – [72 + 46]) Danish approach suggests a "mixed" disorder; a metabolic alkalosis (high pH and BE of +7.6) as well a respiratory acidosis (high $pCO_2$). Some clinicians would interpret high $pCO_2$ as an attempt at "compensation"! However, a metabolic alkalosis (compensated or not) is not in keeping with the clinical picture of fecal peritonitis and septic shock! So, the question: "Why does this patient not exhibit a metabolic acidosis"?

Stewart (Modern) approach suggests that there is a widened SID of 55.7 [132 – (72 + 4.3)]; affecting BE by +17.7 (55.7 – 38). His albumin is also low at 1.8 mg/dL (18 g/L); affecting BE by 6 ([42 – 18]/4). The combined effect of widened SID and low albumin on actual BE is: 7.6 – (17.7 + 6) = –16.1 mEq/L. Thus, after accounting for a widened SID (due to low Cl because of diuretic therapy) and low albumin (due to sepsis) his actual BE is –16.1 mEq/L, a large number of unmeasured anions are present in keeping with his clinical condition. Unfortunately, this patient became progressively more unstable and sicker and died despite multiple organ support in the ICU. His severe metabolic acidosis was *masked* by a wide SID and low albumin.

## DO WE NEED DIFFERENT APPROACHES FOR ARTERIAL BLOOD GAS INTERPRETATION?

Although all approaches used in this chapter in interpreting ABG results have their followers, it has to be emphasized that none of the approaches is perfect. They all have their shortcomings and faults. It is also argued by many that there is no difference in various approaches in terms of diagnostic accuracy.[3] However, as has been shown, at least in one example (Case 5) in this chapter, Stewart approach combined with BE (Stewart-Fencl approach) is best at solving "mysteries" of ABGs where variations in SID and albumin affect BE (and therefore cause confusion in clinicians' mind) that makes the results wide "off the mark". However, not all authorities agree with this observation![4]

## SALIENT POINTS

- A set of ABG results is only an adjunct to clinical diagnosis; acidoses or alkaloses are not diseases in themselves but only pointers to an ongoing disease process.
- Hypoxemia ($PaO_2$ < 75 mm Hg or 10 kPa) is a killer and must be looked for. Look for it first as there is a very simple step that you can take to resolve hypoxemia—administer oxygen ($O_2$) by face mask or if already on $O_2$, increase the fractional oxygen concentration ($FiO_2$).
- Extreme hypercarbia ($pCO_2$ > 60 mm Hg must be looked for next. Although there is not much one can do about these immediately (unless the patient is on ventilatory support, when it can be adjusted), these abnormalities are not immediately fatal.
- Only then does one try to analyze what the rest of the results tell us about the patient.
- Look at the pH, remembering that pH may not be radically abnormal but will give one an indication of

**Table 5:** Arterial blood gas (ABG) parameters and values of case 5.

| Parameter | Value |
| --- | --- |
| pH | 7.48 |
| $pCO_2$ | 60.2 mm Hg |
| $pO_2$ | 66.7 mm Hg* |
| Bicarbonate | 46.0 mEq/L |
| BE | +7.6 mEq/L |
| Na | 132 mEq/L |
| Cl | 72 mEq/L |
| Albumin | 1.8 g/dL (18 g/L) |
| Lactate | 38.7 mg/dL (4.3 mmol/L)** |

*On 24% oxygen by mask.
**To convert lactate mg/dL to mmol/L divided by 9.

which way the abnormality lies. A pH less than 7.40 indicates acidosis and a pH of more than 7.48 indicates alkalosis.
- Next decide if the primary disturbance is respiratory or nonrespiratory (i.e. metabolic) in nature. If the $PaCO_2$ is more than 40 mm Hg and pH acidotic, then respiratory acidosis is the primary problem. If $PaCO_2$ is normal or reduced but the pH is still acidotic, look at BE.
- If BE is –2.5 or less (i.e. –3.0, –4.5, etc.), then the disturbance is a metabolic acidosis and so on and so forth.
- Shifts in SID and changes in albumin levels affect BE and must be looked for and applied to actual BE to get the true BE which will then give an accurate picture of acid–base disturbance.

These simple steps are easy to follow and will most often be adequate to decide what type of abnormality one is dealing with. Having decided that, one then needs to look at the patient and review history and clinical findings. Decide if the ABG results fit the clinical situation. If they do, the best way to treat any abnormality observed in the results is *to treat the patient* and *not the numbers*.

## REFERENCES

1. Kishen R, Honoré PM, Jacobs R, et al. Facing acid-base disorders in the third millennium—the Stewart approach revisited. Int J Nephrol Renovasc Dis. 2014;7:209-17.
2. Kishen R. (2012). Trouble with Bicarbonate (A brief review of Stewart approach for interpreting acid-base disorders). [online] Available from http://www.theiaforum.org. [Last accessed January, 2019].
3. Rastegar A. Clinical utility of Stewart's method in diagnosis and management of acid-base disorders. Clin J Am Soc Nephrol. 2009;4(7):1267-74.
4. Doberer D, Funk GC, Kirchner K, et al. A critique of Stewart's approach: the chemical mechanism of dilutional acidosis. Intensive Care Med. 2009;35(12):2173-80.

# SECTION 4

# Miscellaneous

37. Enteral and Parenteral Nutrition in the ICU
38. Immunonutrition, Vitamins, and Trace Elements in the ICU
39. Transfusion of Blood Products in Critically ill Adult Patients
40. Care for the Potential Organ Donor in the ICU

# CHAPTER 37

# Enteral and Parenteral Nutrition in the ICU

*Mark W Motejunas, Bethany Menard, Louis Anzalone, Cody M Koress, Mark R Jones, Alan D Kaye*

## INTRODUCTION

Nutritional status has deservedly found a more central role in treatment of the critically ill patient over recent decades. Nutritional supplementation is now regarded as a therapy in and of itself, rather than an adjunct.

Critical illness is a catabolic stress state and presence of systemic inflammatory response leads to rapid decline in nutrition status and malnutrition. Lack of appropriate nutrition during this condition can exacerbate the proinflammatory milieu of the critically ill patient and result in increased infectious complications and higher mortality.[1] Most critically ill patients require a higher protein to energy ratio than healthy persons to heal wounds, support immune function, and maintain lean body mass.[2] Timely and appropriate delivery of nutritional support is therefore crucial to patient outcomes.

Nutritional support can be administered enterally (enteral nutrition, EN) or parenterally (parenteral nutrition, PN), or a combination of both. EN is administered into the lumen of the stomach or the small bowel. PN is administered intravenously when patients cannot tolerate EN or when there exists a contraindication to EN. Partial PN is used when the patient cannot tolerate enough EN to meet caloric or protein goals; in this instance, the patient receives EN and PN simultaneously. EN is preferred over PN in most critically ill patients, and it has been associated with significantly decreased infectious complications when compared to PN.[2] EN maintains gut integrity, which decreases bacterial translocation through the gut.[1] In addition, EN has been associated with a decrease in oxidative stress, attenuation of the systemic immune response, and preservation of gut-associated lymphoid tissue (GALT), each of which is directly impactful in decreasing disease severity.[2]

Timely commencement of EN has a positive impact on outcomes including infection, organ failure, and hospital LOS. Early administration (within 24–48 hours) of EN is associated with lower mortality and infectious complication rates than starting EN after 48 hours. Interestingly, a study of burn patients found that those who received EN within 4 hours of injury displayed a significantly lower incidence of complications, pneumonia, and sepsis than controls on a regular oral diet.[2]

It is abundantly clear, therefore, that nutritional therapy is an effective modality for enhancing clinical outcomes in critically ill patients. This chapter will familiarize the reader with the effective management of a critically ill patient's nutritional needs.

## INDICATIONS FOR THERAPY

The Nutritional Risk Screening and Nutrition Risk in Critically Ill (NUTRIC) scoring system (Table 1) was developed to help identify critically ill patients most likely to benefit from aggressive protein-energy provision.[3] The model aimed to link starvation, inflammation, and outcome (measured by 28-day mortality and ventilator-free days), and ultimately proposed variables that score patients' risk of malnutrition. The scores obtained effectively stratify patients into high and low risk categories in order to aid clinical decision making regarding nutritional therapy. Prior to this study, there was no scoring system for nutritional risk in the ICU setting.

### Nutritional Risk Screening

Patients who have NUTRIC scores of six or greater are likely to benefit from aggressive nutritional treatments and are at high risk for both malnutrition and poorer clinical outcomes. If IL-6 testing is not available, the scoring system

**Table 1:** Nutrition Risk in Critically Ill (NUTRIC) score.

| Variable | Range | Points |
|---|---|---|
| Age | <50 | 0 |
| | 50–<75 | 1 |
| | ≥75 | 2 |
| APACHE II Score | <15 | 0 |
| | 15–<20 | 1 |
| | 20–28 | 2 |
| | ≥28 | 3 |
| SOFA Score | <6 | 0 |
| | 6–<10 | 1 |
| | ≥10 | 2 |
| Number of comorbidities | 0–1 | 0 |
| | ≥2 | 1 |
| Number of days from hospital to ICU admission | 0–<1 | 0 |
| | ≥1 | 1 |
| IL-6 | 0–<400 | 0 |
| | ≥400 | 1 |

(APACHE II: acute physiology and chronic health evaluation II[4]; SOFA: sequential organ failure assessment; IL-6: interleukin-6)
*Source:* Heyland DK, Dhaliwal R, Jiang X, et al. Identifying critically ill patients who benefit the most from nutrition therapy: the development and initial validation of a novel risk assessment tool. Crit Care. 2011;15(6):R268.

**Table 2:** Disease processes requiring total parenteral nutrition in the ICU by patient population.

| Patient population | Disease processes |
|---|---|
| Neonate | Congenital gastrointestinal anomalies—gastrointestinal fistula, inadequate absorption resulting from short bowel syndrome, anorectal malformations, gastrointestinal atresia, microvillus inclusion disease, congenital chloride diarrhea, tufting enteropathy |
| Pediatric | • Severe malnutrition<br>• Prolonged diarrhea |
| Pediatric/adult | • Bowel obstruction<br>• Significant weight loss and/or hypoproteinemia when enteral therapy is not possible<br>• Short bowel syndrome due to surgery<br>• Necrotizing enterocolitis<br>• Burns<br>• Multiorgan failure |
| Adult | • Preoperative UGI cancer<br>• Hepatic encephalopathy (branched-chain amino acid-enriched solutions)<br>• Prolonged bowel rest (Crohn's disease, pancreatitis, some stages of ulcerative colitis, and with prolonged bouts of diarrhea) |

(ICU: intensive care unit; UGI: upper gastrointestinal)

may be revised to assume a score of five or greater may be indicative of patients requiring urgent nutritional therapy.

The indications for enteral and parenteral therapy vary widely within patient populations. Malnourished patients requiring parenteral therapy generally lack the necessary gastrointestinal (GI) capacity to absorb nutritive substances or are at significant risk for obstruction (Table 2). The indications for malnourished patients requiring enteral therapy can be even wider, though aspiration with oral nutrition is a common adverse event that would lead a clinician to prescribe enteral therapy. Enteral therapy preserves the mucosal barrier and can be delivered to the stomach or postpyloric in the event of recurrent aspiration of gastric contents, esophageal dysmotility with a history of regurgitation, or significantly delayed gastric emptying.

## ENTERAL NUTRITION

The nutritional needs of a patient will vary widely based on multiple factors that dictate metabolic energy requirements such as weight, temperature, current medications, surgeries, or procedures and are therefore patient specific. For this reason, EN formulations and delivery methods must be tailored for the needs of each patient. The current gold standard for calculating the metabolic requirements in the critically ill setting is the use of indirect calorimetry (IC). This method works via metabolic calculations based on the volumes and concentrations of a patient's inspired and expired carbon dioxide and oxygen. This "metabolic cart" is expensive and not feasible for many locations. Furthermore, like all tests, it is not without flaws. Anything that can artificially affect the carbon dioxide and oxygen concentrations or volumes can lead to erroneous IC calculations. Continuous renal replacement therapy (CRRT), chest tubes, supplemental oxygen, mechanical ventilation, and even anesthesia will all affect these metrics, and patients that require ICU level care more often than not exhibit one or more of these interventions as a part of their care.[2]

There are various proposed calculations for estimating one's metabolic needs. The goal of these equations is simple—to calculate a patient's metabolic requirements based on patient specific comorbidities. However, as previously mentioned, the multiple nonstatic variables render this task exceedingly difficult. The American Society of Parenteral and Enteral Nutrition (ASPEN) has undergone a thorough investigation regarding the accuracy of many of these equations, concluding that no specific formula demonstrates proven superiority.[1] Additionally, when compared to the current gold standard of caloric estimation, IC, these equations demonstrated suboptimal accuracy rates of just 40–75%.[2]

Given the complexity of predicting a patient's anticipated nutritional requirements, clinicians frequently initiate therapy based on a simple weight-based formulas such as 25–30 cal/kg/day and titrate their dietary regimens from there (Table 3). There are multiple EN formulas on the market. For the majority of ICU level patients, a standard polymeric isotonic 1–1.5 kcal/mL formula is well tolerated.[2] As electrolyte abnormalities present themselves, titrations of the formula may be made or an alternative selected. There have been multiple studies examining disease specific enteral formulations for patients with chronic liver failure, kidney failure, or acute pancreatitis, but none of the data have illustrated a significant correlation with improvement of morbidity or mortality.[2]

One aspect of the nutritional calculation inappropriate protein supplementation. Adequate protein supply has been directly correlated with a patient's ability to maintain a healthy immune system and intact wound healing pathways.[2] Weight-based estimates for calculating a patient's protein consumption are most commonly used and are estimated at 1.2–2.0 g/kg/day. Certain disease states and treatments such as obesity or CRRT will alter these calculations and require additional supplementation. For instance, in the obese population supplementation with 2.0–2.5 g/kg/day of ideal body weight is suggested, and for patients on CRRT up to 2.5 g/kg/day is often supplemented given the significant amino acid loss (10–15 g/day) associated with CRRT.[1,2] Clinically, serum protein markers such as albumin, prealbumin and CRP are often trended and correlated as indicators of protein homeostasis. However, in contrast to their frequent use, studies have not validated the accuracy of these methods, and many discourage the use of such metrics to dictate therapy.

No matter the formula or starting dose, consistent literature illustrates the morbidity and mortality benefits of initiating enteral supplementation within the first 24-48 hours of hospitalization, particularly in ICU level patients.[1,2,5] Most commonly enteral feeds are initiated at continuous doses of 10–20 cc/hour and advanced by an additional 10–20 cc/hour until the calculated metabolic requirement is met. In the acute setting the feeds are delivered most easily to the stomach via a nasogastric or orogastric tube. However, if long-term supplemental nutrition is anticipated (>4 weeks), a gastrostomy or jejunostomy tube may be indicated.[1] These devices allow both ease of access to the GI tract in addition to decreasing the risk of aspiration and pneumonia.[5]

It is estimated that less than half of patients in the ICU ever reach their target goal energy intake.[2] For this reason, the rate of delivery and frequency of diet advancement has drawn increased scrutiny from the medical community. A recent study performed by Heyland et al. compared patient outcomes of those that were started at goal EN rates versus patients who were graduated to goal from 15 cc/hour continuous infusions. In traumatic brain injury, they reported that those started on early aggressive enteral feeding regimens had fewer infectious complications and overall more rapid recovery times.[5] This method of starting patients at goal rates has unfortunately not demonstrated the same statistical benefit when applied to other patient populations.

Intolerance to feeds is a leading cause of suboptimal nutritional supplementation and is largely a clinical diagnosis. Gastrointestinal symptoms such as abdominal distention and diarrhea are key indicators, but gastric residual volumes are most often utilized as evidence of feeds intolerance. The heavy reliance on gastric residual volume calculations is illustrated most clearly by a study conducted by Metheny et al., which illustrated that 97% of nurses assess enteral intolerance solely by increased residual volumes.[1] The fear of potential complications such as aspiration and the sequelae of such an event is the

**Table 3:** General caloric and components estimates.

| Energy/components | Goals |
|---|---|
| Total caloric (not protein) intake needs | Enteral and/or parenteral:<br>• 25–30 cal/kg/day |
| Target protein intake | Enteral:<br>• Standard starting replacement dose: 1.2–2.0 g/kg/day<br>• Obesity: 2.0–2.5 g/kg/day of ideal body weight<br>• CRRT 2.5 g/kg/day<br>Parenteral:<br>• Standard starting replacement dose: 0.8–1 g/kg/day |
| Target lipid supplementation | Enteral:<br>• Standard starting supplementation of fats will equate to 30% of total caloric intake<br>Parenteral:<br>• Standard starting replacement dose: 1 g/kg/week<br>• TPN most commonly prescribed having 10% or 20% lipid emulsion formulas. |

(CRRT: continuous renal replacement therapy TPN: total parenteral nutrition)

largest contributor to the vigilant monitoring of residual volumes. However, recent studies have demonstrated no statistical increased aspiration risk or worse patient outcomes when residual volumes of 200 cc were compared to those of 400 cc.[2,6] This study's findings correlate with many others; superior nutritional supplementation without worsening patient morbidity or mortality is achievable by simply foregoing residual volume monitoring altogether.[1,2] Based on this data, the ASPEN published guidelines dissuading the use of gastric residual volumes of less than 500 cc with no other signs of enteral intolerance as a sole reason to interrupt tube feedings. Instead of discontinuing feeds, they suggest utilizing a prokinetic agent such as metoclopramide or erythromycin to improve tolerance and maintain nutrition.

## PARENTERAL NUTRITION

Certain disease states make enteral feeds impracticable, leaving nutritional replacement via venous total parenteral nutrition (TPN) as the only option. Similar to enteral formulations, proper TPN supplementation needs to be personalized based on a patient's functional status, comorbidities, and organ health. Formulas that provide 20–35 kcal/kg/day are most often chosen as initiating doses. The energy sources of the formula are similar to those of enteral feeds and include amino acids, fat emulsions, and carbohydrate-based nourishment. Currently, all commercially available formulations provide all nine essential amino acids (histidine, isoleucine, leucine, lysine, methionine, phenylalanine, threonine, tryptophan, and valine) in varying concentrations in order to maintain robust biochemical pathways.[7] Regardless of the concentration, the provided amino acids should ideally equate to roughly 0.8–1 g/kg/day of protein. Lipid emulsion supplementation is usually initiated at 1 g/kg/week as to avoid intestinal failure associated liver disease from over administration of fatty acids.[7] These lipid formulas include linoleic acid and α-linoleic acid which are essential fatty acids that cannot be synthesized by humans. Without external supplementation of these essential fatty acids (EFAs), an EFA deficiency may develop with serious potential neurological and hematological side effects, including death.[7]

Given the numerous complications and side effects of intravenous metabolic replacement, all other possibilities need to be explored prior to initiating therapy. The ASPEN guidelines propose the use of either the Nutrition Risk Screening (NRS-2002) or the NUTRIC calculator to determine the need for peripheral nutrition supplementation. Based on the results of these calculations, TPN may be initiated, deferred, or contraindicated.

For low nutrition risk patients, defined as patients with NRS-2002 of less than or equal to 3 or a NUTRIC score of less than or equal to 5, PN ought to be held for the first 7 days of an ICU admission even if enteral feeds are not a treatment option.

For high-risk nutrition patients defined as patients with a NRS-2002 of greater than or equal to 5 or a NUTRIC score of greater than or equal to 5, TPN therapy should be initiated as soon as possible during an ICU admission.

Finally, those patients receiving less than 40% of their calculated caloric or protein requirements by enteral feeds after 7–10 days of optimal treatment may require TPN supplementation. Initiation prior to this 7–10-day period does not effectively improve outcomes and may contribute to patient morbidity.

## ADJUNCTIVE THERAPIES

### Fiber

The supplementation of fiber to enteral feeds has been shown to significantly improve gut function, immunity, and structural health, and decrease endotoxin translocation.[8] Similarly, studies have demonstrated fiber's positive impact on gut microbiota by increasing the proportion of *Bifidobacteria* and *Lactobacillus* present in the colon while also acting as a bulking agent via increased intestinal water absorption.[8] Despite these reported physiologic benefits, conflicting evidence remains regarding the benefits of fiber supplementation in the critically ill. Furthermore, with case reports associating fiber administration with bowel ischemia and obstruction, current guidelines deter the use of routine supplementation.[1,2] If diarrhea is present, which for patients on enteral feeds has a reported incidence of 2–95%, then fiber supplementation is clinically indicated.[8] Guidelines suggest the use of fermentable, soluble fiber (e.g. fructooligossaccharides and inulin) at doses of 10–20 g/day for noninfectious diarrhea. The ASPEN guidelines promote the use of soluble fiber rather than mixed fiber formulas in order to minimize the risk of bowel obstruction.

### Probiotics

Hospitalized patients incur a variety of etiologies behind disrupted bowel microbiota. The most common offender is the frequent use of broad-spectrum antibiotics. Probiotics, as viable microorganisms, are often given as adjuncts to nutritional supplementation in hopes of equilibrating the bowel microflora. A healthy balance of certain bacterial species such as *Lactobacillus* and *Bifidobacteria* have demonstrated beneficial effects such as decreased infectious complications, particularly ventilator associated pneumonia.[2] Similarly, patients with feeding intolerances were found to frequently having imbalances of *Staphylococcus* species in their feces and were more prone to bacteremia.[2] It would follow from this information that providing probiotic supplementation would be clinically beneficial. However, while the use of probiotics appears to be safe, there is minimal evidence demonstrating their benefits. According to many investigators, the confounding and frequent antibiotic use in addition to the variability in probiotic dosing makes statistically significant benefit difficult to prove.

### Antioxidants and Trace Minerals

Antioxidants such as vitamins E and C, along with trace minerals such as selenium, zinc, and copper, are frequently added to patient's nutrition regimens. There are no standardized doses for micronutrient and antioxidant supplementation, and doses vary by institution. A recent meta-analysis performed by McClave et al. found a statistically significant mortality reduction in ICU patients, particularly burn patients and mechanically ventilated patients.[2] There was no statistically significant effect on hospital length of stay or infectious complications.

### Glutamine, Arginine, and Fish Oils

Glutamine, arginine, and fish oils have also been found to be frequently added as nutritional supplements to patient's enteral feeding regimens with varying levels of statistical support. Glutamine, most often given parenterally at a dose of 20-40 g/day, has shown some correlation with improved patient outcomes. Evidence exists to support that burn victims receiving glutamine supplementation experience significant reductions in mortality.[5] Other studies have demonstrated trends toward reductions in infectious complications and hospital length of stays, but lacked statistical significance. The supplementation of arginine has been investigated for mortality and infectious benefits, but the data was equivocal. Current ASPEN guidelines do not promote the routine administration of either supplement. Fish oils have displayed statistical benefits in patients with ARDS by significantly decreasing mortality, ventilatory requirements, organ failures, and days in the ICU.[5] However, the study that found these trends used Oxepa®, an enteral formula with fish oils, antioxidants, beta-carotene, taurine, and L-carnitine. A meta-analysis performed by Lu et al., consisting of 1,239 patients, did not find a statistical significance in the mortality benefit of fish oil supplements in patients with sepsis. This study did find low quality evidence that fish oils decreased total ICU length of stay and ventilatory requirements, but these results are reportedly overturned by multiple sensitivity analyzes.[9]

## DRUG INTERACTIONS

Drug interactions with EN/PN and various medications, whether administered via intravenous or enteral route, can prove a complex entity for physicians juggling these medications with feeding requirements. Enteral and parental nutrition cause an altered GI environment, unpredictable absorption of other medications, and incite unintended medication interactions, in addition to problems with the feeding tube itself such as clogging or dislodgement.[1] Some medications require either an alkaline or an acidic environment for absorption; therefore, the location of the feeding catheter tip should be considered when administering certain medications. Locations of the tube can include the gastric region, duodenum, or jejunum depending on desired environmental pH.[6,10] Any time the feeding tube is accessed, it should be flushed with at least 15 mL of water prior to and after any medication administered. A medication should not be mixed into the enteral formal.[11] The preferred formulation for medications given enterally is liquid consistency. Solid medications that can be crushed should be mixed with water prior to administration. Any capsules made of gel need to be dissolved in water to minimize risk of aspiration.[12] Oftentimes feeding catheter can become clogged. Gastric tubes have the largest lumens and are less likely to become occluded. If using a jejunostomy tube, only liquid formulations should be used.[13]

A number of medications exhibit known interactions with EN that may cause deleterious side effects or result in decreased absorption and efficacy of the medication. When administering these medications, EN should be held 1 hour prior and 1 hour after the medication is given.[6] If the medication has measurable data such as serum drug levels (e.g. phenytoin or theophylline) or markers of drug effect (e.g. thyroid hormone levels or prothrombin time), these measurements should be taken to ensure adequate delivery and absorption to allow for drug dosing and titration.[1]

There are a number of interactions between commonly administered medications and enteral feeding formulations. Proton pump inhibitors (PPIs) are typically available as enteric-coated delayed-release granules or tablets. When mixed with an acidic liquid, granules remain intact until reaching duodenum.[14] PPIs can be mixed with alkaline suspension (8.4% sodium bicarbonate) to dissolve granules to avoid occluding the feeding tube, especially small bore tubes.[10] When administering theophylline with enteral feedings, its levels can be decreased by up to 30%.[15] Levothyroxine administration has the potential to bind to the feeding tube itself, causing decreased drug absorption.[16] A commonly studied interaction involving warfarin and enteral feeding discovered that proteins in the enteral formula can bind warfarin and reduce its bioavailability, thereby decreasing its anticoagulant effects.[17]

Extensive research has elucidated the interaction of enteral feedings with several anti-epileptic drugs. Carbamazepine, an anti-epileptic with a narrow therapeutic window, can bind to the polyvinyl chloride in the tubing material, leading to decreased drug delivery.[10] Phenytoin can also bind to the tube itself, again causing decreased delivery. Further, proteins in enteral formulations may decrease phenytoin absorption by 70%.[6,10] Commonly, patients receiving EN have either severe malnutrition or critical illnesses that lead to hypoalbuminemia. With low levels of albumin, levels of free fractioned phenytoin are increased. Free phenytoin levels should therefore be carefully monitored in such clinical scenarios, especially when albumin levels are less than 3 g/dL.[18]

Many antibiotics are also susceptible to pharmacokinetic alteration by enteral feeds. Fluoroquinolones, particularly ciprofloxacin, experience up to a 60% reduction in bioavailability through chelation of divalent cations in enteral feedings.[19] Penicillin can have up to an 80% decrease in bioavailability when given with food or other nutritional support.[6]

It has been established that administering levodopa in combination with food can decrease its absorption. There has been shown to be a potential drug-nutrient interaction with enteral feeding, particularly those with high protein levels, which leads to a decreased level of levodopa.[20]

Propofol, a lipid-based emulsion, is commonly used in intensive care settings and can provide a significant amount of calories leading to both hypertriglyceridemia and overfeeding. Care should be taken when using propofol in patients that are also receiving EN, and daily calorie intake should be closely monitored.[21]

The interaction between EN and vasoactive substances has been studied extensively amongst critical care physicians and researchers. Often, critically ill patients receive some form of vasoactive drug to improve their hemodynamic status along with their overall outcome. Enteral nutrition is also commonly started early in these patients to maintain GI structure and function. In order for nutrients to be absorbed, there must be adequate GI blood flow. Enteral nutrition promotes GI blood flow, yet it remains controversial exactly when to time EN delivery.[22] Common practice dictates that EN be held in hemodynamically unstable patients or those receiving vasoactive substances. This is based on the idea that EN will increase splanchnic oxygen demand which may not be met in a patient with a low-flow state, potentially leading to ischemia and further necrosis. Bowel necrosis is a feared complication of EN, often presenting with abdominal pain, high nasogastric output, and intestinal ileus.[23] Since no evidence currently exists to guide EN use in hemodynamically unstable patients, EN should be used with extreme caution in this patient population. Some evidence suggests that EN can be safely used in patients with noncardiogenic hemodynamic instability, but more evidence is required.[24] Clinicians should always maintain vigilance when monitoring for signs of feeding intolerance, and recognize intolerance or instability in patients requiring higher vasoactive dosages, increased ventilator support, or worsening hemodynamic instability.

## SIDE EFFECTS AND COMPLICATIONS

Given the numerous risks associated with both EN and PN, clinicians must gage patients' personal needs by the appropriate route of administration for that specific patient and clinical circumstance. A systematic review by Gramlich et al. in 2004 examined 13 studies to investigate whether EN resulted in better outcomes compared to PN in critically ill adults. This review showed that EN again was associated with fewer infections, but reported no difference in mortality between the forms of nutrition. This study also showed no difference in hospital length of stays or ventilator-free days in the groups receiving either EN or PN. The PN population had higher rates of hyperglycemia. EN was shown to be cost-effective in four of the studies reviewed. The authors therefore concluded that EN should be a clinician's first choice for nutritional therapy in critically ill states.[25] More recently, a 2016 meta-analysis by Elke and colleagues analyzed 18 randomized controlled trials involving 3,347 critically ill patients. They reviewed routes of nutrition, EN versus PN, and compared clinical outcomes. Neither route of nutrition exhibited a higher mortality rate. EN had a significantly lower rate of infectious complications and less days spent in the ICU. However, no difference was found in hospital length of stays or days mechanically ventilated. This meta-analysis again demonstrated that EN is preferred over PN in critically ill patients needing nutrition therapy.[26] An overview of side effects and complications of EN and PN are described in Table 4.

| Table 4: Complications with enteral and parenteral nutritional replacement. | |
|---|---|
| Complication | Description |
| Clogging of the feeding tube | • Feeding sites ought to be flushed with at least 15 mL of water prior to and after any medication administration. The preferred formulation for medications given enterally is liquid consistency. Any capsules made of gel need to be dissolved in water to minimize risk of aspiration.[12]<br>• Gastric tubes have the largest lumens and are less likely to become occluded.[13]<br>• PPIs can be mixed with alkaline suspension (8.4% sodium bicarbonate) to dissolve granules to avoid occluding the feeding tube, especially small-bore tubes.[10] |
| Renal failure | • Concern arises in patients with renal failure receiving enteral nutrition, as the high protein content in enteral nutrition can increase blood urea nitrogen and potentially worsen renal function. Renal patients should receive a special derived, low protein renal formula.[6] |
| Hemodynamic instability | • Immune-modulating formulas commonly contain arginine, which when metabolized can increase nitric oxide production and cause hemodynamic instability.[2] |
| Parenteral Nutrition Associated Liver Disease (PNALD) | • Large range of presentations including gallstone formation, cholestasis, steatosis, and even cirrhosis if not recognized and treated appropriately.[27] PNALD develops through a variety of mechanisms, including overfeeding, hepatotoxic effects of parental nutrition (PN), and lack of enteral stimulation. Clinicians should manage PNALD by switching to enteral or oral formulation if possible, avoid overfeeding, or turning PN off for 8–10 hours per day.[27] |
| Aspiration | • Risk of gastroesophageal reflux increases with enteral nutrition delivery to the stomach. Patients that have a significant risk of aspiration or have not tolerated gastric feeds in the past should be deferred to jejunal tube placement.[28,29] |
| Hyperglycemia and Hypertriglyceridemia | • The most common side effect of PN is hyperglycemia. Hyperglycemia is more pronounced with parental versus enteral nutrition even when equal amounts are administered.[30] Patients receiving PN should have blood glucose closely monitored and receive insulin as needed.<br>• ASPEN recommends that the daily carbohydrate rate for diabetic and critically ill patients should not exceed 4–5 mg/kg/min.<br>• Hypertriglyceridemia may lead to pancreatitis and worsened immune function.[31] The intravenous fat emulsion also poses a risk for patients with soy or egg allergies, as the emulsion contains egg phospholipids and soy proteins.[31] |
| Infection | • Parenteral nutrition poses a high risk of infection, including a higher risk of central line infection, pneumonia, and abdominal abscesses.[27] Central lines should have a dedicated port for PN and proper handling should be used. If an infection is suspected, consider delaying PN administration or holding it temporarily until the infection is cleared.[6] |

(ASPEN: American Society of Parenteral and Enteral Nutrition; PPIs: proton pump inhibitors)

## CONCLUSION

As correlations regarding outcomes such as infections, hospital length of stay, and even survival have been firmly associated with malnutrition, it becomes increasingly evident that nutritional supplementation must be considered a pillar of proper patient care. Consideration of the patient's continuously changing metabolic requirements, comorbidities, and current medications must all be taken into account in order to optimize therapy. Moreover, like any treatment or intervention performed in the clinical setting, the risks and benefits of supplementation must be continuously analyzed. Enteral and parenteral nutrition administration is not without side effects and complications. Therefore, the physician prescribing the nutritional regimen ought to be comfortable diagnosing these complications and act to mitigate them when able. However, the physician, while a core component of the treatment team, is not alone in providing care. The overall complexities of optimal supplementation truly mandate that the delivery of treatment ultimately involves a multidisciplinary team composed of nurse specialists, dietitians, pharmacists, and gastroenterologists. A properly trained team will be most able to detect suboptimal supplementation and complications, which, in turn, may improve patient outcomes.

## SALIENT POINTS

- Malnutrition is associated with morbidity and mortality in the hospital setting.
- Nutritional supplementation is a standard of appropriate care for best practices standards.
- Consideration of the patient's continuously changing metabolic requirements, comorbidities, and current medications all play an important role to optimize therapy.

- Enteral and parenteral nutrition administration has potential side effects and complications.
- Any physician prescribing nutritional regimen must be comfortable diagnosing these complications and act to mitigate them.
- A multidisciplinary team composed of nurse specialists, dieticians, pharmacists, and gastroenterologists will benefit the delivery of supplemental nutrition and identification of potential complications.

## REFERENCES

1. Elhassan AO, Tran LB, Clarke RC, et al. Total parenteral and enteral nutrition in the ICU: evolving concepts. Anesthesiol Clin. 2017;35(2):181-90.
2. McClave SA, Taylor BE, Martindale RG, et al. Society of Critical Care Medicine; American Society for Parenteral and Enteral Nutrition. Guidelines for the provision and assessment of nutrition support therapy in adult critically ill patient: Society of Critical Care Medicine (SCCM) and American Society for Parenteral and Enteral Nutrition (A.S.P.E.N.). JPEN J Parenter Enter Nutr. 2016;40(2):159-211.
3. Heyland DK, Dhaliwal R, Jiang X, et al. Identifying critically ill patients who benefit the most from nutrition therapy: the development and initial validation of a novel risk assessment tool. Crit Care. 2011;15(6):R268.
4. Knaus WA, Draper EA, Wagner DP, et al. APACHE II: A severity of disease classification system. Crit Care Med. 1985;13(10):818-29.
5. Heyland DK, Dhaliwal R, Drover JW, et al. Canadian Critical Care Clinical Practice Guidelines Committee. Canadian clinical practice guidelines for nutrition support in mechanically ventilated, critically ill adult patients. JPEN J Parenter Enteral Nutr. 2003;27(5):355-73.
6. Kaye AD, Kaye AM, Urman RD (Eds). Essentials of Pharmacology for Anesthesia, Pain Medicine, and Critical Care. New York: Springer; 2015.
7. Pironi L, Arends J, Bozzetti F, et al. Home Artificial Nutrition and Chronic Intestinal Failure Special Interest Group of ESPEN. ESPEN guidelines on chronic intestinal failure in adults. Clin Nutr. 2016;35(2):247-307.
8. Kamarul Zaman M, Chin KF, Rai V, et al. Fiber and prebiotic supplementation in enteral nutrition: A systematic review and meta-analysis. World J Gastroenterol. 2015;21(17):5372-81.
9. Lu C, Sharma S, McIntyre L, et al. Omega-3 supplementation in patients with sepsis: a systematic review and meta-analysis of randomized trials. Ann Intensive Care. 2017;7(1):58.
10. Williams NT. Medication administration through enteral feeding tubes. Am J Health Syst Pharm. 2008;65(24):2347-57.
11. Bankhead R, Boullata J, Brantley S, et al. A.S.P.E.N. Board of Directors. Enteral nutrition practice recommendations. JPEN J Parenter Enteral Nutr. 2009;33(2):122-67.
12. Belknap DC, Seifert CF, Petermann M. Administration of medications through enteral feeding catheters. Am J Crit Care. 1997;6(5):382-92.
13. Powell KS, Marcuard SP, Farrior ES, et al. Aspirating gastric residuals causes occlusion of small-bore feeding tubes. JPEN J Parenter Enteral Nutr. 1993;17(3):243-6.
14. Howden CW. Review article: immediate-release proton-pump inhibitor therapy—potential advantages. Aliment Pharmacol Ther. 2005;22 (Suppl 3):25-30.
15. Gal P, Layson R. Interference with oral theophylline absorption by continuous nasogastric feedings. Ther Drug Monit. 1986;8(4):421-3.
16. Smyrniotis V, Vaos N, Arkadopoulos N, et al. Severe hypothyroidism in patients dependent on prolonged thyroxine infusion through a jejunostomy. Clin Nutr. 2000;19(1):65-7.
17. Dickerson RN, Garmon WM, Kuhl DA, et al. Vitamin K - Independent warfarin resistance after concurrent administration of warfarin and continuous enteral nutrition. Pharmacotherapy. 2008;28(3):308-13.
18. Au Yeung SC, Ensom MH. Phenytoin and enteral feedings: Does evidence support an interaction? Ann Pharmacother. 2000;34(7-8):896-905.
19. Magnuson BL, Clifford TM, Hoskins LA, et al. Enteral nutrition and drug administration, interactions, and complications. Nutr Clin Pract. 2005;20(6):618-24.
20. Cooper MK, Brock DG, McDaniel CM. Interaction between levodopa and enteral nutrition. Ann Pharmacother. 2008;42(3):439-42.
21. Lowrey TS, Dunlap AW, Brown RO, et al. Pharmacologic influence on nutrition support therapy: Use of propofol in a patient receiving combined enteral and parenteral nutrition support. Nutr Clin Pract. 1996;11(4):147-9.
22. Kang W, Kudsk KA. Is there evidence that the gut contributes to mucosal immunity in humans? JPEN J Parenter Enteral Nutr. 2007;31(3):246-58.
23. Schunn CD, Daly JM. Small bowel necrosis associated with postoperative jejunal tube feeding. J Am Coll Surg. 1995;180(4):410-6.
24. Allen JM. Vasoactive substances and nutrition in critical care. In: Diet and Nutrition in Critical Care. Springer; 2015. pp. 473-82.
25. Gramlich L, Kichian K, Pinilla J, et al. Does enteral nutrition compared to parenteral nutrition result in better outcomes in critically ill adult patients? A systematic review of the literature. Nutrition. 2004;20(10):843-8.
26. Elke G, van Zanten AR, Lemieux M, et al. Enteral versus parenteral nutrition in critically ill patients: An updated systematic review and meta-analysis of randomized controlled trials. Crit Care. 2016;20(1):117.
27. Kudsk KA, Croce MA, Fabian TC, et al. Enteral versus parenteral feeding. effects on septic morbidity after blunt and penetrating abdominal trauma. Ann Surg. 1992;215(5):503-13.
28. Heyland DK, Drover JW, MacDonald S, et al. Effect of postpyloric feeding on gastroesophageal regurgitation and pulmonary microaspiration: Results of a randomized lcontrolled trial. Crit Care Med. 2001;29(8):1495-501.
29. Lien HC, Chang CS, Chen GH. Can percutaneous endoscopic jejunostomy prevent gastroesophageal reflux in patients with preexisting esophagitis? Am J Gastroenterol. 2000;95(12):3439-43.
30. Buchman AL, Ament ME. Comparative hypersensitivity in intravenous lipid emulsions. JPEN J Parenter Enteral Nutr. 1991;15(3):345-6.
31. Safe practices for parenteral nutrition formulations. National Advisory Group on Standards and Practice Guidelines for Parenteral Nutrition. JPEN J Parenter Enteral Nutr. 1998;22(2):49-66.

# CHAPTER 38

# Immunonutrition, Vitamins, and Trace Elements in the ICU

*Samir Samal, Shakti Bedanta Mishra, Snigdha Ipsita*

## INTRODUCTION

The nutritional requirements in critically ill patients are complex. Acute physiologic response to stress and illness leads to increased resting energy expenditure, increased catabolism, loss of lean body weight, reduced protein synthesis, fluid retention, and dysregulation of trace elements levels. The other factors which contribute to malnutrition are pre-existing illness, delayed initiation of nutritional support, underfeeding or overfeeding, gastrointestinal disturbances, and other medical and surgical factors. Malnutrition impairs defense mechanisms and increases the susceptibility to infections. Coupled with inflammatory response and oxidative stress, it worsens the outcome in critically ill patients, thereby increasing the intensive care unit (ICU) morbidity, mortality, and length of stay. Hence, besides the conventional goals of preserving lean body mass and reducing infectious or metabolic complications, nutritional support in critically ill patients is now days more directed toward modulation of immune response and prevention of oxidative injury.

## IMMUNONUTRITION

Certain key nutrients, if provided in excess of daily requirements, exert a modulation of immune and inflammatory pathways.[1] This gives rise to the concept of immunonutrition or pharmaconutrition. Immunonutrition is the practice of delivering immunomodulatory agents in therapeutic doses so that they exert a pharmacological effect in selected class of patients.

Studies have been conducted on amino acids like arginine and glutamine, fatty acids, selenium, vitamin A, C, E, ribonucleotides, and some other trace elements. But they differ with respect to the formulas, physiologic actions, and have different outcomes depending upon the underlying disease states. The prediction of dose-response relationship is difficult due to varied composition, different routes of administration, and our lack of knowledge on immune system. Hence, evidence in support of use of these agents is still lacking.

Meta-analysis by Heyland et al. demonstrated that enteral supplementation with immunonutrients decreases the infections complications and length of stay in ICU with no effect on mortality.[2] A multicenter trial involving 597 mixed ICU patient populations compared enteral supplementation of formula containing glutamine, arginine, and omega-3 fatty acids with a non-isonitrogenous, isocaloric enteral formula and found no difference in outcome, ICU morbidity, mortality, or length of stay.[3] The Metaplus trial evaluating the effect of combined use of macronutrients like glutamine, fish oil, and micronutrients like selenium, vitamin C, E, and zinc on infections as primary end point demonstrated no benefit and rather there was an increased long-term mortality.[4] But in these studies, multiple nutrients were used in heterogeneous patient population and hence, the benefit or harm could not be attributed to any particular agent.

The inflammatory response to injury is a double-edged sword. There exists a fragile balance between increased inflammatory response and immune dysfunction. The critically ill patients usually have an exaggerated inflammatory response, increased reactive oxygen species, and oxidative injury. The use of pharmaconutrients with proinflammatory properties like arginine may further stimulate the inflammatory response and may be detrimental. On the other hand, patients in early stage of illness or elective surgical patients have some degree of suppression of cellular defense and use of immune-nutrients may prove beneficial. Patients with increased risk of infection and impaired cellular defense and without fulminant infection like trauma, burns, or postsurgical patients are appropriate candidates for pharmaconutrition.

## MACRONUTRIENTS

### Glutamine

First studied by Fürst P et al. in 1986,[5] glutamine is an alpha amino acid with a molecular weight of 146 Dalton, and molecular formula $C_5H_{10}N_2O_3$. It is synthesized from glutamine and ammonia by glutamine synthetase in muscles and small amounts by lung and brain. It is consumed by kidney cells, intestinal epithelial cells, immune cells, and cancer cells.[6,7]

#### Recommended Dietary Allowance

Glutamine is the most abundant free amino acid in blood and plasma level is 0.5–0.8 mmol/liter, the intracellular to extracellular ratio being 30:1. Endogenous synthesis is 60–80 g/day. Glutamine being a nonessential amino acid, no estimated average requirement or recommended dietary allowance (RDA) is formulated for it. The optimal glutamine dose is still unknown but doses up to 0.5 g/kg/day are safe.[8,9] No adverse effects of glutamine have been found with doses up to 50–60 g/day. However, these values have been derived from short-term studies in adult patients only. Thus, a definite daily allowance cannot be made up for chronic supplementation in healthy individuals.[9]

#### Source

Bone broth, whey protein, beef, Spirulina, cabbage, asparagus, broccoli, organic poultry.

#### Physiology

Glutamine serves to carry ammonia from periphery to the liver; is a precursor of glutathione, arginine, glucosamine, and taurine; helps in regulation of acid-base balance; and is an energy substrate for cells with high demand like intestinal mucosa, macrophages, and lymphocytes.[10] *In vitro* studies show decreased phagocytosis by macrophages in glutamine depleted media.[11] Glutamine prevents cellular apoptosis and preserves tissue metabolic functions and adenosine triphosphate (ATP) levels in sepsis and shock, prevents ischemia reperfusion injury, improves nitrogen balance,[12,13] improves glycemic status, reduces infectious complications,[14,15] and reduces insulin resistance[16] (Table 1).

**Table 1:** Daily dose and functions of macronutrients.

*Macronutrients*

| Macronutrient | Daily Dose | Function | Deficiency |
|---|---|---|---|
| Glutamine | No RDA/EAR as nonessential<br>• Up to 0.5 g/kg/day | • Carry ammonia from periphery to the liver<br>• Precursor of glutathione, arginine, glucosamine, and taurine<br>• Regulation of acid-base balance<br>• Energy substrate for cells with high demand like intestinal mucosa, macrophages, and lymphocytes<br>• Helps in phagocytosis<br>• Prevents cellular apoptosis and preserves tissue metabolic functions and ATP levels in sepsis and shock<br>• Reduces insulin resistance<br>• Reduces infectious complications<br>• Anti-inflammatory effect by reducing the expression of cytokines | • Increased mortality in critically ill patients<br>• *Kegg disease:* Congenital systemic glutamine deficiency |
| Arginine | • No RDA/EAR as nonessential<br>• Up to 25 g/day* | • Facilitates the cytotoxic effect of macrophages via iNOS pathway<br>• Promotes wound healing—via TH2 pathway | |
| Fish oil | AI†1.6 g/day<br>0.5–2% of daily energy intake‡ | • Components of cell membrane<br>• Synthesis of hormonal substances and regulation of immune functions<br>• Beneficial impact on the regulation of cytokines | Delayed growth, skin lesions, and neurological symptoms |

*Well tolerated by trauma patients
†Adequate intake
‡WHO recommendation
(ATP: adenosine 5'-triphosphate; EAR: estimated average requirement; iNOS: inducible nitric oxide synthase; RDA: recommended dietary allowance; TH2: T helper 2; AI: adequate intake; WHO: World Health Organization)

Glutamine also exerts an anti-inflammatory effect by reducing the expression of cytokines like NF-κB (nuclear factor kappa-light-chain-enhancer of activated B cells) and prevents the degradation of its inhibitor.[17] Enhanced heat shock protein (HSP) 70 expression and protection against lung injury have been demonstrated in laboratory animals given glutamine supplementation.[18] Glutamine by enteral or parenteral route has a sustaining effect on enterocytes and stimulates the gut-associated lymphoid tissue.[8]

## Glutamine in ICU

Glutamine is a nonessential amino acid. But in catabolic states like sepsis, polytrauma, major burns, and postsurgery, there is profound depletion of glutamine in plasma and skeletal muscles and hence, it becomes conditionally essential.[10] Low plasma level of glutamine is associated with increased mortality.[19] Hence, exogenous glutamine supplementation may be considered in critically ill patients. But as glutamine has limited stability and solubility, the administration of high-dose glutamine may be difficult, particularly in patients with volume restrictions.

Various studies comparing the enteral and parenteral routes of glutamine supplementation yield conflicting results. A meta-analysis by Novak et al. showed the greatest benefit was derived from at least 6 days of glutamine supplementation in patients with gastrointestinal failure and receiving total parenteral nutrition.[20] Enteral supplementation should be considered in burn and trauma patients.[21] A recent posthoc analysis on 1,223 mechanically ventilated patients in 40 ICUs of Europe and North America demonstrated increased mortality with high-dose glutamine particularly in patients with baseline renal dysfunction.[22]

REDOX (REducing Deaths due to OXidative Stress) and SIGNET (Scottish Intensive care Glutamine or seleNium Evaluative Trial) trials also voiced concern about the use of high-dose glutamine in critical care setting with REDOX trial showing higher mortality rate associated with glutamine (p = 0.02), whereas the SIGNET trial showing no outcome benefit regarding sepsis complications or mortality.[23,24]

## Deficiency

Because the body creates its own glutamine, deficiency of this amino acid is rare. However, it is seen that low levels of glutamine make a person prone to infections. Weight loss and change in bowel habits have also been noted. Increased mortality is seen in ICU patients with low glutamine levels. Congenital systemic glutamine deficiency is also known as Kegg disease.

## Toxicity

Several studies involve glutamine as enteral or parenteral adjunct but none showed any adverse effects or toxicity even with plasma levels more than 2 mmol/L. However, there were few instances of acute liver failure accompanied with high glutamine levels though no literature states that high levels of glutamine are associated with acute liver failure symptoms.[25]

## Guidelines

American Society for Parenteral and Enteral Nutrition (ASPEN) guidelines suggest not to routinely add glutamine to enteral or parenteral nutrition regime in critically ill patients (Quality of evidence: Moderate).[26] Though, addition of glutamine to enteral nutrition regimen did reduce mortality in a study in burn patients by Garrel et al.[27]

# Arginine

Arginine is a semiessential dibasic amino acid. It may be obtained from diet or synthesized in kidneys. It acts as a substrate for nitric oxide production and a secretagogue for insulin, prolactin, and growth hormone. It is also a substrate of histidine, nucleic acid, and polyamine.

## Recommended Dietary Allowance

United States Food and Drug Administration (US-FDA) has not fixed any RDA for arginine as such, although up to 25 g/day has been seen to be tolerated well by trauma patients without side effects (Table 1).

## Source

Nuts (walnut, hazelnut, almond, cashew), seeds (sesame, sunflower), oats, cereals, legumes, dairy products, meat.

## Physiology

Arginine is broken down by arginase I in liver into urea and ornithine and by arginase II in mitochondria into proline and ornithine. Proline is converted into hydroxyproline and collagen and helps in wound healing. The other pathway involves the activation of inducible nitric oxide synthase (iNOS) and generation of nitric oxide.

The preferential activation of arginase or inducible nitric oxide synthetase depends upon the immune status of the patient. In sepsis, there is release of interleukins, T helper 1 (TH1) cytokines, interferon gamma, and tumor necrosis factor alpha (TNF α). This induces the expression of iNOS and there is extensive nitric oxide (NO) production which facilitates the cytotoxic effect of macrophages. But in trauma patients, the TH2 response predominates with release of transforming growth factor beta (TGF β), IL 4, 10. This increases arginase expression which promotes wound healing.[28] Hence, Arginine supplementation may be beneficial in trauma patients but is detrimental in critically ill septic patients (Table 1).[29]

### Arginine in ICU

The endogenous production of arginine is reduced in trauma and sepsis.[30] The earlier studies showed enteral supplementation of arginine (25 g/day) was associated with increased TH cell and lymphocyte and monocyte proliferation.[31] Arginine supplementation reverses increased intestinal permeability and maintains barrier function in experimental intestinal reperfusion injury models.[32] A 7-day course of arginine with a dose of 12–25 g/day may provide benefit in trauma or postsurgery.

### Deficiency

Arginine deficiency is a very rare entity and not much literature is available regarding the same. Growth failure and rashes were seen in children with low arginine levels because of deficient carbamyl phosphate synthetase. In an experimental study, arginine deficiency was seen to be involved in thrombocytopenia and immunosuppression in severe fever with thrombocytopenia syndrome [severe fever with thrombocytopenia syndrome (SFTS) virus—bunyavirus].

### Toxicity

Arginine supplementation in critically ill patients with sepsis or SIRS leads to negative inotropic effects, impaired coagulation, cytotoxic effects, and refractory hypotension associated with vascular dilatation.[33-35] Data pertaining to use of intravenous arginine is controversial.

### Guidelines

ASPEN 2016 guidelines say immune modulating enteral formulations containing arginine, eicosapentaenoic acid (EPA) and docosahexaenoic acid (DHA), glutamine should not be used routinely; but may be used in traumatic brain injury patients and perioperative patients in surgical ICU (Quality of evidence: Very low).[26] Routine use of arginine in patients with severe sepsis is discouraged. (Quality of evidence: Moderate).

## Fish Oil (n-3 Polyunsaturated Fatty Acids)

Fatty acids are a variable length carbon chain with methyl terminus and carboxylic acid head. The n-3 polyunsaturated fatty acids (PUFAs) contain more than one double bond.[36] Depending on the position of first double bond from the methyl terminus, PUFA may be classified as n-3, 6, or 9. Double bond at third carbon from methyl terminus is an n-3 PUFA.

### Recommended Dietary Allowance

Adequate intake for adults is around 1.6 g/day as per Food and Nutrition Board of the US in 2002. The World Health Organization recommends n-3 fatty acid to be 0.5–2% of daily energy intake (Table 1).

### Source

Fish oil contains mostly omega-3 fatty acids, i.e. EPA and DHA. Terrestrial n-3 fatty acid is found in some vegetables, e.g. rape seed and nut (walnut) oils. Flaxseed, soya bean, and canola oils are also good source.

### Physiology

Polyunsaturated fatty acids are important components of cell membrane and they help to promote optimal function and fluidity of the membranes. Besides, they also act as energy sources, help in synthesis of hormonal substances, and regulation of immune functions. The omega-6 fatty acids are proinflammatory and increased levels lead to development of many chronic disorders. Omega-3 fatty acids have a beneficial impact on the regulation of cytokines and immune response. Deficiency of n-3 fatty acids leads to delayed growth, skin lesions, and neurological symptoms (Table 1).

### PUFA in ICU

Increasing the ratio of n-3: n-6 fatty acids may improve outcome in critically ill patients. A high dose of n-3 fatty acids (8 g/day) has anti-inflammatory effects.[37] The PUFA either act as secondary messengers or enters the cyclo-oxygenase pathway. The EPA-derived thromboxane A2 has less platelet aggregating activity; LTB5 decreases chemotaxis. There is reduced production of NF-κB and activator protein 1 (AP-1) activation and TNFα downregulation. Omega-3 fatty acids reduce serum cholesterol, low-density lipoprotein (LDL), and triglyceride levels.

It reduces the ventilator requirements and reduces mortality and length of ICU stay in acute respiratory distress syndrome (ARDS) and sepsis patients.[38] Fish oil reduces autoimmune disease and T lymphocyte IL 2 production. N-3 fatty acids are protective against ischemia reperfusion injury and hence may be used for ischemic preconditioning.[39] They reduce the heart rate, improve the lipid profile, and reduce postoperative atrial fibrillation in coronary artery bypass grafting (CABG) patients except those with high phospholipid levels.[40] N-3 fatty acids also reduce cancer cachexia and improve blood viscosity.

The saturation level of DHA and EPA is 12–13%. So, supplementation with fish oil of patients with high phospholipid levels does not provide much benefit. The 'Enteral Omega-3 Fatty Acid, γ-Linolenic Acid, and Antioxidant Supplementation in Acute Lung Injury (OMEGA-EN)' trial conducted to evaluate the effect of Omega-3 fatty acid supplementation in ARDS patients was terminated due to increased mortality.[41]

### Deficiency

As PUFAs are crucial for structural and functional integrity of neural cells, neurological disturbances are seen on its deficiency. Higher incidences of schizophrenia, Alzheimer disease, depression, hyperactive disorders, dyslexia, and bipolar disorders are attributable to lower levels of PUFA. Delayed growth and skin lesions can also be associated with PUFA deficiency (Table 1).

### Toxicity

Very high doses of n-3 fatty acids increase the risk of bleeding. Gastrointestinal disturbances are common side effects. Some studies suggest that high doses may lead to increased risk of macular degeneration whereas some studies state otherwise. An analysis suggested increased risk of prostate cancer with higher intake.

### Guidelines

In 2009, the European Food and Safety Authority (ESFA) recommended an n-3 fatty acid intake of 2 g/day alpha linoleic acid and 250 mg/day DHA and EPA. US and WHO recommendations have been mentioned previously.[42]

The 2016 ASPEN guidelines could not make recommendations for use of fish oil in ARDS patients because of conflicting data, although it may be used routinely in surgical ICU patients who require enteral nutrition.[26]

## MICRONUTRIENTS: VITAMINS

### Vitamin C

Vitamin C, also known as ascorbic acid, is an essential water soluble vitamin necessary for various metabolic functions in our body. It is a six carbon compound related to glucose. Chemical composition is $C_6H_8O_6$ (Table 2).

### Recommended Dietary Allowance

The current RDA for vitamin C is 60–90 mg/day for healthy, nonsmoking adults. RDA for smokers is around 100 mg/day. Pregnant and lactating women have an RDA of 80–100 mg/day. The tolerable upper intake level is well beyond 2 g/day.[43]

### Source

Guava, black currant, red pepper, kiwi, green peppers, orange, lemon, papaya, broccoli, tomato, potato.

### Physiology

The body pool is around 1,500 mg. It is assumed that there is 85% absorption of the total intake. Vitamin C acts as a cofactor for enzymes in synthesis of collagen, carnitine, neurotransmitters, and catecholamine.[44] It also has a role to play in cholesterol metabolism. It is a very good antioxidant and scavenges reactive oxygen species.[45] It is also hypothesized that vitamin C has a role to play in prevention of chronic diseases and cancer.[46] It has also got antiviral and antibacterial activity.

### Vitamin C in ICU

Sepsis is associated with an exaggerated inflammatory response, increased production of reactive oxygen species, NF-κB activation, and oxidative injury. Patients with sepsis have reduced levels of ascorbate and increased glutathione values.[47] So, administration of antioxidants like vitamin C may help to attenuate the inflammatory reaction, increase responsiveness to vasopressors, and maintain endothelial integrity.

Paul Marik et al. in a retrospective before-after clinical study studied the outcome and clinical course of 94 consecutive septic patients; out of which 47 were treated with vitamin C, hydrocortisone, and thiamine during a 7-month period. They found significant reduction in mortality rates, slowing of progression of organ failure, and faster weaning period off vasopressor therapy in the treatment group.[48]

Similar results regarding mortality and better radiological improvement were noted in patients with severe pneumonia who received vitamin C, hydrocortisone, and thiamine in a propensity score-based analysis of a before-after cohort study by Won-Young Kim et al.[49] Higher incidences of acute kidney injury or superinfection were not noted in patients receiving the treatment.

A systematic review and meta-analysis of vitamin C in critically ill by Michael Zhang and David F Jativa studying effect of isolated use of vitamin C in critically ill patients [four randomized controlled trials (RCTs) and one retrospective trial] did not find any mortality

**Table 2:** Daily dose and function of vitamins.

*Micronutrients—vitamins*

| Vitamin | Daily dose | Function | Deficiency |
|---|---|---|---|
| Vitamin C (ascorbate) | • 60–90 mg/day, adults<br>• 80–100 mg/day, pregnancy<br>• 100 mg/day, smokers | • Cofactor for enzymes in synthesis of collagen, carnitine, neurotransmitters, and catecholamine<br>• Very good antioxidant and scavenges reactive oxygen species<br>• Prevention of chronic diseases and cancer<br>• Antiviral and antibacterial activity | Scurvy, gingivitis, poor wound healing |
| Vitamin D (cholecalciferol) | • <12 years, 400 IU<br>• 12–70 years, 600 IU<br>• >70 years, 800 IU | • Bone mineralization<br>• Barrier function of epithelium* and has antimicrobial action<br>• Activates innate immunity<br>• Anti-inflammatory action | • Rickets, osteomalacia |
| Vitamin B1 (thiamine/aneurin) | • 1.1 mg/day, women<br>• 1.2 mg/day, men<br>• 1.4 mg/day, pregnancy/lactation | • Antioxidant properties<br>• Glucose regulation<br>• Erythropoietic and mood modulating activities<br>• Necessary for neuronal well being | • Dry and wet beriberi<br>• Wernicke encephalopathy, Korsakoff psychosis |
| Vitamin B12 (cyanocobalamin) | 0.5–3 mcg/day<br>+1 mcg/day, pregnancy | • Hematopoiesis<br>• Neural development<br>• Nucleic acid synthesis<br>• Assists folic acid in choline synthesis | • Pernicious anemia, megaloblastic anemia<br>• Subacute combined degeneration of spinal cord (SACD) |
| Vitamin K | • AI 90–120 mcg/day, adults<br>• AI 90 mcg/day, pregnancy and lactation<br>• AI 2–2.5 mcg/day, infants<br>• AI 30–75 mcg/day, 1–18 years of age | • Complete synthesis of certain proteins that are pre-requisite for blood coagulation<br>• Synthesis of proteins necessary for binding of calcium in bones and other tissues<br>• Antidote for warfarin and coumarin poisoning | • Coagulopathy, bleeding disorders<br>• Hypoprothrombinemia<br>• Increased prothrombin time<br>• Osteoporosis and coronary heart disease are associated with lower levels of K2 |
| Vitamin B6 (pyridoxine) | • 1.3–1.7 mg/day, adult male<br>• 1.2–1.5 mg/day, adult female<br>• 1.9–2.0 mg/day, pregnancy and lactation<br>• 0.1–0.6 mg/day, newborn to 8 years<br>• 1 mg/day, 9–14 years | • Macronutrient (glucose, amino acid, and lipid metabolism)<br>• Neurotransmitter (cofactor for serotonin, dopamine, epinephrine, norepinephrine, and gamma amino butyric acid) synthesis, histamine synthesis, hemoglobin synthesis and function<br>• Gene expression | • Seborrheic dermatitis like eruption<br>• Atrophic glossitis with ulceration, angular cheilitis, conjunctivitis<br>• Neurologic: somnolence, confusion, neuropathy<br>• Sideroblastic anemia (impaired heme) |

*Via cathelicidins
(AI: adequate intake; IU: international units)

benefit.[50] However, there was definite reduction in need for vasopressor and decreased duration of mechanical ventilation in patients receiving vitamin C.

A double blind, placebo controlled adaptive RCT is going on to investigate the efficacy of combined use of vitamin C, hydrocortisone, and thiamine in reducing mortality and improving organ function in critically ill patients with sepsis [VICTAS (VItamin C, Thiamine And Steroids in Sepsis) Trial] with an expected enrollment of around 2,000 patients.

Such large scale RCTs will go a long way in helping us understand the role of vitamin C in patients with severe sepsis admitted in ICUs.

Ascorbate levels of 100–200 μM have antitumor activity due to increased collagen synthesis and increased production of hydrogen peroxide and are particularly concentrated in solid tumors. It also has antiviral and antibacterial action.

When vitamin C is given orally, plasma concentrations are limited to less than 100 μM. Increasing the dose further leads to increased renal excretion and increased metabolism. Intravenous administration, on the other hand, results in very high plasma concentrations. The low levels of ascorbate in sepsis may be corrected with a dose of more than 3 g/day.

### Deficiency

Deficiency of vitamin C leads to scurvy. Deficiency leads to fatigue and lethargy. There is weakening of collagenous structures leading to tooth loss, joint pains, and bone and connective tissue disorders. Vitamin C deficiency may also gingivitis and bleeding of gums.

### Toxicity

The use of vitamin C is contraindicated in patients with glucose-6-phosphate dehydrogenase (G6PD) deficiency, hemochromatosis, or those with oxalate nephropathy. High dose also leads to increased intestinal iron absorption and raised urinary excretion of iron, manganese, and calcium. The toxic plasma level of ascorbate in human beings is 25 mM.[51] Doses up to 150 g/day have been safely used in different clinical studies.

### Guidelines

The ASPEN guidelines 2016 suggest that combination of antioxidant vitamins (vitamin C and E) and trace minerals (selenium, zinc, copper) may improve outcome in burn, trauma, and critical patients requiring mechanical ventilation.[26] Fifteen trials were studied and they demonstrated there was a significant reduction in overall mortality ($p = 0.001$) in patients receiving antioxidants and trace elements supplementation (Quality of Evidence: Low).[26] The 2016 ASPEN guidelines have chosen not to recommend trace elements and antioxidant supplementation in sepsis due to many conflicting studies (Level of evidence: Moderate).

## Vitamin D

Known as cholecalciferol, it is also a steroid hormone. It is produced in skin on exposure to ultraviolet rays present in sunlight or is obtained from dietary sources. Its active form calcitriol is necessary for calcium and phosphorus metabolism and mineralization of bones. Its molecular formula is $C_{27}H_{44}O$.

### Recommended Dietary Allowance

The daily amount needed for children up to 12 years of age is 400 IU, 600 IU for up to 70 years, and 800 IU for people above 70 years of age.

### Source

Sunlight exposure (skin), fish liver oil, red meat, liver, egg yolk, fortified foods.

### Physiology

Vitamin D functions both as a vitamin and a hormone. Vitamin D is carried to the receptors in form of 25(OH)D and 1,25(OH)2D bound to vitamin D binding protein and albumin. Activation of toll-like receptors in human macrophages promotes conversion of vitamin D into its active form, interaction with the vitamin D receptors, and upregulates the production of cathelicidins. Cathelicidins promote the barrier function of epithelium and has antimicrobial action. Vitamin D also activates innate immunity and NLRP3 inflammasome. In conditions of immune system hyperactivity, it has an anti-inflammatory action by regulation of p65, ERK½, and toll-like receptors.

The receptors for vitamin D are present in a wide variety of cells and it has a vital role to play in cellular metabolism, gene expression, cytokine production, and histone acetylation.

### Vitamin D in ICU

The effect of vitamin D however depends upon the rate of synthesis, metabolism, gene polymorphism and protein binding, and receptor affinities which are dysregulated in critically ill patients.

In sepsis, the levels of vitamin D and vitamin D binding protein are reduced and are associated with increased mortality.[52] Vitamin D levels less than 15 ng/mL increase the risk of sepsis and acute kidney injury.[53] The 'Effect of High-Dose Vitamin $D_3$ on Hospital Length of Stay in Critically Ill Patients With Vitamin D Deficiency (VITdAL ICU)' trial conducted in 475 critically ill mixed ICU patients with a single 540,000 IU dose of vitamin D orally and 100,000 IU monthly showed improved mortality in patients with vitamin D deficiency and no adverse outcomes except mild hypercalcemia in some cases.[54]

In critically ill patients, a dose of 120,000 IU of vitamin D over 1 week is recommended. The serum level achieved depends upon various factors like gastrointestinal integrity, gene polymorphisms of vitamin D carrier protein, and albumin levels. No parenteral formulation of vitamin D is available yet. Evidence-based recommendations for the use of vitamin D in critically ill patients, epigenetics, deficiency levels, dose, and route of administration are still lacking.

### Deficiency

Deficiency of vitamin D leads to rickets and osteomalacia in adults. These conditions are a result of defective mineralization during new bone formation.

### Toxicity

The toxic concentration of vitamin D3 is 160–200 ng/mL. Hypervitaminosis D results with intake more than 50,000 IU daily. Symptoms are a result of hypercalcemia leading to dehydration, polyuria, nausea, vomiting, bone pain, and muscle cramps. Renal dysfunction, nephrocalcinosis, and seizures may occur in severe form.

### Guidelines

No specific guidelines are currently present for vitamin D in critically ill.

## Vitamin B1 (Thiamine)

Thiamine, also known as vitamin B1 or aneurin, was the first vitamin B to be discovered. It is an essential, water soluble vitamin discovered by Umetaro Suzuki in Japan.[55] Thiamine was discovered while studying the role of rice bran in treatment of beriberi. Chemically, it is a substituted pyrimidine and thiazole rings linked by methylene bridge.

### Recommended Dietary Allowance

Recommended dose is 1.1 mg/day for women and 1.2 mg/day for men. The RDA rises to 1.4 mg/day for pregnant and lactating mothers. RDA up to 12 months is 0.2–0.3 mg/day. Higher doses are necessary in burn patients, alcoholics, patients with neurologic disorders, intestinal disorders, sepsis, malnutrition, and people on high carbohydrate diet. EAR is 0.9 mg/day for women and 1 mg/day for men.

### Source

Brewer's yeast, pork, ham, liver, whole grain, peas, beans, milk.

### Physiology

Thiamine, an essential vitamin, has antioxidant properties and helps in glucose regulation. In addition to these, it has erythropoietic and mood modulating activities. It helps in the functioning of cardiovascular system, nervous system, and digestive system. It has a pivotal role in glucose metabolism in our body. Pyruvate dehydrogenase and alpha ketoglutarate require thiamine pyrophosphate (TPP) for their activity as a coenzyme. TPP is also needed in the pentose phosphate pathway. Thiamine inhibits arterial smooth muscle proliferation by inhibiting action of glucose and insulin on them. It has been also seen that thiamine is necessary for neuronal well-being with deficiency leading to selective neuronal death. Neuronal death due to its deficiency can be attributed to increased free radical production and oxidative stress.

### Thiamine in ICU

Patients in septic shock are in a state of increased metabolic demand. Several studies have showed patient in ICU being deficient in thiamine, which was further associated with poor outcomes. Some studies though failed to corroborate the findings. It is hypothesized that thiamine deficiency leads to reduction of pyruvate supply for Krebs cycle leading to lactic acid production in patients with normal liver function.

A two center, randomized double blind trial to study effect of thiamine on lactate levels in septic shock patients with lactate levels more than 3 mmol was carried out. Patients were given 200 mg thiamine or placebo twice daily for 7 days. There was no significant difference in primary outcome of lactate concentration at 24 hours between groups.[56] Moreover, there was no significant difference in time to shock reversal, SOFA (sequential organ failure assessment) score at 24 hours, mortality rate, and ICU length of stay. However, there was a significant difference in time to death in favor of thiamine group (p = 0.047). Thus, it can be argued that thiamine supplementation in septic shock patients with severe thiamine deficiency (< 7 mmol/L) could be advantageous.

Nonetheless, this study had several drawbacks with regards to sampling and there was no mention of the way of septic shock management in patients. There was also no data showing plasma thiamine levels at 24 hours.

Other trials and studies regarding the role of thiamine in ICU have already been discussed under vitamin C.

### Deficiency

Deficiency of Thiamine is known to cause beriberi which is found in two forms—(1) dry and wet beriberi leading to neurological and (2) cardiovascular disorders. Acute confusion and delirium can be seen in chronic alcoholics called as Wernicke encephalopathy. Untreated, this may lead to permanent brain damage. Severe deficiency for a prolonged period may result in Korsakoff psychosis which is most commonly seen in alcoholics.

### Toxicity
Symptoms of toxicity generally mimic that of a hyperthyroid with restlessness tremors, rapid pulse, and nervous hyperirritability. There are chances of anaphylaxis on faster administration of the drug intravenously.

### Guidelines
The European Society for Clinical Nutrition and Metabolic guidelines for parenteral nutrition (ESPEN Guidelines) in intensive care recommends thiamine supplement of 100–300 mg/day during first 3 days in ICU for all patients with any level of suspicion for thiamine deficiency.[57] There have been reported cases of anaphylaxis while administration, thus the drug has to be administered over 15–30 minutes.

Vitamin B12 also helps in immune function by regulating the production of NF-κB and nitric oxide. But, there are no randomized trials with regard to the dose, route, or mortality benefit of vitamin B12 supplementation in critically ill patients.

## Vitamin B12
Vitamin B12 is an essential water soluble vitamin, which is also known as cyanocobalamin which can be artificially produced. It is a cobalt compound produced by intestinal organisms and is also found in soil and water.

### Recommended Dietary Allowance
Recommended allowance for cyanocobalamin is 0.5–3 mcg/day, the requirement being higher by 1 mcg during pregnancy.

### Source
All animal products are good source of vitamin B12. Fish, meat, poultry, eggs, milk, and meat products are rich sources. It is generally absent in plant foods. Fortified vegetarian products can be consumed though.

### Physiology
Cyanocobalamin needs to be combined with intrinsic factor for absorption. It aids in hematopoiesis, neural development, and nucleic acid synthesis. It also assists folic acid in choline synthesis. It also helps in carbohydrate metabolism and protein synthesis. Dietary turnover rate of vitamin B12 is 0.05–0.2% of total body stores. Vitamin B12 is excreted in human breast milk and is easily transferred to fetus.

### Vitamin B12 in ICU
There have not been many randomized trials with regards to dose, route, or mortality benefit of vitamin B12 supplementation in critically ill patients.

### Deficiency
Vitamin B12 levels less than 200 pg indicate vitamin B12 deficiency. Deficiency leads to pernicious anemia, megaloblastic anemia, and/or neurological disorders. Megaloblastic anemia and neurologic damage is seen with vitamin B12 levels less than 100 pg/mL.

### Toxicity
No toxic or adverse effects have ever been observed with doses as high as 2 mg daily orally.

### Guidelines
No specific guidelines are currently present for vitamin D in critically ill.

## TRACE ELEMENTS
Trace elements are minerals present in living tissues in small amounts. They are necessary for various metabolic functions in our body as catalysts in enzyme system, as cofactors, transport of oxygen, and many more (Table 3).

## Selenium
Selenium is a trace element that is needed in our body for functioning of the enzyme glutathione peroxidase which protects from oxidative damage of deoxyribose nucleic acid (DNA), proteins, and membrane lipids.

### Recommended Dietary Allowance
A committee of the National Research Council set the estimated and adequate daily intake of selenium at 50–200 mcg/day for adults above 11 years of age.

### Source
Pork, beef, turkey, sea foods, lean meats, poultry, egg, legumes, nuts, soy products.

### Physiology
Selenium is a trace element and is a constituent of glutathione peroxidase and selenoproteins. It also plays a vital role in iodine metabolism. When given in bolus dose, selenium initially has a pro-oxidant action. But, it is rapidly utilized for the synthesis of selenoproteins and has an antioxidant and anti-inflammatory effect.

**Table 3:** Daily dose and function of trace elements.

*Micronutrients—trace elements*

| Trace element | Daily dose | Function | Deficiency |
|---|---|---|---|
| Selenium | • AI* 50, 200 mcg/day | • Constituent of glutathione peroxidase and selenoproteins<br>• Iodine metabolism<br>• Antioxidant and anti-inflammatory effect | • Keshan disease<br>• Kashin-Beck disease[†] |
| Zinc | • 11 mg/day, male adult<br>• 8 mg/day, female adult<br>• 11–12 mg/day, pregnancy<br>• 12–13 mg/day, lactation | • Innate and adaptive immunity<br>• Free radical scavenger<br>• Anti-inflammatory action<br>• Cofactor of antioxidant enzymes like glutathione peroxidase, catalase, and superoxide dismutase | • Infections, hypogonadism, weight loss, emotional disturbance, anhedonia, impaired learning, delayed wound healing, alopecia, acrodermatitis enteropathica, delay in age-related macular degeneration |
| Chromium | • AI 20–25 mcg/day, adult female<br>• AI 30–35 mcg/day, adult male<br>• AI 30 mcg/day, pregnancy<br>• AI 45 mcg/day, lactation | • Enhance the action of insulin<br>• Reduce insulin resistance in PCOS | • Severely impaired glucose tolerance<br>• Weight loss<br>• Peripheral neuropathy and confusion |
| Copper | • 0.9 mg/day (WHO, 1.3 mg/day)<br>• 1 mg/day, pregnancy<br>• 1.3 mg/day, lactation | • Cellular energy production (cytochrome C oxidase)<br>• Crosslinking of collagen and elastin (lysyl oxidase); maintains integrity of connective tissue in heart and blood vessels and also in bone<br>• Iron metabolism (iron mobilization and RBC formation) as a part of multicopper oxidases or ferroxidases (oxidize ferrous to ferric form) and ceruloplasmin<br>• Formation and maintenance of myelin sheath<br>• Conversion of dopamine to norepinephrine<br>• Synthesis of melanin (tyrosinase)<br>• Antioxidant (superoxide dismutase and ceruloplasmin)<br>• Regulation of gene expression | • Uncommon<br>• Anemia unresponsive to iron supplementation, myelodysplastic syndrome<br>• Neutropenia<br>• Loss of pigmentation<br>• Neurological symptoms and impaired growth<br>• Osteoporosis, osteoarthritis, rheumatoid arthritis<br>• Symptoms as in Menkes disease (kinky hair, growth failure, and nervous system deterioration) |
| Manganese | • AI 1.9-2.3 mg/day<br>• AI 2 mg/day, pregnancy<br>• AI 2.6 mg/day, lactation | • Constituent of superoxide dismutase—principal antioxidant enzyme n mitochondria<br>• Metabolism of carbohydrates (gluconeogenesis)<br>• Amino acid metabolism (urea cycle)<br>• Synthesis of proteoglycans (healthy cartilage and bone mineralization)<br>• Activation of prolidase (collagen synthesis); wound healing | • Impaired growth, impaired glucose tolerance<br>• Bone demineralization |

*Adequate intake
[†]Atrophy, degeneration, and necrosis of cartilage tissue in the joints
(AI: adequate intake; PCOS: polycystic ovary syndrome; RBC: red blood cell)

## Selenium in ICU

The severity of sepsis is inversely related to the levels of the selenium dependent enzyme glutathione peroxidase.[58] Glutathione peroxidase is a tetrameric enzyme, each of which contains a selenocysteine component.

The level of selenium in patients with severe sepsis is 40% lower than patients without sepsis and is associated with increased mortality.[59] Selenium supplementation improves outcome in postcardiac arrest patients and postoperative patients with multiorgan failure.[60] It also reduces infectious complications in burn patients. Hence, selenium supplementation in critically ill patients may provide benefit but the study results till date are inconclusive.

Data from nine studies regarding parenteral selenium found no difference between patients and controls with regards to ICU length of stay, hospital length of stay, or duration of mechanical ventilation. However, meta-analysis of nine trials by Huang et al. showed a significant reduction in mortality with higher dose of selenium in critical illness.[61]

Selenium is available in both enteral and parenteral formulations (sodium selenite). However, the appropriate route and dose-response relationship is yet to be decided. A dose of 5 mcg/kg/day may be used but trials have used a dose of 4,000 mcg in 24 hours or a cumulative dose of 13 mg with no adverse effects.[62]

### Deficiency

Selenium deficiency along with Coxsackie virus infection may lead to a fatal Keshan disease which is characterized by myocardial necrosis (Table 3). Along with iodine deficiency, it leads to Kashin-Beck disease resulting in atrophy, degeneration, and necrosis of cartilages. Deficiency of selenium may also cause symptoms of hypothyroidism as it is necessary for conversion of thyroxine (T4) to more active T3.

### Toxicity

Selenium toxicity may result in abdominal cramps, arrhythmia, and muscle spasms.

### Guidelines

Discussed under vitamin C. The recommended optimal acute selenium dose for critically ill patients may range between 500 mcg/day and 750 mcg/day for about 1–3 weeks depending on the severity of illness.

## Zinc

Zinc is also a trace mineral that plays a significant role in different physiologic processes.

### Recommended Dietary Allowance

The RDA for zinc is 11 mg/day for adult male and 8 mg/day for an adult female. Normal diet supplies around 12.3 mg of the daily requirement of zinc.

### Source

Shellfish, oysters, beef, red meats, poultry, eggs, milk, yogurt, legumes, nuts, and whole grain cereals.

### Physiology

Zinc helps in innate and adaptive immunity, acts as a free radical scavenger, and has anti-inflammatory action. It is a cofactor for antioxidant enzymes like glutathione peroxidase, catalase, and superoxide dismutase. Zinc deficiency is common in vegetarians, chronic alcoholics, elderly, diabetics, and patients with chronic disorders.

### Zinc in ICU

In critical illness, there is increased excretion of zinc due to muscle catabolism, tissue loss, and hyperglycemia.

During, acute infection or inflammation, zinc gets sequestered into different compartments of body for various physiologic functions. Hence, plasma zinc level falls and measurement of plasma concentration of zinc does not reflect the zinc content of the body. Lower levels of zinc are associated with increased levels of IL 6 and 8 and worsen outcome in critically ill patients.[63]

Studies pertaining to zinc supplementation in trauma and burn patients showed 12–37.5 mg of parenteral zinc lowered the infectious complications and improved outcome.[64,65]

### Deficiency

Zinc deficiency affects a wide range of systems in our body (Table 3).
- *Immune system:* Impair macrophage and neutrophil functions, natural killer (NK) cells, and complement activity. Zinc is necessary for synthesis and activation of T lymphocytes.
- *Connective tissue and wound healing:* Zinc deficiency may lead to acne, xerosis, stomatitis, seborrheic dermatitis, or alopecia. Patients with chronic leg ulcers are supplemented with zinc for better healing.

- *Diarrhea:* Zinc supplementation helps in reducing episodes and duration of acute childhood diarrhea in zinc deficient or malnourished children. WHO and United Nations Children's Fund (UNICEF) recommend zinc supplementation for the same.[66]
- *Vision:* Age Related Eye Disease Study (AREDS) recommends that zinc and antioxidants delay the progression of age related macular degeneration.[67]
- *Neurological:* Cognitive function such as learning is impaired in zinc deficiency. Behavioral abnormalities, lethargy, irritability are also seen in zinc deficiency. Schizophrenia, in some studies, has been linked to low zinc levels.
- *Reproductive system:* Zinc deficiency can lead to lower circulating testosterone, hypogonadism, and delayed puberty.
- *Acrodermatitis enteropathica:* It is an inherited deficiency of zinc carrier protein; it presents with growth retardation, diarrhea, and hair loss and skin rash. Opportunistic candidiasis and other bacterial infections may also occur.

## Toxicity

However, overdose of zinc should be avoided as zinc toxicity leads to hypocupremia, leucopenia, lipid abnormalities, hypotension, diarrhea, and oliguria.

## Guidelines

The 2012 ASPEN guidelines recommended the daily zinc oral intake 11 mg in males and 8 mg in females, 11–19 mg by enteral route, and 2.5–5 mg in parenteral route. Patients with diarrhea, intestinal fistulas, burns, and those with known zinc deficiency may have increased requirements. Doses higher than the recommended dose may be administered for a period of 1–2 weeks.

## REFERENCES

1. Grimble RF. Immunonutrition. Curr Opin Gastroenterol. 2005;21:216-22.
2. Heyland DK, Shaun M, Keefe L, et al. Total parenteral nutrition in the critically ill patient: a meta-analysis. JAMA. 1998;28(3):2013-9.
3. Kieft H, Roos AN, van Drunen JD, et al. Clinical outcome of immunonutrition in a heterogeneous intensive care population. Intensive Care Med. 2005;31:524-32.
4. van Zanten AR, Sztark F, Kaisers UX, et al. High-protein enteral nutrition enriched with immune-modulating nutrients vs standard high protein enteral nutrition and nosocomial infections in the ICU: a randomized clinical trial. JAMA. 2014;312(5):514-24.
5. Fürst P, Albers S, Stehle P, et al. Parenteral use of L-alanyl IL-glutamine (Ala-Gln) and Glycyl L-tyrosine (Gly-Tyr) in postoperative patients. Clin. Nutr. 1988;7:S41.
6. Gouw AM, Toal GG, Felsher DW. Metabolic vulnerabilities of MYC-induced cancer. Oncotarget. 2016;7(21):29879-80.
7. Corbet C, Feron O. Metabolic and mind shifts: from glucose to glutamine and acetate addictions in cancer. Curr Opin Clin Nutr Metab Care. 2015;18(4):346-53.
8. Sacks GS. Glutamine supplementation in catabolic patients. Ann Pharmacother. 1999; 33(3):348-54.
9. Garlick PJ. Assessment of the safety of glutamine and other amino acids. J Nutr. 2001;131(9):2556S-2561S.
10. Andrews FJ, Griffiths RD. Glutamine: essential for immune nutrition in the critically ill. BJN. 2002;87(Suppl 1):S3-8.
11. Parry-Billings M, Evans J, Calde P, et al. Does glutamine contribute to immunosuppression after major burns? Lancet. 1990;336:523-5.
12. Hammarqvist F, Wenerman J, Ali R, et al. Addition of glutamine to total parenteral nutrition after elective abdominal surgery spares free glutamine synthesis in muscle, counteracts the fall in muscle protein synthesis and improve nitrogen balance. Ann Surg. 1989;205:455-61.
13. Morlion BJ, Stehle P, Wachtler P, et al. Total parenteral nutrition with glutamine dipeptide after major abdominal surgery: a randomized double blind, controlled study. Ann. Surg. 1988;227:302-8.
14. Fuentes-Orozco C, Ananya-Prado R, Gonzalez-Ojeda A, et al. L-alanyl-L-glutamine-supplemented parenteral nutrition improves infectious morbidity in secondary peritonitis. Clin Nutr. 2004;23(1):13-21.
15. Houdijik AP, Rijnsburger ER, Jansen J, et al. Randomised trial of glutamine enriched enteral nutrition on infectious morbidity in patients with multiple trauma. Lancet. 1998;352(9130):772-6.
16. Déchelotte P, Hasselman M, Cynober L, et al. L-alanyl L-glutamine dipeptide supplemented total parenteral nutrition reduces infectious complications and glucose intolerance in critically ill patients: the French controlled, randomized, double-blind, multicentre study. Crit Care Med. 2006;34(3):598-604.
17. Singleton KD, Beckey VE, Wischmeyer PE. Glutamine prevents activation of NF-KappaB and stress kinase pathways, attenuates inflammatory cytokine release, and prevents acute respiratory distress syndrome (ARDS) following sepsis. Shock. 2005;24(6):583-9.
18. Singleton KD, Serkova N, Beckey VE, et al. Glutamine attenuates lung injury and improves survival after sepsis. Role of enhanced heat shock protein expression. Crit Care Med. 2005;33:1206-13.
19. Oudemans-van Straaten HM, Bosman RJ, Treskes M, et al. Plasma glutamine depletion and patient outcome in acute ICU admissions. Intensive Care Med. 2001;27:84-90.
20. Novak F, Heyland DK, Avenell A, et al. Glutamine supplementation in serious illness: a systematic review of the evidence. Crit Care Med. 2002;30:2022-9.
21. Heyland DK, Dhaliwal R, Drover JW, et al. Canadian clinical practice guidelines for nutrition support in mechanically

ventilated, critically ill adult patients. J Parenter Enteral Nutr. 2003;27:355-73.
22. Heyland DK, Elke G, Cook D, et al. Glutamine and antioxidants in the critically ill patient: a post hoc analysis of a large-scale randomized trial. J Parenter Enteral Nutr. 2015;39:401-9.
23. Heyland DK, Dhaliwal R, Day AG, et al. Canadian Critical Care Trials Group. REducing Deaths due to OXidative Stress (The REDOXS Study): Rationale and study design for a randomized trial of glutamine and antioxidant supplementation in critically-ill patients. Proc Nutr Soc. 2006;65(3):250-63.
24. Andrews PJ, Avenell A, Noble DW, et al. Randomised trial of glutamine and selenium supplemented parenteral nutrition for critically ill patients. Protocol Version 9, 19 February 2007 known as SIGNET (Scottish Intensive care Glutamine or seleNium Evaluative Trial). Trials. 2007;8(9):25.
25. Clemmesen JO, Kondrup J, Ott P. Splanchnic and leg exchange of amino acids and ammonia in acute liver failure. Gastroenterology. 2000;118(6):1131-9.
26. McClave SA, Taylor BE, Martindale RG, et al. Guidelines for the Provision and Assessment of Nutrition Support Therapy in the Adult Critically Ill Patient: Society of Critical Care Medicine (SCCM) and American Society for Parenteral and Enteral Nutrition (A.S.P.E.N.). J Parenter Enteral Nutr. 2016;40(2):159-211.
27. Garrel D, Patenaude J, Nedelec B, et al. Decreased mortality and infectious morbidity in adult burn patients given enteral glutamine supplements: a prospective, controlled, randomized clinical trial. Crit Care Med. 2003;31(10):2444-9.
28. Bansal V, Ochoa JB. Arginine availability, arginase and the immune response. Curr Opin Clin Nutr Metab Care. 2003;6:223-8.
29. Heyland DK, Samis A. Does immunonutrition in patients with sepsis do more harm than good? Intensive Care Med. 2003;29(5):669-71.
30. Barbul A. Arginine and immune function. Nutrition. 1990;6:53-8.
31. Cerra FB, Lehman S, Konstantinides N, et al. Effect of enteral nutrient on in vitro tests of immune function in ICU patients: a preliminary report. Nutrition. 1990;6:84-7.
32. Kubes P. Ischemia-reperfusion in feline small intestine: a role for nitric oxide. Am J Physiol. 1993;264:G143-G149.
33. Lowenstein CJ, Dinerman JL, Snyder SH. Nitric oxide: a physiologic messenger. Ann Intern Med. 1994;120:227-37.
34. deFraaf JC, Banga JD, Moncada S, et al. Nitric oxide functions as an inhibitor of platelet adhesion under flow conditions. Circulation. 1992;85:2284-90.
35. Lorente JA, Landin L, DePablo R, et al. L-arginine pathway in the sepsis syndrome. Crit Care Med. 1993;21:1261-3.
36. Salem N. Introduction to polyunsaturated fatty acids. Backgrounder. 1999;3(1):1-8.
37. Mehra MR, Lavie CJ, Ventura HO, et al. Fish oils produce anti inflammatory effects and improve body weight in severe heart failure. J Heart Lung Transplant. 2006;25:834-8.
38. Calder PC. Rationale and use of n-3 fatty acids in artificial nutrition. Proc Nutr Soc. 2010;69:565-73.
39. Arakawa K, Himeno H, Otomo F, et al. N-3 polyunsaturated fatty acids as a predictor of ischemia/reperfusion injury immediately after myocardial reperfusion in patients with ST elevation acute myocardial infarction. Eur Heart J. 2013;34:1299.
40. Skuladottir GV, Heidarsdottir R, Arnar DO, et al. Plasma n-3 and n-6 fatty acids and the incidence of atrial fibrillation following coronary artery bypass graft surgery. Eur J Clin Invest. 2011;41:995-1003.
41. Rauch B, Schiele R, Schneider S, et al. OMEGA Study Group. OMEGA, a randomized, placebo-controlled trial to test the effect of highly purified omega-3 fatty acids on top of modern guideline-adjusted therapy after myocardial infarction. Circulation. 2010;122(21):2152-9.
42. Agostoni C, Bresson JL, Fairweather-Tait S, et al. Scientific opinion on dietary reference values for fats, including saturated fatty acids, polyunsaturated fatty acids, monounsaturated fatty acids, transfatty acids, and cholesterol. EFSA Journal. 2010;8(3):1461.
43. Carr AC, Frei B. Toward a new recommended dietary allowance for vitamin C based on antioxidant and health effects in humans. Am J Clin Nutr. 1999;69(6):1086-107.
44. Institute of Medicine (US) Panel on Dietary Antioxidants and Related Compounds. Dietary Reference Intakes for Vitamin C, Vitamin E, Selenium, and Carotenoids. Washington (DC): National Academies Press (US); 2000.
45. Halliwell B. Vitamin C: antioxidant or pro-oxidant in vivo? Free Radic Res. 1996;25(5):439-54.
46. Bendich A. Vitamin C safety in humans. In: Packer L, Fuchs J (Eds). Vitamin C in Health and Disease. New York: Marcel Dekker Inc.; 1997. pp. 367-9.
47. Long CL, Maull KL, Krishman RS, et al. Ascorbic acid dynamics in the seriously ill and injured. J Surg Res. 2003;109:144-8.
48. Marik PE, Khangoora V, Rivera R, et al. Hydrocortisone, Vitamin C, and Thiamine for the Treatment of Severe sepsis and Septic Shock: A Retrospective Before-After Study. Chest. 2017;151(6):1229-38.
49. Kim WY, Jo EJ, Eom JS, et al. Combined vitamin C, hydrocortisone, and thiamine therapy for patients with severe pneumonia who were admitted to the intensive care unit: Propensity score-based analysis of a before-after cohort study. J Crit Care. 2018;47(10):211-8.
50. Zhang M, Jativa DF. Vitamin C supplementation in the critically ill: A systematic review and meta-analysis. SAGE Open Med. 2018;6:2050312118807615.
51. Ohno S, Ohno Y, Suzuki N, et al. High-dose vitamin C (ascorbic acid) therapy in the treatment of patients with advanced cancer. Anticancer Res. 2009;29(3):809-15.
52. Lee P, Eisman JA, Center JR. Vitamin D deficiency in critically ill patients. N Engl J Med. 2009;360:1912-4.
53. Braun AB, Litonjua AA, Moromizato T, et al. Association of low serum 25 hydroxyvitamin D levels and acute kidney injury in the critically ill. Crit Care Med. 2012;40:3170-9.
54. Amrein K, Schnedl C, Holl A, et al. Effect of high dose Vitamin D3 on hospital length of stay in critically ill patients with vitamin D deficiency: the VITdAL-ICU randomized clinical trial. JAMA. 2014;312:1520-30.
55. National Center for Biotechnology Information. PubChem Compound Database; CID=1130. [online] Available from

https://pubchem.ncbi.nlm.nih.gov/compound/1130. [Accessed April, 2019].

56. Donnino MW, Andersen LW, Chase M, et al. Randomized, Double-blind, Placebo-Controlled Trial of Thiamine as a Metabolic Resuscitator in Septic Shock: A Pilot Study. Crit Care Med. 2016;44:360-7.
57. Singer P, Berger MM, den Berghe GV, et al. ESPEN guidelines on parenteral nutrition: intensive care. Clin Nutr. 2009;28:387-400.
58. Forceville Z, Aouizerate P, Guizard M. Septic shock and selenium administration. Therapie. 2001;56:653-61.
59. Angstwurm MW, Gaertner R. Practicalities of selenium supplementation in critically ill patients. Curr Opin Clin Nutr Metab Care. 2006;9:233-8.
60. Stoppe C, Schalte G, Rossaint R, et al. The intraoperative decrease of selenium is associated with the postoperative development of multiorgan dysfunction in cardiac surgical patients. Crit Care Med. 2011;39:1879-85.
61. Huang TS, Shyu YC, Chen HY, et al. Effect of parenteral selenium supplementation in critically ill patients: A systematic review and meta-analysis. PLoS ONE. 2013;8(1):e54431.
62. Forceville X, Laviolle B, Annane D, et al. Effects of high doses of selenium, as sodium selenite, in septic shock: a placebo-controlled, randomized, double-blind, phase II study. Crit Care. 2007;11:R73.
63. Besecker BY, Exline MC, Hollyfield J, et al. A comparison of zinc metabolism, inflammation and disease severity in critically ill infected and noninfected adults early after intensive care unit admission. Am J Clin Nutr. 2011;93:1356-64.
64. Berger MM, Spertini F, Shenkin A, et al. Trace element supplementation modulates pulmonary infection rates after major burns: a double blind, placebo controlled trial. Am J Clin Nutr. 1998;68:365-71.
65. Young B, Ott L, Kasarskis E, et al. Zinc supplementation is associated with improved neurologic recovery rate and visceral protein levels of patients with severe closed head injury. J Neurotrauma. 1996;13:25-34.
66. World Health Organization and United Nations Children Fund. Clinical management of acute diarrhoea. WHO/UNICEF Joint Statement, August, 2004.
67. Age-Related Eye Disease Study Research Group. A randomized, placebo-controlled, clinical trial of high-dose supplementation with vitamins C and E, beta carotene, and zinc for age-related macular degeneration and vision loss: AREDS report no. 8. Arch Ophthalmol. 2001;119:1417-36.

# CHAPTER 39

# Transfusion of Blood Products in Critically Ill Adult Patients

Armin Ahmed

## INTRODUCTION

Like many other therapies in critically ill, our recent understanding of blood product transfusion has shown the role of less is more. Packed red blood cells (PRBCs) transfusion trigger has decreased from 9 g/dL to 7 g/dL and indiscriminate use of fresh frozen plasma (FFP) for correction of coagulopathy in nonbleeding patients is no more indicated. However, one size does not fit all and there are certain subgroups of patients who have their specific requirements. This chapter deals with current concepts in blood product transfusion in critically ill.

## PACKED RED BLOOD CELLS

Critically ill patients suffer anemia due to hemorrhage, hemodilution, frequent blood sampling, and reduced red cell production due to inflammation.[1] Rationale behind PRBC transfusion is thought to be correction of anemic hypoxia by increasing oxygen transport. The exact level of hemoglobin beyond which anemia shows deleterious effects remains unknown and largely varies from patient to patient depending upon the rapidity of onset of anemia, compensatory mechanisms at work, patient's cardiorespiratory reserves, and his/her own unique disease pathophysiology. A detailed description of oxygen delivery and consumption is beyond the scope of this chapter. Key indications and trials related to PRBC transfusion are discussed below.

### Preparation and Storage

Blood components can be separated by *centrifugation* as they differ in their specific gravities with PRBCs having the highest specific gravity followed by leucocytes, platelet, and plasma respectively.[2] After collecting 350 or 450 mL of whole blood in a CPDA-1 (citrate phosphate dextrose, adenine solution) bag, the components are separated within 5–8 hours via centrifugation. PRBC is stored in ADSOL (adenine, dextrose, sorbitol, sodium chloride and mannitol) or SAGM (saline-adenine-glucose-mannitol) solution for up to 42 days at 4 ± 2°C. During preparation of blood components, most leucocytes are contained in buffy coat. Discarding buffy coat gives a leucoreduced product. Such products have greatly reduced febrile nonhemolytic transfusion reaction. Leukocyte removal is best achieved by filtration, which gives a leucodepleted blood product. Leucodepleted PRBC is used in patients with ongoing requirement of transfusion, in order to prevent alloimmunization to leukocyte antigens. One unit of PRBC is expected to increase Hb by 1–1.3 g%.

### Indication

Packed red blood cell transfusion is indicated for management of following conditions:
- Acute hemorrhage in hemodynamically unstable patient
- Treatment of anemia (depending upon the clinical scenario).

### Transfusion Trigger

Over past two decades the role of restrictive transfusion practice has been emphasized. Currently the recommended threshold for PRBC transfusion is 7–8 g/dl but it is unclear whether same threshold is appropriate for patients with cardiac disease (Flowchart 1). Landmark studies in the field are discussed below:
- *TRICC trial (Lower versus Higher Hemoglobin Threshold for Transfusion in Septic Shock)*
  Hebert et al. in their landmark multicenter randomized controlled trial (RCT) showed a restrictive transfusion

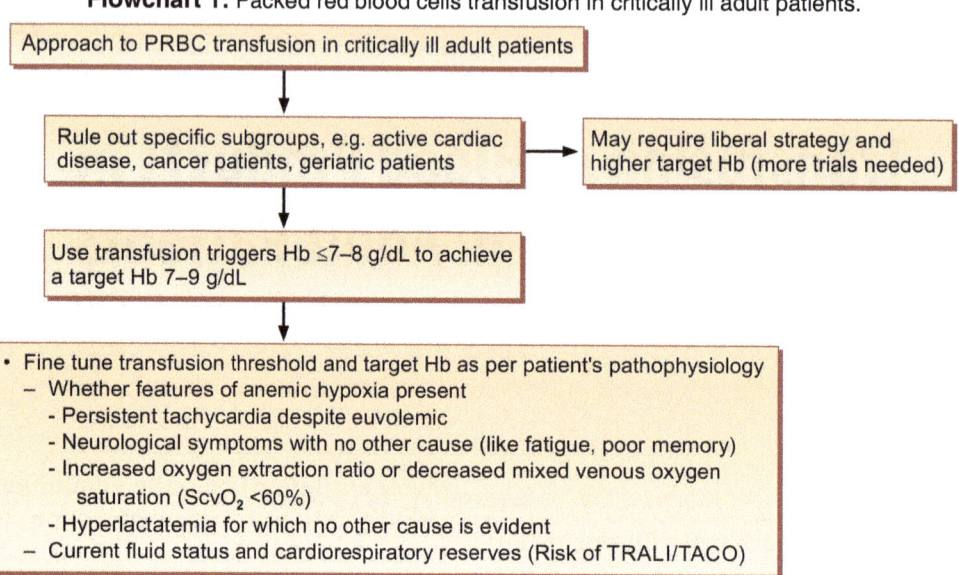

Flowchart 1: Packed red blood cells transfusion in critically ill adult patients.

(PRBC: packed red blood cells; TRALI: Transfusion-related acute lung injury; TACO: Transfusion-related circulatory overload)

strategy where trigger for PRBC transfusion was taken as hemoglobin 7 g/dL (target Hb 7–9 g/dL) was at least as effective or possibly superior to liberal transfusion strategy where transfusion threshold was taken as hemoglobin 9 g/dL (target Hb 10–12 g/dL) in critically ill patients with the exception of patients with active cardiac disease.[3]

- *CRIT trial (Anemia and blood transfusion in the critically ill current clinical practice in the United States)* Corwin et al. conducted a prospective multicenter observational study including 4,892 patients across 284 intensive care units (ICUs) of United States.[4] Authors reported number of RBC transfusion was an independent predictor of increased mortality, longer ICU stay, and increased length of hospital stay.
- *TRISS trial (Lower versus Higher Hemoglobin Threshold for Transfusion in Septic Shock)* Holst et al. randomized septic shock patients to low hemoglobin threshold group (trigger for transfusion Hemoglobin 7 g/dL) and high hemoglobin threshold group (trigger for transfusion Hemoglobin 9 g/dL).[5] Patients in the lower threshold group received a median of 1 unit leukopoor PRBC while those in the higher threshold group received a median of 4 unit leukopoor PRBC. Ninety-day mortality, rate of ischemic events and use of life support were similar in the two groups.

### Transfusion Triggers in Specific Population

Currently, most trauma and critical care guidelines recommend a target Hb of 7–9 g/dL.[6-8] Certain subgroups requiring special mention are:

- *Traumatic brain injury (TBI)*: Cerebral tissue oxygenation remains well maintained even in anemic patients via activation of compensatory mechanisms, i.e. increased cardiac output, increased cerebral blood flow, increased cerebral oxygen extraction, vasodilation, decreased viscosity, and improved microcirculation. These compensatory mechanisms begin to fail beyond a critical threshold (generally 5–6 g/dl of Hb) when maximum vasodilation and oxygen extraction has been achieved and cannot increase any further. In traumatic brain injury patients these compensatory mechanisms are blunted as cerebral autoregulation gets impaired. As a result, theoretically TBI patients are at risk of anemia-induced brain dysfunction. However, observational studies have shown conflicting results and high-quality evidence is lacking in this field. Most guidelines recommend a hemoglobin target of 7–9 g/dL for TBI patients, with fine tuning to higher targets (up to 9 g/dL) in patients with features of cerebral ischemia.[8] Results of a few ongoing RCTs (HEMOTIO; HEMOglobin Transfusion Threshold in Traumatic Brain Injury OptimizatioN, TRAIN; TRansfusion Strategies in Acute Brain INjured Patients) are likely to increase our knowledge regarding optimal threshold for PRBC transfusion in TBI patients.[9,10]
- *Cardiovascular disease*: Anemia has been found to be associated with worse outcome in cardiac patients in observational studies, but high-quality evidence to support higher hemoglobin targets in this subgroup is lacking in literature.[11] Most guidelines recommend transfusion threshold of 8 g/dL and target

Hb of 8.0–10.0 g/dL in acute coronary syndrome (ACS) patients.[6,7] Results of MINT (myocardial ischemia and transfusion) trial is awaited to shed more light in this area. A meta-analysis including 11 trials comparing liberal vs. restrictive transfusion strategies in cardiac disease patients in noncardiac surgery settings showed increased risk of new ACS when restrictive transfusion thresholds were used, however, 30 days mortality was not different between the two groups.[12]

- *Geriatric patients*: Murphy et al. conducted a meta-analysis of studies looking at PRBC transfusion in geriatric patients.[13] They found increased risk of 30 days and 90 days mortality with restrictive strategy as compared to liberal transfusion strategy. The paper has been criticized for biases and including trials with younger patients in the cohort. More research is needed in this field before clear recommendations can be made.
- *Adult respiratory distress syndrome patients*: It is recommended not to use PRBC transfusion as a method to facilitate weaning from mechanical ventilation. PRBC transfusion should be avoided in patients with acute respiratory distress syndrome (ARDS) once resuscitation is complete.[7]

## Age of PRBC

Recently, age of stored RBC has been a matter of concern in critically ill patients as erythrocytes acquire "storage lesions" with passage of time even with currently used improved preservation methods. During storage of RBC, there is gradual depletion of 2,3-diphosphoglycerate (2,3-DPG) and adenosine triphosphate (ATP). RBCs become less deformable and show increased osmotic fragility. Bioreactive substances accumulate in the storage medium and may play role in activation of inflammatory pathway after transfusion.

Literature has shown conflicting results in this field. Most of the studies showing harmful effects of stored RBC are observational, retrospective and subject to bias while large RCTs have not shown such findings. Results of large RCTs are described below. Interpretation of these studies should be done with caution as many patients received leukopoor PRBC which is not a routine practice in many developing countries.

- *ABLE trail (Age of Transfused Blood in Critically Ill Adults)*: Lacroix et al. conducted a multicenter study including 64 centers across Canada and Europe.[14] Critically ill patients were randomized to receive either fresh PRBC [mean storage (±SD) of 6.1 ± 4.9 days] or standard PRBC (mean storage 22.0 ± 8.4 days). The study showed no difference in mortality or other secondary outcomes in the two groups.
- *RECESS trial (Effects of Red-Cell Storage Duration on Patients Undergoing Cardiac Surgery)*: Steiner et al. evaluated the effect of PRBC storage in patients undergoing complex cardiac surgery.[15] The median PRBC storage time was 7 days in short-term storage group and 28 days in long-term storage group. There was no difference in mortality and multiple organ dysfunction syndrome between the two groups.
- *TRANSFUSE trial (Age of Red Cells for Transfusion and Outcomes in Critically Ill Adults)*: Cooper et al. randomized 4,994 *critically ill adult* from 59 centers in Australia and New Zealand to short PRBC storage group and long PRBC storage group.[16] There was no difference in mortality in the two groups and secondary outcome.
- *INFORM trial (Effect of Short-Term vs. Long-Term Blood Storage on Mortality after Transfusion)*: Heddle et al. studied the effect of RBC storage in *general hospital population* by randomizing 31,497 patients to receive either short-storage PRBC or long-storage PRBC.[17] There was no significant difference in mortality between the two groups.

## Alternatives to PRBC Transfusion

Intravenous ferric carboxymaltose with or without erythropoietin has been used to decrease the need for PRBC transfusion in critically ill patients. Literature in this field is confounded by heterogeneity in study design. Meta-analysis of five RCTs including 665 critically ill patients did not show reduction in RBC transfusion requirement with iron supplementation.[18] Litton et al. conducted a well-designed multicenter RCT (*the Intravenous Iron or Placebo for Anemia in Intensive Care: IRONMAN*) involving four Australian ICUs to study intravenous iron replacement and need for PRBC transfusion in 140 critically ill anemic patients.[19] They did not find any significant decrease in median number of PRBC units transfused in intervention group (IV ferric carboxymaltose supplementation group) as compared to placebo group but hemoglobin at discharge from hospital was significantly higher in the intervention group. The study has been criticized for its poor generalizability due to large number of surgical patients and means unit PRBC transfusion being just 1.9.

## FRESH FROZEN PLASMA

Fresh frozen plasma transfusion is classically used for three indications; stop bleeding in patients with coagulopathy, plasmapheresis, and prevent bleeding in patients with coagulopathy who are undergoing invasive procedure. Out of the above three indications prophylactic FFP transfusion is least supported by evidence and remains one the most important causes of irrational use of FFP transfusion. Stanworth et al. studied the FFP transfusion practice in UK. A total 4,969 FFP transfusion in 190 hospitals were evaluated.[20] The study showed high use of FFP transfusion (43%) for prophylaxis purpose before intervention or surgery in patients with deranged coagulation profile and many of these patients had international normalized ratio (INR) equal to or less than 1.5. There was marginal change in the coagulation parameters after FFP transfusion. The study raised many questions regarding rationale use of FFP transfusion.

## Preparation and Storage

- *Preparation*: Plasma is the noncellular component of the blood. It contains all coagulation factors but no red cells, white cells or platelets. Plasma is prepared by centrifugation of whole blood or apheresis. The term *fresh frozen plasma* is used when plasma is frozen within 8 hours of collection and stored at –25°C or lower temperature to maintain the activity of labile coagulation factors. FFP can be stored for up to 1 and a half years at this temperature.[2]
- *Quality monitoring*: Factor VIII, being the most labile coagulation factor is used for quality monitoring of FFP. At least 75% of the units should have 0.7 IU/mL of factor VIII immediately after thawing.
- *Thawing*: Fresh frozen plasma is thawed via methods like dry heat, microwave ovens, and water bath. Each of these methods has their own advantages and disadvantage. Ideally FFP should be provided in double pack container so that the inner plasma pack does not come into direct contact with the thawing devices. Hospitals should have their thawing protocol and cleaning and maintenance records of the thawing devices.

While using water bath for thawing it is important to have a vacuum seal overwrap to prevent bacterial contamination, as there can be invisible pin holes or cracks in the plastic pack. FFP is kept in water bath at 33–37°C for 20–30 minutes. If it is not used immediately thawed FFP can be stored at room temperature for 4 hours and in refrigerator provided the temperature is maintained at 2–6°C and infusion is complete within 24 hours of thawing. Thawed FFP when stored for more than 24 hours has reduced concentration of labile factors (factor V and VIII), due to degradation of these factors if plasma is stored in liquid state. FFP should be transfused within 4 hours of removal from controlled temperature.

Prethawed FFP can be stored for up to 120 hours at 2–6°C. Once out of controlled temperature environment, prethawed FFP can be accepted back in temperature controlled storage if done only once for less than 30 minutes.

- *ABO compatibility*: Different blood groups have their antigens on the red cells while plasma contains the respective antibodies. Therefore plasma derived from blood group A will have anti-B antibodies and vice versa. Plasma from blood group O will have both anti-A and anti-B antibodies while plasma from AB blood group will have no antibodies. This makes AB plasma as universal donor which is vice versa of PRBC. The Rh status does not matter for plasma as anti-D antibodies are destroyed during manufacturing stage.

## Indications

There is wide variation in indication for FFP transfusion among critically ill patients. As already discussed indications for FFP transfusion can be classified into three major groups:

1. Therapeutic transfusion in bleeding patients
2. Plasmapheresis
3. Prophylactic transfusion in nonbleeding patients with coagulopathy.

Massive transfusion and warfarin-related intracranial bleed are two indications supported by evidence. Most of the other indications for FFP transfusion require more robust data to establish clear benefit. But epidemiological studies show that a large number of FFP transfusions are done prophylactically. Clinicians should be aware of the potential adverse effects of FFP transfusion.

In nonbleeding patients FFP is used prophylactically when an invasive procedure or surgery is planned or to prevent spontaneous bleeding in patient with deranged coagulation parameters. There is limited evidence to support the practice of FFP transfusion in nonbleeding patients.[21,22]

Muller et al. studied prophylactic FFP transfusion in nonbleeding critically ill patients with coagulopathy (INR 1.5–3.0) undergoing invasive procedures (central venous line placement, tracheostomy, thoracocentesis, and abscess drainage).[23] Eighty one coagulopathic patients were randomized to receive or not receive single dose of 12 mL/kg FFP. There was no difference in bleeding complications among the two groups regardless of FFP use.

It is recommended to take personal history and family history of bleeding tendency, drug history, and assessment of bleeding risk involved with planned procedure as key practice point as abnormal coagulation parameters [PT (prothrombin time) and APTT (activated partial thromboplastin time)] are poor predictors of bleeding risks.

### Liver Disease and FFP

Both chronic and acute liver disease is associated with deranged coagulation parameters (PT and APTT) but these findings should be interpreted with caution as there is concomitant reduction of pro- and anticoagulants leading to rebalanced hemostasis. Prophylactic FFP transfusion should not be used in low bleeding risk procedures like paracentesis.

According to AASLD (American Association for the Study of Liver Diseases), correction of INR by FFP transfusion is not recommended in patients with portal hypertensive bleed as it does not represent the coagulation status correctly in cirrhosis patients and over enthusiastic transfusion can lead to increased portal pressure and rebleed.[24]

### Dose

The optimal dose of FFP in nonbleeding patients with coagulopathy remains controversial as most studies do not show clinical benefit of prophylactic transfusion. If transfusion is planned before a surgical/invasive procedure in high-risk patients (family history/personal history of bleeding tendency, concomitant thrombocytopenia etc.) a starting dose of 15 mL/kg can be considered.

In patients with massive transfusion hemostatic resuscitation is recommended to prevent dilutional coagulopathy.

- *Initial resuscitation*: For initial resuscitation (i.e. from arrival in emergency to availability of coagulation parameters) fixed ratio shock packs are used, where PRBC and FFP are transfused in fixed ratio (1:1 or 2:1) as per local massive transfusion protocol. This is plasma-based resuscitation strategy.[8]
- *Goal directed*: Further resuscitation is goal directed (i.e. as per the coagulation parameters in standard laboratory testing or point of care thromboelastographic or thromboelastometry studies).

## CRYOPRECIPITATE

### Preparation

Cryoprecipitate is prepared from FFP by slow thawing at 4°C. This causes precipitation of cryoproteins, i.e. factor VIII, von Willebrand factor, factor XIII, fibrinogen, and fibronectin.[2] The cryoproteins are separated through centrifugation and then suspended in small amount of plasma (around 50 mL). The quality is monitored by measuring fibrinogen and factor VIII level which should be 140 mg and 70 IU respectively in at least 75% packs. Cryoprecipitate is stored at less than or equal to – 25°C for a maximum period of one and a half years.

### Dose

- Prophylactic use of cryoprecipitate remains controversial. If transfusion is planned before a surgical/invasive procedure in high-risk patients (positive family history/personal history of bleeding tendency, concomitant thrombocytopenia etc.) a dose of 2–5 packs of cryoprecipitate can be considered if fibrinogen is less than 1.0 g/L.
- Low fibrinogen level is a frequent and early finding in trauma patients with major bleed. European guidelines suggest 3–4 g fibrinogen supplementation (= 15–20 single donor units of cryoprecipitate OR 3–4 g fibrinogen concentrate) during initial resuscitation (fibrinogen-based strategy) along with PRBC.[8] Further replacement is done goal directed as per the results of viscoelastic monitoring and standard laboratory coagulation studies.

### Pathogen Inactivation of Plasma and Cryoprecipitate

Pathogen inactivation systems licensed in Europe are methylene blue, amotosalen, and riboflavin. All systems work well against enveloped viruses but activity against nonenveloped viruses (Parvovirus B19 and Hepatitis A and E viruses) is variable. All pathogen inactivation systems reduce the level of coagulation factors and their inhibitors especially factor VIII, fibrinogen, and factor XI.

Solvent detergent treated plasma (SDFFP) includes a prion reduction step.

## PROTHROMBIN COMPLEX CONCENTRATE

Prothrombin complex concentrate (PCC) is prepared from cryoprecipitate supernatant via ion exchange chromatography. It is mainly used for replacement of Vitamin K-dependent clotting factors. Different techniques are used to produce three factor (II, IX, X) and four factor (II, VII, IX, X) concentrates. PCC also contains balanced concentration of vitamin K-dependent anticoagulants, i.e. protein C and protein S. Clotting factor concentration in

PCC is 25 times higher than normal plasma. It is available in lyophilized form and can be reconstituted in small volume. PCC has been shown to be superior to FFP in reversal of warfarin toxicity in various studies. As compared to FFP it does not require large volume for infusion and has reduced risk of TACO (TRANSFUSION-related Circulatory Overload) and TRALI (Transfusion-related Acute Lung Injury).[25]

Prothrombin complex concentrate has also been used in combination with tranexamic acid, for management of life-threatening bleed in patients on direct oral anticoagulants—factor Xa inhibitors (rivaroxaban, apixaban, edoxaban) and thrombin inhibitor (dabigatran). European guidelines suggest monitoring of drug levels in order to ascertain the extent of coagulation parameter derangement attributed to the drug before giving PCC. Idarucizumab is the antidote and drug of choice for reversal of dabigatran.

Prothrombin complex concentrate administration is associated with increased risk of thromboembolism. Therefore, thromboprophylaxis should be started earliest possible once hemostasis has been achieved.

## PLATELET TRANSFUSION

### Preparation and Storage

Platelets are prepared either by buffy coat method (BC) or platelet rich plasma (PRP) method. Out of these two, the former is superior and requires automation while later can be done manually and is relatively cheap.[2] Such methods produce random donor platelets. Platelets are also prepared by apheresis, which is a procedure of collection of single or more blood component via centrifugation or filtration and returning rest of the components back to the donor. Similar to PRBCs, platelets can also be leucoreduced or leucodepleted to decrease febrile nonhemolytic reaction or prevent alloimmunization to leucocyte antigens respectively. Platelets are stored at 20–24°C with continuous gentle agitation for 1–5 days depending upon the collection system.

Indications and contraindications are given below.[26]

### Indications

- *Prophylactic transfusion*:
  - Prophylactic transfusion is done to maintain a platelet count at or above $10 \times 10^9$/L in nonbleeding patients with reversible bone marrow failure. If additional risk factors for bleeding are present threshold should be increased to between 10 and $20 \times 10^9$/L. Same strategy is followed for nonbleeding critically ill patients also.
  - Recommended dose of prophylactic platelet transfusion is 1 unit single donor platelet.
  - In asymptomatic patients with chronic bone marrow failure prophylactic platelet transfusion is not indicated unless they are undergoing intensive therapy.
  - Prophylactic transfusion before interventions; routine prophylactic transfusion is not indicated before bone marrow biopsy, insertion of PICC (peripherally inserted central catheters) line, cataract surgery or removal of tunneled central line. Recommended platelet count thresholds are described in Table 1.
  - Platelet transfusion should be avoided in renal failure as the transfused platelets will also acquire platelet dysfunction. Other factors like anemia and uremia should be corrected and if needed preprocedural desmopressin or estrogen can be used.
- *Therapeutic transfusion*: Recommended therapeutic targets are described in Table 2.

### Contraindications

- Prophylactic platelets should not be transfused in patients with autoimmune thrombocytopenia. If platelet transfusion is needed for life-threatening bleeding, simultaneous intravenous immunoglobulin should be given.
- In heparin-induced thrombocytopenia (HIT) and thrombotic thrombocytopenic purpura (TTP) platelet transfusion should be used only in life-threatening bleeding.

**Table 1:** Recommended platelet levels for different invasive procedures.

| | |
|---|---|
| Central line placement under USG guidance | $>20 \times 10^9$/L |
| Lumbar puncture | $>40 \times 10^9$/L |
| Epidural catheter placement or removal | $>80 \times 10^9$/L |
| Major surgery | $>50 \times 10^9$/L |
| Neurosurgery or ophthalmic surgery (posterior segment) | $>100 \times 10^9$/L |
| Percutaneous liver biopsy | $>50 \times 10^9$/L |
| (USG: ultrasound) | |

**Table 2:** Recommended platelet levels to be maintained in different clinical conditions.

| | |
|---|---|
| Severe bleeding | $>50 \times 10^9$/L |
| Polytrauma, trauma brain injury and spontaneous intracerebral hemorrhage | $>100 \times 10^9$/L |
| Non-life-threatening bleed | $>30 \times 10^9$/L |

## MASSIVE TRANSFUSION

Uncontrolled blood loss is an important cause of death in young adults. Postpartum hemorrhage is the most common cause of maternal death across the globe while exsanguination is responsible for 35–40% trauma-related deaths. Most of these patients are young and potentially salvageable. Management of patients with massive hemorrhage requires team approach, protocol-based management and collaboration between clinicians and transfusion services.[27,28]

Massive transfusion can be required in trauma as well as nontrauma patients (gastrointestinal bleed, obstetric bleed, surgical bleed). In adults, it is defined as presence of any of the following:
- Transfusion of more than 10 PRBCs or total blood volume within 24 hours
- Transfusion of more than 4 PRBCs within 1 hour with anticipation of continued need
- Replacement of more than 50% of total blood volume within 3 hours.

Patients undergoing massive transfusion frequently develop multifactorial hemostatic defects which includes acute coagulopathy of trauma, hyperfibrinolysis, dilutional coagulopathy, thrombocytopenia, and disseminated intravascular coagulation.[29] Hypocalcemia, citrate toxicity, hypothermia, and metabolic acidosis due to hypoperfusion further damage normal hemostasis. Therefore, identifying the high-risk group and early activation of massive transfusion protocol is essential to improve outcome. Institutions should develop their own massive transfusion protocols which include using scoring system to trigger activation of protocol, transfusion of shock packs with 1:2 or 1:1 FFP-PRBC ratio, use of adjuncts to transfusion, e.g. tranexamic acid, avoiding and correcting hypothermia, metabolic acidosis, and other transfusion-related complications.

## BLOOD TRANSFUSION REACTION

### Transfusion-related Acute Lung Injury

It is defined as ARDS occurring within 6 hours of transfusion in the absence of other risk factors.[30] Delayed TRALI is defined as onset of respiratory distress from 6 hours to 72 hours after blood product transfusion. All blood products can cause TRALI, but products with higher amount of plasma are more frequently involved. FFP has 6.9 times higher risk of TRALI as compared to PRBC transfusion. Patients at risk include those on mechanical ventilation, critically ill, cardiac surgery patients, patients requiring massive transfusion and those in sepsis. The true incidence of TRALI remains unknown as it is indistinguishable from ARDS caused by other causes like sepsis or lung contusion.

The pathogenesis of TRALI has been explained by two hit theory. The initial hit is generally caused by sepsis or any other condition causing increased adherence of primed neutrophils to pulmonary capillary endothelium. The second hit results from chemical mediators in blood transfusion-induced activation of endothelial cells and primed neutrophils leading to capillary leakage. TRALI can be antibody mediated and nonantibody mediated. In antibody-mediated TRALI, antibodies against human leukocyte antigen (HLA) class I and class II as well as human neutrophil antigens (HNAs) in the donor play key role in activation of already primed neutrophils. Non–antibody-mediated TRALI is linked with accumulation of proinflammatory chemical mediators during storage of blood products.

Transfusion-related acute lung injury can occur even in healthy individuals with no previous predisposition, if the second hit (i.e. the quantity of antibodies in the transfused blood product) is very large.

Clinically TRALI presents as tachypnea, hypoxemia, and respiratory distress. Chest X-ray may show bilateral diffuse opacity. Laboratory testing may show transient leucopenia due to antineutrophil antibodies. TRALI should be differentiated from pulmonary edema due to fluid overload; sepsis-induced respiratory distress and anaphylactic reaction due to blood product transfusion. Treatment is mainly supportive and includes oxygen therapy, restrictive fluid strategy, and mechanical ventilation.

Transfusion-related acute lung injury can be prevented by following restrictive transfusion strategy which includes using a lower threshold of hemoglobin as a trigger for transfusion, delaying transfusion till the acute inflammation has settled in nonemergent situations, conducting regular audits to evaluate and bring down the use of blood products. TRALI should be reported to blood bank for identification of donors with antibodies and further restriction of donation by such individuals. High-risk donors include multiparous women and donors with history of blood transfusion.

### Transfusion-related Circulatory Overload

This condition presents as respiratory distress and pulmonary edema during or following transfusion of blood products. Clinically, it is difficult to differentiate from TRALI. Predisposing factors for development of TACO include extremes of age, cardiac, respiratory, and renal disease. Piccin et al. reported human error as an important cause of

TACO in their hemovigilance report of transfusion reactions occurring over 10 years period in Ireland.[31] Limited clinical supervision of junior doctors, knowledge deficit on the part of clinical staff, poor compliance of hospital transfusion policy, and failure to recognize impending fluid overload status of the patient are some of the contributors to TACO. Treatment includes oxygen therapy, diuretics, and continuous positive airway pressure. TACO patients with cardiovascular disease are associated with worse outcome.

### Hemolytic Transfusion Reactions

They occur due to incompatible blood transfusion.[32] ABO incompatibility causes immediate reactions while delayed reactions are due to minor blood group incompatibility like Rhesus and Kidd.

- *Immediate reactions*: Antigens on the surface of donor RBC reacts with antibodies in the recipient's plasma. Even small amount of ABO incompatible blood transfusion can precipitate severe life-threatening reactions. Severity of reaction depends upon the antibody titer in recipient's body. Clinical features include head, chest and flank pain, fever, rigors, hypotension, dyspnea, hemoglobinuria, acute kidney injury, and disseminated intravascular coagulation. Management is mainly supportive and directed toward maintaining oxygenation and adequate perfusion.
- *Delayed reactions*: Classically they present as unexplained hemoglobin drop, unconjugated hyperbilirubinemia and positive direct Comb's test. It is difficult to prevent delayed transfusion reaction as pretransfusion screening might be negative due to low antibody titers. Further exposure to the antigen at the time of transfusion can cause increased antibody production due to amnestic response. Hemolysis is extravascular and transfused cells are destroyed between 1 and 3 weeks duration after being coated with IgG.

### Febrile Nonhemolytic Reactions

They are caused by antileukocyte antibodies in the recipient or cytokines released from leukocytes in the stored blood component.[33] Though they are clinically not significant, they should be differentiated febrile hemolytic reactions and septic reactions. Using leucoreduced products minimize these reactions.

### Allergic (Urticarial Reactions)

They occur in 1–3% of all transfusions. Clinically present as urticaria, mild wheezing, flushing, and pruritus. They are caused due to antibodies to donor plasma proteins.

### Anaphylactoid or Anaphylactic Reactions

These are caused by antibodies to donor plasma proteins (haptoglobin, IgA, C4) and are relatively rare. Symptoms are much severe as compared to allergic reactions and characterized by bronchospasm, angioedema with or without hypotension.[33] These reactions are more common with FFP and platelets. Treatment included epinephrine, steroids, and antihistaminics.

### Graft versus Host Disease

It is rare but usually fatal complication of transfusion. Viable lymphocyte from donor engrafts and proliferates within the recipient. This can be prevented by using irradiated blood product.

## SALIENT POINTS

- Recent research in the field of transfusion medicine has emphasized the importance of judicious and restrictive use of blood products.
- Currently recommended transfusion trigger in critically ill general patient population is Hb less than or equal to 7 g/dL (target Hb 7–9 g/dL).
- Specific subgroups require special consideration, e.g. active cardiac disease, cancer patients, geriatric patients. These patients may require liberal strategy and higher target Hb (more trials needed).
- Age of PRBC has not been shown to be associated with increased mortality in randomized control trials. Most of these trails have used leukopoor PRBC.
- Prophylactic transfusion of FFP in nonbleeding patients with coagulopathy is not supported by evidence. Such transfusions should be individualized and done only if invasive procedure/surgery is planned.
- Initial resuscitation in hemorrhagic shock patients is done using fixed PRBC:FFP:Platelet ratios in order to avoid dilutional coagulopathy. Further resuscitation is guided by point of care viscoelastic tests (thromboelastography thromboelastometry) or traditional tests of coagulation.
- Institutes should develop their own massive transfusion protocols for management of hemorrhagic shock.

## REFERENCES

1. Hayden SJ, Albert TJ, Watkins TR, et al. Anemia in critical illness: insights into etiology, consequences, and management. Am J Respir Crit Care Med. 2012;185(10):1049-57.
2. Basu D, Kulkarni R. Overview of blood components and their preparation. Indian J Anaesth. 2014;58(5):529-37.

3. Hébert PC, Wells G, Blajchman MA, et al. A multicenter, randomized, controlled clinical trial of transfusion requirements in critical care. Transfusion Requirements in Critical Care Investigators, Canadian Critical Care Trials Group. N Engl J Med. 1999;340(6):409-17.
4. Corwin HL, Gettinger A, Pearl RG, et al. The CRIT Study: Anemia and blood transfusion in the critically ill-current clinical practice in the United States. Crit Care Med. 2004;32(1):39-52.
5. Holst LB, Haase N, Wetterslev J, et al. Transfusion requirements in septic shock (TRISS) trial – comparing the effects and safety of liberal versus restrictive red blood cell transfusion in septic shock patients in the ICU: Protocol for a randomised controlled trial. Trials. 2013;14:150.
6. Carson JL, Guyatt G, Heddle NM, et al. Clinical Practice Guidelines From the AABB: Red Blood Cell Transfusion Thresholds and Storage. JAMA. 2016;316(19):2025-35.
7. Napolitano LM, Kurek S, Luchette FA, et al. Clinical practice guideline: red blood cell transfusion in adult trauma and critical care. Crit Care Med. 2009;37(12):3124-57.
8. Rossaint R, Bouillon B, Cerny V, et al. The European guideline on management of major bleeding and coagulopathy following trauma: rourth edition. Crit Care. 2016;20:100.
9. East JM, Viau-Lapointe J, McCredie VA. Transfusion practices in traumatic brain injury. Curr Opin Anaesthesiol. 2018;31(2):219-26.
10. Lelubre C, Bouzat P, Crippa IA, et al. Anemia management after acute brain injury. Crit Care. 2016;20(1):152.
11. Docherty AB, Walsh TS. Anemia and blood transfusion in the critically ill patient with cardiovascular disease. Crit Care. 2017;21(1):61.
12. Docherty AB, O'Donnell R, Brunskill S, et al. Effect of restrictive versus liberal transfusion strategies on outcomes in patients with cardiovascular disease in a non-cardiac surgery setting: systematic review and meta-analysis. BMJ. 2016;352:i1351.
13. Simon GI, Craswell A, Thom O, et al. Outcomes of restrictive versus liberal transfusion strategies in older adults from nine randomised controlled trials: a systematic review and meta-analysis. Lancet Haematol. 2017;4(10):e465-74.
14. Lacroix J, Hébert PC, Fergusson DA, et al. Age of transfused blood in critically ill adults. N Engl J Med. 2015;372(15):1410-8.
15. Steiner ME, Ness PM, Assmann SF, et al. Effects of red-cell storage duration on patients undergoing cardiac surgery. N Engl J Med. 2015;372(15):1419-29.
16. Cooper DJ, McQuilten ZK, Nichol A, et al. Age of red cells for transfusion and outcomes in critically ill adults. N Engl J Med. 2017;377(19):1858-67.
17. Heddle NM, Cook RJ, Arnold DM, et al. Effect of short-term vs. long-term blood storage on mortality after transfusion. N Engl J Med. 2016;375(20):1937-45.
18. Shah A, Roy NB, McKechnie S, et al. Iron supplementation to treat anaemia in adult critical care patients: a systematic review and meta-analysis. Crit Care. 2016;20(1):306.
19. Litton E, Baker S, Erber WN, et al. Intravenous iron or placebo for anaemia in intensive care: the IRONMAN multicentre randomized blinded trial: A randomized trial of IV iron in critical illness. Intensive Care Med. 2016;42(11):1715-22.
20. Stanworth SJ, Grant-Casey J, Lowe D, et al. The use of fresh-frozen plasma in England: high levels of inappropriate use in adults and children. Transfusion. 2011;51(1):62-70.
21. Gajic O, Dzik WH, Toy P. Fresh frozen plasma and platelet transfusion for nonbleeding patients in the intensive care unit: benefit or harm? Crit Care Med. 2006;34(5 Suppl):S170-3.
22. Roback JD, Caldwell S, Carson J, et al. Evidence-based practice guidelines for plasma transfusion. Transfusion. 2010;50:1227-39.
23. Müller MC, Arbous MS, Spoelstra-de Man AM, et al. Transfusion of fresh-frozen plasma in critically ill patients with a coagulopathy before invasive procedures: a randomized clinical trial (CME). Transfusion. 2015;55(1):26-35.
24. Garcia-Tsao G, Abraldes JG, Berzigotti A, et al. Portal hypertensive bleeding in cirrhosis: Risk stratification, diagnosis, and management: 2016 practice guidance by the American Association for the study of liver diseases. Hepatology. 2017;65(1):310-35.
25. Franchini M, Lippi G. Prothrombin complex concentrates: an update. Blood Transfus. 2010;8(3):149-54.
26. Estcourt L, Birchall J, Allard S, et al. Guidelines for the use of platelet transfusions. Br J Haematol. 2017;176(3):365-94.
27. McDaniel LM, Etchill EW, Raval JS, et al. State of the art: massive transfusion. Transfus Med. 2014;24(3):138-44.
28. Pham HP, Shaz BH. Update on massive transfusion. Br J Anaesth. 2013;111 Suppl 1:i71-82.
29. Kushimoto S, Kudo D, Kawazoe Y. Acute traumatic coagulopathy and trauma-induced coagulopathy: an overview. J Intensive Care. 2017;5:6.
30. Vlaar AP, Juffermans NP. Transfusion-related acute lung injury: a clinical review. Lancet. 2013;382(9896):984-94.
31. Piccin A, Cronin M, Brady R, et al. Transfusion-associated circulatory overload in Ireland: a review of cases reported to the National Haemovigilance Office 2000 to 2010. Transfusion. 2015;55(6):1223-30.
32. Strobel E. Hemolytic transfusion reactions. Transfus Med Hemother. 2008;35(5):346-53.
33. Pandey S, Vyas GN. Adverse effects of plasma transfusion. Transfusion. 2012;52 (Suppl 1):65S-79S.

# CHAPTER 40

# Care for the Potential Organ Donor in the ICU

*Pranav Jetley, Kapil Dev Soni*

## INTRODUCTION

Improvements in surgical techniques, intensive care unit (ICU), anesthesia care, and immunosuppressive therapies, have helped organ transplantation become the mainstay management for many end-stage organ diseases. These advances have produced new demands for solid organs, which are severely undermet by a diminutive organ donor pool. An ideal organ donor rate is described as 50 donors per million (DPM) people. Most modern western societies have quoted a rate of 18–20 DPM, whereas it may stand as low as 0.34 DPM in developing countries.[1] To reduce disparity between supply and demand, it is imperative to maintain health in the donor, even after brain death. Advances in intensive care management of the deceased donor have improved the chances of a successful outcome for the recipient. This chapter describes the various aspects of intensive care for the potential organ donor in the ICU and highlights recent research.

## DONATION AFTER NEUROLOGICAL (BRAIN) DEATH

Ever since its inception, organ transplantation has been based on the premise of donor death. Before modern medicine had developed, death was simply defined as cessation of heart and lung function. Unfortunately, it was difficult to obtain viable organs from so defined "cadavers". In 1968, the Harvard Medical School revised the definition of death in a way that would help make more patients with catastrophic neurological injury eligible for organ transplantation under the dead donor rule.[2] Presently, the bulk of donated organs come from deceased donors after determination of brain death using the below stated neurological criteria (commonly referred to as "brain death"). Most of the countries with an active organ transplantation program have their own set of criteria for the diagnosis of brain death (Flowchart 1 and Table 1). In 1971, Finland was the first country to acknowledge brain death as a legal form of death. Many fundamental initial steps toward the definition and recognition of brain death were taken in Europe[3,4] but after the Harvard Medical School definition in 1968, and further debate centering

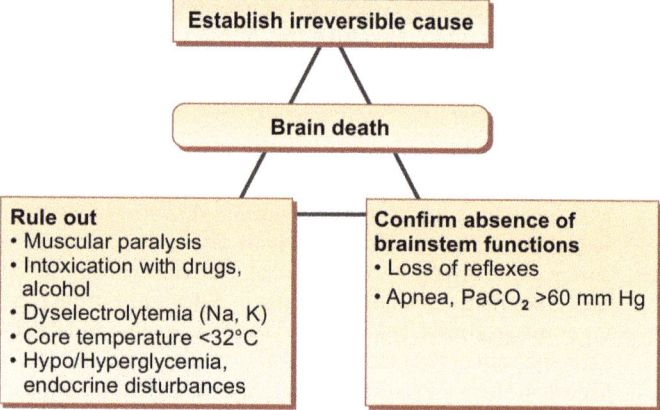

**Flowchart 1:** Requirements for the diagnosis of brain death.

**Table 1:** Guidelines for the diagnosis of brain death.

| Region | Society | Website link |
| --- | --- | --- |
| Australia and New Zealand | Australia and New Zealand Intensive Care Society, 2013 | www.anzics.com.au |
| United Kingdom | Academy of Medical Royal Colleges, 2008 | www.aomrc.org.uk |
| United States | American Academy of Neurology, 1995 | www.aan.com |
| WHO | World Health Organization, 2012 | www.who.int/patientsafety/montreal-forum-report.pdf |

in America, most countries have taken guidance from the criteria formalized by the American Academy of Neurology in a summary statement in 1995.[5] The following are the specific guidelines for approaching the diagnosis of neurological *death* included in the consensus statement given by the Society of Critical Care Medicine (SCCM), American College of Chest Physicians (ACCP), and Association of Organ Procurement Organizations (AOPO) regarding the management of the potential organ donor in the ICU, which was first laid down by the American Academy of Neurology.[6]

## Prerequisites: Immediate Cause Known and Irreversible

- Clinical or imaging evidence of acute CNS catastrophic injury expected to cause brain death
- Excluding confounding conditions (dyselectrolytemia, acid-base imbalance, endocrine dysfunction)
- Exclude intoxication or poisoning
- The core temperature should be more than 32°C (90°F).

## Coexistence of Absent Brainstem Reflexes, Coma, and Apnea

- *Coma or unresponsiveness*: No motor response to pain in all four extremities (demonstrable by nail bed pressure or supraorbital pressure)
- *Absent brainstem reflexes*:
  - *Pupils*:
    - Nonresponsive to light
    - Size: 4–9 mm
  - *Ocular movement*:
    - Absence of oculocephalic reflex (should be tested only when cervical spine fracture or dislocation has been safely excluded)
    - Absence of oculovestibular reflex (no deviation of eyes when 50 mL of cold water is irrigated in the vestibular canal)
  - *Facial sensation and motor response*:
    - Absent corneal reflex
    - Absent jaw reflex
    - Absent grimacing on application of deep pressure on nail bed, supraorbital ridge, or temporomandibular joint
  - *Pharyngeal and tracheal reflexes*:
    - Absent response on stimulating the posterior pharynx with a tongue blade
    - Absent cough reflex when stimulating with a tracheal suction catheter

- *Apnea—testing should be performed as follows*:
  - *Prerequisites*:
    - Exclude hypothermia—confirm a core temperature more than or equal to 36.5°C or 97°F
    - Acceptable systolic blood pressure more than 90 mm Hg
    - Ensure euvolemia
    - Ensure a normal $PCO_2$. It may be advisable to maintain an arterial $PCO_2$ greater than 40 mm Hg
    - Ensure a normal $PaO_2$. Preoxygenation with 100% oxygen to a $PaO_2$ more than 200 mm Hg
    - It is prudent to obtain baseline arterial blood gas (ABG) measurement.
  - After ensuring adequate monitoring, the pulse oximeter should be disconnected.
  - Oxygen should be delivered at a rate of 6–10 L/min. This can be done by placing a cannula at the level of the carina.
  - Respiratory movements like abdominal movements or chest excursions should be observed.
  - An ABG measurement should be done after 8 minutes.
  - *The apnea test is positive if*:
    - There is an increase in arterial $PaCO_2$ by more than 20 mm Hg from baseline or it increases to more than 60 mm Hg. If these values are not achieved a repeat test should be considered.
    - Respiratory movements are not observed. In case they are present, a repeat test should be performed.
  - In case the blood pressure falls to less than a 90 mm Hg systolic reading, or any tachy- or bradyarrhythmia develops, the test should be aborted and repeated after hemodynamic stability is achieved.

## Drawbacks in the Diagnosis of Brain Death

In case the following conditions complicate the patient condition, confirmatory tests area advised.
- Severe facial trauma
- Preexisting pupillary abnormalities
- *Drugs*: Aminoglycosides, tricyclic antidepressants, anticholinergics, antiepileptic drugs, chemotherapeutic agents, or neuromuscular blocking agents
- Chronic retainers of $CO_2$ like chronic airway disease patients or in case of obstructive sleep apnea

## Observations Congruent to Brain Death

Certain clinical signs may occasionally manifest, but should not confound the diagnosis:

- Spontaneous limb movements different from pathologic flexion or extension response
- Movements imitating respiration like shoulder adduction and elevation, arching of the back, nonpurposeful intercostal expansion
- Tachycardia, sweating or blushing
- Blood pressure not requiring vasopressors, and sudden swings in blood pressure
- Diabetes insipidus not present
- Presence of deep tendon reflexes or superficial reflexes, triple flexion response
- A positive Babinski reflex

### Confirmatory Laboratory Tests

The diagnosis of brain death is a clinical one, although in certain clinical settings, the use of adjunct tests may become mandatory. These tests are listed below in order of most sensitive first. It is worth noting that these tests may be positive in catastrophic brain injuries even when the clinical signs of brain death have not appeared.

- *CT angiography shows following signs*: There is absence of intracerebral filling at the level of the carotid bifurcation or at the level of circle of Willis. The external carotid artery and circulation remains patent, and filling of the superior longitudinal sinus may be delayed.
- Electroencephalography shows absence of electrical activity during at least 30 minutes of recording.
- Transcranial Doppler ultrasonography shows complete absence of flow. But, it is important to remember that up to 10% of the population may not have adequate intonation windows. A very high intracranial pressure (ICP) shows small systolic peaks with reverberating flow pattern.
- *Technetium-99m hexamethylpropyleneamine oxime brain scan*: There is absent uptake into the brain parenchyma (hollow skull phenomenon).
- *Somatosensory evoked potentials*: There is bilateral absence of the N20-P22 response while stimulating the median nerve.

### Documentation

It is important to document the following aspects of the patient's condition when diagnosing brain death:
- Etiology and irreversibility of the patient's condition
- Absent brainstem reflexes
- Absent motor response to pain
- A positive apnea test as indicated by the require $PCO_2$ rises
- Whether a confirmatory test was required and its result
- A repeat neurological examination within an arbitrary interval (most commonly 6 hours) and its result.

There have been no reported cases of return of brain function after the diagnosis of brain death by the above criteria.[7] Despite their sturdiness, widespread variation in their implementation exists. As per the American Association of Neurology guidelines, clinical diagnosis is sufficient. The use of ancillary tests is optional, limited to cases in which preconditions for brain-death testing are not met. In Europe, ancillary testing is mandatory in up to 11 countries and is also employed to shorten observation periods. A prerequisite for brain death diagnosis in Japan requires the identification of "irreversible" lesions on a CT-scan. Also, major variations occur worldwide regarding the number of physicians required, the experience and specialization of these doctors, and number of examinations and intervals between subsequent examinations.[8] The WHO guidelines for the Determination of Death analyzes and suitably summarizes the key points common to all brain death diagnostic systems and also lists the areas where variation exists. It is a step in the direction of global consensus regarding the definition of death in general and acts as a base on which future guidelines may be formulated.[9]

## DONATION AFTER CARDIAC DEATH

To address the unmet need for donor organs, an alternative donor pool has been utilized. These include donors who satisfy circulatory, rather than neurological criteria for death. When a patient or the patient's proxy wishes to discontinue life support but opts to donate organs, this option may be used, or sporadically when there is unanticipated circulatory death of a viable brain dead organ donor. After life support is discontinued or after resuscitative attempts have ceased, once circulation permanently stops, the patient is declared dead. After cessation of circulation, the patient is observed for 5 minutes but a minimum of 2 minutes prior to surgical recovery of organs. This time period is to confirm that patient circulation does not spontaneously restart. Such a donor has also been termed a nonheart-beating organ donor, donor after determination of cardiac death, and such a donation is also known as donation after circulatory determination of death (DCDD). Circulatory death can be said to occur in two settings: In an *uncontrolled* setting when there is unanticipated circulatory arrest; and in a *controlled* setting, when there is deliberate withdrawal of life support. With DCDD, transplants may have to accept longer warm ischemia times, greater rates of primary graft failure and often delayed graft function. Albeit, when delayed graft function occurs, DCDD kidneys have similar long term outcomes to DNDD kidneys in studies.[10,11] Though in one study, the 3 year and 6 year graft survival was better in DCDD kidneys as compared to DNDD kidneys, still more research in this respect is warranted.[12] Majority of DCDD liver transplants have been failure with poorer graft survival in DCDD livers.[13,14]

A significant number of brain dead donors may die from cardiac arrest in the ICU before transplantation. In such a setting, DCDD donations may provide viable organs for transplantation.

## EFFECTS OF BRAIN DEATH

The onset of brain death is followed by a period of instability in the health of the potential donor, which is proportional to the time period between brain death and organ procurement.[15] This period is associated with profound systemic effects (Table 2). Maintenance of physiology should be actively pursued during this period, leading to greater graft success rates and better outcomes for the recipient.

### Hemodynamic Effects

The hemodynamic effects of brain death are a consequence of an ischemic process in the brainstem. Raised ICP causing cerebral herniation through the tentorium cerebelli and the loss of brainstem activity usually follows. The mechanisms responsible for the cardiovascular effects are complex, arising from neurohumoral, hormonal, and proinflammatory pathways. Brain death comprises of two distinct phases—when the herniation is occurring and the ischemic process is ongoing, the brainstem compensates by trying to increase its perfusion. This is known as the progressive brainstem ischemia phase. This is followed by the brainstem death completion phase, which marks the conclusion of the ischemic process.

In the first phase, increased ICP causes compensatory rise in mean arterial pressure via a sympathetic surge. This sympathetic surge acts synergistically with a loss of vagal cardio-motor nucleus function in the medulla oblongata leading to an unopposed massive sympathetic stimulation and loss of baroreceptor control.[16,17] A several fold increase in baseline values of noradrenaline, dopamine, and adrenaline occurs resulting in an acute rise in systemic vascular resistance, central redistribution of blood volume, hypertension, tachycardia, arrhythmias, and acute myocardial dysfunction (a takatsubo-cardiomyopathy like state). Myocardial necrosis occurs due to cyclic adenosine monophosphate (cAMP)-dependant calcium influx, which is compounded by oxygen derived free radical species induced myocyte injury. This pattern of cardiac injury is similar to that seen in subarachnoid hemorrhage, pheochromocytoma, or severe emotional stress. The fall in cardiac output (CO) and a biventricular failure with left atrial enlargement and mitrial regurgitation often ensues.

During the second phase of brainstem death completion, coinciding with the terminal herniation of the brainstem, there is intense vasodilatation leading to a state of relative hypovolemia. This causes fall in preload reserves, myocardial dysfunction, and reduced afterload. In dogs, this phase has been shown to be accompanied by spinal cord ischemia and a shut down of the sympathetic system, motor tone loss, a decrease in serum catecholamine levels, and impaired cardiac stimulation.[18] A variety of other conditions aggravate the myocardial dysfunction. The pituitary ischemia and initial brain injury cause diabetes insipidus and stimulation of inflammatory pathways, producing leaky capillaries (due to cytokine upregulation—IL-6, TNF-α, IL-1β) resulting in a state of absolute hypovolemia. These phenomena compound myocardial dysfunction and culminate in total circulatory failure. Hyperosmolar fluid therapy such as hypertonic saline, loop diuretics, or mannitol administered to decrease ICP aggravates fluid loss. Concomitant abnormalities like acidosis, anemia, sepsis, and adrenal insufficiency additionally affect the hemodynamic status.[19]

### Respiratory Effects

Pulmonary edema is observed in these patients due to an increased pulmonary capillary hydrostatic pressure and often gets aggravated by endothelial damage due to raised

**Table 2:** Common derangements in brain dead patients.

| System | Effect | Pathophysiology |
| --- | --- | --- |
| Cardiovascular | Hypotension, arrhythmias | Vasodilatation, hypovolemia, cardiac injury and dysfunction, catecholamine surge during increased ICP |
| Temperature homeostasis | Hypothermia | Catecholamine surge leading to hypothalamic injury, vasodilatation, decreased metabolism |
| Coagulation | Disseminated intravascular coagulation | Tissue factor release (e.g. traumatic brain injury), coagulopathy due to trauma, concomitant sepsis |
| Endocrine | Diabetes insipidus | Posterior pituitary damage |
| Pulmonary | Pulmonary edema | Catecholamine surge leading to capillary endothelium damage |

norepinephrine and epinephrine levels. In addition, there are frequent respiratory complications associated with ICU stays like atelectasis, ventilator acquired pneumonias, pneumothorax, aspiration pneumonias which can develop in these patients. These are also cited as common reasons for the low rate of lung procurement for transplantation.[20]

### Endocrine, Metabolic, and Stress Response

Animal studies have shown that anterior and posterior pituitary ischemia frequently occur after brain death. However, posterior pituitary dysfunction is relatively commoner than anterior and manifests as central diabetes insipidus. The underlying mechanism is not fully understood. However, it is postulated that it is due to differential ischemia and shift from aerobic to anerobic metabolism.[21] Anterior pituitary circulation is variably preserved and anterior pituitary failure is relatively uncommon.[22]

Thyroid dysfunction is also observed frequently and is similar in pathology to the "sick euthyroid syndrome" seen in non-brain dead ICU patients. Low levels of thyroid hormones may further damage mitocondrial function, the ability to utilize a metabolic substrate, and ATP generation.[23,24] Insulin resistance, decreased serum insulin levels, and hyperglycemia are also frequently seen after brain death.[25,26]

Hypothalamic failure also causes loss of temperature homeostasis and may result in hyper- or hypothermia depending upon phase of brain death. Hyperthermia occurs initially followed by hypothermia due to a decreased metabolic rate, peripheral vasodilation, and decreased muscular activity.

An injured brain releases excess inflammatory mediators that get aggravated by associated trauma or critical illness.[27] A global ischemia–reperfusion injury may occur in vital organs causing metabolic derangements. Coagulopathy is also commonly seen after brain injury. Brain tissue injury and necrosis release tissue thromboplastin and may lead to a disseminated intravascular coagulation like state.[28]

## MANAGEMENT OF POTENTIAL ORGAN DONOR AFTER BRAIN DEATH

The pathophysiology of brain death is so severe that up to a quarter of donors may have a loss of organ function during or after brainstem death, making them unsuitable for transplantation.[29]

The goals of hemodynamic resuscitation and maintenance are to maintain a desirable blood pressure for optimal organ perfusion, to achieve normovolemia, to maintain an optimum CO despite the cardiovascular changes of brain death, and to achieve these targets with the minimal use of vasopressor or inotropic drugs.

**Table 3:** Suggested goals for active management of brain dead donor.

| Parameter | Target |
|---|---|
| Cardiovascular | Heart rate 80–120 beats/minute |
| | SBP ≥ 100 mm Hg, mean pressure ≥ 70 mm Hg |
| | JVP of 6–10 mm Hg |
| | Invasive cardiac monitoring goals: PCWP of 6–10 mm Hg Cardiac index of 2.4 L/min/m² SVR 800–1,200 dyn-s/cm⁵ |
| Electrolytes | Serum Na 130–150 mmol/L Normal K, Ca, Mg, phosphate |
| Urine output | 0.5–3 mL/kg/h |
| Blood glucose | 4–8 mmol/L |

(JVP: jugular venous pressure; PCWP: pulmonary capillary wedge pressure; SBP: systolic blood pressure; SVR: systemic vascular resistance)

It has been shown that with aggressive management to achieve hemodynamic physiology, organs that were initially considered unsuitable for transplantation may achieve viability. In a multicenter study it was shown that all organs benefit from an aggressive approach toward treatment, and improved cardiac function translates into an improvement in the function of all organs, and hence organ yield.[30,31] The study validated a "Critical Pathway for the Organ Donor", which was first proposed by the United Network for Organ Sharing (UNOS) in 1999, and was endorsed by the American Society of Transplant Surgeons (ASTS), the American Society of Transplantation (AST), the North American Transplant Coordinators Organization (ATCO), and the AOPO.

The Crystal City consensus of 2002 delineated targets, management strategies, and monitoring guidelines for cardiac donors.[32] It encouraged targeted cardiovascular management, invasive CO monitoring, and propagated pulmonary artery catheterization. The Canadian multidisciplinary forum on organ donor management also advised a similar strategy with specific goals for treatments, and areas for further research (Table 3).[33]

There is still significant variation in the adaptation of guidelines, targets, and strategies between institutions. Overall, it has been established that the protocol-based management of the organ donor leads to better organ procurement rates and higher number of transplantable organs.[34]

### Hemodynamic Support

The main aim of fluid management is to optimize perfusion and hence organ preservation, which can be achieved by ensuring normovolemia and an adequate CO. IV fluid therapy and hemodynamic management should be guided by invasive or noninvasive monitoring techniques targeting optimal conditions. Dynamic measurements are more reliable than static measurements and offer better chances of organ preservation. Although these devices have not been investigated in donor subjects, they may be considered accurate based on the results of studies from other cohorts. These include devices predicting fluid responsiveness based upon stroke volume variation or pulse pressure variation. Other devices such as a central venous catheter and/or pulmonary artery catheter (PAC) may be considered if available but they may be inaccurate in providing information about fluid status [central venous pressure (CVP)] or require proficiency in interpretation (PAC). Pulmonary artery catheters are often considered gold standard in expert hands, they provide additional information, e.g. pulmonary artery occlusion pressure (PAOP), CO, and cardiac index. Most hemodynamic goals are based on consensus statements like the Crystal City consensus statement guidelines which are also accepted by UNOS. The same guidelines also form part of the recent consensus statement given jointly by the SCCM, ACCP, and AOPO Societies, published in 2015.[6]

These recommendations are summarized as follows:
- Hypovolemia must be addressed promptly.
- Hemodynamic monitoring tools should be employed to guide volume status and response to therapy. These may include invasive or noninvasive methods. Transthoracic echocardiography for continuous CO monitoring is the modality of choice. Transesophageal echocardiography may be employed if TTE is not possible.
- Guidelines for adequate IV fluid resuscitation are:
  - Mean arterial pressure more than 60 mm Hg
  - Urine output more than 1 mL/kg/hour
  - Left ventricle ejection fraction more than 45%
  - Employ a low vasopressor dose (dopamine ≤10 μg/kg/min).
- Serial monitoring of CVP, PAOP, acid-base balance, base deficit, mixed venous oxygen saturation, and lactate is recommended.

A management dilemma arises in the donation of both lung and kidney, where resuscitation goals may be antagonistic. It has been traditionally thought that a liberal fluid strategy benefits kidney procurement whereas a conservative fluid strategy benefits the procurement of lungs. Minambres et al. noted that a conservative CVP target did not affect graft survival or development of delayed graft function.[35] A CVP target of 10 mm Hg which incorporated hormone replacement therapy for heart and lung donors also increased the yield of donor kidneys.[36]

## Choice of Fluid Therapy

The initial choice for resuscitation of the organ donor is an isotonic crystalloid.[6] Normal saline and lactated Ringer's remain the first choice, though there is absence of evidence guiding management in this specific setting. Hyperchloremic acidosis may be aggravated by normal saline, though the debate continues about its physiological and clinical significance. Similarly, hypoosmolar solutions like Ringer's lactate may not be suitable for some donors, especially with coexisting diabetes insipidus which is widely prevalent in this population.

Colloid solutions may be used for rapidly expanding intravascular volume. Albumin 20% and hydroxyethyl starch (HES) are commonly available colloids. HES is associated with acute kidney injury and coagulopathy, and often leads to acute volume overload, which compromises right ventricular performance. It has also been implicated in cases of graft organ dysfunction in the form of delayed graft function and graft failure.[37] Rapidly degradable low-molecular-weight HES solutions have shown better safety profile in a study, which compared 130-kDa HES with 200-kDa HES and resulted in lesser instances of delayed graft function.[38] The 2015 guidelines do not advise the routine use of HES, but if required the infused volume should be restricted to 500–1,000 m.[6]

## Vasoactive Drugs

The hemodynamic effects of brain death are initially due to a catecholamine surge which is followed by a vasoplegic state and relative hypovolemia. The brainstem ischemia phase of brain death is a compensatory mechanism to increase cerebral perfusion in the setting of high ICP. It denotes impending herniation, but brain death has not yet occurred. Strategies to decrease ICP like hyperosmotic therapies or decompressive procedures like placement of an extraventricular drain or craniotomy/craniectomy should be employed to prevent herniation. The catecholamine surge observed during this are associated with deleterious cardiac effects like catecholamine induced tachycardia, increased oxygen consumption, and can be limited with the use of adrenergic antagonists like esmolol.[39]

In the settings of circulatory shock, vasopressor use is recommended when volume resuscitative measures have failed and CO cannot be maintained. Vasoactive support should be escalated to achieve hemodynamic targets, especially in presence of left ventricular dysfunction. The diagnosis of stress cardiomyopathy should prompt the early institution of invasive and noninvasive hemodynamic monitoring.

Vasopressors with alpha agonistic properties predispose to increased extravascular lung water due to increased pulmonary capillary permeability. These vasopressors may also induce coronary and renal vasoconstriction prior to organ retrieval. Dopamine has traditionally been the favored drug due to its ionotropic and vasopressor activities. It may also protect against reperfusion injury and inflammation through induced heme oxygenase-1.[40] Kidneys procured from donors who have been maintained on dopamine also have lower dialysis requirements.[41]

Vasopressin increases vasomotor tone and effectively reverses diabetes insipidus (DI) reducing fluid loss and vasopressor requirement. It acts on vascular V1a receptors, closes potassium channels and nitric oxide signaling pathways. In a randomized controlled trial, authors evaluated the use of hormone replacement therapy (vasopressin along with T3) which showed improvement in cardiac performance by reducing norepinephrine requirement.[42] Moreover, the use of vasopressin in brain dead organ donors has been shown to improve organ yield.[43] Other vasopressors like noradrenaline, adrenaline may be added when dopamine doses exceed 10 μ/kg/min, but have been associated with poor outcomes for the recipient.[44]

## Hormone Replacement Therapy

Posterior pituitary dysfunction is commonly observed in the brain dead patients, seen in up to 80%.[21] It may manifest before brain death in the setting of increased ICP or traumatic brain injury as a state of diabetes insipidus. Anterior pituitary dysfunction, which manifests as hypocortisolism and thyroid hormone hyposecretion is rarely reported. Many studies have shown benefit when hormone replacement therapy (HRT) is incorporated into management protocols.

The UNOS pathway first incorporated HRT which consisted treatment comprising methylprednisolone, vasopressin, and triiodothyronine (T3), or L-thyroxine.[45]

Vasopressin is advocated when hypotension persists despite adequate fluid resuscitation, or in the following settings, which make the diagnosis of diabetes insipidus likely.
- Observed polyuria as indicated by a urine output more than 3–4 L/d or 2.5–3.0 mL/kg/hour.
- A normal or increased serum osmolality in the setting of decreased osmolarity dilute urine (specific gravity <1.005, urine osmolality <200 mOsm/kg $H_2O$).
- Hypernatremia ($Na^+$ >145 mmol/L).

A dose of 0.03–0.04 IU/min of arginine vasopressin not only improves cardiovascular parameters but also reduces inotropic requirements in donors.[46] Desmopressin may be considered in the hemodynamically stable hypernatremic patient. After an initial 1–4 μg bolus, 1–2 μg is administered 6 hourly, depending upon urine output and sodium levels. Its selective $V_2$ agonism does not produce vasoconstriction or hypertension.

The injured brain also triggers a cascade of proinflammatory and immunologic mediators. Mega doses of methylprednisolone are frequently recommended to decrease inflammatory reactions and improve graft outcome. This is administered as a bolus 250 mg followed by an infusion at 100 mg/hour. It is important that this is done after blood is drawn for cross matching because methylprednisolone may alter HLA expression and interfere in matching.

The evidence for thyroid hormone supplementation is conflicting. Animal studies show decreases in T3 and T4 levels and enforce the physiological basis for its administration[21] whilst randomized studies have failed to show benefits.[47] It seems reasonable to add thyroid hormone in patients whose CO is not improving despite optimal treatment and also in cardiac donors with abnormal left ventricular ejection fraction (<45%). Both T3 and T4 are acceptable for HRT. One protocol advocate administration of T4 IV with a 20-μg bolus, followed by an infusion at 10 μg/hour, or administration of T3 IV with a 4.0-μg bolus, followed by an infusion at 3 μg/hour.[6]

Data regarding the effects of hyperglycemia on organ procurement outcome are scant. Hyperglycemia may cause an osmotic diuresis and aggravate hypovolemia. As in the ICU setting, it seems prudent to manage hyperglycemia as for non-brain dead patients with intravenous insulin, according to institutional protocols. It is also recommended to avoid dextrose containing solutions.

## Ventilatory Management

Ventilator-induced lung injury is widely prevalent in ICU patients.[48] UNOS initially suggested tidal volumes of 10–12 mL/kg with a PEEP of 5 cm$H_2O$. However, lower tidal volume ventilation has been associated with improved outcomes in acute lung injury and is now the widely accepted practice in ICU. Its implementation to donor management with lower tidal volumes and PEEP levels to prevent derecruitment has been associated with increased numbers of transplantable lungs.[49] Avoiding high inspired oxygen concentrations may decrease incidence of bronchiolitis obliterans syndrome in lung recipients. Also, nursing in the head up position along with ensuring other VAP prevention bundles is imperative. A fluid conservative approach, although difficult to achieve in the brain dead patient, is advised and diuretics should be used to treat fluid overload.

## Other Management Issues

As previously mentioned, the brain dead patient has impaired heat conservation due to hypothalamic dysfunction overlaying vasodilatation related heat loss. Temperature monitoring and active heating is advisable to maintain a core temperature more than 35°C.

Coagulopathies are common in the brain dead population.[50] Causes of active bleeding should be investigated and promptly corrected. Thromboprophylaxis should also be continued.

Nutrition of the brain dead patient should be continued, either by feeding or glucose infusions to target blood glucose less than 180 mg/dL.

## CONCLUSION

Management of the brain dead patient poses several challenges. Evidence currently favors an aggressive approach, guided by invasive monitoring, and has been shown to increase organ yields and improve recipient outcomes.

Many crucial management decisions right from the diagnosis of brain death, the counseling of family members, to the maintenance of donor health, and hence organ health, are taken in the ICU. The impacts of these decisions are felt in terms of organ procurement rates, as well as long-term outcomes for the recipient. The intensive management of the brain dead donor gains even more significance in the face of a diminutive donor pool, which is pressured by an ever-growing demand for solid organs. An in-depth knowledge of management strategies as well as legal and ethical issues regarding the brain-dead potential donor would therefore serve any intensivist well.

## SALIENT POINTS

- Brain death certification must include essential prerequisite of known irreversible cause with absent brainstem reflexes.
- Confirmatory tests may be needed in selected cases such as facial trauma, patients on multiple drugs mimicking brain death or patients with severe airway diseases.
- Circulatory death is an viable alternative to increase organ donor pool.
- Brain death causes severe alterations in multiple organs of the body including systemic hemodynamic effects, profound endocrine changes and metabolic stress.
- Hemodynamic support is the mainstay of therapy for potential organ donors along with selective hormone replacement and ventilation support.

## REFERENCES

1. Indian Transplant Newsletter. (2014-2015). 14(43). [online] Available from https://www.edqm.eu/sites/default/files/newsletter_transplant_2015.pdf [Last accessed January, 2019].
2. A definition of irreversible coma. Report of the Ad Hoc Committee of the Harvard Medical School to examine the definition of brain death. JAMA. 1968;205(6):337-40.
3. Mollaret P, Goulon M. The depassed coma (preliminary memoir). Rev Neurol (Paris). 1959;101:3-15.
4. Wertheimer P, Jouvet M, Descotes J. Diagnosis of death of the nervous system in comas with respiratory arrest treated by artificial respiration. Presse Med. 1959;67(3):87-8.
5. Practice parameters for determining brain death in adults (summary statement). The Quality Standards Subcommittee of the American Academy of Neurology. Neurology. 1995;45(5):1012-4.
6. Kotloff RM, Blosser S, Fulda GJ, et al. Society of Critical Care Medicine/American College of Chest Physicians/Association of Organ Procurement Organizations Donor Management Task Force. Management of the potential organ donor in the ICU: Society of Critical Care Medicine/American College of Chest Physicians/Association of Organ Procurement Organizations Consensus Statement. Crit Care Med. 2015;43(6):1291-325.
7. Wijdicks EF, Varelas PN, Gronseth GS, et al. Evidence-based guideline update: determining brain death in adults: report of the quality standards subcommittee of the American Academy of Neurology. Neurology. 2010;74(23):1911-8.
8. Wijdicks EF. Brain death worldwide: Accepted fact but no global consensus in diagnostic criteria. Neurology. 2002;58(1):20-5.
9. World Health Organization. (2012). International Guidelines for the Determination of Death - Phase 1. Montreal Forum Report. [online] Available from https://www.who.int/patientsafety/montreal-forum-report.pdf [Last accessed January, 2019].
10. Nicholson ML, Metcalfe MS, White SA, et al. A comparison of the results of renal transplantation from non-heart-beating, conventional cadaveric, and living donors. Kidney Int. 2000;58(6):2585-91.
11. Tojimbara T, Fuchinoue S, Iwadoh K, et al. Improved outcomes of renal transplantation from cardiac death donors: A 30-year single center experience. Am J Transplant. 2007;7(3):609-17.
12. Brook NR, White SA, Waller JR, et al. Non-heart beating donor kidneys with delayed graft function have superior graft survival compared with conventional heart-beating donor kidneys that develop delayed graft function. Am J Transplant. 2003;3(5):614-8.
13. Mateo R, Cho Y, Singh G, et al. Risk factors for graft survival after liver transplantation from donation after cardiac death donors: An analysis of OPTN/UNOS data. Am J Transplant. 2006;6(4):791-6.
14. Abt PL, Desai NM, Crawford MD, et al. Survival following liver transplantation from non-heart-beating donors. Ann Surg. 2004; 239(1):87-92.
15. Nygaard CE, Townsend RN, Diamond DL. Organ donor management and organ outcome: a 6-year review from a Level I trauma center. J Trauma. 1990;30(6):728-32.

16. Bittner HB, Kendall SW, Campbell KA, et al. A valid experimental brain death donor model. J Heart Lung Transplant. 1995;14(2):308-17.
17. Novitzky D. Detrimental effects of brain death on the potential organ donor. Transplant Proc. 1997;29(8):3770-2.
18. Shivalkar B, Van Loon J, Wieland W, et al. Variable effects of explosive or gradual increase of intracranial pressure on myocardial structure and function. Circulation. 1993;87(1):230-9.
19. Wood KE, Becker BN, McCartney JG, et al. Care of the potential organ donor. N Engl J Med. 2004;351(26):2730-9.
20. Reilly PM, Grossman MD, Rosengard BR, et al. Lung procurement from solid organ donors: role of fluid resuscitation in procurement failures. Chest. 1996;110:222S.
21. Novitzky D, Cooper DK, Rosendale JD, et al. Hormonal therapy of the brain-dead organ donor: experimental and clinical studies. Transplantation. 2006;82(11):1396-401.
22. Tien RD. Sequence of enhancement of various portions of the pituitary gland on gadolinium-enhanced MR images: correlation with regional blood supply. AJR Am J Roentgenol. 1992;158(3):651-4.
23. Gramm HJ, Meinhold H, Bickel U, et al. Acute endocrine failure after brain death? Transplantation. 1992;54(5):851-7.
24. Novitzky D, Cooper DK, Wicomb W. Hormonal therapy to the brain-dead potential organ donor: the misnomer of the "Papworth Cocktail". Transplantation. 2008;86(10):1479-80.
25. Bugge JF. Brain death and its implications for management of the potential organ donor. Acta Anaesthesiol Scand. 2009;53(10):1239-50.
26. Smith M. Physiologic changes during brain stem death—lessons for management of the organ donor. J Heart Lung Transplant. 2004;23(Suppl 9):S217-22.
27. Barklin A. Systemic inflammation in the brain-dead organ donor. Acta Anaesthesiol Scand. 2009;53(4):425-35.
28. Barklin A, Tønnesen E, Ingerslev J, et al. Coagulopathy during induced severe intracranial hypertension in a porcine donor model. Anesthesiology. 2009;110(6):1287-92.
29. Mackersie RC, Bronsther OL, Shackford SR. Organ procurement in patients with fatal head injuries. The fate of the potential donor. Ann Surg. 1991;213(2):143-50.
30. Wheeldon DR, Potter CD, Oduro A, et al. Transforming the 'unacceptable' donor: outcomes from the adoption of a standardized donor management technique. J Heart Lung Transplant. 1995;14(4):734-42.
31. Rosendale JD, Chabalewski FL, McBride MA, et al. Increased transplanted organs from the use of a standardized donor management protocol. Am J Transplant. 2002;2(8):761-8.
32. Zaroff JG, Rosengard BR, Armstrong WF, et al. Consensus conference report: maximizing use of organs recovered from the cadaver donor: cardiac recommendations, March 28-29, 2001, Crystal City, Va. Circulation. 2002;106(7):836-41.
33. Shemie SD, Ross H, Pagliarello J, et al. Pediatric Recommendations Group. Organ donor management in Canada: recommendations of the forum on medical management to optimize donor organ potential. CMAJ. 2006;174(6):S13-32.
34. Klein AS, Messersmith EE, Ratner LE, et al. Organ donation and utilization in the United States, 1999-2008. Am J Transplant. 2010;10(4 pt 2):973-86.
35. Miñambres E, Rodrigo E, Ballesteros MA, et al. Impact of restrictive fluid balance focused to increase lung procurement on renal function after kidney transplantation. Nephrol Dial Transplant. 2010;25(7):2352-6.
36. Abdelnour T, Rieke S. Relationship of hormonal resuscitation therapy and central venous pressure on increasing organs for transplant. J Heart Lung Transplant. 2009;28(5):480-5.
37. Cittanova ML, Leblanc I, Legendre C, et al. Effect of hydroxyethylstarch in brain-dead kidney donors on renal function in kidney-transplant recipients. Lancet. 1996;348(9042):1620-2.
38. Blasco V, Leone M, Antonini F, et al. Comparison of the novel hydroxyethyl starch 130/0.4 and hydroxyethyl starch 200/0.6 in brain-dead donor resuscitation on renal function after transplantation. Br J Anaesth. 2008;100(4):504-8.
39. Audibert G, Charpentier C, Seguin-Devaux C, et al. Improvement of donor myocardial function after treatment of autonomic storm during brain death. Transplantation. 2006;82(8):1031-6.
40. Hoeger S, Gottmann U, Liu Z, et al. Dopamine treatment in brain-dead rats mediates anti-inflammatory effects: The role of hemodynamic stabilization and D-receptor stimulation. Transpl Int. 2007;20(9):790-9.
41. Schnuelle P, Gottmann U, Hoeger S, et al. Effects of donor pretreatment with dopamine on graft function after kidney transplantation: A randomized controlled trial. JAMA. 2009;302(10):1067-75.
42. Venkateswaran RV, Steeds RP, Quinn DW, et al. The haemodynamic effects of adjunctive hormone therapy in potential heart donors: A prospective randomized double-blind factorially designed controlled trial. Eur Heart J. 2009;30(14):1771-80.
43. Plurad DS, Bricker S, Neville A, et al. Arginine vasopressin significantly increases the rate of successful organ procurements in potential donors. Am J Surg. 2012;204(6):856-1.
44. Stoica SC, Satchitahananda DK, White P, et al. Noradrenaline use in human donor and relationship with load-independent right ventricular contractility. Transplantation. 2004;78(8):1193-7.
45. Rosendale JD, Kauffman HM, McBride MA, et al. Aggressive pharmacologic donor management results in more transplanted organs. Transplantation. 2003;75(4):482-7.
46. Pennefather SH, Bullock RE, Mantle D, et al. Use of low dose arginine vasopressin to support brain-dead organ donors. Transplantation. 1995;59(1):58-62.
47. Venkateswaran RV, Steeds RP, Quinn DW, et al. The haemodynamic effects of adjunctive hormone therapy in potential heart donors: a prospective randomized double-blind factorially designed controlled trial. Eur Heart J. 2009;30(14):1771-80.
48. Wheeler AP, Bernard GR. Acute lung injury and the acute respiratory distress syndrome: a clinical review. Lancet. 2007;369(9572):1553-64.
49. Mascia L, Pasero D, Slutsky AS, et al. Effect of a lung protective strategy for organ donors on eligibility and availability of lungs for transplantation: a randomized controlled trial. JAMA. 2010;304(23):2620-7.
50. Hefty TR, Cotterell LW, Fraser SC, et al. Disseminated intravascular coagulation in cadaveric organ donors. Incidence and effect on renal transplantation. Transplantation. 1993;55(2):442-3.

# Index

Page numbers followed by *b* refer to box, *f* refer to figure, *fc* refer to flowchart, and *t* refer to table.

## A

Abdomino-thoracic index, calculation of 259*f*
Abscess drainage 390
Acetate 244
Acid-base
    abnormalities 350, 351
    component of 331
    disorder 330, 350
        metabolic 329
        primary 329
    disturbance 349, 352, 353, 355, 358, 361
    homeostasis 325
    status 351
Acidemia 336
Acidic drugs 246
Acidic liquid 369
Acidosis 294, 348, 360
    acute respiratory 41, 326, 331
    chronic respiratory 326, 331, 344, 346
    compensation, chronic respiratory 327*f*
    hypercapnic 343, 344
    state of 350
*Acinetobacter* 190
Acrodermatitis enteropathica 384
Activated clotting time 205
Activated partial thromboplastin time 205
Acute coronary syndrome 335, 389
Acute hypercapnic respiratory failure 35
Acute hyponatremia 282, 282*b*
    causes of 279*fc*
Acute lung injury, transfusion-related 388, 392, 393
Acute respiratory distress syndrome 3, 29, 49, 74, 88, 121, 138, 151, 197, 216, 220, 224, 269, 272, 376, 389
    pathophysiology of 85
    severe 198
Adenine 387
    monophosphate 307
Adenosine
    monophosphate 44
    triphosphate 307, 374, 389
Adrenaline 402
Adult respiratory distress syndrome 389
Advanced cardiac life support 24, 32
Aerosolized therapy 192
Air 66, 71
    embolism 218
    entrainment
        devices 21
        nebulizers 22
        mask 19, 22*f*
    humidification, degree of 181
    trapping 82
        exhale causing 108
Airway 87
    access, type of 184
    anatomy 181
    burns, context of 4
    clearance
        mechanisms 182
        system 229*f*
    collapse, volume related 11
    disease
        chronic 397
        severe 403
    management equipment 227
    obstruction of 61
    occlusion pressure 142, 166
    pressure 137, 152, 220
        release ventilation 121-123
    protection of 61
    resistance 144
Albumin 251, 350, 367
    concentration of 330
    low 43
    parathyroid hormone 309
Albuterol sulfate 183
Alcohol 315
    abuse 307
    dehydrogenase 334
Alkalemia 338
Alkaline suspension 369
Alkalosis 332, 346, 356, 360
    acute respiratory 328, 328*f*, 331
    chronic respiratory 328, 331
    diuretic-induced 338
    state of 350
Allen test 348
Allergic reactions 394
Alveolar arterial oxygen gradient 29, 39
Alveolar capillary
    boundary 119
    membrane 28
    perfusion 10
Alveolar dead space 10
Alveolar epithelial cells 8, 14
Alveolar gas equation 28, 29
Alveolar oxygen
    content 30
    tension ratio 30
Alveolar plateau phase 119*f*
Alveolar pressure 82, 151
Alveolar recruitment maneuvers 105
Alveolar ventilation 10, 36, 342
    inadequate 342
Alveoli, functional cellular anatomy of 9*f*
American Thoracic Society 85, 172, 177
Amino acid 373, 375
Aminoglycosides 284
Ammonium chloride 340
Amphotericin B 190, 284
Amylopectin 248
Anaerobic metabolism 245
Anaphylactic reactions 394
Anaphylaxis 253
Anemia 43, 388
Anesthesia
    epidural 241
    ventilators 71
Angiotensin converting enzyme 3, 240
    inhibitors 294
Angiotensin receptor blockers 294
Anion gap
    approach 351
    metabolic acidosis, normal 330
    normal 335
Antibiotics 190, 308
Anticholinergics 254
    bronchodilator 41
Anticonvulsants 308
Antidiuretic hormone 239, 276, 278
    level 277*fc*
Antidotes 41
Antigen presenting cells 3
Antineutrophil antibodies 393
Antioxidant 369
    supplementation 369
Anxiety 346
Apixaban 392
Apnea 397
    hypopnea index 42
    test 397
Arginine 369, 373-375
    deficiency 376
    physiology 375
    source 375
    toxicity 376
    vasopressin 255, 275

Arrhythmias 291, 299, 399
Arterial blood
   care and transport of 348
   gas 35, 48, 207, 254, 311, 346, 348, 355, 356t-359t, 360, 360t
      analysis 32, 39, 254
      interpretation, basics of 348
      values 311t
   pressure 251
   samples 348
Arterial cannulation 215
Arterial carbon dioxide
   partial pressure of 36
   tension 176
Arterial gas embolism 25
Arterial oxygen
   content 27, 30
      saturation 27, 176
         measurement of 115
      tension 42, 176
Arterial puncture 349
Arteriovenous pumpless system 214
Artificial airway 181, 183
Artificial colloid 247
Aspartate aminotransferase 312
Aspiration 371
   pneumonia 85
   protection from 6
   risk of 226, 367
Aspirin 246
Assist control ventilation 69, 147
Asthma 50, 334, 342, 346
   comprise of 77
   severe 78, 79t
   treat 289
Asynchrony
   index 107
   types of 108
Ataxia 315
Atelectasis 29, 33
Atelectrauma, prevention of 155
Atmospheric pressure 151
Atrial fibrillation 333
Atrial natriuretic peptide 241
Atrial pressure, right 129f
Autoimmune polyglandular syndrome 298
Auto-positive end-expiratory pressure 78, 108
Aztreonam 190

## B

Bacteremia, gram-negative 309
Bacteria, gram-negative 190
Bacterial colonization 8
Bacterium leuconostoc mesenteroides 248

Bag mask
   device 24, 24f, 31
   ventilation 19, 33
Balanced colloid solution 269
Balanced salt solutions 245
Barbiturate 246
Barometric pressure 30, 39
Barotrauma 109, 220
   predisposes to 85
Bartter's syndrome 290, 315, 316, 338
Basal pressure 91
Basic acid-base physiology 349
Basolateral membrane 283
Baydur test 141
Beer's law 114
Beta-adrenergic blockers 293
Bicarbonate 246
   therapy 301
Bifidobacteria 368
Bilevel positive airway pressure 35, 59, 60, 69
Bilirubin 115
Bioelectrical impedance analysis 238, 261
Bio-med devices 73
Biotrauma 9
Bisphosphonates 304, 305t
Bivaluridin 205
Bleeding 254
   tendency, history of 391
Blood
   flow 122, 323
   gas
      analysis 333
      partial pressure of 117
   glucose 237
   loss, exceptional anemia from 25
   pressure 53, 54, 176, 211, 240, 348, 400
   products, transfusion of 387
   transfusion 388
      reaction 393
   urea 237
      nitrogen 35, 276
   volume index 261
Body fluid 238
   compartments 235
      composition of 236
      volume of 237t
   distribution of 236f
   homeostasis 235, 266
   spaces, measurement of 237
Body mass index 35, 207, 216
Bone resorption, prevent 304
Boston rules 329
Bowman's glands 3
Boyle's law 24
Bradycardia 319

Brain
   death 396, 397
      diagnosis of 396fc, 396t, 397
      effects of 399
      pathophysiology of 400
   dysfunction 388
   injury 271
   natriuretic peptide 241, 254
Brainstem
   death 400
   reflexes 397
      absent 397
Breath stacking 78
Breathing 107
   cycle 55
   pattern of 21
   trial failure
      signs of spontaneous 176t
      symptoms of spontaneous 176t
   work of 14, 48, 53
Brewer's yeast 380
Broad-spectrum antibiotics 368
Bronchial asthma 77
Bronchial smooth muscle, role of 8
Bronchioles 8
Bronchoconstriction 182
Bronchodilatation 105
Bronchodilator
   receptors 181
   role of 41
   therapy, effect of 104
Bronchopleural fistula 83, 94
   etiologies of 83t
   harmful effects of 84t
   management of 84
   preventive strategies for 84
Bronchoscopy, fiberoptic 83
Bronchospasm 70, 78, 100, 184
Bubble reduction 24
Bulbar dysfunction 43

## C

Calcimimetics 305
Calcitonin 296, 297
Calcium 244, 296
   chloride 301
   functions of 296b
   gluconate 295, 301
   metabolism 297f
   sensing receptor 315
Cannula
   sizes 203t
   variety of 203t
Capillary blood flow 3
Capillary endothelium destruction 25
Capillary leak index 254

Capnograph 118
Carbamazepine 239, 370
Carbohydrates, oxidation of 235
Carbon dioxide 35, 47, 71, 119, 213, 217
    clearance 222
    concentrations 114
    measurement 117
    monitoring 40
    partial pressure of 209, 342
    tension in blood, measurement of 117
Carbon monoxide
    intoxication 334
    poisoning 18
        severe 25
Carbonic acid 350
Carboxyhemoglobin 117
Cardiac chambers, volume of 131
Cardiac disease 387
    active 394
Cardiac dysfunction 144
Cardiac index 258
Cardiac output 18, 27, 115, 198
    syndrome, low 197
    total 30
Cardiac surgery, protective ventilation in 125
Cardiac tamponade 32, 253
Cardio-abdominal-renal syndrome 261
Cardiogenic pulmonary edema, management of 135
Cardiovascular disease 388
Cardiovascular disorders 380
Cardiovascular system 130, 177, 240, 299, 319
Carpopedal spasm 300
Cartilage, long teardrop-shaped 5
Catabolic stress 365
Caudal ventrolateral medulla 239
Cavities, abdominal 161
Cefotaxime 190
Ceftazidime 190
Cell structures, part of 307
Cellular
    acidosis 334
    defense 373
    dysfunction 309
    metabolism 307
Central nervous system 37, 177, 199, 206, 278
    disorders 225
    dysfunction 199
    toxicity 25
Central respiratory depression 31
Central venous pressure 132, 251, 258, 268, 401

Cerebral
    attack 335
    edema 245, 271
    ischemia 246
    salt-wasting syndrome 271
    tissue oxygenation 388
Cerebrospinal fluid 37
Cervical spine injuries, high 31
Cetuximab 315, 317
Chest
    deformations 50
    physiotherapy 92, 105
    radiograph 40
    trauma 83
    tube 366
        management 84
        occlusion, intermittent inspiratory 84
        placement 83
    wall 12, 78
        diagnosis of 343
Chloride 244
    levels of 269
    responsive metabolic alkalosis 338
Chloroquine toxicity 40
Cholecalciferol 379
Cholera, physiology of 243
Chromium 382
Chronic obstructive pulmonary disease 13, 36, 49, 82, 92, 164, 181, 190, 216, 217, 225, 289, 338, 344
Chvostek's sign 300
Circulatory system, medications performance of 48
Cisplatin 284
Citrate phosphate dextrose 387
Clark electrode 116
Claustrophobia 25
Clofibrate 239
Clostridial myonecrosis 25
Colitis 319
Colloid 247
    oncotic pressure 237, 254
    osmotic pressure 268f
    solutions 401
Colored nail varnish 115
Coma 397
Complete blood count 33, 40, 205
Compressed gas storage system 5
Consciousness
    decreased level of 4
    depressed level of 77, 239
Continuous positive airway pressure 49, 91, 121, 174, 224
Conventional ventilatory support 196
Core body temperature 4

Cormack-Lehane descriptive system 5
Coronary artery bypass grafting 376
Cortical collecting tubule 294
Corticosteroids 284
Cough
    ineffective 61
    reflex, trachea in 3
    strength 144
C-reactive protein 254
Creatine phosphokinase 40
Cricoid cartilage 5
Critical care myopathy 173
Critical illness polymyoneuropathy 162
Crystalloid 243, 249, 271
    solutions 243, 271
Cumulative fluid balance 253
Cushing's syndrome 290
Cyanosis 179
Cycled air, humidity of 181
Cystic fibrosis 182
Cytokines 86
Cytotoxic drugs 308

## D

Dabigatran 392
Decompression sickness 25
Dehydration 253
Demeclocycline 284
Dental barotrauma and pain 25
Dephlogisticated air 17
Depressed mental status 176, 179
Dextran 243, 248
Dextransucrase 248
Dextrose 294, 387
    containing fluid 245, 246
Diabetes insipidus 240, 283, 285, 402
Diabetes mellitus 284
    acute complication of 335
Diaphoresis 179
Diaphragm 67, 162
    activity, monitor 166
    anatomy 161
    dysfunction 162
        development of 163fc
        diagnostic of 166
    electric activity 165
    electrical activity of 73, 148
    excursion of 147
    function 161
    inactivity 164
    pressure generation, ratio of 165
    protective ventilation concepts 166
    thickness 147
    ultrasound 147
Diaphragmatic dysfunction, ventilator-induced 147, 161, 163, 167

Diarrhea 253, 254, 271, 384
   chronic 308, 315
Diastolic function 256
Diethylene glycol 334
Diodes, light-emitting 114
Dipalmitoylphosphatidylcholine 9
Disinfectant solution 227
Disinfection techniques 229
Distal nephron function, abnormal 291
Disulfiram 247
Dizziness 346
Dobutamine 289
Docosahexaenoic acid 376
Domiciliary ventilators 227
Dorsal chest 122
Double gap acidosis 334
Driving pressure 95, 141, 156
Drug
   dose 183
   formulation 183
   interactions 369
   properties of 181
Dry cold gas 5
Dry powder inhalers 184
Duchenne muscular dystrophy 37
Duodenum 307
Dynamic hyperinflation 47, 78, 85, 107
   hemodynamic consequences of 79
Dynamic occlusion test 148
Dysplasia, bronchopulmonary 220
Dyspnea 39, 48
   sudden onset of 83
Dyssynchrony 85

## E

Echocardiography 208
Edema 241
   cardiogenic pulmonary 49, 226
   pulmonary 135$fc$
Edoxaban 392
Effective circulatory fluid volume 279, 280
Eicosapentaenoic acid 376
Eisenmenger's syndrome 30
Ejection fraction 251
Electrical impedance tomography 261
Electrocardiogram 35
Electroencephalogram 38
Electrolyte 255
   abnormalities 317
   balance 330
   compartments of 235
   disturbance 144, 357
      management of 312
      severe 173
Electromagnetic stimulation 147
Electromyography 40, 166

Emergency medical services 71, 73
End-diastolic volume 129, 257, 259
End-expiratory collapse 124
End-expiratory lung volume 78, 152
End-expiratory occlusion 258
   button 138
   technique 80
   test 135, 261
End-inspiratory muscle pressure 142
Endobronchial intubation 32
Endoluminal bronchial secretions 182
Endothelial cells, cytoskeleton of 9
Endothelial glycocalyx 252
Endothelial nitric oxide production 122
Endotracheal intubation 6
Endotracheal tube 94, 157, 184, 186
End-tidal carbon dioxide analyzer 118
Enteral nutrition 366, 370
Epidermal growth factor 314, 315
Epiglottic cartilage 5
Epiglottis 4
Epilepsy 315
Epithelial cells, cytoskeleton of 9
Eplerenone 294
Esophageal Doppler monitoring 257
Esophageal manometry 124
Esophageal pressure 80, 141, 146, 148, 157, 161
Esophageal region, fresh fixations in 61
Esophagus 145
Estimated glomerular filtration rate 199
Ethanol 284
Ethylene 334
Ethylenediaminetetraacetic acid 293, 298
European Respiratory Society 172, 177
Euvolemia 253, 272
Expiratory flow
   limitation 82, 99$f$
      consequences of 82
   obstruction, causes of 84
   until downstream water 82
Expiratory muscles, activation of 82, 112$f$
Expiratory positive airway pressure 52, 57
Expiratory sensitivity 111$f$
Extracellular fluid 235, 236, 238, 275, 307
   composition and volume, regulation of 238, 240
   volume 240$fc$
      regulation of 240
Extracellular space 243
Extracellular water 262
Extracorporeal blood flow rate 215
Extracorporeal carbon dioxide removal 196, 200, 213
Extracorporeal cardiopulmonary resuscitation 203

Extracorporeal circuit configuration 214$f$
Extracorporeal Life Support 199
   Organization 196, 198
Extracorporeal membrane
   carbon dioxide removal 213
   oxygenation 43, 87, 88, 196, 197, 197$t$, 197$f$, 198, 200, 201, 206, 209, 210
Extracorporeal membrane oxygenation
   cannulation 207, 211
   contraindication for 197, 198
   management of 202
Extracorporeal therapy 215$t$
Extravascular lung water 258, 259
   index 261
Extubation failure, risk factors for 43$b$

## F

Face mask 51, 52
   simple 19, 20$f$
Face tent aerosol mask 23$f$
Facial
   edema 87
   hair, thick 52
   sensation 397
   skeleton, trauma of 61
Fanconi's syndrome 308
Fast oxygen delivery 72
Fatal metabolic alkalosis 350
Fatty acids 373, 376
   essential 368
Febrile nonhemolytic reaction 392, 394
Femoral artery, left 204$f$
Femoral vein cannula, simultaneous left 201$f$
Fistula 84
   arteriovenous 302
Fluid 253
   adverse effects of 268
   and Catheter Treatment Trial 269
   and electrolytes 233
   balance 32, 252, 254
   bolus therapy 269
   choice of 285$t$
   classification of 243
   disturbance 357
   homogeneous 243
   interstitial 236, 236$f$, 237
   loss 253
      during surgery 241
   osmotic properties of 243
   responsiveness 253, 258
      predictor of 256
   resuscitation, history of 266
   therapy 266, 270, 401
      goals of 266$fc$
      maintenance 269
   unresponsiveness 260$f$

Forced vital capacity 35
Fresh frozen plasma 204, 206, 389
　indications 390
　preparation 390
　storage 390
Functional residual capacity 8, 11, 78, 94, 130, 152
　concept of 78
Furosemide 294, 319

## G

Galactosemia 308
Gamblegram 337$f$
Gas
　exchange 144, 215
　　catheters 214, 215
　　　pathophysiology of 197
　mixture, volume of 21
　partial pressure 349
　supply 66
　trapping 78
Gastric
　catheter 148
　contents, aspiration of 366
　mucosal pH measurement 120
　pressure 146, 161
　tonometer 120$f$
　tubes 52
Gastrointestinal failure 375
Gastrointestinal tract 241, 296, 314
Gelatin 248
　solutions, types of 248
Gilbert index 165
Gitelman's syndrome 290, 291, 315, 317
Global ejection fraction 258
Global end-diastolic volume index 258
Glomerular filtration rate 240
Glucocorticoids 305
Gluconate 244, 369, 373-375
Glutamine
　deficiency 375
　high-dose 375
　in ICU 375
　physiology 374
　source 374
　supplementation 375
Glutathione depletion 334
Glycogen storage diseases 308
Graft versus host disease 394
Granulomatous diseases 302
Guillain-Barre syndrome 31, 37, 343

## H

Haldane effect 36
Hans Rudolph half mask 51$f$
Harlequin syndrome 203, 204$f$
Hartmann's solution 245
Headaches, cluster 18
Heart
　failure 32, 39, 254, 266, 289, 299
　　chronic 177
　　congestive 278, 279
　　decompensated chronic 197
　function 396
　lung interaction 128
　　clinical applications of 131
　　determinants of 128
　rate 18, 54, 134, 258, 348
　rhythm 134
Heat
　and moisture exchanger 52, 184
　exchange malfunctions 218
Hemiplegia 38
Hemodynamic monitoring 258
　techniques 256
Hemodynamic support 202, 400
Hemoglobin 198, 350, 387
　bound oxygen 27
　concentration 18, 27, 115, 117
　deoxygenated 117
　oxygen dissociation curve 343
Hemolysis 218
Hemolytic transfusion reactions 394
Hemorrhage, intra-alveolar 25
Henderson-Hasselbalch equation 119, 351
Heparin, unfractionated 204-206
Hepatocyte nuclear factor 315
Hepatorenal syndrome, development of 272
Hernia, congenital diaphgramatic 223
High anion gap metabolic acidosis 333
High expiratory flow rate 59
High frequency oscillatory ventilation 88, 121, 123, 220, 222
　advantages of 222
　disadvantages of 222
　indications 220
　initiation of 220
　weaning from 222
High-flow devices 21
High-frequency oscillation ventilation 43
Home-based ventilation 178, 225, 226, 230
　classification of 226$t$
　disinfection of 229
Homeostasis 235
Hormone
　replacement therapy 402
　role of 241
Human albumin 247
　fluids 247
　half-life of 247
Human immunodeficiency virus 298
Human leukocyte antigen 393
Human nasal hair differs 4
Human neutrophil antigens 393
Human serum albumin 272
Humidification 57
　nose in 3
　poor 8
Hungry bone syndrome 298, 315
Hydrochlorothiazide 315
Hydrogen ion 36
Hydrostatic pressure 122, 243
　effect 241
Hydroxyapatite 296
Hydroxyethyl starch 244, 248, 249, 401
Hyoepiglottic ligament 5
Hyperbaric oxygen 24
　therapy 19, 24, 24$b$
　　effect of 24$f$
　　physiologic effects of 24
　　side effects of 25, 25$b$
　　uses of 25$b$
Hyperbilirubinemia 311
Hypercalcemia 247, 296, 302, 304$fc$, 330
　clinical effects 303
　clinical presentation of 303$t$
　etiology 302, 302$b$
　evaluation 303
　management 303
　mild 302, 303
　severe 303
Hypercalciuria 315
Hypercapnia 35, 40$fc$, 217
　acute 37, 38
　advantages of 38
　chronic 38
　common causes of 39$fc$
　disadvantages of 38
　effects of 37$t$, 343
　evaluation of 39
　impact of 43
　management of 35
　mechanism of 36
　prognosis of 35
　symptoms of 39
Hypercapnic respiratory failure 42, 47
　differential diagnosis of 39
Hypercarbia, managing 222
Hyperglycemia 254, 371, 400
　control 308
Hyperglycemic syndromes, severe 272
Hyperinflation, mechanism of 78
Hyperkalemia 247, 288, 291, 292$f$, 294, 295, 312
　cause of 293
　clinical effects 294
　differential diagnosis of 292$t$

etiology 291
evaluation 294
management 294
mechanism 291
treatment of 294t, 295
Hyperlactatemia 245, 357
Hypermagnesemia 314, 318, 319, 319t, 330
clinical effects 319
etiology 318
evaluation 319
management of 319, 320
mechanism 318
Hypernatremia 254, 275, 283, 284fc, 285fc
causes of 283t
chronic 284
clinical features 283
drugs causing 284t
etiology 283
management of 286
Hyperoncotic albumin solutions 272
Hyperoxia 24
effects of 25
Hyperoxygenation 24
Hyperparathyroidism
primary 302
tertiary 305
Hyperphosphatemia 307, 310, 311, 311t, 312
cause of 310
etiology 310
management 312
Hyperpnea 284
Hypertension 399
arterial 333
Hyperthermia, malignant 311
Hypertonic saline 282
Hypertonicity 294
Hypertriglyceridemia 371
Hyperventilation 118
physiological effects of 85
Hypervitaminosis 284
Hypervolemia 135, 253, 277
Hypervolemic hypernatremia, diagnosis of 285
Hypoalbuminemia 266
Hypocalcemia 37, 296-298, 300fc, 301, 306, 312, 316
clinical presentation of 299t
etiology 298, 298b
evaluation 300
management 300
mechanism 298
mild 300
pearls in managing 301
severe 300
symptomatic 300, 312
treatment of 300, 301b

Hypocapnia 346
Hypochloremia 330
Hypoglycemia 25
Hypokalemia 37, 288-290, 317
causes of 289, 290
clinical effects 290
development of 295
differential diagnosis of 290t
etiology 288
evaluation 290
management 291
mechanism 288
Hypomagnesemia 37, 310, 314, 315, 315t, 316, 317, 318fc
amplification loop of 316fc
causes of 315, 315b
familial 315
Hyponatremia 275-277, 277fc, 278, 280, 281fc, 282b, 330
category of 277
causes of 280, 282, 282b
chronic 280, 281fc
diagnostic evaluation of 279fc
etiologies for 278
evaluation of 278
hypertonic 277
management of 282
pathogenesis of 277
pathophysiology of 278fc
rapidly corrected 282
therapy of 280
true 277
Hypoperfusion, treatment of 266
Hypophosphatemia 37, 307, 307t, 308-310
clinical effects 309
drug-induced 308t
etiology 307
management 309
severe 309
severity of 309
treatment of 309
X-linked 308
Hypotension 83, 122, 310, 319
Hypothalamic disease 239
Hypothyroidism 40
Hypotonic solutions 271
Hypoventilation 30, 32
Hypovolemia 241, 251-253, 255, 262, 277, 284
absence of 338
absolute 241
causes of 241t
clinical signs of 254b
consequences of 253
etiology of 253
hemodynamic parameters in 258b

laboratory biomarkers for 254b
signs of 256b
situations of 85
Hypoxemia 27, 32, 33, 35, 346
absence of 17
classification of 18t
differential diagnosis of 32fc
managing 221
mechanism of 29
mild 18
moderate 18
severe 18, 356
symptoms of 17
Hypoxia 18, 27, 346
types of 19, 19t
Hypoxic blood 10
Hypoxic pulmonary vasoconstriction 28

I

Immune system 383
Immunity, humoral 3
Immunoglobulin molecules 3
Immunonutrition 373
Impair diaphragm muscle function 162
Indocyanine green 115
Infection 144, 206
Inferior vena cava 134, 200, 256
Inferior vena collapsibility index 257f
Inflammation 37
Inspiratory air, humidification of 58
Inspiratory flow 84
rate 156, 183
Inspiratory muscle pressure index 142
Inspiratory muscle training 168
role of 168
Inspiratory oxygen fraction 176
Inspiratory positive airway pressure 52, 57
Inspiratory pressure 138, 142
generation 146
maximal 54, 174, 179
Inspired air, humidity of 4
Inspired oxygen, fraction of 18, 29, 35, 48, 69, 73, 153, 156, 186, 192, 197, 202
Insulin 294
deficiency 294
plus glucose 294, 295
Intellivent-adaptive support ventilation 73
Intensive care unit 5, 28, 40, 42, 66, 114, 144, 161, 172, 196, 207, 224, 238, 248, 251, 269, 288, 342, 355, 366, 373
Interleukin 8 156
Internal jugular vein 200
Intestinal disorders, primary 308
Intestinal malabsorption 308
Intra-abdominal pressure 122, 129, 252, 261

Intracellular fluid 236, 236f, 238, 275, 307
Intracellular water 261
Intracranial pressure 243
Intrapleural pressure, application of 84
Intrathoracic pressure 129
    effect of 129, 130fc
    hemodynamic effects in 129
Intravenous ferric carboxymaltose 389
Intravenous fluid 243, 269
Invasive mechanical ventilation, sedation in 43
Ipratropium bromide 41
Ischemia reperfusion injury 400
Ischemic central nervous system lesions 31
Isothermic saturation boundary 5
Isotonic bicarbonate solution 245, 247
Isotonic crystalloid 401
Isotope dilution techniques 262

## J

Janus Kinase-signal transducer 166
Jaw thrust 4
Jejunostomy tube 369
Jejunum 307
Jet entrainment 22f
Jet nebulizer 185, 188
Jugular venous pressure 254, 400

## K

Ketoacidosis, diabetic 272, 311
Kidney 206
    disease 253
        chronic 249, 295, 299, 302, 311, 333
    dysfunction 255
    failure 367
        chronic 333
    injury, acute 261, 269, 293, 295, 312, 357
Krebs cycle 334
Kussmaul's breathing 85
Kussmaul's sign 132
Kyphoscoliosis 40, 225

## L

*Lactobacillus* 368
Lamina densa 9
Laryngeal nerve 6
Laryngeal sensory chemoreceptors 6
Laryngoscopy 5
Laryngospasm 6
Larynx 5
    anatomy of 5, 6f
Leakage compensation 55, 56
Left vein cannulation 204f
Left ventricular
    ejection 135
    failure 359
    outflow tract 256
Levodopa, level of 370
Levothyroxine administration 370
Life-threatening bleed, management of 392
Limb ischemia 204
Lipid metabolism, incomplete 325
Liquid consistency 369
Lithium 246, 284
Liver
    disease 272, 368, 371, 391
        acute 391
        chronic 272
    failure 272
        chronic 367
    function tests 33
Loop diuretics 284
Loop expresses airway resistance 91
Loop system flow, leakage in 104
Loops analysis 100
Low pressure region 151
Low serum osmolality 277
Low tidal volume
    strategy 84
    ventilation 86
Lowe's syndrome 308
Low-pressure receptors, mechanism of action of 239fc
Lumbar vertebrae 161
Lung 86
    aeration 182
    capacity, total 11
    compliance 134
    consolidation, effects of 13
    disease, interstitial 40
    elastic recoil 98
    function 396
    hyperinflated 257
    injury
        acute 85, 334
        prevention 41
        ventilator-induced 86, 121, 124, 151, 172, 217, 402
    parenchyma 12
        compression of 122
    protective
        one-lung ventilation 125
        ventilation 43, 88
    recruitment
        evaluation of 140
        high potential of 140f
        low potential of 140f
        maneuvers 121, 125
        maneuvers, advantages of 123t
        maneuvers, disadvantages of 123t
        methods 121b
    regions, aeration of 181
    stress and strain 141
    surface area increase 157
    transplant 218
    volume 124
        and capacities 11
        at end-expiration 79
        hemodynamic effects to changes in 130
    zones of 10
Lymphatic system 241
Lymphoid tissue, gut-associated 365

## M

Macronutrients 374
    functions of 374t
Magnesium 244, 299
    homeostasis 314
        clinical effects 316
        etiology 315
        management 317
        mechanism 315
Mainstem bronchi 183
Malate 244
Malnutrition 365
Manganese 382
Manitol 284
Mask 51, 54
    designs 22
    non-rebreather 19, 21, 21f
Mass median aerodynamic diameter 182
Massive transfusion 393
Maximum inspiratory flow 68
Maximum inspiratory pressure 144, 146, 165
McCune-Albright syndrome 309
Mean airway pressure 138, 211, 214
Mean arterial blood pressure 210, 258, 261, 267
Mean systemic filling pressure 128, 129
Mechanical challenges 218
Mechanical energy 156
Mechanical insufflation-exsufflation 229
Mechanical oscillation, high frequency 229
Mechanical power and intensity 157
Mechanical ventilation 19, 33, 61, 90, 114, 137, 153, 161, 178, 198, 210, 220, 228, 231
    controlled 164
    conventional 223
    evolution of 73
    graphic analysis of 90
    invasive 24, 35, 42
    mode of 181
    noninvasive 216
    weaning from 50, 172

Mechanical ventilator 65, 90, 109f
  circuit 108, 181
  models of 92
  related equipment 227
  settings 154f
Meconium aspiration 223
Medical air 66
Medical gases 66
Medical Research Council Score 162
Membrane lung 199
Mental retardation 315
Mesenchymal tumors 309
Metabolic abnormality 350
Metabolic acidosis 246, 311, 329, 331, 333, 335, 351, 360, 361
  causes of 333, 335, 358
  hyperchloremic 247
  normal response for 328
  primary 355
  severe 84
Metabolic alkalosis 329, 331, 337, 338, 352
  causes of 338, 338b
  mild 356
  normal response for 328
Metabolic cart 366
Metabolic causes 179
Metabolic disorders 328
Metabolic disturbances 37
Metabolic rate, estimate 200
Metabolic regulation 297
Metabolic system 177
Metabolism 37
Methemoglobin 117
Methemoglobinemia 18, 115
Methylene blue 115
  test 83
Methylprednisolone 402
Microvascular blood flow 267
Microvascular injury 162
Middle ear barotrauma 25
Milk-alkali syndrome 302, 311
Mineralocorticoid excess, primary 338
Modafinil 43
Molecular diffusion 221
Monarchtm airway clearance system 229
Motor neuron disorders 226
Mucosal cells 119
Mucosal edema 78
Mucous
  glands 3
  plugging 32, 33, 34
Multidisciplinary team 227
Multiorgan dysfunction 9
Multiorgan failure 253, 383
Multiple organ dysfunction syndrome 389
Mural alveoli 8

Muscle
  action, direction of 161f
  damage 107
  dome-shaped 161
  fatigability 343
  pressure 137
  weakness 50, 108, 284
Muscular dystrophy 31
Myasthenia gravis 31
Myocardial dysfunction, acute 399
Myocardial infarction 197, 211
Myocardial necrosis 399
Myocardial stress 135
Myocarditis 197
Myoinositol 283
Myopia, hyperoxic 25

## N

Nail varnish 115
Narcotic overdose 33
Nasal airflow, turbulence of 4
Nasal airway resistance 58
Nasal cannula 18, 19, 20f, 177
  high flow 19, 23, 23f, 177, 192
  receiving high-flow 192
Nasal catheter 19, 20
Nasal mask 51, 54
Nasal mucosa 4
Nasal pillow masks 51
Nasal prongs 18
Nasopharyngeal mucosa 5
Nasopharynx 4
Natriuretic peptides 238
Natural colloid 247
Near infrared spectroscopy 117
Nebulizers 187
  ventilator-compatible 187f
Neovascularization 24
Nerve 162
  conduction studies 37
Nervous system 299
  sympathetic 238
Neural control 8
Neurologic complications 334
Neurologic diseases, acute 173
Neurologic symptoms 37
Neurological injury 271
Neuromuscular
  blocking agents 162
  causes 162, 179
  coupling 165
  disease 37
  disorder 225
    progressive 225
  efficiency 149
  junction, dysfunction of 343
  weakness 32, 38

Neurophysiological causes 179
Nitric oxide
  extensive 375
  generation of 375
  inhaled 191
  synthase 374
Nitroprusside test 335
Nitrous oxide 71
Nocturnal hypoventilation 55
Nonconventional ventilatory techniques 44
Noninvasive ventilation 19, 24, 41, 47, 48, 49t, 51, 53, 56, 57b, 60, 68, 177, 224, 226
  contraindications for 60, 61, 61b
  efficacy, signs of 54t
  failure, causes of 54
  implementation technique 53b
  indications for 48b
  proper qualification for 57
  qualification for 61
  rebreathing during 58
  receiving 191
Nonrenal potassium loss 288-290
Nonstatic variables, multiple 366
Nonsteroidal anti-inflammatory drugs 292, 293
Noradrenaline 402
Normal anion gap metabolic acidosis, causes of 335b
Normovolemia 277
Nucleus tractus solitaries 239
Nutrition
  high-risk 368
  risk in critically ill score 366t
  status 365
Nutritional risk screening 365
Nutritional therapy 365

## O

Obesity hypoventilation syndrome 31, 42, 50
Obstructive airway diseases 77
Obstructive sleep apnea 51, 225, 226
Oncotic pressure, reduced 241
Operation theater 238
Oral
  cavity, motor innervation of 4
  fluids 269
Organ donor after brain death, management of potential 400
Organ dysfunction 288
  assessment of 261b
Organ function, monitoring of 262
Organum vasculosum of lamina terminalis 239, 283

Orofacial injuries 52
Oropharyngeal pathway, reduced trauma to 178
Osmosis 236
Osmotic concentration 236
Osmotic demyelination syndrome 280
Osmotic regulation 276*fc*
Osteoblastic metastasis 299
Osteopenia 314
Osteoradionecrosis
    prevention of 25
    treatment of 25
Overhydration 253
Oxidative injury, prevention of 373
Oxidative stress 162, 163, 168
Oxygen 17
    administration 41
        equipment 227
    arterial saturation of 18
    concentration 8
        analyzers 116
    consumption of 27, 198
    content of 198, 199
    continuous measurement of 114
    delivery 18, 27, 115
        devices 17, 18, 19*t*
    flush 72
    hoods and tents 24
    in alveolus, pressure of 29
    in arterial blood, pressure of 27, 29
    low concentration of 18
    mask 177
    measurement 114
    partial pressure of 197, 198
    saturation 18, 25, 114, 122
    source 31
    species, reactive 24, 154, 156, 163
    tank 60
    tension in blood, measurement of 115
    therapy 17, 57, 60
        father of 17
        goals of 17
        history of 17
    to tissues, low delivery of 18
Oxygenated hemoglobin, concentration of 117
Oxygenation, targeted 124
Oxyhood (infants) 19

## P

Packed red blood cell 206, 387, 388
    transfusion 387, 388*fc*
Palliative ventilation 224, 230
Pancreatitis
    acute 299, 367
        alcoholic 337
    chronic 307

Paranasal trauma 25
Parathyroid
    adenoma 306
    glands 298
        surgical removal of 304*b*
    hormone 296, 298, 300, 304, 309, 314, 316
    secretion 296
Parenteral nutrition 368, 371
    replacement 371*t*
    total 310, 367
Partial pressure
    arterial oxygen 48
    carbon dioxide 48
Partial rebreathing mask 19-21, 21*f*
Partial thromboplastin time 196
Passive leg raising test 260
Passy Muir valve 228
Patient-ventilator
    asynchrony 42, 107
    dyssynchrony 164
    synchrony 148
    system 94
Peak airway pressure 210
Peak and plateau pressure 137
Peak expiratory flow 98
Peak inspiratory
    flow 103, 144
    pressure 95, 138
Pendelluft 13, 153
Perfusion pressure, abdominal 261
Peripartum cardiomyopathy 197
Peripheral and central chemoreceptors, role of 36
Peripheral capillary oxygen saturation 28, 54, 210
Peripheral nervous system 177
Permissive hypercapnia 37, 42, 44, 217
Persistent pulmonary hypertension 223
pH homeostasis 325*f*
Pharyngeal reflex 397
Phenytoin 284, 369
Philips Respironics face mask 51*f*
Phlegm in airways, volume of 54
Phosphate
    excretion 311
    homeostasis 307
    internal redistribution of 308
    load 310
    renal loss of 308
Phospholipid 9
Phrenic nerve stimulation 147
Physical drug properties 182
Pickwickian syndrome 31
Pillows 51
Plasma 271

    colloid oncotic pressure 255
    osmolality 239, 255
        effective 275
        normal 239
    osmolar substances in 236*f*
    osmotic pressure of 239
    pathogen inactivation of 391
    proteins, compartments of 235
    renin 291
    sodium 283, 283*fc*, 284
        levels 255
    volume 236, 238
    water 275
Plasma-Lyte 246
Plateau airway pressure 80, 84, 87
Plateau pressure 95, 122, 137, 156
    end-inspiratory 138
Platelet
    inhibitor cytochalasin 206
    levels 392*t*
    rich plasma 392
    transfusion 392
        contraindications 392
        indications 392
        preparation and storage 392
Pleural effusion 33
Plicamycin inhibits 305
Pneumonectomy 83
Pneumonia 33, 43, 98, 346
    community-acquired 43, 346
    necrotizing 83
    reduction in rates of 178
    risk of 367
    ventilator-associated 50, 172, 226
Pneumothorax 18, 33, 34, 94
    with chest tube 83
Poiseuille's law 13
Polymethylpentene 213
Polyunsaturated fatty acids 376
Portal vein, entry of 134
Positive end expiratory pressure 11, 42, 55, 68, 83, 88, 121, 125, 138, 152, 155, 173, 184, 202, 220, 228, 254
    intrinsic 37
    selection of 82
Positive expiratory pressure 65
Positive fluid balance 269
Positive pressure ventilation 129, 132, 220, 225
    effects of 130*fc*, 135*fc*
    noninvasive 23, 24, 191
Postextubation ventilatory failure
    treatment 50
Postural hypotension 284
Potassium 244, 296
    homeostasis 288, 314

Potato starch 248
Potential airway obstructions 173
Prealbumin 367
Pressure assist control ventilation 69
Pressure carbon dioxide 54
Pressure continuous mandatory
　　ventilation 69
Pressure control 93
　　ventilation 103$f$, 104
Pressure measurements 165, 166
Pressure of air, total 349
Pressure sores 87
Pressure support 71, 92
　　ventilation 66, 70, 84, 142$f$, 147, 174
　　　　mode 71$f$
Pressure trigger 67, 146
Pressure ulcers 87
Pressure-controlled
　　mode 110
　　ventilation 92
Pressure-targeted
　　ventilation 53, 55, 56, 56$f$
　　ventilators 56
Pressure-variable ventilation 60
Pressurized metered-dose inhaler 183, 185
Procainamide myopathy 40
Proinflammatory cytokines 162
Prophylactic transfusion 392
Propylene 334
Prostanoids 191
Protein catabolism 325
Proteolytic pathways, activation of 162
Prothrombin complex concentrate 391
Proton pump inhibitor 315, 316, 369
Pseudohyperkalemia 291, 292, 293
Pseudohyperphosphatemia 311
Pseudohypokalemia 288, 290
Pseudohyponatremia 277
*Pseudomonas* 190
Psychosis 239
Pulmonary anatomy 182
Pulmonary arterial vasodilation 346
Pulmonary artery 259
　　catheter 401
　　occlusion pressure 132, 258, 259
Pulmonary capillary 10
　　wedge pressure 400
Pulmonary circulation, pathophysiology
　　of 9
Pulmonary compliance 47, 95
Pulmonary complications 226
　　postoperative 155
Pulmonary drug delivery 185
Pulmonary edema 25, 33, 346, 399
　　negative pressure 132
　　of weaning 135

Pulmonary embolism 132, 253, 346
Pulmonary embolus 29, 39
Pulmonary fibrosis 13, 31
Pulmonary function tests 35
Pulmonary gas exchange 28
Pulmonary hyperinflation 78
Pulmonary interstitial emphysema 223
Pulmonary lymphatics 10
Pulmonary oxygen toxicity 25
Pulmonary recruitment maneuver 125
Pulmonary vascular
　　permeability 259
　　resistance 129, 130
Pulmonary vasculature 122
Pulmonary venous return 131
Pulmonary vessels 10
Pulsatil oxygen saturation 74
Pulse
　　oximeter 114, 114$f$
　　oximetry 114, 115$t$
　　oxygen saturation 42
　　pressure variation 128, 131, 133, 134,
　　　　134$t$, 258, 260
　　　　calculation of 133$f$
　　rate 114
Pulsus paradoxus 131
Pump flow rate 199
Pump in circuit 215
Pump system 214
Pumpless system 214
Purulent fluid, expectoration of 83
Pyrexia, low-grade 358

### R

Radical oxygen species 25
Randomized controlled trial 49, 88, 174,
　　217
Rapid shallow breathing 14
　　from pain 33
　　index 173, 174
Rebreathing, minimize issue of 59
Recruitment maneuvers
　　advantages of 123
　　disadvantages of 123
　　methods of 121
Red blood cell 31, 236, 271
Reflex, hepatojugular 254
Refractory osteomyelitis 25
Regional respiratory mechanics 140
Rehabilitation 178
Renal ammoniagenesis 327$f$
Renal disease, end-stage 198, 336
Renal failure 300, 336, 371
　　acute 199
　　chronic 199
Renal function 255
　　normal 318$fc$

Renal loss 315
Renal outer medullary potassium 315
Renal potassium
　　excretion, disorders of 293
　　loss 288, 290
Renal regulation 314
Renal replacement therapy 309, 335, 366
　　continuous 367
Renal response 326
Renal symptoms 38
Renal tubular acidosis 291
Renin angiotensin
　　aldosterone system 238, 254, 255, 292
　　system 276
Reproductive system 384
Reservoir cannula 19
Reservoir devices 19
　　low-flow 20
Resmed nasal mask 51$f$
Respiration 3
Respiratory acidosis 84, 328, 329, 331, 342,
　　343, 356
　　acute-on-chronic 346
　　causes of 342$t$
　　clinical effects 343
　　etiology 342
　　management of 344
　　normal response for 326
Respiratory alkalosis 328, 329, 331, 342,
　　346, 347, 355
　　causes of 346
　　management of 346
　　normal response for 327
Respiratory arrest 77
Respiratory bronchioles 3, 8, 182
　　microscopic 3
Respiratory center 31
Respiratory compensation 336, 357
Respiratory cycle 56, 118, 137, 139
　　total 82
Respiratory dialysis 214, 216
Respiratory disorder 225, 326, 350
Respiratory distress syndrome 344
Respiratory duty cycle 82
Respiratory effects 399
Respiratory epithelia, structure of 4$f$
Respiratory failure
　　chronic 351
　　etiologies of 173
　　severe 344
Respiratory frequency 176
Respiratory insufficiency 309
Respiratory mechanics 12, 178
　　pathophysiology of 12
Respiratory mucosa 5
　　damage, risk of 184

Respiratory muscle 54, 328
 fatigue 82, 172
 forceful contraction of 6
 less fatigued 48
 weakness of 37, 82, 168
Respiratory physiology 181
Respiratory portion 3
Respiratory rate 21, 36, 53, 54, 67, 79, 153, 155, 174, 179
 effect of 192
Respiratory response 326
Respiratory support 41
Respiratory system 12f, 48, 90, 177, 299, 328
 compliance 12, 55, 97, 137
  monitor static 84
 elastic recoil of 14
 end-inspiratory elastic load of 137
 physiological pressures of 139f
 plateau pressure 156
 pressures of 138f
 resistance 137
Respiratory tract, structural elements of 3
Resting lung volume 78
Restlessness 284
Resuscitation
 cardiopulmonary 92, 197
 fluids 251
Retrolental fibroplasia 25
Ribonucleotides 373
Right ventricular
 ejection fraction 258
 end-diastolic
  area 223
  volume 257
Ringer's lactate solution 243
Ringer's solution 245
Rivaroxaban 392

## S

Salbutamol 289
Saline, normal 245
Sclerosis, amyotrophic lateral 226
Secreted albumin remains 247
Sedation with noninvasive ventilation 42
Selenium 373, 381, 382
 deficiency 383
 guidelines 383
 in ICU 383
 physiology 381
 source 381
 toxicity 383
Sensorineural deafness 315
Sensory systems 4
Sepsis
 pathophysiology of 270fc
 severe 334

Septal dyskinesia 252
Septic shock 270, 360
 management of 270
Serotonin release assay 205
Serum
 bicarbonate 335
  level 329
 calcium 309
 chemistry 39
 electrolytes 309
 magnesium levels 319t
 osmolality 279
 phosphate 309, 311
 potassium 316
 sodium 237, 279
 sodium concentration 283
  regulation of 275
Severe adult respiratory failure 196
Severe hypercalcemia, classification of 302
Shock 253, 334
 hemorrhagic 271
 hypovolemic 271
Short bowel syndrome 289, 290, 366
Shunt 29
 blood flow 30
 equation 30
 fraction 11, 30
 physiology 28
 right-to-left 29
Sick eucalcemia syndrome 301
Sick euthyroid syndrome 400
Sickle cell crisis 18
Sinus 25
Sjögren's syndrome 308
Skeletal disorders 225
Skeletal muscle weakness 31
Sleep disorders 107
Smoke inhalation 25
Smoking 115
Snoring 38
Society of Critical Care Medicine 85
Sodium 244, 285
 acetate 246
 bicarbonate 283-285, 294, 369
 chloride 283-285, 293, 387
  concentrations of 246
  solution 245
 concentration 335
 polystyrene sulfonate 294, 295
 reabsorption of 296
Solvent detergent treated plasma 391
Sophisticated transport ventilators 73
Sorbitol 387
Speaking valve 228
Spectroscopy, bioimpedance 238
Spinal anesthesia 241

Spinal cord, traumatic transection of 40
Spironolactone 294
Splanchnic blood flow 120
Spontaneous bacterial peritonitis 272
Spontaneous breathing 55, 151
 trial 144, 172, 174, 179
  protocol 175fc
Spontaneous ventilations 103
Squamous cell tumors 302
*Staphylococcus species* 369
Static and dynamic hyperinflation 78
Static transdiaphragmatic pressure, maximum 83
Sterofundin 246
Stewart's approach 331, 354
Stewart's equations 331
Stewart-Fencl approach 351, 352, 355, 360
Stiff lung syndrome 310
Stomach 145
Stomatitis 254
Stress 141
 index 124
 raisers, mechanism of 153f
Stroke 40
 inspiratory down 119f
 volume 258
  variation 131, 133, 134, 134t, 260
Subclavian artery cannula with graft, right 201f
Subcutaneous emphysema 83
Subglottic larynx 6
Sublingual microcirculation 262
Succinylated gelatin 248
Superior vena cava 134, 200, 256
Supraventricular arrhythmia 320
Surgical emphysema 342
Surrogates 253
Sustained inflation 121, 123
Symptomatic hypercalcemia, severe 302
Syndrome of appropriate deficiency 281
Syndrome of inappropriate antidiuretic hormone 278-280, 282
Systemic vascular resistance 400
Systolic blood pressure 400
Systolic pressure variation 131, 133, 258

## T

Tachycardia 284, 399
Tachypnea 41, 43, 48, 78
Tank respirator 65
Tank ventilator 226
Taurine 283
Tension pneumothorax 253
Theophylline 289, 369
Theoretical osmolarity 244

Therapeutic transfusion 392
Thiamine 380
    deficiency of 380
Thiazide diuretic 315, 317
Thompson portable respirator 66
Thrombin inhibitor 392
Thrombocytopenia, heparin-induced 198
Thrombocytosis 302
Thromboelastometry, rotational 206
Thromboelastogram 206
Thrombotic thrombocytopenia, heparin induced 205
Thyroid
    dysfunction 400
    function tests 40
Tidal volume 21, 36, 79, 86, 122, 134, 137, 152, 154, 176, 183
Timed inspiratory effort 146
Tonic-clonic seizures 276, 282
Tonicity 237
    regulation of 239
Toxic glycolic acid 334
Toxicology screen 40
Trace elements 381
    function of 382$t$
Trach collar mask 23$f$
Trachea 183
Tracheal reflex 397
Tracheobronchial lymph nodes 10
Tracheobronchial tree 157
Tracheostomy 43, 178
    tube, speaking with 228
Tractus solitaries, nucleus of 239
Tranexamic acid 392
Transbronchial biopsy 83
Transdiaphragmatic pressure 54, 148, 161, 166
Transdiaphragmatic twitch pressure 147
Transesophageal cardiac ultrasound 257
Transfusion trigger 387
Transient receptor potential melastatin 314
Translocational hyponatremia 277
Transmural pressure 128
    maintains 129
Transpulmonary
    pressure 128, 139, 141, 148, 151, 157
    thermodilution 259
Transrespiratory pressure 151
Transthoracic
    echocardiogram 125
    echocardiography 256
    pressure 151
Transtracheal catheter 19, 20
Traumatic brain injury 245, 342, 367, 388
Triiodothyronine 402

Trousseau's sign 300
Tubular necrosis, acute 315
Tubular phosphate reabsorption 311
Tumor 40
    lysis syndrome 299, 319
Twitch airway pressure 147
Tympanic membrane, rupture of 25
Tyrosine kinase inhibitor 308

## U

Ulcer disease, active 319
Upper airway 4
    in humidification, role of 4
    mucosa 5
    obstruction 32
    trachea 14
Upper respiratory tract, mucosa of 3
Urinalysis 255
Urinary phosphate
    excretion 308
    measurement of 312
Urinary potassium
    assessment of 290
    wasting, causes of 295
Urine
    osmolality 279
    sodium concentration 280
Urticarial reactions 394

## V

Vagus nerve 6
Vancomycin 190
Vascular injury 218
Vascular pressures 122
Vasoactive drugs 401
Vasopressin
    clinical aspect of 240
    mechanism of action of 239
    receptor inhibitors 284
    secretion 239
Vasopressors 173
Vena caval variation 134
Venoarterial venous 200
Venous blood gas 41
Venous collapsibility index 256
Venous flow 10
Venous oxygen
    content, mixed 30
    saturation 270
Venovenous 196, 215, 216
    pulmonary artery 200
    pump system 215
Ventilation 1, 28, 206, 215
    brief historical recall of 65
    continuous mandatory 68, 69
    dyshomogeneities, detection of 140

    high frequency 84
    intermittent mandatory 174
    long-term 50, 225$t$
    manual 83
    minute 21, 36, 174, 179
    modalities of 225
    mode and settings 181
    monitoring during 79
    negative-pressure 226
    parameters, adjustment of 57, 61
    plus, proportional assist 73
    pressure controlled 93
    reduces comfort of 54
    scintigraphy 83
    strategies 86
    volume targeted 53, 56, 56$f$
    with intentional leak 60$f$
Ventilation-perfusion 36
    mismatch 191
Ventilator 31, 109
    assist, neurally adjusted 73, 146, 148, 149, 166
    asynchrony 149
        auto-triggering 108
        delayed cycling 112
        double triggering 107, 108
        flow asynchronies 108, 110
    breathing circuit 52, 60
    circuit 181, 183
        disinfection 230
        humidification of 183
    equipment, care of 229
    first-generation 226
    induced diaphragm dysfunction
        concept of 162
        diagnosis of 165
    mid-level ICU 67
    modern 103
    operation 55
    patient asynchrony 57
    patient synchrony 55
    second-generation 226, 231
    selection 225
    settings 183
    supported patients 188
    variables 158
Ventilator-assisted patients, long-term 224
Ventilator-induced diaphragm dysfunction
    pathophysiology of 163
    prevention of 166
Ventilatory failure
    after extubation, development of 50
    treating acute 49$t$
Ventilatory management 402
Ventilatory modes 69$t$
Ventilatory muscles, fatigue of 47

Ventilatory support at night 225
Ventricular assist device 197
Ventricular fibrillation 199
Ventricular function 129
Ventricular interdependence 131
Ventricular septal defect 29
Ventricular tachycardia 199
Vertigo 346
Vibrating mesh nebulizer 188
Vigorous exercise 253
Vili, pathophysiology of 152
Vision 384
  changes 25
Vital capacity 48
Vital signs 32
Vitamin 373, 377
  A 302, 373
  B1 378, 380
  B12 378, 381
    deficiency 381
    physiology 381
    source 381
    toxicity 381
  B6 378
  C 369, 373, 377, 378
    deficiency of 379
    meta-analysis of 377
    physiology 377
    source 377
    use of 379
  D 296, 297, 302, 309, 378, 379
    deficiency 298, 300, 379, 380
    guidelines 380
    physiology 379
    severe 301
    source 379
    toxicity 380
  E 369, 373
  function of 378$t$
  K 378, 391
    dependent anticoagulants 391
Vocal cords 5, 6
Volotraumatismes 65
Volume assist-control 35
Volume continuous mandatory ventilation 69
Volume control 93
  mode 110
  ventilation 96, 101-103
Volumetric capnography 119
Volutrauma 83, 141
Vomiting 253, 254, 271, 291, 308

## W

Wall and gas turbine 67$f$

Water
  balance 275, 276, 276$fc$
  compartments of 235
  deficit, primary 283
  diffuses 236
  loss 283
  vapor 5
    pressure 39
Weaning failure 148, 172
Weaning noninvasive ventilation 42
Weaning success 172
Wernicke encephalopathy 380
Whisper-Swivel connector 59
White blood cell 35
Wilson's disease 308
Winter's formula 353
Winters' rules 329
Wound healing 383

## X

Xerostomia 254

## Z

Zinc 382, 383
  deficiency 383
  physiology 383
  source 383
  toxicity 384

EU GSPR Authorised Reprsentative
Logos Europe, 9 rue Nicolas Poussin
1700, La Rochelle, France
Phone: +33 (0) 6 67 93 73 78
E-mail: contact@logoseurope.eu

www.ingramcontent.com/pod-product-compliance
Ingram Content Group UK Ltd.
Pitfield, Milton Keynes, MK11 3LW, UK
UKHW051847210426
5322IPUK00019B/290